MOSBY'S
FRONT
OFFICE
SKILLS
FOR THE
Medical
ASSISTANT

MOSBY'S
FRONT OFFICE SKILLS

FOR THE

Medical
ASSISTANT

De A. Eggers, MBA
CEO/President
De A. Eggers & Associates
Sonoma, California

Anne M. Conway, CMA
Medical Assisting Instructor
National Career Education
Citrus Heights, California

with 195 illustrations

Mosby

An Affiliate of Elsevier

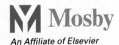
Mosby
An Affiliate of Elsevier

Editor: Adrianne Williams
Developmental Editor: Sarahlynn Lester
Project Manager: Patricia Tannian
Senior Production Editor: Anne Salmo
Design: Kangrga Design Inc.
Design Coordinator: Renée Duenow

Mosby, Inc.
11830 Westline Industrial Drive
St. Louis, Missouri 63146

Library of Congress Cataloging in Publication Data
Eggers, De A.
    Mosby's front office skills for the medical assistant / De A.
Eggers, Anne M. Conway.
        p.   cm.
    Includes bibliographical references and index.
    ISBN 0-8151-2386-8
    1. Medical assistants.   2. Medical offices.   I. Conway, Anne M.
II. Title.   III. Title: Front office skills for the medical
assistant.
    [DNLM: 1. Office Management.   2. Medical Secretaries.   W 80 E295m
    1999]
R728.8.E36   1999
651'.961--dc21
DNLM/DLC
for Library of Congress   99-23139
                                                                      CIP

9 8 7 6 5

Reviewers

Chris Kientzle
Medical Assisting Program
Sanford-Brown College
Hazelwood, Missouri

Sharon McCaughrin
School Director
Ross Medical Education Center
Clinton Township, Michigan

Vicki Prater, CMA, RMA, RAHA
Medical Program Director
Concorde Career Institute
Colton, California

Susan Schilling, BS, CMA
Allied Health Programs Director
Bryant and Stratton
Syracuse, New York

Dolly Swanson, RMA
Student Services Advisor
Stockton, California

Susan K. Zolvinski, LPN
Medical Assisting Instructor
Commonwealth Business College
LaPorte, Indiana

I wish to dedicate this book to my grandfather,
Thomas Jefferson Roberts,
history professor, author, theologian, parent, and wonderful, encouraging grandparent,
who always maintained that no matter your career choice, always do your best.
He who, long before it was considered appropriate, supported equality for women.
Thank you, Grandpa!

D. A. E.

Preface

Today's administrative medical assistants work in a variety of health care settings, whether that setting is a typical physician's office, a clinic, a free-standing surgery center, or an inpatient or outpatient center. *Mosby's Front Office Skills for the Medical Assistant* was created with the idea that the medical office is a business, and that the role of today's front office medical assistant is to ensure the smooth and successful operation of that business. It incorporates all of the relevant concepts and skills necessary for training students to understand and adapt to the demands of any of these health care environments.

Any front office textbook must include the latest standards and procedures, particularly for billing and completing health insurance claims. These topics have been given broad coverage in this text, particularly electronic claims submission, since government requirements are enhanced to have as many claims submitted electronically as possible. Information for computer systems, as well as details on how to obtain and implement computerized systems for the front office, also are a necessary component of front office training and have been given ample discussion. In addition, managed care is increasingly governing how health care is being delivered in this country, which is why a separate chapter on this influential topic encompasses the most up-to-date information available regarding managed-care programs and their influence on the American public. The information included about computer systems, managed care, and many other topics extends above and beyond current requirements, to prepare students for the future.

This author team is uniquely prepared to offer students an inside look into the world of front office medical assisting. De A. Eggers is owner and president of De A. Eggers & Associates, a company providing education, medical billing and collection, consulting, and training in the health care field. She is in the field every day, solving problems and instructing physicians and their staffs in appropriate office procedures. This enabled her to write a text that is very practical and linked to real-world experiences. Anne M. Conway is a longtime instructor of medical administrative assisting and laboratory assisting at National Career Education School. She is a certified medical assistant and a very experienced educator. She knows what it means to be a medical assistant and how to prepare students, and has added many special features to the text.

Boxed information throughout the book summarizes key procedures in a step-by-step format that is easy for students to follow and retain. Other boxed information highlights real-life applications, practical on-the-job tips, and nice-to-know information. In addition, each chapter includes challenge exercises designed to develop critical thinking and decision-making skills, as well as practical, real-world activities that include a myriad of practice forms for completion. An enhanced full-color design and full-color artwork throughout provide an engaging environment, while helpful tables summarize important concepts in an attempt to give students every advantage for learning and retaining key theory and skills.

A widely used medical office computer software program, Stratford Healthcare Management System, is available for free to instructors of programs using this book. Appendix B provides guidance on how to use the program and exercises to be used with the program on the computer. This Y2K-compatible software will provide students the opportunity to practice scheduling, forms completion, and electronic claims submission in an engaging and realistic manner.

Chapters are organized in a logical order of increasing complexity, helping the student develop a solid foundation of knowledge and information required to perform the ever-growing number of skills required to successfully manage the front office operations of a busy medical practice. Supporting each chapter are exercises in a separate workbook that will greatly assist in reinforcing key content and competencies, and will help prepare students for the certification examination, as well as for a career as a front office medical assistant.

It is intended that the information in this textbook will be practical, easy to understand, and applicable as a future reference guide and that the student will find it a challenging and practical source for preparing to work in this increasingly complex area of health care.

Acknowledgments

We wish to express our most sincere thanks to the many friends, family, colleagues, and other personnel in the health care field for their support, encouragement, inspiration, and assistance while this book was being written. Special appreciation and recognition are due to our outstanding publishing team for their expertise, patience, support, and guidance. A very special thanks to close friends, colleagues, and employees whose very special love and support helped make this book a reality.

De A. Eggers   **Anne M. Conway**
Sonoma, California   **Citrus Heights, California**

Contents

9   Patient/Medical Records Management, 214

10   Filing, 246

11   Medical Office Management, 264

MOSBY'S

FRONT
OFFICE
SKILLS

FOR THE

Medical

ASSISTANT

The Professional Administrative Medical Assistant

OUTLINE

On completion of Chapter 1 the administrative medical assistant student should be able to:

1. Define the key terms listed in this chapter.

2. Describe specialties in the health care field.

3. List basic skills needed in administrative medical assisting.

4. List and discuss at least eight areas of responsibility that apply to administrative medical assisting.

5. List professional organizations available to the administrative medical assistant.

6. Explain how medical knowledge can be kept current.

KEY TERMS

Administrative medical assistant	Trained medical assistant who carries out management, secretarial, and supervisory duties, and participates in activities designed to educate and improve health standards of the community (also known as a *front office assistant*).
American Academy of Procedural Coders (AAPC)	National association involved in promoting professional standards and recognition for procedural coders.
American Association for Medical Transcription (AAMT)	National association of medical transcriptionists; membership is limited to practicing or former transcriptionists and students in medical transcription programs.
American Association of Medical Assistants, Inc. (AAMA)	National association of medical assistants, medical assistant students, and medical assistant educators with both state and local chapters; recognized by the American Medical Association.
American Medical Association (AMA)	National association and professional society of physicians.
American Medical Technologists (AMT)	National association that features a registered medical assistant program for certification as well as student membership.

Continued

KEY TERMS

(Continued)

American Medical Women's Association (AMWA)
National association of women physicians and medical students dedicated to improving the professional well-being of its members and increasing the influence of women in all aspects of the medical profession.

Association of Medical Technologists
National association for certifying personnel for laboratories.

Certified medical assistant (CMA)
Individual who receives certification after completing appropriate training and passing an examination administered by the American Association of Medical Assistants, Inc.

Medical Group Management Association (MGMA)
National association dedicated to providing a strong professional network for health care office managers, group managers, and ongoing professional education.

Paraprofessional
Individual who may or may not possess educational training, hands-on training, certification, and on-the-job experience, who functions in a specific health or human services care role, under supervision.

Professional Association of Health Care Office Managers (PAHCOM)
National association dedicated to providing a strong professional network for health care office managers.

The Role of the Administrative Medical Assistant

The administrative medical assistant is an integral part of modern medical practice (see the box about the importance of the administrative medical assistant). Increasingly, administrative medical assistants are necessary in medical offices to perform specialized tasks. Medical assisting is a career, not just a job. As an administrative medical assistant, you will work as an integral part of a health care team to deliver medical services to the public. Your chosen career has changed greatly over the years. Medical assistants used to be general helpers for physicians. Now, some medical assistants perform specific tasks that no one else in the medical office is responsible for, to keep the office running smoothly.

Depending on the size of the office in which you work, you may be able to choose what area of specialty you might like to pursue. You could manage the front office, handle all of the office correspondence and medical records, be in charge of all of the office's insurance coding needs, keep the office appointment

PERSPECTIVES IN MEDICAL ASSISTING

The Importance of the Administrative Medical Assistant

Michael is a new physician who, several years ago, tried to set up a new practice with two partners. The three developed a careful business plan, even hiring a market analyst to assess meticulously the health care needs of the community in which they hoped to practice. They chose a suburban location and hired a registered nurse and a receptionist to help with appointments, answering telephones, managing patient records, and office traffic. Finally, the clinic opened its doors.

"That's when our troubles began," Michael said. "At first everything was under control, but then, as our clientele built up, I'd hear the phone ringing constantly. One day I stepped into the hall to discover that the receptionist was near tears and patients were frustrated. She had no training in how to handle referrals or medical records, and medical insurance is tricky business. So in addition to normal patient calls, she was trying to deal with all these issues—including complaints that she wasn't handling things right. We still have no idea how many new-patient calls we missed while she was wrestling with this stuff.

Another problem was that nobody was coordinating our use of outside services—labs, radiology, hospital liaisons—even basic supplies were not being monitored by anyone. The receptionist did her best but confessed to me that even the terminology, let alone procedures, was an overwhelming stumbling block. And as for coding, billing, and processing claims? Forget that! *None* of us knew what we were doing.

Probably the problem that scared me the most, though, was insurance. I remember the day a very professional-looking woman I'd been treating asked me, 'How can I get my insurance to cover this? I have no idea what to do.' I looked at her with surprise and was embarrassed to admit that I had no idea either. I remember thinking, after she left, that *we must look really bad. We must look really unprofessional.*

Besides all this, we had one more problem, and it was a big one. Few people realize that in a practice like ours, the partners don't get paid until everything else—and everyone else (employees, leasing companies, you name it)—gets paid first. Because we were in over our heads as far as management issues were concerned, nobody was getting paid, nobody was watching out for insurance issues, and so—even though enough business was coming in—my partners and I were not getting paid. We literally did not know how to go about paying ourselves! We were too worried about responding to creditors and insurance companies. We were in big trouble and we knew it."

The solution?

Michael smiled and rolled his eyes. "We kept the receptionist, but we let her do her job and stopped expecting her to do something she had no training in. We hired an administrative medical assistant and she saved our necks."

FIGURE 1.1

The solo administrative medical assistant's job includes all of the responsibilities discussed in this book.

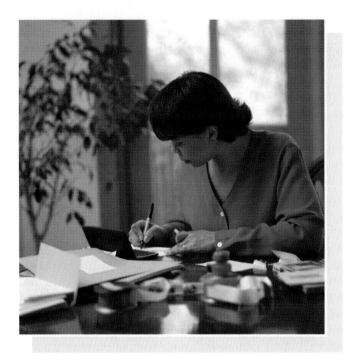

book, handle referrals, coordinate the office's use of outside medical services, order supplies, or control the office billing practice. In some offices, you might be responsible for doing several or even all of these things.

Administrative medical assisting is the business portion of the medical assisting profession. The administrative medical assistant works in that part of a facility commonly referred to as the *front office,* or *business office,* handling the business portion of the practice or facility. The size of a practice and number of patients seen determines the number of assistants necessary to perform the administrative duties. The solo administrative medical assistant's job will include all of the responsibilities discussed in this book (Figure 1.1). In an office or other health care facility that employs more than one administrative medical assistant, the responsibilities will be divided among these individuals. The administrative medical assistant often sets the tone for an efficiently run facility and creates the public's initial impression of the facility.

General Responsibilities

As you can see from the case scenario about Michael, the new physician who attempted to establish a practice, the administrative medical assistant is much more than a receptionist or even more than the typical office manager. Key business responsibilities expected of an administrative medical assistant may include any or all of the following:

- Managing patient registration and communication
- Scheduling and referral management
- Managing correspondence
- Patient or medical records management

- File system management
- Office, equipment, and financial management
- Specific aspects of medication handling
- Coding, billing, and claims processing
- Insurance responsibilities
- Working with managed care plans
- Credit, billing, and collection
- Computer operations
- Banking
- Accounting and bookkeeping

This book provides the administrative medical assistant with broad knowledge of these basic issues—knowledge that will be crucial to possess when working in any medical facility. Besides these topics, discussions on medical law and medical ethics and how they influence the practice of medicine also are included. These, too, are significant features of the why and how of medical office practices.

Patient Education

As a member of a health care team, the administrative medical assistant also has the opportunity to perform patient education. This vital service not only benefits the patient but also reflects the good will of the provider. An informed patient generally is more relaxed and cooperative than an uninformed patient when receiving any medical care. As an educator, the administrative medical assistant provides valuable information to the patient about medical care facilities and providers, such as laboratories, therapeutic agencies, and hospitals, with which the patient may come in contact.

To realize the value of this service, put yourself in the position of the patient. The anxiety and stress of being in a medical setting is only intensified when the patient does not understand why a procedure is necessary, how it will be accomplished, whether his or her carrier authorizes it, how it will be billed to the insurance company, or what payment amounts are expected from the patient.

A receptive environment will provide the patient with a comfortable atmosphere in which to ask questions, and as an information source, you can anticipate patient needs for this information and provide it without being asked.

Anticipating the patient's needs is especially essential when providing basic information about appointment schedules, billing, insurance services, telephone hours, the physician's office hours, hospital affiliation, and reaching the physician after regular office hours. You can go a long way toward inspiring confidence by emphasizing the office policy on confidentiality, saying, for example: "Mr. Jones, if you ever need copies of your records sent anywhere else at any time, I will need to have you sign a release of records. We are very careful to protect our patients' confidentiality."

You also may be responsible for providing information about services and facilities outside of the immediate area to patients who are referred to other health care facilities. You may be called on to provide information about support services, such as transportation, hotels, traffic directions, parking facilities,

PERSPECTIVES IN MEDICAL ASSISTING

Origin of the Administrative Medical Assistant

The country doctor treated patients in their homes. His only assistants were members of the patient's family. As time went on, the physician set up his practice in part of his house, and patients came to see him there. He perhaps trained his wife to help him in his office. Eventually the physician established an office outside his home to handle an increased patient load and separate homelife from work. At this time he trained a person—almost always a woman—to assist him. As medicine became more sophisticated, he needed someone in the back office as well as the front to run his practice. In today's age of specialization, many doctors prefer to have a trained person—the administrative medical assistant—handle the front, or business, office, that is, appointments, telephone, insurance, computer systems, and physician transcription.

and visiting-nurse services, available in the community. It may also be necessary to assist the patient or patient's family in obtaining financial assistance for medical services through public medical assistance or in obtaining billing and insurance policy answers or authorization from the insurance carrier for these referred services. This readily available information will reassure the patient that such referrals are routine.

As an administrative medical assistant you will be a public representative of the physician or health care facility. Often you will even be the patient's *first* contact with your medical office, as well as the first contact for physicians and staff of other facilities, salespersons, and supply company, pharmaceutical, and service representatives. Courtesy, patience, and effective communication skills will help you present a positive public image of the physician's office or the health care facility and its staff. These skills also will establish you as an asset to your employer.

Work Environment

In the case scenario presented earlier, we glimpsed the value of the administrative medical assistant to one clinic. Clearly, in Michael's case, a skilled, highly trained administrative medical assistant made all the difference in both good patient care and a well-run medical office. However, opportunities are not limited to the physician's private practice. In its brief history, the medical assisting profession has undergone a remarkable transition (see the box about the origin of the administrative medical assistant). From a humble beginning as the physician's general helper, the medical assistant has evolved to be a special member of the health care team. Administrative medical assistants have found that they have many choices and opportunities to expand their range of professional experiences because their skills are needed in various locations and allied health fields.

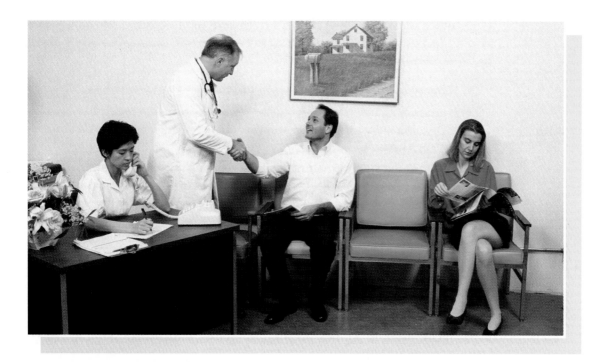

FIGURE 1.2

Today's administrative medical assistant can choose from various work environments and specializations.

Today's administrative medical assistant can choose among various work environments and specializations as well (Figure 1.2).

Outpatient vs. Inpatient Facilities

One of the first decisions an administrative medical assistant may want to make when considering either that first position or a subsequent job change is whether to choose an inpatient or outpatient setting. What is the difference between these two, and how do we determine how a specialty fits in these two categories?

Outpatient services are a range of basic health care services excluding hospitalization; this includes all levels of clinical diagnostic evaluation, testing, and treatments for all age groups. Outpatient services are available for patients who are ambulatory and able to go to a physician's office, clinic, or health care center for required medical services; they also may apply to patients who are cared for at home. All of these facilities require numerous administrative medical assistants.

Inpatient care is provided in hospitals, skilled nursing facilities, nursing homes, or hospices in which the patients reside temporarily or permanently. All necessary medical services are provided through these facilities. The professional administrative medical assistant can select a position from among several opportunities in outpatient and inpatient facilities.

Another way of breaking down health care services is the three-level care system. In this system, health care services are provided in three basic types of facilities as follows:

- Primary care level—the solo or multiphysicians' office or clinic
- Intermediate care level—requiring certified staff supervised by more senior personnel (i.e., the surgery center, skilled nursing facility, patient's home)
- Hospital setting—providing a complete range of either primary care services (outpatient) or surgery/hospitalization treatment (inpatient services)

How do work environments vary within these levels? In outpatient care, alternatives to the private practice include positions in an ancillary care setting, a general or specialty clinic, surgery center, an agency, a health maintenance organization (HMO), or a hospital-based care plan. However, if you think you might enjoy working in an inpatient facility, you might consider a position in an admissions department, billing department, business office, medical records department, walk-in clinic, urgent care center, accredited surgical center, trauma center, or burn unit.

These are only a few examples of the employment opportunities available to administrative medical assistants. Roles are increasing as the options in health care expand. In addition, awareness is increasing among the rest of the medical community regarding the role and function of the administrative medical assistant. Physicians, administrators, nurses, therapists, and technicians recognize a well-trained administrative medical assistant as a vital part of the health care team.

The Health Care Team

Regardless of the field chosen, an administrative medical assistant inevitably works with a team of professionals and must be familiar with their distinctive roles (Figure 1.3). This means working with various services, coordinating their use, and frequently acting as a liaison between them and the primary facility he or she represents. For example, someone must monitor the access, use, and financial arrangements between the primary facility and any outside laboratory services. Even in this small part of the administrative medical assistant's relationships, a range of terminology and procedures must become second nature. In the case of crucial tests needed in an especially timely fashion (e.g., perhaps the physician is waiting for a specific test result before determining the next step in a patient's treatment), someone has to monitor scheduling, delivery of specimens, prompt reporting, and channeling of insurance payments. Juggling these responsibilities means having frequent communication with other members of the health care team.

The health care team is a group of individuals, each with a different function, that coordinates their efforts to accomplish a specific goal. This team concept has evolved to cope with the complex environment of health promotion, maintenance, treatment, and rehabilitation. A health care team is made up of

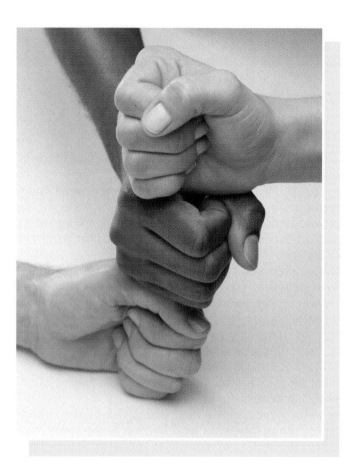

FIGURE 1.3

Regardless of the field chosen, the administrative medical assistant works with a whole team of professionals.

various health care providers whose primary concern is the health and welfare of each individual patient. Table 1.1 lists the many types of medical professionals who may possibly be part of a health care team. The medical assistant is an essential member of this team.

In the typical outpatient health care facility, administrative medical assistants will work with other administrative personnel such as bookkeepers, insurance clerks, and receptionists, as well as the clinical personnel, and this is in addition to working with health care team members employed in various other outpatient and inpatient settings. All of these team members can be considered extensions of the medical office staff, since the services they provide must be coordinated with the services provided in the physician's office. These services may include medical testing facilities (laboratory, radiology), rehabilitative services (physical therapy, occupational therapy), support services (home health care, transportation), and hospital facilities (outpatient surgery, surgery, admission). The administrative medical assistant's relationship with other ancillary medical services personnel begins when it is necessary to refer patients for these services.

The administrative medical assistant employed in an outpatient setting can expect some patients to require hospitalization. He or she will communicate with hospital admitting clerks, unit secretaries, and nurses as necessary when arranging for the patient's hospital admission, during the course of the patient's hospital stay, and when the patient is about to be discharged.

TABLE 1-1

Health Care Team Members

Personnel	Duties
Electrocardiogram (ECG) technician	Obtains ECG tracings from patients and prepares tracings for interpretation by the physician
Licensed practical nurse (LPN)	Provides clinnical care and support under the supervision of a physician
Licensed vocational nurse (LVN)	Provides clinical care and support under supervision of a physician
Medical assistant	Certified to conduct the business portion of the medical practice or facility
Medical technologist	Obtains, prepares, and examines samples of body tissues and fluids to assist in the determination of the presence of disease processes
Medical transcriptionist	Prepares reports, records, and correspondence from the physician's dictation
Nuclear medicine technologist	Under the direction of a physician-specialist, obtains diagnostic data or treats disease processes with radioactive nuclides
Nurse practitioner	Certified to provide specified diagnostic evaluations and/or treatment plans under the supervision and assumed responsiblity of a physician in certain specialty areas
Occupational therapist	Under the direction of a physician-specialist, designs and executes a program to retrain patients for new or expanded jobs
Orthotist	Under the direction of a physician-specialist, designs braces or equipment to assist patients in regaining, as much as possible, previous levels of personal or job functioning after a debilitating injury
Physician	Certified to direct and monitor health care services
Physician assistant (PA)	Certified to conduct specified diagnostic evaluations and/or treatment plans under the supervision and assumed responsiblity of a physician in certain specialty areas
Psychiatric technician (PT)	Under the direction of a psychiatrist, works one-on-one to bring patients back to their previous level of social functioning
Registered dietitian (RD)	Plans therapeutic nutrition programs and develops sample menus as guides
Registered nurse (RN)	Administers treatment under the direction of a physician and plans and organizes nursing procedures for health maintenance, rehabilitation, and prevention of complications
Registered physical therapist (RPT)	Under the direction of a physician-specialist, designs and executes therapy designed to rehabilitate patients to their previous functional levels
Respiratory therapist	Obtains diagnostic information on a patient's respiratory functions and prepares data for interpretation by the physician; treats patients with respiratory conditions under the physician's orders
Work hardening therapist	Under the direction of a physician-specialist, works with patients in their actual work environment to retain them to previous levels of functioning after a disabling injury
X-ray technician	Obtains x-rays from patients and prepares x-ray film for interpretation by the physician

AT WORK TODAY

About Jobs

Undoubtedly you are interested in what type of jobs will be available to you as an administrative medical assistant. Examples of classified advertisements you may pursue are:

Medical—Front Office
Accounts receivable. High-volume office. Knowledge of computers, Medicare/Medicaid, managed care, insurance billing/claims. Fax resume to (916) 555-3990.

Medical Front Office/FT
Computer scheduling, busy phones. Competitive salary and benefits, Equal Opportunity Employer. Fax resume to (916) 555-4492.

Professionalism in the Medical Environment

To work effectively with such a diverse group of services and individuals, a high degree of professionalism is required. Professionalism reflects both an attitude and an image. As an administrative medical assistant, your professional manner can create the impression that the office procedures, medical attention, and the standard of practice at your facility surpass that of any other. Such an impression is easy to generate if you are knowledgeable and confident in technical areas as well as in public relations; if you show that you care about and are committed to your clients' needs; and if you maintain a professional demeanor and appearance.

Adhering to the following standards can help the administrative medical assistant develop professionalism:

- Support the physician and other staff members in discussions with or about patients (Figure 1.4). When staff members disagree and the patient becomes aware of this, his or her confidence in the entire facility is undermined. Disagreements should be held in private, away from patient observation.

- First and foremost, always protect the patient's right to confidentiality. In fact, the personal and professional lives of the physician, co-workers, and patients should always be kept confidential. The best policy is to leave office information in the office.

- Accept constructive criticism from the physician, co-workers, or patients without displaying defensive behavior. By contrast, when the administrative medical assistant is defensive, angry, or nonresponsive, professionalism is lost.

- Encourage the patient to ask questions and discuss needs and concerns. Frequently, a patient is dissatisfied with treatment results or information about

FIGURE 1.4

The professional administrative medical assistant must support the physician and other staff members.

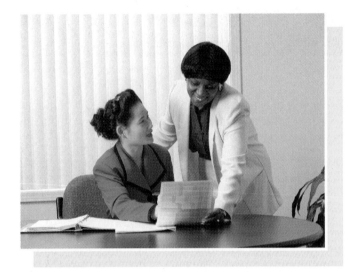

a financial situation but feels too intimidated or uncomfortable to ask the physician a question. When this happens, the administrative medical assistant becomes the patient representative or spokesperson. This allows the physician to provide competent and comprehensive care.

• Resist personal prejudice in patient relations. Be aware of your particular biases regarding race, religion, national origin, and political or sexual orientation, and the need to prevent these biases from interfering with the patient's health care.

• Be aware of the importance of individual presentation; observe the manner and dress of other professionals and strive to present the same professional image. Doing this can set the tone for the entire office. A neat, clean appearance and an efficient and personable presentation can make the patient feel at ease with the care provided. An office with unkempt personnel or personnel who clearly are not interested or committed can completely undermine the patient's confidence in the entire facility.

• Participate in professional organizations that contribute to career enhancement. The assistant should maintain certification and continue to participate in educational programs.

• Become highly motivated and apply self-management principles. The administrative medical assistant cannot always depend on other co-workers or the physicians to prioritize work assignments. Instead, a true professional can manage and prioritize his or her own work, setting goals and becoming proficient in time management.

Personal Attributes, Basic Technical Skills, and Education

Balancing all of the responsibilities of an administrative medical assistant requires specific personal attributes, basic technical skills, and education.

PERSONAL ATTRIBUTES OF THE SUCCESSFUL ADMINISTRATIVE MEDICAL ASSISTANT

Ability to communicate clearly with others	Empathy
Common sense	Tolerance
Diplomacy	Sense of humor
Honesty	Consideration
Interest in helping others	Attentiveness to personal appearance
Integrity	Calm manner
Dependability	Courtesy

WHAT DO YOU THINK?

Evaluate yourself. What are your personal qualifications?
1. Do you enjoy people and can you interact with the public empathetically while answering telephones, handling requests, and scheduling for large numbers of patients?
2. Do you strive for excellence in any job that you do?
3. Can you be flexible, innovative, and responsive to change?
4. Can you have a caring and positive attitude about your job, the people you work with, and with patients?

Personal Attributes

Try to remember a time when you required the services of a physician. Whether you were having a routine examination or you were ill and seeking care, you may recall that you perceived yourself as the most important person in the process. Regardless of your reason for being in the medical setting, your attention was directed toward your own well-being, and you expected the employees of the facility to treat you in a professional and caring manner.

The administrative medical assistant often is the first and last health care professional to interact with the patient as a representative of the facility; thus, it is important to leave the patient with a good impression. Evaluate your skills against those listed in the box about personal attributes to determine whether you possess qualifications compatible with those recognized as important for success in this profession.

Basic Technical Skills

Personal attributes must be developed over time through family and interpersonal relationships, experience, and education. Essential technical skills required of the administrative medical assistant can be acquired through a sequence of courses designed to meet the needs of the student and the medical community (Figure 1.5). The required professional skills (both cognitive and

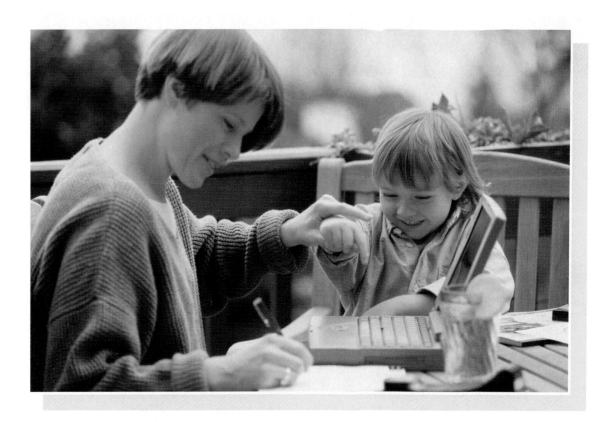

FIGURE   1.5

Essential technical skills can be acquired through a sequence of courses designed to meet the needs of the student and medical community.

performance related) are presented throughout this book. Basic technical skills that will enhance the medical assistant student's success are listed in the box on the facing page.

Education

In the recent past, medical care was relatively simple and little, if any, training was required of the few people who were paraprofessionals. As medical science progressed, new knowledge, advanced equipment, and complex treatment techniques developed. In addition, the means of providing care for increasing numbers of patients changed from basic one-physician offices to sophisticated medical practices, clinics, and hospitals.

Health care providers, particularly physicians, now rely on various personnel to deliver medical services. Medical assistants have emerged as unique among allied health professionals because of their broad scope of training for administrative or clinical positions. Administrative medical assisting is a career, not just a job, and the administrative medical assistant is a valued member of the various teams formed to provide necessary health care.

The concept of training personnel specifically for work in the physician's office was initiated by Dr. M. Mandl, a biologist and former teacher in the New York City public schools. Dr. Mandl established the first school for medical

TECHNICAL SKILLS OF THE SUCCESSFUL ADMINISTRATIVE MEDICAL ASSISTANT

Mathematics
Bookkeeping and Banking
Grammar
Computers and keyboarding
Written communication
Transcription
Spoken communication and telephone skills
Medical terminology
Knowledge of human behavior
Appointment scheduling/referrals

assistants in 1934. Today there are many private schools and public community colleges throughout the country with programs for training medical assistants for diverse positions and career opportunities.

Methods of training

An administrative medical assistant can be educated through on-the-job training or training at a proprietary (private) school, junior college, or community college. At one time, on-the-job training was the most common way of learning the duties and skills needed in a medical office. After an individual acquired a position, he or she would learn how to assist the physician and perform other duties as the occasion arose. Today, on-the-job training rarely is the only preparation needed to work as a medical assistant. More common today is attendance at either a proprietary school or community college. Once a program of training is completed and the graduate obtains a position, he or she receives limited on-the-job training. At this time, the new employee is introduced to the specific needs and requirements of the medical practice at which he or she will work.

After acquiring the necessary theoretical foundation, the medical assistant student may be eased into the work environment through a student work experience program. This program allows the student to observe and participate as a member of an actual health care team. This concept is discussed further in Chapter 20.

Expanding Your Professional Development

For the administrative medical assistant, education does not stop after permanent employment. In most fields, an employee is not required or expected to seek information about how similar jobs are conducted elsewhere. However, medical assistants and other health care professionals must continuously learn about current and new practices in other localities as well as advances in medical assisting and changes in medicine itself. A number of powerful organizations are available for continuing education as well as for the opportunity to seek and share information with other professionals.

The American Association of Medical Assistants

In 1959, about 25 years after the founding of the first school for medical assistants, the American Association of Medical Assistants (AAMA) established national headquarters in Chicago. Since its founding, the AAMA has grown to a present membership of thousands of dedicated medical assistants. As a nationwide organization, the AAMA has the advantage of monitoring the needs and status of medical assistants throughout the country. In an effort to serve its membership, the AAMA participates in the accreditation of training programs and supports continuing education. It also has developed a mechanism for certifying the professional medical assistant. State and local divisions of the AAMA serve as links between the medical assistant and the national organization by distributing information about decisions made at the national level and providing information to the AAMA on local and regional needs.

Accreditation Responsibilities

Training programs for medical assistants are accredited and periodically reevaluated by a joint team from the AAMA and the American Medical Association (AMA). After careful examination of all aspects of a program seeking accreditation, the accreditation team makes a recommendation to the Independent Committee on Allied Health Education and Accreditation of the AMA. A favorable recommendation will result in the accreditation of the proprietary or community college program.

Certification Examination

In 1966, in an effort to standardize the quality of medical assistants' knowledge, the AAMA developed a national examination for certifying graduates of accredited training programs or individuals with documented work experience. These examinations are given in January and June in more than 100 cities throughout the United States. A medical assistant need not be a member of the AAMA to be eligible for the examination. A state or local branch of the AAMA will be able to assist a candidate for examination by providing application forms and information about the examination site. Successful completion of the basic examination will result in the award of the title certified medical assistant (CMA). After the basic CMA examination has been passed, specialty-area examinations are available. These examinations and subsequent credentials include the following:

- Administrative (CMA-A)
- Clinical (CMA-C)
- Combined administrative and clinical (CMA-AC)
- Pediatric (CMA-P)

A priority of the AAMA is continuing education for medical assistants. This is accomplished through professional publications, annual meetings, and accredited continuing education courses.

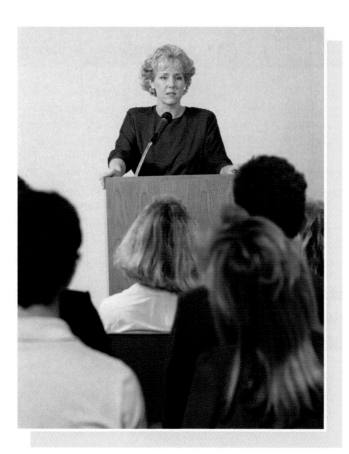

FIGURE   1.6

In addition to specialty training, medical assistants may participate in various professional organizations.

Professional Affiliations

In addition to specialty training, medical assistants may participate in various professional organizations and subscribe to one or more publications (Figure 1.6). Some of the most prominent organizations and publications are listed in the box on p. 18. Unless otherwise indicated, all the publications listed are monthly.

The Health Care System Today and Tomorrow

Health care has been changing for hundreds of years; however, never before have the changes occurred as rapidly as they are today. These recent changes include:

- Increased use of computers and high-tech communications systems
- Computer-assisted diagnosis and treatment
- A changing patient population
- Progress in disease management

WHAT DO YOU THINK?

Profession—A vocation or calling; usually one that involves some branch of advanced learning or science
Professional—Of or belonging to a profession; having or showing the skill of a professional; competent
Professionalism—The qualities or typical features of a profession or of professionals, especially competence or skill

You will represent the physician(s) for whom you work and your profession. You will need to be a good example of the medical assisting profession at all times, whether at the reception desk or talking on the telephone. Professionalism will need to be evident in everything about you—your appearance, what you do and say—both on and off the job. It will be a challenge to become a professional, and you will need to continue practicing and perfecting it. Are you capable of doing the job?

PROFESSIONAL ORGANIZATIONS AND PUBLICATIONS FOR MEDICAL ASSISTANTS

Organizations

American Academy of Procedural Coders (AAPC)
2144 Highland Drive, Suite 100
Salt Lake City, UT 84106

American Association of Medical Assistants (AAMA)
20 North Wacker Drive
Chicago, IL 60606

American Association for Medical Transcription (AAMT)
P.O. Box 576187
Modesto, CA 95457

Medical Group Management Association (MGMA)
104 Inverness Terrace
Englewood, CO 80112

Professional Association of Health Care Office Managers (PAHCOM)
461 East 10 Mile Road
Pensacola, FL 32504-7355

Registered Medical Assistant (RMA) or (AMT)
170 Higgins Road
Park Ridge, IL 60068

Publications

The Professional Medical Assistant
American Association of Medical Assistants, Inc.
20 North Wacker Drive
Chicago, IL 60606

Medical Economics
1 Paragon Drive
Montvale, NJ 07645

Physicians' Magazine
One East First Street
Duluth, MN 55802

Vital Signs
RMA Newsletter (quarterly)
710 Higgins Road
Park Ridge, IL 60068

The Doctor's Office
P.O. Box 10488
Lancaster, PA 17605-0488

Professional Collections Manager
P.O. Box 10488
Lancaster, PA 17605-0488

Journal of the American Association for Medical Transcription
P.O. Box 576187
Modesto, CA 95357

Computers and Communication

Satellites, modems, cellular telephones, and pagers make it possible to take advanced medical diagnoses and treatments to rural areas not previously serviced (Figure 1.7). Satellites and video cameras now are used with patients in remote areas who have various diagnoses. The most commonly known program is one for Parkinson's disease. This program was implemented by physicians at the University of Kansas. Someday, advances in the diagnosis and treatment of many diseases may be made available by link-ups from medical centers and physician offices to the rural and urban high-risk patient's home.

Patient information, such as medical billing and clinical data, now can be transferred by telephone and computer systems (for example, the transfer of patient information from outlying areas to specialists in large, urban regional facilities). Two factors may help to increase future use of electronic data transmission for the transfer of patient information: (1) more advanced computer systems and hardware in provider locations such as hospitals, clinics, physician offices, and laboratory facilities throughout the health care industry; and (2) a universal computer language. The federal government and various private agencies and organizations are working to establish such a universal language. Although some standards for electronic data transmission exist in the areas of medical billing, laboratory, and radiology, for instance, much more emphasis now will be focused on the other more clinical parts of a patient medical record. This increase in electronic transmission is expected to be considerably more accurate and cost effective as it develops, eliminating the transfer and storage of paper. Further standardization may provide 24-hour on-line access to critical patient information.

Electronic data communication advances also have led to the transfer of data to insurance carriers for reimbursement of claims. Now it also may be capable of transferring the operative report and clinical records regarding the

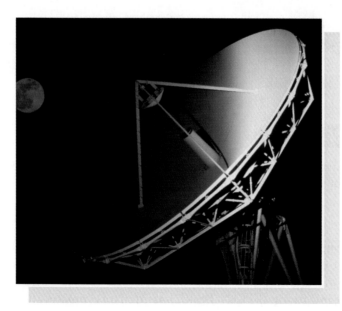

FIGURE 1.7

Satellites, modems, and video take advanced medical diagnoses and treatments to remote areas.

AT WORK TODAY

Computerized Medical Records

Medical records will become completely computerized in the future, saving time and the problems related to paper charts. A touch screen shows any aspect of a patient's chart with a few touches from your finger to the screen. Screens show the information and options needed to complete each step of the patient's visit. For example, an office-status screen might show the name of the patient in each examining room, the service that each patient requires (for example, examination, vital sign measurements, specific tests, immunizations), how long each patient has been waiting for each service, the number of patients in the waiting room, and the number of patients checked out that day. Another touch takes you to information on patients' previous visits to the office.

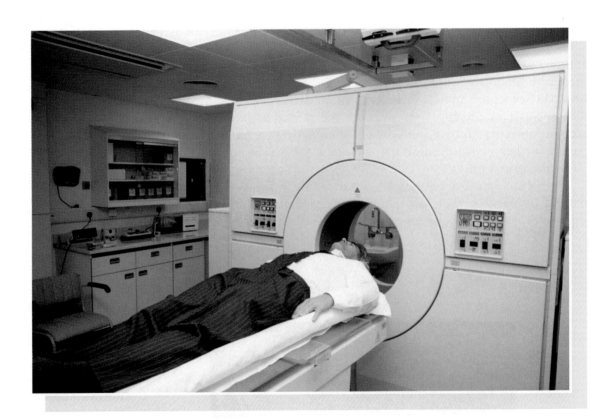

FIGURE   1.8

The CT scan and MRI have replaced many diagnostic procedures because they make it easier to locate abnormalities.

patient, to support payment of the claim. The government has completed development of systems to return the reimbursement of a claim to the physician office via on-line banking systems. Other major carriers, preferred provider organizations (PPOs), health maintenance organizations (HMOs), and others are currently developing this same mechanism.

Computer-Assisted Diagnosis and Treatment

Specialized devices are used to diagnose and treat patients in physician offices, hospital outpatient facilities, and hospitals. The computed tomography (CT) scan and magnetic resonance imaging (MRI) have replaced many diagnostic procedures; not only do these devices obtain the traditional x-ray information but also, with the assistance of a computer, they provide three-dimensional images represented by "slices," making it easier to locate even minute abnormalities throughout the body (Figure 1.8). The gamma knife, developed by Lawrence Berkeley Laboratory, uses the Cyclotron for stereotactic radial surgery. The proton beam, developed by Loma Linda University, irradiates inoperable brain tumors. Computers of the future may interact with human physiology for extended periods, formulating and assisting dynamic explanations of the functioning body systems, such as cardiovascular and nervous systems, and the experience of pain. These highly advanced technologies are expected to solve many of the mysteries associated with current medical problems. Many of these treatment-based computer functions most likely will be accomplished with the use of microcomputers, which probably will be based with the patient.

In the future it is anticipated that in many cases the physician will serve as an orchestrater of the high-tech world of medicine, utilizing a far greater number of computer technicians for diagnosis and treatment. More than likely, there will be a greater educational and training distinction between the primary care physician or diagnostician and the computer-trained physician.

Patient Population Changes and Disease Trends

With the influx over the past 15 years of immigrants of many nationalities to the United States, new diseases and culture-based medical treatments have been embraced. At the same time, cancer, heart disease, and many other diseases are now being treated with far greater success than previously. It is not difficult to imagine that many of the diseases currently being treated (for example, diabetes, Parkinson's disease, and multiple sclerosis) may someday be eradicated just as measles, smallpox, and diphtheria have been. By the same token, new and even more troubling diseases that are immune to current medications and treatments no doubt will be discovered, and subsequently new treatments will be created.

Finally, the average life span of the population is expected to increase within the next 20 years, bringing new medical challenges. In the past, a person was considered old at age 60 or 70; however, now a less frail, more competent, and active senior population is emerging. A large portion of the aging population will remain productive, active, and vital at a much older age. As a result, the current aging population has begun to reject the traditional constraints of aging.

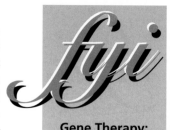

Gene Therapy: The Future?

Like grains of sand or snowflakes, each of us is different and possesses many distinctive characteristics. Each of these characteristics is determined by our genetic makeup, and until recently this makeup has been controlled entirely by nature. It is now possible for parents to influence the gender of their child. In the future, genetics may be able to be manipulated so that parents can choose other characteristics for their children. Genetic manipulation may mean that diseases can be prevented in their children as well as in themselves and others. Research is ongoing to genetically alter genes that contribute to life-threatening or debilitating diseases such as cystic fibrosis, Alzheimer's disease, and cancer. This process will allow scientists to alter the gene responsible for the disease before disease sets in.

Growth of the Administrative Medical Assistant Field

Over the past several decades, the health care industry's job market has expanded even further than expected. The roles of physician, nurse, and technician have changed dramatically, and the supply cannot meet the demand for

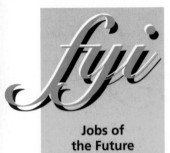

Jobs of the Future

Health technology will be one of the fastest growing job markets of the future. The jobs in this field range from the home health aide to the administrative medical assistant to the genetic engineer. Educational requirements range from specific training to 4-year degrees to graduate degrees. Your strengths and skills, such as the ability to be flexible, work as a team, practice effective communication, and be a leader, will be valuable. The use of technology and the ability to manipulate and analyze computerized data will be important in the future work world so it is vital that you learn and sharpen your computer skills.

nonphysician health care professionals. The growth trends are most often linked to increased demands for health care by an aging population, but another strong factor is advanced technology. In addition, socioeconomic trends and shortages of health care personnel also have brought changes in the delivery of health care services. These changes include the following:

- Insurance and payment plans are creating the most significant changes. A wide variety of health insurance plans are available to the general public, creating an enormous amount of paperwork for medical assistants. The requirements to keep up with each plan's regulations, authorizations, coding, preadmission requirements, and primary care physician (PCP) approval force front office personnel to constantly evaluate data from each carrier. In addition, medical facilities will make increased demands for coding specialists. In fact, this need has been realized: carriers are already forcing nonpayment when coding for procedures and diagnoses do not correlate or when the procedure was not specifically authorized by the carrier.

- The need for ambulatory care centers to deliver immediate, outpatient care has increased steadily for the past 10 years. The impact of these centers on the medical assisting profession has been to create more and more jobs; in the future, even more assistants will be needed. The emphasis on health maintenance in ambulatory care settings will only increase in an effort to reduce the need for expensive inpatient hospital services. Salaries for the medical assistant are likely to increase because of a shortage of assistants.

- Patient expectations have changed. Patients are demanding more available service, more information on wellness and preventive medicine, staff members who are knowledgeable about insurance, and more information on and/or referral to community resources. More front office personnel will be needed to meet the increased demands for these health care services as well.

The Medical Assistant's Role in Current and Future Health Care

The medical assistant must function as a professional member of the health care team, understand the ever-changing patterns of treatment, and participate in the overall delivery of services within the health care system. The medical assistant will need to help educate the patient, while understanding, and many times accepting, the lifestyle changes brought about by illness. The medical assistant may work with the patient to explain current trends in health care delivery, helping the patient cope with the frustrations of newer restrictions on access to health care, as well as coping with ill health, and achieving an optimum of wellness.

Conclusion

Individuals who choose a career in medical assisting will find themselves in a challenging and ever-changing profession, with numerous opportunities to demonstrate acquired skills. In return, the administrative medical assistant will receive personal satisfaction and enhanced self-esteem for a job well done. Becoming part of a health care team is a rewarding experience. As a member of that team, the administrative medical assistant can anticipate an ever-increasing level of responsibility as medical science and medical professionals continue to advance.

Review QUESTIONS

1. Why is health care considered a team effort?

2. Describe the method of training you are using to become an administrative medical assistant. Compare and contrast your method with other available methods.

3. What is the purpose and functions of the American Association of Medical Assistants (AAMA)?

4. How can personal attributes affect your work as an administrative medical assistant?

5. List and describe the duties of five members of a health care team.

6. What responsibilities can you expect to assume throughout your career with regard to co-workers, patients, and public relations contacts?

7. What personal rewards do you expect to acquire from a career in health care?

SUGGESTED READINGS

American Medical Association: *Winning ways with patients,* Chicago, 1990, The Association.
CCMA: *The medical assistant,* Chicago (monthly publication).

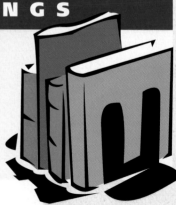

Medical Practice and Specialization

OUTLINE

- **Primitive Medicine**
- **Medical Concepts of the Ancients**
- **Medicine in the Dark and Middle Ages**
- **Effects of the Renaissance (1350–1650)**
- **Post-Renaissance Contributions**
- **Development of Surgery**
- **Advancement of Nursing**
- **Twentieth-Century Achievements**
- **Modern Medical Practices**
  Basic Medical Education
  Licensure
  Organizational Forms
  Development of Specialization
  Specialty Categories
- **Medical Associations**
  General Medical Associations

OBJECTIVES

On completion of Chapter 2 the administrative medical assistant student should be able to:

1. Define the key terms listed in this chapter.

2. Describe the role of superstition in primitive medicine.

3. Discuss the medical contributions of the ancient Greeks and Romans.

4. Name six scientists of the post-Renaissance period, and discuss their contributions to medicine.

5. Discuss the two major contributions that allowed the advancement of surgery.

6. Name the three women responsible for modern nursing techniques, and discuss their influence on medical care.

7. Describe basic medical education and the two methods of obtaining a medical license.

8. Discuss the development of medical specialization and the requirements of specialty education.

9. List the 5 primary care specialties, the 25 consultative specialties, and the 10 surgical specialties.

10. Discuss the concept of continuing medical education.

KEY TERMS

Disposition The act of managing or distributing; placement or arrangement.

Disseminate To spread, circulate, or disperse.

Immunology The science or study of the protective mechanisms of the body against disease; the mechanisms may be natural or acquired.

Internist A common term for the physician who practices internal medicine; a specialist who has completed an internship and a residency in internal medicine after completing medical school.

Internship Period of practical study, usually 1 year, immediately after medical school; the physician is called an intern during this time, a term not to be confused with internist.

Microbiology The science or study of microscopic plants and animals.

Operative Pertaining to surgical procedures.

Continued

(Continued)

Primitive   Belonging to the earliest ages in time.

Residency   A 3- to 5-year period of study after internship during which the physician prepares for the practice of a specialized field in medicine.

Today's health care consumer is accustomed to a great number of services for all types of health care. Consumers have high (and sometimes unreasonable) expectations of the health care provider. Patients are accustomed to a vast array of diagnostic and treatment modes, numerous preventive and curative medications, and a readily available variety of health care providers. Many patients cannot remember a time when antibiotics did not exist, even though penicillin was not refined or produced in quantity until World War II. Surgery is common, relatively safe, and painless today, yet a little more than 100 years ago, it was dangerous and painful because of the lack of knowledge about bacterial infection and anesthesia.

Progress in medical science has led to the specialization of physicians and medical practice. Allied health professionals also may choose to specialize. The administrative medical assistant who develops a foundation of knowledge and theory will be prepared to make an intelligent decision about employment opportunities in the diverse health care field.

Primitive Medicine

In the earliest days of civilization, mystery, magic, and medicine were synonymous. Without sufficient knowledge to explain cause-and-effect relationships, primitive peoples attributed many phenomena they could not explain to supernatural powers. Superstition played a dominant role in the healing arts, and witch doctors were believed to have special powers to drive away evil spirits. The effective tribal doctor was able to rid patients of the spirits responsible for their symptoms. In performing this function, the primitive physician inadvertently discovered and used substances that are components of some of our modern medicines (Figure 2.1). For example, early practitioners accidentally discovered that chewing the leaves of the foxglove plant could slow and strengthen the heartbeat; because of this discovery, we now have digitalis, a cardiac stimulant. The bark of the cinchona tree was found to control fever and muscle spasms; quinine, an antimalarial drug, is derived from that source. Juice from the belladonna plant (deadly nightshade) was found to relieve abdominal

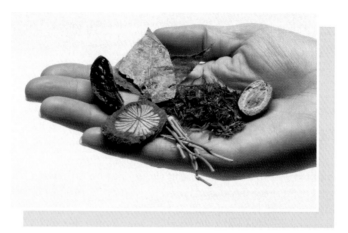

Early physicians inadvertently discovered and used substances that are components of some of our modern medicines.

pain and intestinal cramps; atropine, a modern drug used for this type of abdominal problem, is one of several medicines made from that plant. Some varieties of the poppy plant produce opium, now used as the medication morphine to relieve severe pain.

As the centuries passed and tribal organizations developed, the medicine man grew in importance as both priest and physician, maintaining a link between the spiritual world and the role of healer. Even before people discovered the means to control and use fire, the tribal physician recognized the relaxing or stimulating qualities of some plant roots used for nourishment. By isolating or combining these substances, the witch doctor was able to control people, and he often used this power to assume a position of tribal leadership.

Medical Concepts of the Ancients

The earliest civilization of which we have an extensive knowledge is that of the Egyptians. The medicine of the Egyptians was a combination of superstition, religion, and practical considerations. The gods were invoked to heal, but early Egyptian physicians also administered medicines to the sick and used splints to heal fractures. Egyptian physicians were adept in the diagnosis and treatment of numerous diseases, and even performed surgery as sophisticated as trephination to relieve intracranial pressure.

The ancient Greeks made the first step toward scientific inquiry and away from the pure superstition and mysticism of the primitives. The ancient Greeks attempted to study nature objectively by considering the human body and its disease without resorting to supernatural explanations. The Greeks became the first people to proclaim the value and principles of scientific medicine, including the importance of research. They removed mystery from medicine, making medicine a practice of common sense, observation, and logical reasoning.

PERSPECTIVES ON MEDICAL ASSISTING

Hippocrates

Hippocrates was an excellent observer. This is demonstrated by his "Aphorisms," or advice, to physicians:

When sleep puts an end to delirium, it is a good sign.
When on a starvation diet, a patient should not be fatigued.
In every disease it is a good sign when the patient's intellect is sound and he enjoys his food—the opposite is a bad sign.
Old men generally have less illness than young men but such complaints as become chronic in old men last until death.
All diseases occur at all seasons, but some diseases are more apt to occur and be aggravated at certain seasons.
Those who are attacked by tetanus either die in four days or, if they survive, recover.

Hippocrates, often referred to as the father of medicine, lived during the golden age of Greek culture (circa 400 BC) and developed great skill in diagnosis. He enhanced the scientific approach by carefully noting and recording signs and symptoms associated with various diseases. Hippocrates also is credited with establishing a standard of ethics, known as the Oath of Hippocrates (see the box on p. 53), which serves as the foundation for modern principles of medical ethics.

Religious custom prevented the Greeks from gathering information on anatomy and physiology through dissection of the body after death. Instead, Greek physicians derived their knowledge from bedside observation of patients, noting the signs, symptoms, and eventual outcome of the patient's condition. They tried to correlate the information they observed with the experiences of their previous patients.

The Romans drew upon this knowledge and developed it further. The Greeks established the importance of personal hygiene, and the Romans derived from this concept principles of public health. From a medical standpoint the greatest contributions of the Roman era were in sanitation. Even without knowledge of microorganisms, the Romans recognized the need for a system of sanitary engineering, drained swamps, built aqueducts to carry fresh water to their cities, and constructed a system of sewers to carry off wastewater.

Surgery apparently was a well-accepted practice in the Roman Empire, as substantiated by an archeological find of more than 200 surgical instruments in the ruins near Pompeii. Postmortem dissection of the human body, however, was still considered a sacrilegious act and was forbidden. The advancement of anatomy and physiology during this period is credited to Galen, a Greek physician who worked and taught in Rome (see the box on the facing page).

PERSPECTIVES ON MEDICAL ASSISTING

Medicine in Ancient Times

Egypt is one of the oldest civilizations on earth and from there came Imhotep, one of the earliest named physicians. He was the author of the oldest known script about surgery. Ancient Egyptians had an amazing range of clinical practices, from rational thinking and clinical observations to pure magic and religion. A document on papyrus has been excavated that includes information on very logical accounts of when to stitch wounds and how to apply splints and bandages. It discusses complications related to wound care, such as infection and tetanus, and suggests treatments for them.

Greece's earliest source of medical knowledge and description of medical practices is the poems of Homer. The *Iliad* covers part of the tenth and final year of the Trojan War and mentions nearly 150 different wounds with surprising anatomical accuracy.

Rome's Galen succeeded Hippocrates in the advancement of medical science. Galen believed that knowledge of anatomy was essential for a physician, and he was a master of dissection (probably animals). He was viewed as a learned authority at the end of the second century, and his works and ideas were the sole basis of medical knowledge for the next 14 centuries.

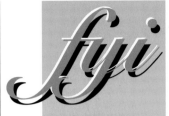

The Church: The First Hospital

The Dark Ages was a time of hunger, pestilence, and war, and there was a desperate need for a place for the sick and wounded to go. The one institution that was willing and able to offer and ensure asylum was the Catholic Church. Persons who needed medical help would go to the monasteries, where monks kept lists of medicinal herbs.

It is recorded that the monastery of St. Gall in 820 AD had a medicinal herb garden, rooms for six sick people, a pharmacy, and special lodging for a physician. (The monastery appears to be the first example of a hospital in Western Europe.)

Medicine in the Dark and Middle Ages

After the fall of the Roman Empire, the progress of medical science came essentially to a halt. During the 400 years of the Dark Ages (circa 400 AD to 800 AD) and the 600 years of the Middle Ages (circa 800 AD to 1400 AD), medicine was practiced only in the great monasteries and convents. Treatments consisted chiefly of custodial care and the use of herbal medication. The monks' greatest contributions to medical science were the collection and translation of the works of Greek and Roman physicians. During this period a breakdown of public health practices resulted in the tragic spread of communicable diseases, especially the bubonic plague, which killed an estimate 20 million people in Europe (see the box on p. 30).

Effects of the Renaissance (1350–1650)

The Renaissance, which occurred roughly between 1350 AD and 1650 AD, is considered an era of great cultural and scientific activity. Four main developments during this time influenced the future of medical science. First, universities and associated medical schools were founded, providing an environment in which research and instruction in the medical arts could take place more sys-

PERSPECTIVES ON MEDICAL ASSISTING

"This is the End of the World"

The quote above is from the Siena Chronicle, which was written in 1354 to describe what people said and believed about the plague. Over a period of 2 years, the plague had spread throughout most of Europe, and in some places entire populations succumbed. The following is a quote about the plague from Boccaccio's Decameron:

"How many grand places, how many stately homes, how many splendid residences, once full of retainers, of lords, of ladies, were now left desolate of all, even to the meanest servant! How many brave men, how many fair ladies, how many gallant youths . . . broke fast with their kinsfolk in the morning and when evening came supped with their forefathers in the other world!"

tematically. Second, a transition occurred in human understanding from unquestioning acceptance to the challenging of existing beliefs and the exploration of new horizons. Third, the invention of the printing press allowed the rapid dissemination of information, including advances made in medical science. Fourth, the stigma attached to the dissection of the dead dissipated with the realization that knowledge of anatomy and physiology would be advanced only through organized scientific examination. The combined effect of these four factors influenced the future of the art and science of medicine.

Post-Renaissance Contributions

The seventeenth and eighteenth centuries were characterized by a tremendous increase in the accumulation of technical facts. Once physicians understood the structure of the human body, they were able to turn their attention to the functioning of its systems. Knowledge of physiology remained in the embryonic stages until the 1600s, when William Harvey (1578–1657), an English physician, accurately described the way blood circulates through the body. Experimenting with animals, he actually witnessed and felt a heart beating. Harvey's great contribution to medical knowledge helped substantiate the interdependence between the structure of the body and its internal workings.

The discovery of the microscope provided scientists with the tool necessary to examine life-forms not visible to the naked eye (Figure 2.2). Anton van Leeuwenhoek (1631–1723), a Dutch lens maker and scientist, produced the earliest forerunner of today's microscope. He was able to identify bacteria and recognize variations among microorganisms, confirming the presence of numerous forms of microscopic life. (However, the role of bacteria in the cause of disease was not recognized until 150 years later.)

Although Leeuwenhoek and other seventeenth-century pioneers described various forms of microscopic life, the real significance and origin of these

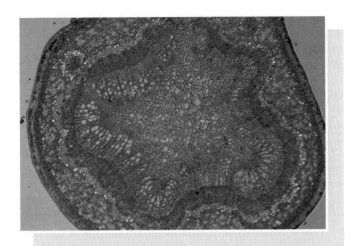

FIGURE **2.2**

The discovery of the microscope provided scientists with the tool necessary to examine life-forms not visible to the naked eye.

bodies were not understood until they were investigated by Louis Pasteur (1822–1895). Pasteur was a French bacteriologist and chemist whose work paralleled that of a German physician, Robert Koch (1843–1910). The research of both men showed that bacteria exist everywhere and that sterilization kills bacteria. Although his study of the fermentation process helped the French wine industry, Pasteur most commonly is associated with the process of heating food to prevent the growth of bacteria. This process, called pasteurization, is still used today. Koch generally is credited with discovering the tubercle bacillus. Although he was unable to find a cure for the disease it causes, tuberculosis, he developed laboratory aids, such as culture plates and dried, fixed, and stained slides of bacteria, for microscopic examination.

Edward Jenner (1749–1823) of England made one of the greatest contributions toward the prevention of disease when he discovered a small pox vaccination. Jenner's discovery led to the science of immunology and eventually to public health preventive medicine.

Medicine progressed rapidly during the nineteenth century. Great discoveries in chemistry and physics were applied to research in physiological problems. The medical advances of the nineteenth century, particularly those arising from the demonstration of the bacterial cause of infection, made medicine a social necessity and a guiding force in modern civilization.

Continuing the work of the pioneers in microbiology, Paul Ehrlich (1854–1915) facilitated the identification and classification of various organisms. His techniques of staining bacteria and cells provided the means for differential analysis.

Development of Surgery

Although surgery has been performed since ancient times, it was not until the late eighteenth century that it was elevated to the status of a medical science. Often referred to as the father of modern surgery, John Hunter (1728–1793) developed surgical techniques that were founded on knowledge of anatomy

FIGURE 2.3

Newly acquired knowledge about the existence of bacteria and their relationship to infection introduced the concept of antisepsis.

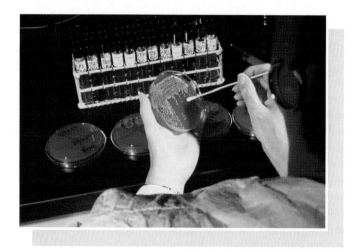

PERSPECTIVES ON MEDICAL ASSISTING

The Founder of Scientific Surgery

John Hunter was born in 1728 in England. He learned dissection from his brother, William, and then acquired extensive knowledge of gunshot wounds in the army. After retiring from the army, he practiced surgery and lectured on anatomy and surgery. His surgical procedures were based on sound knowledge of pathology. He also was the first to study teeth scientifically. He inserted the first gastric feeding tube. He trained at least two important medical men, William Shippen Jr. and Edward Jenner, in surgery.

and physiology and the diagnosis of pathological conditions. The English School of Surgery, founded by Hunter, still exists (see the box above).

Recognizing the need for surgery and developing effective surgical techniques solved many problems associated with surgery. The remaining problems involved pain and wound infection. Joseph Lister (1827–1912), using the newly acquired knowledge about bacteria and determining the relationship between bacteria and infection of operative wounds, introduced the concept of antisepsis (Figure 2.3). Lister searched for a substance that would kill bacteria on wounds, prevent the entrance of other bacteria, and not cause injury to the tissue. His experiments with carbolic acid proved his theory of the bacterial cause of infection. He eventually expanded the use of carbolic acid, developing a spray for the operation room before surgery, a bath for the surgical instruments, and a washing solution for the surgeon's hands. Lister's development of surgical asepsis proved to be one of the greatest contributions to modern surgery.

Until the early 1840s, physicians emphasized the speed of surgery to reduce pain and shock. However, the development of anesthesia allowed physicians to concentrate on accuracy and precision, two hallmarks of modern surgery. In the United States, Dr. Crawford Long, a physician, and Dr. William Morton,

PERSPECTIVES ON MEDICAL ASSISTING

The Nightingale Pledge

The Nightingale Pledge, below, was written at the old Harper Hospital in Detroit, Michigan, and was used by its graduating class of nurses in the spring of 1893. It is an adaptation of the Hippocratic Oath taken by physicians (Florence Nightingale probably had no knowledge of its content).

I solemnly pledge myself before God and in the presence of this assembly, to pass my life in purity and to practice my profession faithfully. I will abstain from whatever is deleterious and mischievous, and will not take or knowingly administer any harmful drug. I will do all in my power to maintain and elevate the standard of my profession, and will hold in confidence all personal matters committed to my keeping and all family affairs coming to my knowledge in the practice of my calling. With loyalty will I endeavor to aid the physician in his work and devote myself to the welfare of those committed to my care.

a dentist, helped make anesthesia safe for surgery. Working independently, both began to use ether as a general anesthetic. The use of anesthetics made possible many operations that previously were avoided, thereby providing the means to cure many diseases.

The alleviation of pain and the reduction of wound infections combined to advance surgical technique rapidly. With the need for speed eliminated by general anesthesia, surgical operations could last longer, and the surgeon could devote time to precision and care.

Advancement of Nursing

The recognition of nurses as qualified health care providers began in the nineteenth century. Florence Nightingale (1820–1910) received what was considered formal training at the first hospital-based school for nurses in Kaiserwerth, Germany. Recognizing that educated nurses had more to offer patients than hygiene and hand-holding, Nightingale mobilized people in support of her cause. Her efforts during the Crimean War (1850–1853) did a great deal to alleviate the suffering of the ill and wounded and establish credibility for her theories of training. After many disappointments and a long struggle, Nightingale succeeded in getting public support for her efforts to improve the care of the sick. The principles she established have served as a fundamental guide for nursing progress, and the school she established at St. Thomas Hospital in London has served as the model for subsequent nursing schools.

Clara Barton (1821–1912) was an American nursing pioneer during the American Civil War. The difficulties of tracing the whereabouts of injured or dead soldiers led to Barton's role in the formation of the Federal Bureau of Records. The problems of procuring supplies in battle and disaster situations and her exposure to the Red Cross organization in Europe resulted in Barton's establishment of the American Red Cross in 1881. She served as the president of the organization until 1904, 8 years before her death at age 91.

The third outstanding contributor to the advancement of nursing was Lillian Walt (1867–1940), a graduate of the New York Hospital Training School. She is credited with placing public health nursing on a firm and rational foundation. She championed the idea that the health needs of patients were closely related to their social needs. She was instrumental in founding the Henry Street Settlement House in 1893 in New York City. This establishment now is famous as the seed of public health nursing.

The development of nursing as an adjunct to physicians' health care practices laid the foundation for future complementary professions. The role of formally trained medical assistants in health care will broaden over time just as the nursing and medical professions have advanced.

Twentieth-Century Achievements

Medicine has made enormous strides since 1900. X-rays, discovered by the German physicist Wilhelm Roentgen, were refined and provided a means to diagnose injuries and disease processes and treat some cancers. The French physicists Marie and Pierre Curie discovered radium as a treatment of malignancies. Radiology has since progressed to include the use of radioisotopes and sound-, heat-, and computer-assisted imaging. Highly technical pieces of imaging equipment, such as the CT scanner and MRI, now are used to view all parts of the body. In addition, the gamma knife can be used to eliminate an inoperable brain tumor by the use of a proton beam. Diagnostic and therapeutic procedures are being discovered and refined at an unprecedented rate. Techniques in laboratory analysis, electrocardiology, and physical therapy provide invaluable assistance to the physician and patient (Figure 2.4).

Modern Medical Practices
Basic Medical Education

Medical students who wish to become physicians receive training for a minimum of 9 years. The basic preparation for practicing medicine is 4 years of college (with a major in premedical studies or a basic science), 4 years of medical school, and 1 year of internship (a period of practical experience). Physicians who do not wish to specialize in one area of medicine may choose a rotating internship, which provides experience in multiple specialty areas throughout the 1-year period. This allows the physician to practice medicine as a general practitioner.

Licensure

In the United States a physician is eligible to practice general medicine in individual states after successful completion of the required medical school cur-

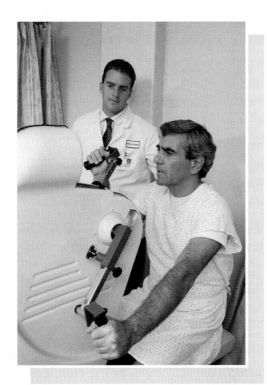

A

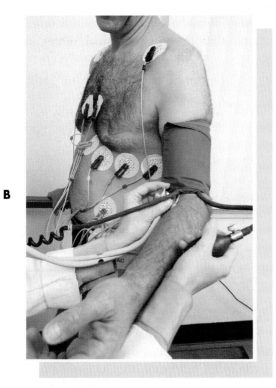

B

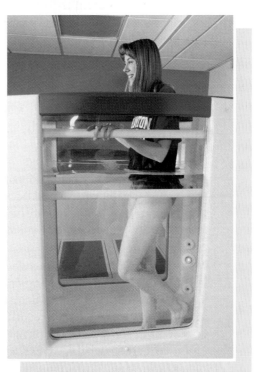

C

Techniques in laboratory analysis (A), electrocardiology (B), and physical therapy (C) provide invaluable assistance to the physician and patient.

WHAT DO YOU THINK?

In the past, when someone made a decision to become a physician, he or she would get the training, hang out the "shingle," and then practice for the rest of his or her life. The physician's practice frequently consumed his or her entire life. Patients were seen whenever necessary, whether during the week, the weekend, holidays, day, or night. Although they sacrificed family time, many physicians could never see themselves in any other profession. They practiced until they no longer could.

Now the physician's life has become much more complicated. Following is an example of working as a physician today:

Dr. Jones is still in private practice, but he now is a provider for a health maintenance organization (HMO) and must practice differently. In his opinion, he can no longer practice medicine in a way that places service first and payment second.

Jim Fletcher, a patient whom Dr. Jones has been seeing, was sitting in the waiting room. Dr. Jones could not call him in for an evaluation because no authorization had been approved by Mr. Fletcher's HMO. Seeing a patient without proper authorization could result in Dr. Jones not being paid for his services. All Dr. Jones could do was check to make sure Mr. Fletcher was not seriously or dangerously ill and wait for approval to see him several weeks later.

What can Dr. Jones do to change this situation? Or, can he change it?

riculum, an internship, and the state's board examination. Most states now accept successful completion of the National Board Examination for licensure in lieu of an individual state examination. Generally the examination is taken just before completion of medical school, and the license is issued after the internship. This license is valid for the physician's lifetime and is renewed periodically with payment of a fee. Physicians who choose to begin private practice at this time are considered general practitioners.

Organizational Forms

Just as science and technology have led to major changes in the practice of medicine, medical, legal, and governmental factors have influenced the way physicians organize their practices. The most common legal forms for medical practices are sole proprietorships, partnerships, professional corporations, and associations. Physicians can provide care in the following legal relationships: employer-employee, association, group, and institutional.

Sole Proprietorship

The physician in a sole proprietorship has total authority and responsibility for all administrative decisions in the practice (Figure 2.5). This physician may choose to employ another physician to assist with clinical duties. Physician-employees are salaried members of the staff and subject to the authority of the physician-owner. Physician-owners in the other practice forms identified here may also employ other physicians in their practices. The physician-owner has the right to all assets and is responsible for all expenses.

Partnership

A partnership is a legal agreement and association of two or more physicians who act as co-owners of the business. Each partner is legally responsible for all professional (clinical) and financial actions of all other partners.

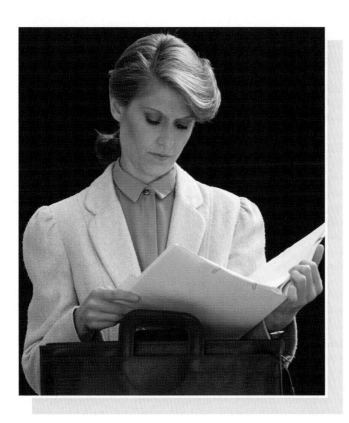

FIGURE   2.5

The physician in a sole proprietorship has total authority and responsibility for all administrative decisions in the practice.

Professional Corporation

During the 10-year period between 1961 and 1971, each state enacted legislation allowing professionals (individually or in groups) to incorporate. A professional corporation gave physician-owners and employees many legal and financial benefits. Until 1985 the majority of medical practices in the United States were incorporated. Congress has since removed many of the advantages of being incorporated, and currently, for the most part, only groups benefit from this legal designation.

Association

An association is a legal agreement and association of two or more physicians who act as co-owners of the business in clearly defined areas. Individual partners are not legally responsible for all professional (clinical) and financial actions of the other partners. Associations usually have weekly or monthly meetings to divide expenses and make decisions regarding the practice.

Practicing in an association is beneficial to physicians, particularly those who wish to have practices in several locations. In this type of practice, physicians usually contribute only to the expenses incurred when they are at that location. Consequently, bookkeeping for this type of practice can be very labor intensive.

Employer-employee

The physician who chooses the position of employee in a medical practice usually is a recent graduate of a training program who is interested in evaluating practice forms, various communities and opportunities, and other methods of practice. In this position, the physician is relieved of the responsibility of administrative decisions and financial burdens (Figure 2.6).

FIGURE 2.6

The physician who
chooses the position of
employee in a medical
practice is relieved of the
responsibility of administrative decisions and
financial burdens.

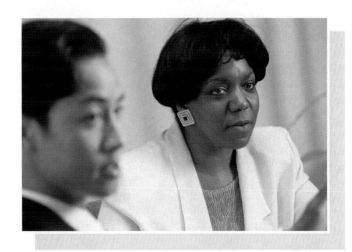

A physician may choose only to work as a locum tenums (employee) or wish to work rural health or at different geographical locations and not be involved in the day-to-day running of the practice. Today, we have physicians who are called "circuit riders," because they are part of transplant teams, rotating one day a month in various small cities or remote rural areas that cannot support specialty physicians.

A physician-employee has less impact with decisions regarding staffing and administration of the practice. For the medical assistant little changes; the physician and assistant both are employees. The assistant still will have the same duties to perform for this physician as she or he does for the others. The physician-employee, however, will not be able to demand certain information and reports regarding the practice from the assistant.

Group Practice

The American Medical Association (AMA) defines a medical group practice as the provision of health care services by a group of at least three licensed physician-practitioners who are engaged full time in a formally organized and legally recognized entity; share the groups income and expenses in a systematic manner; and share facilities, equipment, common records, and personnel, and are involved in both patient care and business management (Figure 2.7). Today, small groups comprise three to eight physicians, usually of the same specialty; a medium group has nine to 50 physicians, usually with various specialists and general practitioners (or what are now known as primary care physicians); and groups from 50 to 150, which are considered large, multispecialty groups.

Institutional Relationships

When physicians choose to practice in an institutional setting, they receive a salary from the institution, whether a medical center or a free-standing health maintenance organization (HMO). The physician assumes no financial responsibility for the overall maintenance of the facility, records, or staff. This is strictly a salaried position.

Development of Specialization

Specialization is a relatively recent phenomenon in the history of medicine. The division of medical functions began about 100 years ago with the indus-

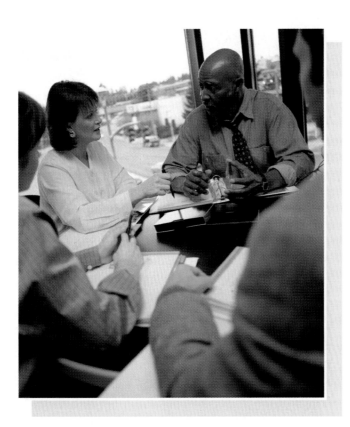

FIGURE 2.7

Medical group practice is the provision of health care services by a group of at least three licensed physician-practitioners.

trial and technological revolution, which accelerated the advancement of the sciences and the development of precision instruments.

Specialty Education

The greatest single factor in advancing medical specialization was World War II. During this period, soldiers sustained unprecedented injuries. Physicians were not sufficiently prepared to use the scientific and technological advancements of the time to treat these patients. The physicians drafted for the war effort had been out of medical school for varying lengths of time, and the new technological discoveries were being applied with such speed that not all the physicians had the necessary skills. The usual educational experience of physicians before World War II was limited to what now is considered basic medical education. The U.S. Army Medical Corps responded to the immediate need for training by organizing brief, intensive courses for its personnel. Subsequently, medical schools and health care facilities developed programs, known as postgraduate study, for physicians interested in developing new skills and knowledge in specific areas.

The selection of a specialty is a highly individual matter for physicians; the choice is dictated by personal preference, interest, and special ability. Physicians who seek out advanced study in one of the specialties tend to restrict their practice to the diagnosis and treatment of ailments falling into that category. Depending on the specialty, the physician who decides to pursue a specialty must plan to spend an additional 3 to 6 years of study after internship. This period is known as residency, and the student is referred to as a resident physician. If physicians wish to extend their knowledge in the chosen specialty, they may pursue a fellowship. The students then are referred to as fellows. Fellowships are difficult to obtain: Only two to four fellows are chosen each year in the teaching facilities that offer this type of program.

Specialty Certification

After residency the physician is prepared to begin practice as a specialist. Each specialty recognized by the AMA has a national board to set standards and certify the competency of its members. The physician applying for certification in a specialty must fulfill certain requirements with regard to education, training, and practical experience and also is expected to pass a written or oral examination. On successful compliance with all board requirements, the physician is awarded a certificate of competency in the specialty and becomes known as a diplomate of the specialty. The common designation of the certified specialist is fellow, as in Fellow of the American College of Surgeons (FACS).

Specialty Categories

Specialists may practice medicine, surgery, or both. Medicine involves treatment by physical or chemical means; surgery involves treatment by manual and operative procedures. Specialty practices also may be classified as primary and consultative care.

Primary Care Specialties

Physicians who practice primary care provide all basic diagnostic, preventive, and treatment services for their patients. The specialties commonly designated as primary care include family practice, gerontology, gynecology, internal medicine, and pediatrics, as well as general practice. Medical assistants who work for a primary care physician will have the opportunity to use almost every facet of their training and preparation. Variety in duties and responsibilities is the rule, not the exception. A brief overview of the primary care specialties will help administrative medical assistants choose the area to which they would prefer to devote their efforts. Primary care practices tend to run at a much faster pace, since most physicians will schedule at least four patients per hour. The assistant who works in primary care will find that each day passes very quickly and there never seems to be enough hours to accommodate every patient and the associated workload. The more patients the practice sees, the more telephone calls there are, the more paperwork that is generated, and so forth.

Family Practice. Family practice resembles internal medicine but differs in that the physician cares for all members of the family unit. Treating the entire family allows the physician to observe and interpret the influence of family relationships in maintaining or restoring the health of individual members.

Gerontology. The gerontologist is prepared to handle the special needs of older patients because of additional training in the evaluation and treatment of diseases related to the aging process.

Gynecology. Gynecology deals with the examination or treatment of the female reproductive organs. It is classified as primary care because the gynecologist often is the only physician a woman sees regularly. Therefore the patient

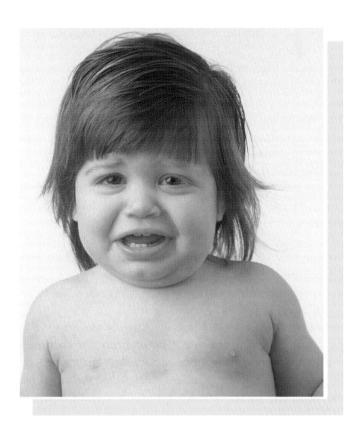

FIGURE 2.8

Pediatrics involves the evaluation and treatment of infants, children, and adolescents.

often seeks advice on matters other than gynecology, and the physician periodically performs screening evaluations.

Internal Medicine. Specialists in internal medicine evaluate and advise the patient about the functioning of internal organs and treat disorders by physical or chemical means.

Pediatrics. Pediatrics involves the evaluation and treatment of infants, children, and adolescents (Figure 2.8). Pediatricians are prepared to deal with the special needs of their patients because of additional training in the growth and development phases of life and the diseases unique to children.

Consultative Specialists: Institutional Settings

Consultative specialists have elected to work within one area of the body and concentrate all efforts toward that specialty. For example, clinical pharmacology works within a pharmacy setting to provide physicians with access to all data regarding drug interactions, as well as patient information. In this way, physicians can avoid prescribing drugs that may result in a serious reaction for the patient either because of his or her illness or other medications he or she may be taking. For example, a patient who has had renal failure should never take the drug ciprofloxacin (Cipro) for bladder or respiratory infections because the drug can shut down the kidneys. Another example is critical care physicians, who work exclusively with critically ill patients within a hospital intensive care unit. Should these patients subsequently become outpatients, these physicians will see them to clear their status for return to the care of their primary care physician.

Emergency medicine, neonatology, nuclear medicine, radiology, and pathology all primarily are hospital-based practices.

Some consultative specialists are best able to practice in institutional settings, including hospitals, educational facilities, and research facilities. Because medical assistants working in these settings have direct or indirect contact with these specialists, a brief description of each follows.

Clinical Pharmacology. Clinical pharmacology involves the treatment of disease with chemical substances. The physician consults on the selection of appropriate medication, drug interactions, and the diagnosis of adverse reactions from the use of drugs.

Critical Care. Specialists in critical care evaluate and treat severely ill, injured, and traumatized patients in the hospital setting. These physicians work in the intensive care unit (ICU) or cardiac care unit/critical care unit (CCU). These physicians treat the most critically ill and injured patients in the hospital and consult with other caregivers.

Emergency Medicine. Specialists in emergency medicine (EM) practice in the emergency rooms of hospitals, trauma centers, or commercial facilities developed to provide intervention in situations involving sudden, serious, and potentially life-threatening illnesses or injuries. Once the crisis has passed, the EM physician refers the patient to the appropriate specialist(s) for continued care.

Neonatology. Specialists in neonatology practice primarily in the hospital setting to evaluate and treat severely ill infants, many of whom are born premature or with congenital defects or drug-related illnesses.

Nuclear Medicine. Specialists in nuclear medicine diagnose and in some cases treat disease processes by means of radioactive substances. These physicians interpret the x-ray images, computed tomographic (CT) scans, and magnetic resonance images (MRIs) that have been taken by the technician. They also determine the amount of radiation that a cancer patient requires at specified areas of the body.

Pathology. Pathology deals with the causes of disease, and the pathologist helps other physicians make a diagnosis by evaluating tissue or fluid taken from the patient. Laboratory tests are used by the pathologist to assist in determining cellular changes that affect the structure or function of the body systems.

Perinatology. Specialists in perinatology provide evaluations and advise patients about possible congenital illnesses of the fetus.

Preventive Medicine. Preventive medicine provides specific counseling with regard to patients' family history of health problems. As the name of the specialty suggests, the focus is on prevention.

Radiology. Radiology is a diagnostic or therapeutic specialty. The diagnostic radiologist assists other physicians in determining a patient's structural or functional status through the use of various imaging techniques. Therapeutic radiologists treat certain disease processes with various radioactive substances.

Consultative Specialists: Private Practice

Consultative specialists who establish private offices provide the most job opportunities for administrative medical assistants (Figure 2.9). Brief

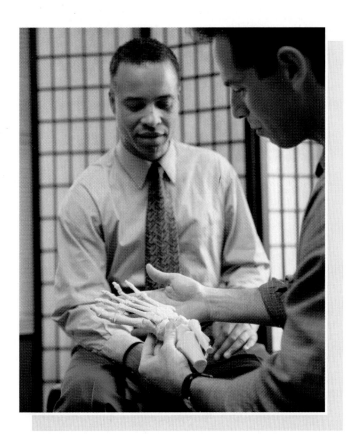

FIGURE 2.9

Consultative specialists who establish private offices provide the most job opportunities for administrative medical assistants.

descriptions of the specialties most commonly encountered in private practice follow.

Allergy. Allergy specialists diagnose and treat allergic reactions that may include internal and external illnesses. A new subspecialty, environmental allergies, involves the evaluation and treatment of patients whose illnesses are caused by the environment in which they live.

Cardiology. Cardiologists evaluate and treat patients with heart conditions, as well as internal and external illnesses.

Dermatology. Dermatologists are concerned with the proper care of the skin and the treatment of disease affecting the skin. Skin disorders may be caused by environmental contact or internal sources. Treatment may be medical or surgical.

Endocrinology. Endocrinology deals with the ductless glands and their disorders. The diseases treated include overproduction or underproduction of hormones by the various glands.

Gastroenterology. The diagnosis and medical or surgical treatment of diseases of the digestive system are the primary concerns of gastroenterologists.

Hepatology. Hepatology deals with the liver and pancreas and their disorders. This involves diagnosis, treatment, and sometimes liver transplants.

Infectious Disease Medicine. The infectious disease specialist diagnoses and treats communicable diseases. The process includes investigation to deter-

FIGURE 2.10

Throughout pregnancy, labor, and birth, the obstetrician has a dual responsibility to the mother and developing fetus or fetuses.

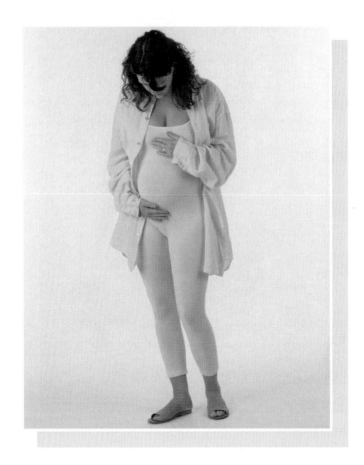

mine the cause, provision of appropriate treatment, and development of a plan to prevent recurrence or spread of the infectious organism.

Legal Medicine. The relatively new field of legal medicine developed as a result of the increasing complexity of the health care field and the growing number of legal cases involving medical situations. A practitioner of legal medicine may be a physician qualified to serve as an expert witness in specific areas of medicine. The legal medical specialist may hold degrees in both law and medicine, choosing either to practice law and specialize in medical cases or to practice medicine and specialize in cases involving legal issues.

Maternal/Fetal Medicine. Specialists in the new field of maternal/fetal medicine treat the fetus in the womb. Their patients are high-risk mothers with a variety of illnesses who are having trouble carrying the baby to full term. Often these specialists also are working with the fetus, who may have some abnormality. These physicians may remove tumors from the fetus and perform heart surgery before delivery. This is a highly specialized field; at this time there are still few training centers for maternal fetal medicine; however, more and more are being established each day, as the need for this type of service is recognized.

Neurology. Neurology involves the diagnosis and treatment of disorders of the central and peripheral nervous systems. These disorders may be caused by injury, disease, or infection. The neurologist is concerned primarily with the diagnosis and treatment of conditions by medical means.

Obstetrics. Often practiced in combination with gynecology, obstetrics relates to the care of women during pregnancy, labor, birth, and the recovery period after birth (usually 6 weeks). Throughout pregnancy, labor, and birth, the obstetrician has a dual responsibility to the mother and developing fetus or fetuses (Figure 2.10).

Ophthalmology. Ophthalmology involves the evaluation of the structure and function of the eye and the medical or surgical treatment of any disorders. The ophthalmologist is a physician and is not to be confused with the optometrist, who is limited to the evaluation of visual ability and the adaptation of the lens, or the optician, who prepares corrective lenses according to the directions of the ophthalmologist or optometrist.

Otorhinolaryngology. Otorhinolaryngology commonly is referred to as ENT because the specialist medically or surgically treats disorders of the ear, nose, and throat.

Physical Medicine and Rehabilitation. This specialty involves the evaluation of an individual's functional status and the development of a treatment plan designed to return the patient to an optimal level of physical performance. Physicians practicing physical medicine and rehabilitation are referred to as physiatrists, and their patients often have organic disorders such as cerebrovascular accident (CVA) or injuries such as quadriplegia caused by an auto accident. The physiatrist works with other health care providers such as physical, occupational, and recreational therapists.

Pulmonary Medicine. Pulmonary medicine deals with the lungs and the respiratory system. Many of these disorders may be caused by injury, disease, or infection.

Psychiatry. Psychiatry deals with the etiology, diagnosis, treatment, and prevention of mental disorders. The foundation of psychiatry is the one-to-one relationship between the physician and the patient. The treatment of more serious psychiatric disorders has been greatly enhanced in recent times by the development of mood-stabilizing drugs.

Oncology. The oncologist treats patients with cancer, using either radiation therapy (megadoses of radiation) or chemotherapy (powerful intravenous drugs).

Surgical Specialties

Surgery is treatment by manual or operative procedures. Combined advances in anesthesia and drugs, physiology, and technology have enhanced the scope and safety of surgical treatment. These advances have created specialized subcategories of surgery. Surgery now includes the use of lasers and the high-powered radiological proton beam, which is called sterlotactic radiosurgery.

Breast Surgery. Breast surgery involves the evaluation and treatment of the breast, which may include taking tissue samples for biopsy to test for cancer, removing the breast, and reconstructing the breast.

Cardiovascular Surgery. Cardiovascular surgery is limited to the heart, heart valves, and the vessels that serve the heart muscle.

Colon and Rectal Surgery. Surgeons who specialize in colon and rectal surgery limit their evaluation and treatment to the lower segment of the digestive system.

General Surgery. General surgery involves the treatment of neoplasms and functional disorders of the abdominal organs, breasts, subcutaneous tissue, and extremities.

Neurosurgery. Neurosurgery involves the invasive treatment of the brain, spinal cord, and peripheral nervous system.

Orthopedic Surgery. The musculoskeletal system is the concern of the orthopedic surgeon. Orthopedic surgery includes treatment of structural or functional disorders of the muscles, ligaments, tendons, bones, and joints.

Plastic Surgery. Plastic surgery involves the repair or restoration of tissue for cosmetic or functional purposes. The specialist may consult on cases involving burns, amputations, or birth defects.

Thoracic Surgery. The thoracic surgeon treats disorders of the structures in the chest such as the lungs, bronchi, esophagus, and diaphragm.

Urological Surgery. The urologist medically or surgically treats diseases and dysfunctions of the urinary tract and the male reproductive system.

Vascular Surgery. Vascular surgery is the invasive treatment of veins and arteries throughout the body.

Relicensure and Recertification

License Renewal. An increasing number of consumer advocates and other interested individuals believe lifetime licensure of physicians is inappropriate and physicians should be required to prove periodically that they are keeping abreast of developments in their field. Most physicians agree that the medical profession should have more public accountability. The report of the 1970 Carnegie Commission of Higher Education pointed out that physicians who do not remain lifelong students "face partial obsolescence in five to ten years." At this writing, no state requires an examination for license renewal.

Specialty Recertification. Increasing concern about medical proficiency also is influencing the 25 medical specialty boards recognized by the AMA. Although practicing a specialty does not legally require board certification, hospitals frequently require it before granting physicians staff privileges in their particular specialty. Many proponents of recertification argue that it promotes higher quality medical care by forcing physicians to maintain their skills and keep up with rapidly changing medical knowledge.

Continuing Medical Education. Continuing medical education (CME) is one way for physicians to remain abreast of medical trends. Some states now require proof of continuing medical education for license renewal. In 1971, New Mexico became the first state to implement a license reregistration law. Physicians in New Mexico lose their right to practice unless they accumulate 150 hours of CME credits every 3 years. As of August 1977, medical practice acts in 19 states authorize the state board of medical examiners to require evidence of CME as a condition of license renewal. Some state medical associations require CME as a condition of membership. However, this trend is progressing at a slow rate. Since 1985, all states require CME credits for medical association membership and license renewal. The effort toward making physicians more accountable is expected to spread. The requirement of CME for recertification and relicensing probably will be a fact of life soon.

Medical Associations

General Medical Associations

Local Medical Societies

Physicians interested in developing relationships with other physicians in the community usually join local medical societies or associations. The size of the local society usually is determined geographically by county. Member-physicians develop policy, establish committees, perform community services, and select representatives to communicate local needs and views to the state and national associations.

State Medical Associations

Associations at the state level establish health care policy, monitor state political activity affecting medical care, assist in the censure of negligent physicians, promote continuing medical education, and provide services specific to the area.

National Medical Associations

State and local medical associations send delegates to the national organization, the American Medical Association (AMA). The AMA establishes guidelines for the ethical practice of medicine, monitors and initiates federal political activity with regard to health standards and legislation, and serves as a representative for state and local organizations of physicians.

In most situations the physician who joins the local society automatically becomes a member of the state and national associations. A portion of the dues paid to the local society is designated to the state and national organizations. If state and national membership is optional, physicians decide the level at which they wish to belong. The structure of the AMA is similar to that of the American Association of Medical Assistants (AAMA).

Specialty Associations

Many physicians choose to maintain membership in organizations established to serve their special interests. Some associations relate to the physician's medical specialty, such as the American College of Surgeons, the American College of Cardiology, the American Academy of Family Practice, and the American Society of Clinical Pathologists. These organizations provide current medical information and serve as the mechanism by which physicians become certified in their specialty. Physicians may also choose to participate in specialty public service organizations such as the American Heart Association, the American Cancer Society, and the Muscular Dystrophy Association.

Conclusion

Modern-day advances in medical science were not even conceivable 100 years ago. Today people are living longer, communicable diseases are being conquered, organs are being transplanted, and joints and limbs are being replaced with prostheses. Technological and scientific advances can be expected to escalate and accelerate progress in the future.

Medical specialization of physicians has become common, and the specialization of ancillary personnel is following this precedent. Medical assistants, laboratory technicians, nurses, and other health care providers may offer unique services designed to meet special needs. Regardless of the setting or specialty, medical assistants will find a growing need for their services in administrative or clinical areas.

Review QUESTIONS

1. What is superstition? What role did it play in primitive medicine?

2. Which drugs do we use today that were discovered in primitive times?

3. How did the ancient Greek and Roman physicians contribute to today's medical care?

4. Name and describe four major developments of the Renaissance period that influenced modern medicine.

5. State the contributions of the following post-Renaissance scientists to modern medicine: William Harvey, Anton von Leeuwenhoek, Louis Pasteur, Robert Koch, Edward Jenner, and Paul Ehrlich.

6. Describe in your own words how modern surgery was made safe.

7. What is the basic education required to practice medicine?

8. How does a physician become a specialist?

9. What is primary care? Which specialists are considered primary care physicians?

10. Briefly describe the relicensure process today and proposed changes.

SUGGESTED READINGS

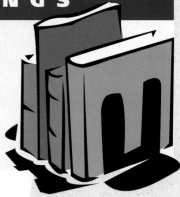

Clendening Logan, MD: *Behind the doctor,* Chicago, 1989, Alfred A. Knof.

Garrison Fielding H, MD: *History of medicine,* ed 4, Philadelphia, WB Saunders, 1929 (reprint).

Major Ralph H, MD: *History of medicine,* New York, 1981, Charles C. Thomas.

Medical Practice and Ethics

OBJECTIVES

On completion of Chapter 3 the administrative medical assistant student should be able to:

1 Define the key terms listed in this chapter.

2 Discuss the historical development of medical ethics.

3 Discuss the development of the American Medical Association Principles of Medical Ethics.

4 List the five sections of the American Association of Medical Assistants Code of Ethics.

5 List the seven sections of the American Medical Association Principles of Medical Ethics, and discuss the application of each section to the medical practice.

6 Discuss the Judicial Council of the American Medical Association and the purpose of the Council Opinions.

7 List and discuss the nine sections of the Council Opinions.

8 Discuss the medical assistant's responsibility to the AMA and AAMA codes of ethics.

KEY TERMS

Bylaw A rule or regulation made by an organization to govern the conduct of business.

Collaboration The act or result of working together with others, especially in literary or scientific work.

Colleague A professional associate.

Confidential Secret or private.

Consent A state of agreement, or to grant approval.

Ethics The science of moral behavior; principles or guides for moral behavior.

Fraud A technique of reaching a goal by deceptive or deceitful means.

HMO Health maintenance organization; a means of providing health care with an emphasis on preventive medicine. All health care is provided for a fixed monthly fee, prepaid by the patient or the patient's employer to the HMO.

IPA Independent Physicians Association; a group of physicians who have enrolled in the IPA to service enrolled patients in a specified area.

Judicial Pertaining to the administration of justice or to the courts of law.

Mandatory Related to or as a part of an official command; compulsory.

Continued

KEY TERMS

(Continued)

Medicolegal Pertaining to the relationship between medicine and law.

Mode The manner or way of accomplishing an activity.

Philosophical Pertaining to the principles that explain events, facts, or a specific system of beliefs.

PPO A preferred provider organization; a means of providing health care to a select group of patients by physicians who have agreed to provide services to that select group. These organizations often allow only a limited number of physicians of any given specialty to join.

Principle A truthful or honest foundation that forms the basis for other truths or laws.

Standard An established quality or degree that is accepted as desirable.

Statute A law enacted by a recognized governing body, such as a state legislature.

*E*thics is a system of correct conduct for an individual or a group with a single objective. The term *ethics* has its origin in the Greek word *ethos,* meaning custom or habitual mode of conduct, and the Latin word *ethics,* meaning related to moral character. Ethical systems primarily are concerned with voluntary acts. It is assumed that individuals responsible to a code of ethics possess sufficient knowledge and freedom of choice to participate in the system.

The ethics of a particular profession is the code by which it attempts to regulate the actions of its members and establish general standards. One of the chief purposes of formulating a professional code of ethics is to elevate the standard of competence in a given field by strengthening the relationships among its members, thereby benefiting the entire community.

Medical Ethics

Historical Development

The earliest known written code of medical ethics dates to 2250 BC. The document, created by the Babylonians, was known as the Code of Hammurabi. It was extremely detailed and not easily adaptable to rapid developments in modern medical science and complex cultural patterns.

In the fifth century BC, when Greece was experiencing a period of intellectual enlightenment, a brief statement of principles that has lasted throughout

PERSPECTIVES ON MEDICAL ASSISTING

OATH OF HIPPOCRATES

I swear by Apollo the physician, and Aesculapius, and Hygeia, and Panacea, and all the gods and goddesses that according to my ability and judgment, I will keep this oath and stipulations:

TO RECKON him who taught me this art equally dear to me as my parents, to share my substance with him, and to relieve his necessities if required; to regard his offspring as on the same footing with my own brothers, and to teach them this art if they should wish to learn it, without fee or stipulation, and that by precept, lecture, and every other mode of instruction, I will impart a knowledge of the art to my own sons and to those of my teachers, and to disciples bound by a stipulation and oath according to the law of medicine, but to none others.

I WILL FOLLOW that method of treatment which, according to my ability and judgment, I consider for the benefit of my patients, and abstain from whatever is deleterious and mischievous. I will give no deadly medicine to anyone if asked, nor suggest any such counsel; furthermore, I will not give to a woman an instrument to produce abortion.

WITH PURITY AND HOLINESS I will pass my life and practice my art. I will not cut a person who is suffering from a stone, but will leave this to be done by practitioners of this work. Into whatever houses I enter I will go into them for the benefit of the sick and will abstain from every voluntary act of mischief and corruption; and, further, from the seduction of females or males, bound or free.

WHATEVER, in connection with my professional practice, or not in connection with it, I may see or hear in the lives of men which ought not to be spoken of abroad I will not divulge, as reckoning that all such should be kept secret.

WHILE I CONTINUE to keep this oath unviolated, may it be granted to me to enjoy life and the practice of the art, respected by all men at all times but should I trespass and violate this oath, may the reverse be my lot.

history was developed. The Oath of Hippocrates, named for the physician who developed it (see the box and text on p. 28), has survived in a statement of ideal for medical practitioners. The Oath of Hippocrates protects the rights of the patient and guides the physician by appealing to moral instincts rather than imposing sanctions or penalties. It also functions as a basic frame of reference for much of the law connected with the practice of medicine.

After the Oath of Hippocrates the most outstanding contribution to the development of medical ethics was made by Thomas Percival, a British physician, author, and philosopher. Percival's interest in the advancement of sociology and his association with the Manchester Infirmary led to the development of a code of conduct based on hospital situations. Percival's *Code of Medical Ethics* was published in 1803.

Development of the American Medical Association Principles of Medical Ethics

The American Medical Association (AMA) held its first official meeting in 1847 in Philadelphia. At that meeting the two major items on the agenda were the establishment of minimum requirements for the education and training of physicians and the creation of a code of medical ethics. The Code of Ethics adopted at that meeting clearly was based on Percival's code.

Although the basic language and concepts of the 1847 code went unchanged over time, some revisions were necessary to reflect the needs of the times. The desire to state the basic concepts in the clearest possible way led to revisions in 1903, 1912, and 1947.

In 1987 the AMA House of Delegates accepted a drastic revision of the principles after wide publication and much discussion among physicians. Preserving the basic principles but stating them in language better suited to clear explanation and practical organization, the AMA reduced the code to a preamble and 10 short sections.

The 1987 version was revised to incorporate contemporary legal standards, and the most recent revision, adopted in 1991, was done at the request of the AMA Judicial Council. This revision eliminated all reference to gender and addressed contemporary medicolegal guides in a preamble and additional principles.

Medical Ethics for the Administrative Medical Assistant

The American Association of Medical Assistants (AAMA) Code of Ethics provides an ethical foundation for the medical assistant. It also provides the latitude necessary to incorporate new information as technological developments occur. The AAMA Code of Ethics has a philosophical link with the code of the AMA. Administrative medical assistants use the AAMA Code of Ethics in their work, but they also must understand the AMA Principles of Medical Ethics. As the physician's representative, the medical assistant must carry out administrative and clinical duties with the guidelines of the AMA Principles of Medical Ethics in addition to the AAMA Code of Ethics.

American Association of Medical Assistants Code of Ethics

The AAMA Code of Ethics serves as a standard of practice for the professional medical assistant. Medical assistants must be familiar with the five specific guides of conduct in their code, reprinted with the permission of the AAMA. The code is included in the Association bylaws. After a review of the AAMA code, the physician's principles are presented and evaluated. Sections of the AMA Principles of Medical Ethics appear in italic type. You will notice the similarities in the two codes. These parallels demonstrate the close alliance of the two professions (see the box about the AAMA Code of Ethics).

PERSPECTIVES ON MEDICAL ASSISTING

AAMA Code of Ethics

The Code of Ethics of the AAMA shall set forth principles of ethical and moral conduct as they relate to the medical profession and the particular practice of medical assisting.

Members of the AAMA dedicated to the conscientious pursuit of their profession, and thus desiring to merit the high regard of the entire medical professional and the respect of the general public which they serve, do pledge themselves to strive always to:

- Render service with full respect for the dignity of humanity
- Respect confidential information obtained through employment unless legally authorized or required by responsible performance of duty to divulge such information
- Uphold the honor and high principles of the profession and accept its diciplines
- Seek to continually improve the knowledge and skills of medical assistants for the benefit of patients and professional colleagues
- Participate in additional service activities aimed toward improving the health and well being of the community

WHAT DO YOU THINK?

Two medical assistants meet for lunch every day in the medical building cafeteria. They like to discuss their daily problems, including the patients. This cafeteria is open to both staff and patients in the building.

1. What type of risks are these two medical assistants taking with their discussions?

2. Is this an ethical problem?

American Medical Association Principles of Medical Ethics

Preamble

The medical professional has long subscribed to a group of ethical statements developed primarily for the benefit of the patient. As a member of this profession, a physician must recognize responsibility not only to patients, but also to society, to other health professionals, and to self. The following Principles adopted by the American Medical Association are not laws, but standards of conduct which define the essentials of honorable behavior for the physician.

Principle I

A physician shall be dedicated to providing competent medical service with compassion and respect of human dignity.

The physician must treat each individual with respect and understanding, without regard to race, creed, sex, or social status. Each patient has the right to expect personal attention and all necessary services within the physician's capabilities.

Principle II

A physician shall deal honestly with patients and colleagues, and strive to expose those physicians deficient in character or competence, or who engage in fraud or deception.

The appropriate channel for dealing with ineffectual, incompetent, or impaired physicians is through the official medical associations, beginning at the local level. Inquiries or complaints about physicians may be made in writing to the professional relations committee of the local medical association. A physician-member contacts the physician in question and if appropriate, secures the records of the patient involved. If the complaint, usually made by other physicians, appears accurate, the committee holds a hearing, makes a determination on the case, and reports its findings to the physician and the complainant. If legal matters are involved, the issue is referred to the state board of medical examiners.

If the professional relations committee determines that the physician is impaired, a different approach is attempted. An impaired physician is one who is incapable of optimally performing professional duties because of substance abuse or mental or physical illness (Figure 3.1). Impaired physicians are offered professional help in an effort to avoid legal difficulties or censure by the association. Many state associations have established committees to approach, educate, and obtain help for the impaired physician.

If the state board of medical examiners initiates the investigation of a physician based on a complaint of a legal or personal nature by a physician, patient, or interested individual, the process is similar to that used by the medical society. Facts are gathered, the physician is allowed to submit information, and formal hearings are held. Once a complaint has been filed with the state board, the information is considered public and a copy of the complaint is forwarded to the appropriate medical society. The society may initiate proceedings to censure the physician.

Principle III

A physician shall respect the law and also recognize a responsibility to seek changes in those requirements which are contrary to the best interests of the patient.

Ethical standards and the law are distinctly related. The standards of conduct established to guide the professional physician never demand less than the law or conflict with established laws. In some cases, the Principles of Ethics require more from the physician than do the state statutes. To reinforce this relationship, the AMA principles direct the physician to respect all laws.

Principle III also emphasizes the responsibility of physicians to work toward the removal of laws that interfere with patients' well-being. Such laws might include those that restrict services for state-supported indigent patients, disclose patients' records inappropriately, and deny sex education to teenagers. Physicians who wish to change the law should work through appropriate channels and support organizations.

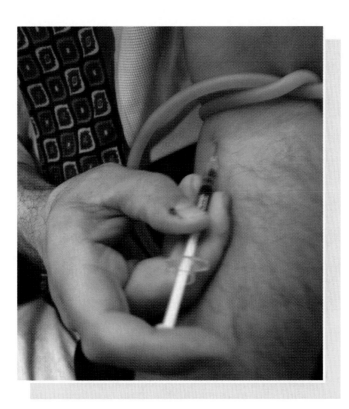

FIGURE 3.1

An impaired physician is one who is incapable of optimally performing professional duties because of substance abuse or mental or physical illness.

Principle IV

A physician shall respect the rights of patients, colleagues, and other health professionals and shall safeguard patient confidences within the constraints of the law.

The first part of Principle IV affirms the physician's responsibility to each individual with whom he or she comes into contact when fulfilling professional duties. The physician must always keep in mind the rights of consumers and other providers of health care services. Mutual respect enhances the end result—effective patient care.

The second part of Principle IV addresses the issue of patient confidentiality. Patients have the right to expect protection of the information acquired by the physician. Professionals must ensure that oral and written communication with and about a client is confidential. By educating the patient on the policy of confidentiality, health care professionals provide the patient with the freedom to reveal all the information necessary for an accurate diagnosis and effective treatment. The release of confidential records or information requires the written consent of the patient except in limited legal situations. Instances that override the need for written submission involve reports required by state and county agencies, patient involvement in a criminal act, and lawsuits instituted by the patient.

Principle V

A physician shall continue to study; apply and advance scientific knowledge; make relevant information available to patients, colleagues, and the public; obtain consultation; and use the talents of other health professionals when indicated.

FIGURE **3.2**

A physician shall continue
to study and obtain
consultation and use the
talents of other health
professionals.

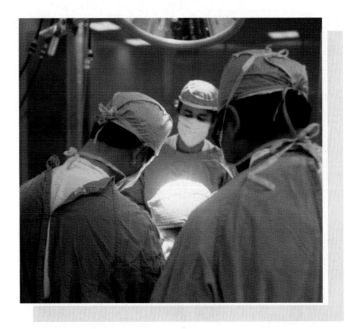

Although the AMA opposes mandatory continuing medical education, this
principle clearly indicates that physicians have a responsibility to remain
abreast of developments in their field and share their skill and knowledge. In
addition, physicians are morally bound to request the collaboration of other
physicians when it will enhance the patient's welfare or hasten the course of
recovery or when the patient requests a second opinion. Physicians should recognize patient's rights and be sensitive to the fact that patients may not realize
their rights or may be too timid to request consultation. If physicians suspect
that patients are feeling insecure, they should offer the opportunity for another
opinion (Figure 3.2).

Finally, Principle V encourages physicians to use the specialized skills of
other health care professionals when such skills will benefit the patient. This
can involve clinical and administrative assistance, and it relates to any individual who can provide necessary health care services.

Principle VI

*A physician shall, in the provision of appropriate patient care, except in emergen-
cies, be free to choose whom to serve, with whom to associate, and the environment
in which to provide medical services.*

Rendering appropriate emergency care depends on the environment in
which the emergency occurs and the equipment that is available or can be
improvised. In any case, physicians are ethically bound to offer whatever assistance they can. Good Samaritan laws in every state protect the physician from
legal recourse if their efforts do not succeed.

Emergency assistance does not establish a physician-patient relationship.
Such a relationship is established when the patient or another physician acting
as the patient's agent requests the services of a physician and the physician
agrees to accept the patient. This relationship is implied once an appointment
has been made for the patient. From an ethical standpoint, physicians who wish

to discontinue a physician-patient relationship must provide the patient with adequate written notice of intent to withdraw from the case and allow appropriate time for the patient to secure the services of another physician.

Although physicians may choose with whom they wish to associate, they may not voluntarily associate with individuals who use unscientific methods of treatment. Associating involves sharing responsibility for the treatment of a patient. An association does not exist when a patient is referred to another physician for care. In this situation the physician who accepts the referral assumes total responsibility for the patient's care. The physician may accept a patient referral from any available source.

Physicians are free to choose the environment in which to provide medical care, including private practice, institutional settings, health maintenance organizations (HMOs), and managed care contracts. The physician's ethical responsibility in making this selection is to choose an environment in which nonmedical considerations do not restrict his or her ability to provide optimal care to patients.

Principle VII

A physician shall recognize a responsibility to participate in activities contributing to an improved community.

Physicians acquire knowledge that is valuable not only to individual patients but also to the general public. Physicians may assist the public by serving on medical association committees, which provide for community needs and educate the public regarding scientific developments or potential health hazards. Voluntary participation in charitable and research organization functions also serves the community.

The Judicial Council of the AMA

Defining the Council

The Judicial Council of the AMA consists of five members nominated by the AMA president and elected by the House of Delegates for a 5-year term. Because one member's term expires each year, a new member is elected at each annual convention. The Judicial Council performs several functions, including the interpretation of the Principles of Medical Ethics. The Council has absolute authority in judicial matters, and its decisions are final.

When a physician is serving on the Judicial Council, the practice may experience numerous interruptions. The administrative assistant may have to reschedule appointments, hold appointments, and handle conference calls and other disruptions to the normal routine of the practice.

The Purpose of the Council Opinions

The Current Opinions of the Judicial Council was published in 1989. It is an appendage to the latest revision of the Principles of Medical Ethics.

The opinions presented by the Judicial Council are guides to responsible professional behavior. The Council insists, however, that its opinions are not strict guidelines on morality but rather are a means to achieve high standards of medical morality. For clarity, the Council's opinions are grouped into nine major headings by number and subject matter. Subheadings are numbered as

WHAT DO YOU THINK?

Nicole has been offered a job in a large clinic as soon she completes her schooling as a medical administrative assistant. Although she interviewed for the job, she was not aware that some doctors at this clinic perform abortions. Nicole morally opposes abortion, but this is her first job offer.

1. Should she work at the clinic until she has some experience?

2. Should she explain to her supervisor her feelings about abortion and find another job?

decimal points of the major numbers; thus 1.00 is the number for the heading "Introduction," and 1.01 is the number of the subheading for terminology.

The numbering for the Council subject headings does not coincide with the numbering of the subject matter covered in the Principles of Medical Ethics. The Current Opinions of the Judicial Council is more detailed than the Principles because the Opinions must address the increasing number of situations unique to the complex medical environment. Only a brief overview of each major subject is presented here.

Council Subjects

1.00 Introduction

Section 1.00, titled "Introduction," deals with the terminology of ethics and the interdependent relationship of law and ethics. This section points out that legal proceedings and censure by a medical organization are conducted separately. However, evidence of a physician's possible criminal action discovered by a medical society must be reported to the proper government authorities.

2.00 Opinions on Social Policy Issues

Section 2.00 is the largest section of the Council Opinions. This indicates the complexity of social, medical, and technological developments. Subjects covered include the following:

Abortion. The physician is not prohibited by ethical considerations from performing a lawful abortion within the guidelines of the law and in consideration of good medical practice.

Abuse. When a physician becomes aware that a patient, parent, or other person is abusing a child, it creates a difficult situation for the physician. The physician is required by law to report the abuse. If the physician does not report the abuse, it may continue, adding an ethical violation on the part of the physician (Figure 3.3).

Allocation of health resources. Society must at times decide who will receive care when it is not possible to accommodate all who need it. For instance, a number of people may need an organ transplant but few donors are available. Who should be the recipient? Kidney dialysis is another situation in which the demand is greater than the supply. This creates a conflict for the physician, who is expected to participate in the decision. The Council Opinion is that priorities should be given to persons who are most likely to be treated successfully or obtain long-term benefit.

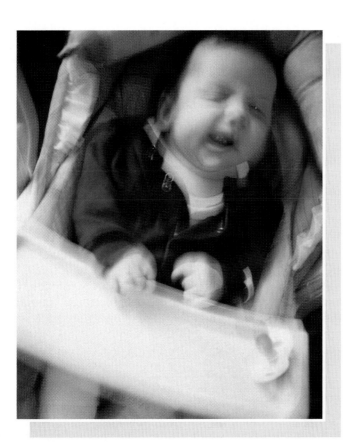

FIGURE 3.3

The physician is required to report any child abuse as he or she becomes aware of it.

Artificial insemination (by standard and test tube methods). The physician is required to obtain consent from both the recipient and the donor. The physician is ethically responsible for complete screening of the donor for any weaknesses or defects that may adversely affect the fetus. The physician may not reveal the identity of the donor to the recipient if they do not already know each other.

Capital punishment. As a member of a profession dedicated to preserving life, the physician should not participate in a legally authorized death; however, the physician may certify death.

Clinical investigation. When participating in clinical investigation of new drugs and procedures, written consent must be obtained from the patient or the patient's legally authorized representative. If the patient is a minor or a mentally disabled adult, additional restrictions apply. Physicians should show the same concern for the welfare and safety of the person involved as would prevail if the participant were a private patient.

Cost. Because of technological developments and new, expensive treatments, the physician must determine the advantages of these treatments for the patient.

Genetic counseling. Counseling for genetic engineering and organ transplant will require personal and ethical decisions concerning the patient's quality of life.

Organ donation. Each physician should encourage donation of organs; however, payments to donors that exceed the reimbursement of expenses

AT WORK TODAY

Organ Donation/Organ Transplantation

All of the states have adopted some form of Uniform Anatomical Gift Act. If the person is of age (18 years) and of sound mind, he or she may donate all or part of his or her body. This gift may be a provision in a will or there may be a witnessed and signed card stating wishes for the donation. In the United States, body parts may not be sold, although this does happen in other parts of the world.

The list for transplant recipients has continued to grow—at the end of 1997 approximately 56,000 people were waiting for organs, and in 1996 only 19,410 transplants were performed, leading to questions regarding who should be on these lists. You may already be aware of the furor that the transplants for some celebrities caused across the country (the inference was that money could get a "quicker" transplant).

A person may move up the list for certain reasons—the status of a patient in critical need of an organ may be elevated, for instance. Some discrepancies have occurred using this method; no perfect method exists at this time.

One of the most influential stories about donated organs is that of Nicholas Green, the 7-year-old boy who was shot by a sniper while traveling through the Italian countryside. His parents donated his organs to seven people in Italy, inspiring millions of people to consider organ donations.

AT WORK TODAY

AUSTRALIA and EUTHANASIA

In July 1996 the northern territory of Australia enacted a law permitting active euthanasia but with certain controls. The first person to take advantage of the new law was 66-year-old Bob Dent, who had been diagnosed with cancer in 1991. In a letter he stated, "If you disagree with voluntary euthanasia, then don't use it, but please do not deny the right to me."

He said that no religious group should "demand that I behave according to their rules, endure unnecessary pain until some doctor decides that I have had enough, and increases the morphine until I die." In the presence of his wife and physician, Dent initiated a process that delivered a lethal drug injection. After his death, the Australian Senate repealed the law even though it was directly against public opinion.

directly related to the removal of the donated organ are considered unethical. The rights of the donor and the recipient must be equally protected. Should the donated organ come from a dead donor, the donor's death must be certified by a physician other than the recipient's physician.

Quality of life. Occasionally the physician must determine the fate of a patient whose future is essentially nonexistent. The physician's primary ethical concern must be what is in the best interest of the patient.

Surrogate mothers. The Council does not endorse surrogate motherhood as an alternative for couples who would otherwise be unable to conceive a child. This opinion is due to the many controversial legal concerns, such as surrogates who refuse to relinquish custody and the plight of severely dis-

WHAT DO YOU THINK?

Do you believe that a competent, terminally ill adult should have the right to ask for a physician's assistance in hastening death if their suffering becomes unbearable? How does it fit with your moral beliefs?

Euthanasia also is referred to as *right-to-die* or *physician-assisted suicide*. Physicians do remove patients from mechanical life support according to their or their families' wishes and they do give large amounts of morphine to patients in the hospital who are terminally ill. This typically is the extent of such measures. However, one physician, Dr. Jack Kevorkian, has advocated assisted suicide for several years for patients who want to die with dignity while they can make their own decisions and before they are in agonizing pain. His actions in connection

with assisted suicide have generated much controversy. The state of Oregon enacted legislation in 1994—the Death with Dignity Act. Several groups are working to have the law repealed.

One well-known case of euthanasia occurred in 1975 and involved a young woman named Karen Ann Quinlan. She was comatose, and her condition was deteriorating. Her parents gave her physicians permission to end life support, but the physicians disagreed on moral grounds and refused to do it. The conflict went to the courts, which initially ruled against the family. The physicians were ordered to meet with the hospital ethics committee regarding Quinlan's prognosis and to determine whether a solution could be found. Quinlan eventually was weaned off the mechanical ventilator and lived without the aid of machines until her death in 1986.

WHAT DO YOU THINK?

Modern technology has changed childbearing with practices such as in vitro fertilization, artificial insemination, and surrogate motherhood. The concept of surrogate motherhood evolved as a means for some women who had exhausted all other means of assisted conception and could not carry a child to become mothers. Most surrogate mothers are paid not only for expenses but also an additional monetary sum for the process.

The so-called Baby M case was the first instance of surrogate motherhood to become generally

known. Although Mary Beth Whitehead-Grould had contracted with a couple named Stern to conceive a child by artificial insemination, to carry the baby to term, and to give it to the Sterns after birth, she decided not to relinquish the infant. The case was settled in a New Jersey courtroom, which first ruled in favor of the biological father and allowed his wife to adopt the baby. The court ruling later was changed, allowing the biological father to retain custody of the child; the surrogate mother was allowed parental rights.

abled children when neither the surrogate nor the adoptive parents will accept custody.

Withholding or withdrawing life-prolonging medical services. The physician is expected to be committed to relieving suffering and saving lives. Occasionally these two intentions are incompatible, and then a choice must be made. If at all possible, the patient should make the decision. Some patients live in states that have living will statutes. A living will is a document that stipulates the patient's wishes in the event of a terminal illness. Normally, patients prepare living wills to prevent heroic life-prolonging measures from being taken when they may be unable or incompetent to make decisions. When there is no preplanning, the physician must act in the best interest of the patient. It is not considered unethical to discontinue life support treatment when the physician has determined that the patient is and will remain permanently unconscious.

These subjects are controversial and can be confusing to the general public. The physician should determine when to discuss such matters with the patient.

3.00 Interprofessional Relations

The interprofessional relations of the physician are primarily governed by ethics; however, some legal restrictions also exist. The physician has many opportunities to request the services of other health care professionals for diagnostic or treatment services. Physicians are responsible for selecting practitioners who will provide competent care in accordance with accepted standards.

4.00 Hospital Relations

The hospital is a necessary facility for the practice of medicine, and physicians are necessary for the continued functioning of the hospital. Many physicians have staff privileges at more than one hospital. The relations between physicians and hospitals should be positive for the ultimate benefit of the patient (Figure 3.4). The Judicial Council developed its opinions on physicians' fees for hospital care, physician ownership of health facilities, physicians as hospital employees, and the organization of hospital medical staff members to enhance education and professional skills. The granting of hospital privileges is based on the training, competence, and experience of the physician

5.00 Confidentiality, Advertising, and Communications Media Relations

Section 5.00 of the Council Opinions involves some very complex issues that have changed recently because of technology and federal regulations.

Confidentiality of patient information is discussed in relation to attorney-physician relations, the potential impact of computers, insurance company representatives, and industrial cases. Advertising and publicity are discussed in relation to the form of communication (print, radio, or television), the content of the advertising, and federal standards for commercial advertising.

The final area covered in Section 5.00 involves the release of information to the press. In routine cases, information regarding a patient's condition, illness, or disease cannot be released to the press without the consent of the patient or the patient's legal representative. The only situation that does not require the patient's authorization occurs when the information is in the public domain. The category of public domain involves births, deaths, accidents, and police cases. In these cases the physician may reveal demographic data such as name, address, age, and sex, the general nature of the accident, the diagnosis, the prognosis, and the patient's present condition.

6.00 Fees and Charges

The basic theme of Section 6.00 is prevention of the charging or collecting of illegal or excessive fees. Fees for medical services must be reasonable, as determined by criteria such as the complexity of the service, the usual and customary fee for the locality, the quality of the services provided, and the experience of the physician.

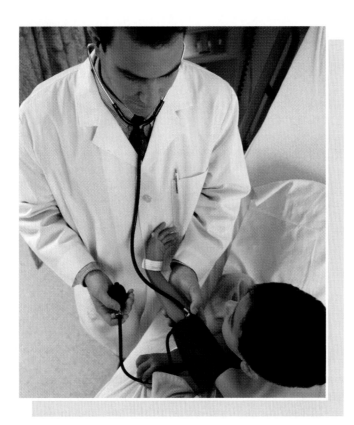

FIGURE 3.4

The relations between physicians and hospitals should be positive for the ultimate benefit of the patient.

Fee splitting (paying another health care provider for only the referral of a patient) is always unethical. This includes payments to the referring physician by other physicians, clinics, laboratories, free-standing surgery centers, and drug companies (for prescriptions written).

Section 6.00 of the Opinions also presents three points regarding charges that involve the medical assistant, the education of patients, and the establishment of office policy: (1) charging for completion of insurance forms, (2) charging interest and finance fees on unpaid balances, and (3) billing for certain outside services. The Council's opinion is that a fee should not be charged for routine, simple insurance forms. A customary fee may be charged for complex forms or those that require billing an excessive number of carriers. Adding interest and finance charges is ethical if the patient is informed in advance. The notice must be in writing and may be accomplished by a posted sign, a patient information pamphlet, or a notice on the statement sent to the patient. However, harsh collection practices are not appropriate. Billing for outside laboratory services is done when a laboratory specimen is collected in the physician's office and sent to a clinical laboratory for analysis (Figure 3.5). In an effort to reduce costs, the laboratory generally does not send statements to individual patients. Instead, the laboratory bills the physician for all services performed each month, itemized by patient and at a reduced rate because of the saved billing fees. The physician's statement to the patient states the actual fee charged by the laboratory and a minimal separate charge for the professional skill required in obtaining the specimen. The latter often is called a *handling fee*. The total charge to patients is less than if they had gone to the laboratory for the services and been billed separately by the laboratory.

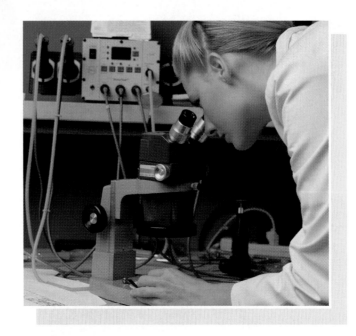

FIGURE 3.5

Billing for outside laboratory services is done when a laboratory specimen is collected in the physician's office and sent to a clinical laboratory for analysis.

One final area in the discussion of fees involves the method of charging for physicians' assistants in surgery. Each physician involved in the surgery should send a separate bill for his or her services. In the rare case in which the primary surgeon bills for all the physicians' (such as an organ transplant team's) services and distributes the fees, the practice is considered ethical if the patient understands the financial arrangement in advance.

7.00 Physician Records

Section 7.00 of the Judicial Council Opinions deals with the ownership and transfer of patient records. The progress notes made in a patient's chart and the data gathered are considered the physician's personal property. The information should not be withheld from other physicians, attorneys, or other persons designated by the patient in writing. Record requests accompanied by an appropriate release may not be denied for any reason, including nonpayment of a bill for medical services.

Many states have enacted laws that give patients access to their medical records. However, some of these laws include a restriction on the availability of psychiatric records. If the patient has a legal right to the record, the physician must supply a copy of the file or a narrative summary, depending on local statute. The physician should never release the actual chart. A reasonable charge may be made to cover the cost of photocopying the records or supplying a narrative report.

On retirement or death of a physician, patients must be notified and their records transferred to the physician of their choice on receipt of written authorization. If the patient does not request a transfer, the records should be retained by an individual legally permitted to act as a custodian of records. If a medical practice is sold, the new physician acquires the furniture, equipment, medical records, and goodwill. The goodwill of a medical practice is the opportunity to continue the care of patients formerly treated by the physician selling the practice. Patients must be notified that their records are to be transferred to a new physician and offered the opportunity to transfer them to a physician of their choice.

8.00 Opinions on Practice Matters

Practice matters are discussed in numerous subsections that cover various subjects. Some are related to the mode of practice and outline the physician's ethical requirements when working for a clinic or under contractual arrangements. Physicians in these situations must be satisfied that all members of the group also practice ethical medicine.

Fees and income are discussed with regard to source and influence. A patient may be charged for a missed appointment or one not cancelled with a 24-hour notice if the patient is fully aware that this charge may be made. Physicians are advised, however, to resort to this tactic infrequently and only after careful consideration of the patient's circumstances. The physician's preferences in drug prescription may not be influenced by any financial interest in a pharmaceutical firm, and the patient should have free choice of where to fill the prescription. Patients should not be discouraged from requesting a written prescription, nor should they be encouraged to patronize a specific pharmacy because the physician has a direct intercom line to that pharmacy.

Other practice matters discussed involve the patient's right to informed consent, to pertinent information about the condition under treatment, and to the attention of the physician. Once a physician-patient relationship is established, the physician may not neglect the patient and must give adequate notice in the event of withdrawal from a case.

Another area discussed under practice matters involves substitution of a surgeon without the patient's knowledge or consent. In popular literature and medical jargon, this is known as "ghost surgery." In all respects, substituting a surgeon without the patient's knowledge violates the patient's right to free choice of physician. Should the surgeon become incapacitated for any reason, the patient must be informed and allowed to decide whether to accept the substitute. An emergency situation may preclude the consent of a patient, and the selection of the surgeon may rest with the health care facility if there is no available next of kin.

9.00 Professional Rights and Responsibilities

The last section of the Council's Opinions deals with the civil rights of physicians and their right to membership in professional associations without regard to race, religion, ethnic origin, or sex. Physicians can expect discipline according to association rules, review by their peers, and the right to due process.

Patients may also exercise their right to free choice of physician or health care plan. They may expect ethical conduct from their physician of choice, whether the physician practices in a private setting, a clinic, an HMO, a group practice, or a closed panel. A closed panel is a relatively new method of practice involving a group of patients who agree to a health care plan with a limited number of physicians from which to choose.

The latest detailed copy of Current Opinions of the Judicial Council of the American Medical Association is available from the following address:

Order Department OP-122
American Medical Association
P.O. Box 10946
Chicago, IL 60610

(When requesting a copy, note that you are an administrative medical assistant student.)

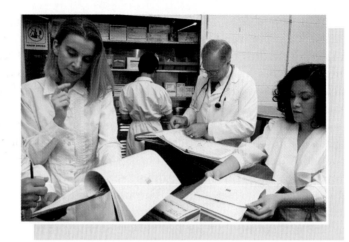

FIGURE 3.6

The medical assistant is expected to conduct business according to the standards set for and expected of physicians.

The Physician and the Medical Assistant

The five sections of the medical assistant's Code of Ethics (see the box on p. 55) are clearly aligned with the physicians' Principles of Medical Ethics. Three of the AMA Principles (III, VI, and VII) deal with matters that can be controlled only by the physician. Responsibility for respecting legal boundaries and working toward changes of inappropriate statutes rests solely with physicians (Principle III). In addition, only physicians can determine who they will serve (Principle VI), the environment in which they will practice (Principle VI), and the activities they can perform to improve their community (Principle VII). Similarly, Section E of the AAMA code, the equivalent of AMA Principle VII, is under the control of the medical assistant.

Aside from the three sections of the Principles that are strictly under the physician's control, you are expected to conduct business and perform skills according to the standards set for and expected of physicians (Figure 3.6). A working knowledge of the AMA Principles will provide the guidelines necessary to avoid an inadvertent error or a breach of ethics. Understanding the AMA Principles also means understanding the AAMA Code of Ethics. The medical assistant is responsible for both.

Conclusion

The medical assistant is bound to ethical practices, as are all health providers. As a professional medical assistant, you will have a responsibility to the patient, the profession, and the community. If you follow the physician's Principles and the medical assistant's Code of Ethics, you will be performing at the highest possible standards. It is rare but possible that a physician or facility will conduct business outside the guidelines established by the professional principles of ethics. If you believe that the codes of ethics are not being upheld in the place where you are working, you should attempt to evaluate the situation objectively. Perhaps you are not aware of all the factors involved or have misunderstood an event. In that case, seek the guidance of a more experienced individual or discuss the situation with the physician. In either case, you should not presume to mention unethical behavior. Instead, state that you do not understand a certain situation and would appreciate help in understanding the basic reasons for it. If the question still is not resolved to your satisfaction, seek the advice of knowledgeable professionals without revealing confidential information. If you determine that unethical practices are taking place, you must decide whether to stay in the practice or seek other employment. If you choose to stay in the hope of changing the situation, remember that others may be equally aware of the unethical conduct. This awareness may reflect negatively on you when you seek employment in another office or agency. If you choose to leave the situation, be discreet in explaining the reason to your present and future employers.

Review QUESTIONS

1. Define the key terms listed in this chapter.

2. How many principles are there in the AMA Principles of Medical Ethics?

3. State in your own words the sections that are similar in the AMA and the AAMA statements on ethical behavior, and briefly interpret both.

4. State the three principles of the AMA code that are under the sole control of the physician.

5. Briefly describe the Judicial Council Opinions on social policy issues, interprofessional relations, confidentiality, fees and charges, and physicians' records.

6. Describe the responsibilities of the medical assistant in relation to medical ethics.

7. Describe your options if you believe that the Principles of Medical Ethics are not being respected in your place of employment.

SUGGESTED READINGS

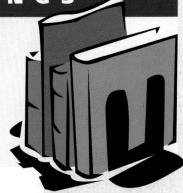

American Medical Association: *Current opinions of the judicial council,* Chicago, 1992, The Association.

American Medical Association: *Medicolegal forms with legal analysis,* Chicago, 1991, The Association.

Lewis MA, Warden CD: *Law and ethics in the medical office, including bioethical issues,* Philadelphia, 1988, FA Davis.

Tomes JP: *Healthcare records: a practical legal guide,* Dubuque, Iowa, 1990, Kendall/Hund Publishing.

Medical Practice and the Law

OBJECTIVES

On completion of Chapter 4 the administrative medical assistant student should be able to:

1. Define the key terms listed in this chapter.

2. Discuss medical practice acts, their purpose, and their relationship to licensure.

3. List the four elements of negligence.

4. Describe physicians' legal responsibility for others.

5. Discuss Good Samaritan acts and their limitations.

6. Discuss briefly the reporting responsibility for births, deaths, communicable diseases, medical examiner cases, and child abuse cases.

7. Discuss informed consent.

8. Discuss patient rights.

KEY TERMS

Binding arbitration A method of settling a dispute in which the facts are heard by a neutral third party and the decision of the arbitrator is final; neither party may subsequently pursue the issue in court.

Civil law The laws concerned with disputes between individuals or groups and those between the government and its citizens.

Criminal law The laws that seek to prevent people from deliberately harming one another or damaging one another's property. Although the victims are individuals (as, for example, in murder or robbery), the crimes are considered to be offenses against society as a whole and are punishable by and in the name of society.

Continued

KEY TERMS

(Continued)

Defamation	An injury to an individual's public image or reputation through deliberate false, misleading, or malicious statements.
Felony	A criminal offense of a serious nature that usually is punishable by imprisonment.
Good faith	Good faith means that physicians have conducted themselves in a manner that involves honesty and competent and conscientious treatment and care. It means that they are honorable and qualified, and that the treatment is safe, fitting, and proper and is valid in the eyes of the community.
Judicial	Pertaining to the administration of the law.
Rule of discovery	The point in time at which a patient realized or should have realized that he or she has been injured; the starting point of the statute of limitations.
Slander	Spoken defamation that results in injury to the reputation of another individual.
Statute of limitations	A period of time established by law during which an individual may file a civil lawsuit. The period, often 1 year, begins at the time an injury occurs or at the time an individual discovers the injury.

*A*dministrative medical assistants find that some basic knowledge of legal responsibilities as they pertain to the medical practice is helpful (Figure 4.1). This chapter covers laws that affect administrative medical assistants and the medical practice in general. All staff must be aware that their actions may cause serious problems for the practice. For example, the administrative assistant must be very careful about discussing patients, their medical problems, or their medications, by their given name. In many practices the front desk is completely open to the reception area, leaving the assistant vulnerable when trying to call in prescriptions or talk with a patient about a bill or sensitive issues such as laboratory results. In such a situation everyone in the reception area can hear who and what about them is being discussed. The patient's right to confidentiality then is violated, making the practice vulnerable to a lawsuit. It is inappropriate for the assistant to discuss patient information where all can hear. When the assistant must discuss a patient with another staff member, they must remember to never use the patient's name. The assistant can be held as responsible as the physician for violating a patient's right to confidentiality.

Medical Practice Acts

The consumer, or patient, is the reason for medical practice acts, which are state laws that regulate methods of providing health care to protect the rights and the

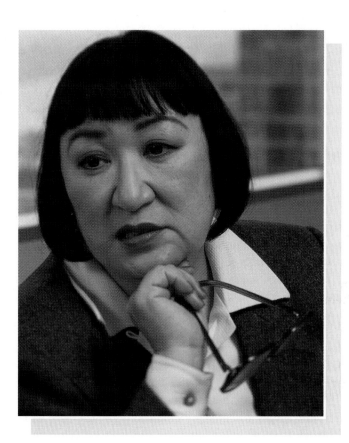

FIGURE 4.1

The administrative medical assistant benefits from having some basic knowledge of the legal responsibilities pertaining to the medical practice.

health of patients. Before the creation of medical practice acts, quackery was common, medical care was inconsistent, and patient welfare was jeopardized. By 1900, medical science was developing at a rapid pace, which increased the risk of exposure to inadequate care. Each state recognized the need to enact laws protecting consumers and develop standards by which the public could be assured of appropriate care. The licensing board in each state receives its authority from the statute or law known as the *medical practice act* and polices the activity of the physicians practicing in the state. All states require that physicians be licensed by the state in which they practice. The medical practice act of each state defines the limitation of medical practice, prescribes the penalties for practicing without a valid license, and specifies the conditions warranting the revocation of a physician's license. Some common reasons for the revocation of a medical license include the following:

- Drug addiction or substance abuse (the physician is considered impaired)
- Felony conviction
- Crime involving moral turpitude
- Prescribing drugs without examining the patient or performing a good-faith examination of the patient
- Insurance claim fraud
- Gross negligence in the care of patients

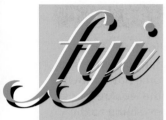

The legalities and ethics of the medical profession are philosophically linked. Medical laws and ethics complement one another and serve as guides toward the same goal: to make the best and safest possible health care available to consumers.

Medical Licensure and Registration

All states and the District of Columbia have licensing statutes, and practicing medicine without a license is illegal throughout the United States. In most states the physician may acquire a license by written examination, endorsement, or reciprocity. Each state medical board provides a written examination for physicians and sets the level of proficiency required for a license to practice. In an effort to develop national standards for the practice of medicine, a National Board Examination was developed and is now taken by most medical students before graduation. In 1990 the Federation of State Medical Boards and the National Board of Medical Examiners agreed to establish a single licensing examination for graduates of accredited medical schools. The new examination, titled the *United States Medical Licensing Examination (USMLE),* was gradually phased in starting in 1992. States now accept a passing national board score in lieu of the state examination and may issue licenses by endorsement. When a state issues a license by endorsement, they are in fact accepting the national board score as valid, and the physician will not have to pass an additional examination. The third method of obtaining a license to practice medicine is by reciprocity. If a physician wishes to change residence from one state to another, the medical licensing board of the new state can grant the physician a license based on successful completion of the USMLE. Regardless of the way physicians acquire their license to practice medicine, they are responsible for fulfilling the obligations outlined in the guidelines of the state's medical practice act.

After the physician is licensed, periodic reregistration is necessary. A physician may be registered in more than one state at the same time. Each state is responsible for notifying the physician when reregistration is due; however, the date and frequency of notification vary among states. Reregistration is necessary annually or biennially (every 2 years); a fee ranging from $15 to $200 is normal. The physician also must complete at least 50 hours per year in continuing education. Continuing Education Units (CEUs) are granted to the physician for attending CEU-approved seminars, lectures, scientific meetings, and courses in accredited colleges and universities. Almost all states require proof of CEUs.

The Administrative Medical Assistant's Role

The administrative medical assistant plays a role in keeping the physician's registration current. You should be aware of deadlines for registration fees, keep paperwork together with the required fee, and submit the necessary materials in a timely fashion, thus preventing a possible lapsing of the registration. You also may be expected to make arrangements for the physician to complete the CEUs required for license renewal.

Law of Contracts

Establishing a Physician-Patient Relationship

Patient care is established by mutual agreement between the physician and the patient. This agreement is a contract, whether it is expressed or implied. An *expressed contract* is a formal contract, usually in distinct written or oral language. Most patient care contracts are *implied;* they are not produced by or documented in an explicit agreement between the physician and the patient. The physician-patient relationship is a contractual agreement resulting from a series of events. First, physicians make their services available. Patients accept those services by requesting treatment. The final step occurs when physicians begin to treat patients. Physicians and patients seldom write, sign, or even discuss a contract between them; however, the contract is recognized and enforceable by law, and both parties have responsibilities as a result.

Patient Expectations

Physicians and medical assistants must remember that most patients are not aware of all the legal fine points of medical care and frequently are distracted or anxious before their appointment. Patients may become restless when diagnostic and treatment plans take longer than expected, or they may make impossible demands (Figure 4.2).

Careful and consistent patient education and the establishment of an open communications system are important. Patients who understand the

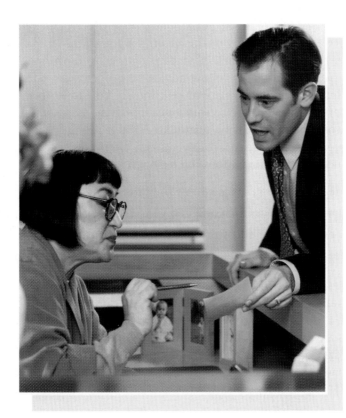

FIGURE 4.2

Patients may become restless when treatment plans take longer than expected, or they may make impossible demands.

reasons that certain procedures are necessary and know what to expect during treatment programs usually are more cooperative and realistic in their expectations.

Third-Party Contracts

The implied contract agreement between physician and patient includes the assumption that the patient is legally responsible for paying for the care received, either through an insurance policy or out of pocket. Sometimes, another individual or company, called a *third party,* may be involved in obtaining care for a patient. This may result from an on-the-job injury for which an employer is responsible. As another example, a friend may bring the patient in with injuries that occurred at the friend's home. Although the friend may express willingness to pay the bill, the physician cannot legally require payment from the friend unless a third-party agreement is signed. If the friend later refuses to pay for the services, the patient is legally responsible; however, it may be nearly impossible to collect the fee. This example shows the importance of obtaining a written agreement from the third party promising to pay for the services the patient receives. The agreement should be signed and witnessed.

Terminating a Contract

A physician enters into an implied contract with a patient as soon as treatment begins. From this point on the physician is legally obligated to provide ongoing care for the patient. If the physician decides to terminate the relationship with the patient, a letter of termination of treatment and services must be written and sent by certified mail to the patient, with a return receipt requested from the postal service. A photocopy of the letter along with the mail receipt should be placed in the patient's chart. The physician may terminate patient care because the patient refuses to follow advice or cooperate in the agreed treatment program or because the patient continually fails to keep appointments. The patient also may choose to terminate care by the physician. The physician-patient relationship also must be terminated when the physician retires, relocates, or discontinues practice for any reason. The patient may charge abandonment unless the physician does the following:

- Provides adequate notification of the intention to terminate care
- Remains available to the patient during the notification period
- Provides competent substitute care when continuing care is necessary
- Cooperates with the new physician by supplying the information necessary to provide appropriate care.

Abandonment also can be charged in less obvious situations. A physician may be sued if a telephone message requesting help is not relayed, if hospitalized patients are not visited daily by the physician or a competent substitute, if on-call coverage is not provided during the physician's absence, or if the patient is not given a way to contact the physician or an associate 24 hours a day in case of emergency.

Terminating the Physician-Patient Relationship

When the dismissal of a patient is necessary for any reason, a predetermined procedure should be followed to prevent missing an important step. Once an effective procedure has been developed, it should be integrated into the office procedures manual and used as needed. A sample letter that might be used in completing the procedure is shown in Figure 4.3. One method of terminating

---

Physician's Name
Street Address
City, State, Zip Code

September 23, 19__

Ms. Jane Doe
123 Main Street
Anywhere, USA 12345

Dear Ms. Doe:

    As we discussed at your last appointment on July 15, 19__, I feel it is very important for you to have diagnostic studies and possible surgery because of your continued abnormal Pap smears, the last being dated June 2, 19__.
    Since you have refused appointments for follow-up care offered by my staff on four separate occasions, it is necessary for me to withdraw as your physician effective October 15, 19__. You require continued medical care, and I urge you to select another physician before that date. On receipt of your written request I will supply your new physician with all information necessary to continue your care.
    If you should require medical care before October 15, 19__, I will be available to you.

Very truly yours,

Physician's Name, M.D.

FIGURE 4.3

Sample dismissal letter.

MEDICAL ASSISTING STEP-BY-STEP

Terminating a Physician-Patient Relationship

Objective: To give written notice of the physician's intent to terminate care of the patient.

Necessary materials:
- Patient chart or file
- Computer or typewriter
- Office policy and procedures manual

Procedural steps:

1. Gather necessary materials.

2. Follow guidelines in office policy and procedures manual to write letter indicating the physician's decision to withdraw from the relationship (see Figure 4.3). The letter should advise the patient of the following:
   The physician's care is being discontinued
   The physician will turn over the patient's records to the patient or to another physician

3. Send the letter by certified mail and request a return receipt.

4. Place a photocopy of the letter in the patient's file.

5. When the receipt is returned, attach it to the photocopy of the letter in the patient's file.

the physician-patient relationship is outlined in the box above. Refer to your employer's policy and procedure manual for specific guidelines.

Standards of Care

Patients expect a certain standard of care, a level of quality that includes professional skill and diligence. In a legal sense the standard of care is determined by the care that would be provided by an average practitioner under the same or similar conditions. In all cases, physicians are expected to fulfill the following obligations:

- Apply their best judgment in diagnosis and treatment
- Refer a patient to a specialist or request consultation when necessary
- Advise patients of their physical condition, limitations, or need for continued care

If a physician becomes involved in a legal dispute over a standard of care, the law presumes that the defendant-physician provided appropriate care. The responsibility for proving that the physician did not meet the standard of care rests with the plaintiff, or patient. If other physicians are used as witnesses in this type of case, they must have training and experience similar to that of the defendant-physician and practice under similar conditions.

AT WORK TODAY

Nazi Prison Camps

The Declaration of Helsinki was not in place during the time Nazi physicians conducted experiments using concentration camp prisoners. Experiments involving freezing/hypothermia were conducted on men to simulate the conditions German armies suffered on the Eastern Front. (Thousands of German soldiers froze to death or were debilitated by the cold.)

Experiments involving freezing/hypothermia were divided into two parts: (1) how long it would take to lower body temperature before death occurred and (2) how to resuscitate the frozen victim. Two main methods were used to freeze victims. They were either put into a vat of icy water or sent naked into the subzero cold.

Experiments involving warming were just as cruel and painful. Victims were placed under sun lamps so hot that their skin would burn or had boiling water forcefully irrigated into their bladder and intestines. Living persons were used to warm up people who had frozen. Hot baths were used in which temperatures gradually were increased.

Experimental Procedures

The first consideration in experimental procedures involves medical ethics. This consideration evolved after the trials at Nuremberg that followed World War II. These trials dealt with Nazi prison camp physicians who performed experimental procedures on human subjects without their consent. When the trials were over, the World Medical Association developed the Declaration of Helsinki, which subsequently was endorsed by the American Medical Association (AMA). With some modification, the Declaration remains the foundation for modern medical ethics regarding experimentation on human beings (see the box above).

Scientific experimentation is classified as either primarily for treatment or for the gathering of scientific knowledge. In general, the latter category does not provide medical benefits to the individual participating in the study but is designed to help a segment of the population eventually. Experimentation for treatment, on the other hand, is used in anticipation of helping an individual recover from or survive an illness. In both situations the physicians working with the experimental process must ensure the safety, health, and welfare of the patient or subject. The patient must give informed consent, especially with regard to risks, expected outcome, and alternative treatment.

An example of uninformed consent is the inhabitants of the German concentration camps of World War II, many of whom were subjected to all forms of experimentation such as drug testing, unusual surgical procedures, surgical procedures without benefit of medication, and deliberately brutal experiments. In the United States, it was found that people were tested for different levels of radiation without their consent or knowledge. Although many of the people in the United States volunteered for the testing, the public was not informed of other select projects.

Today many people throughout the word frequently volunteer for pharmaceutical testing in the hope that a cure may be found for their particular illness

PERSPECTIVES ON MEDICAL ASSISTING

Experimental Procedures

Mary is a 34-year-old female who was diagnosed 4 years ago with relapsing/remitting multiple sclerosis (MS). She states that she had symptoms of the disease for about 9 years but was undiagnosed. She had been treated for anxiety/depression and thyroid disorders before numbness on one side of the face and along her arm prompted her to see a neurologist. A magnetic resonance image showed demyelinated patches in the brain, indicating possible MS.

Her disease progressed to loss of cognitive function, specifically forgetfulness, which interfered with her ability to work as a driving instructor. Eventually she could not walk more than 50 yards and experienced bladder spasms.

In April 1997, she began a 2-year trial of the new drug Avonex (Interferon beta-1a), which she receives as an injection once a week. She was warned that the effects to internal organs were not known and that final results of the treatment were unknown. It was explained that the main side effects are painful flulike symptoms that last for about 24 hours after the injection.

A year later, Mary has less physical pain, experiences fewer spasms, and can walk normally again. Her cognitive functioning improved, and she is attending vocational school daily to become a medical administrative assistant.

such as cancer, acquired immunodeficiency syndrome (AIDS), multiple sclerosis (MS), and respiratory illnesses. A significant number of individuals agree to drug testing in the United States (see the box above).

The Food and Drug Administration (FDA) has established rules to regulate informed consent if drugs are involved in the experiment. Drug experiments are classified as Phase I, Phase II, and Phase III. Written informed consent is required for Phase I and Phase II experiments. A Phase III experiment is the final step before a drug is released to the market, and the physician has the option of obtaining either oral or written consent. However, the responsibility to inform the patient of all relevant information still applies.

Professional Liability

General Law

State laws involve two types of actions and responsibilities: criminal and civil. In very limited terms, *criminal law* deals with actions that are punishable as offenses against the state. *Civil law* involves the actions of individuals against individuals and is covered by the segment of the law known as *tort*. Most lawsuits against physicians, including professional liability determinations, are civil lawsuits.

WHAT DO YOU THINK?

A 16-year-old boy was hit by an automobile while riding his bicycle. He was taken by a parent to the emergency room, where the physician on call looked him over and sent him home. The boy died a few hours later. Autopsy revealed that he had sustained a massive skull fracture.

Was the physician's lack of a thorough examination the cause of the patient's death? Although this was a legal case, what do you think is wrong here?

Cooper v. Sisters of Charity, 272 NE 2d 97 (Oh. 1971)

Defining Professional Liability

Professional liability claims must have the following two components to be valid:

1. The physician fails in his or her duty to a patient as required by the medical practice acts.
2. The failure in duty results in a discernible injury to the patient.

The common term for professional liability is *malpractice,* a word that medical professionals dislike because of its negative connotation. The use of the word *malpractice* should always be avoided when performing professional duties; use the term *medical professional liability* instead.

Liability Insurance

Insurance policies are available specifically to protect the physician's assets in the event that a liability claim is made by or settled in favor of a patient. The number of lawsuits filed against physicians has increased steadily since the early 1960s. Increased technology, the complexity of available medical services, an increase in the population, and the rising expectations of patients all have contributed to the growing number of claims. As claims and the dollar amounts of settlements increased, the cost of liability insurance also increased, until it reached unprecedented proportions in the early 1970s. During 1974 and 1975, some insurance premiums were raised 300% to 400%, which created real problems for physicians. The astronomical increase in insurance premiums was the direct result of high settlement agreements awarded to patients who had suffered various ill effects from treatment. For instance, in some areas insurance premiums for certain specialties increased higher than the average income. For example, insurance premiums for obstetricians-gynecologists jumped to an average of $56,000 a year. Consequently, many family practitioners no longer delivered babies or assisted with surgeries, taking the family physician from the patient and placing the patient squarely in the hands of surgeons. Neurosurgeons and other specialty surgeons experienced massive increases of premiums as well. Premiums have continued to rise but not at the excessive rate of the 1970s.

The cost of professional liability is determined by the potential risk of the medical specialty. The medical practices considered at lowest risk include

FIGURE   4.4

Obstetrics is among those specialties at high risk for professional liability.

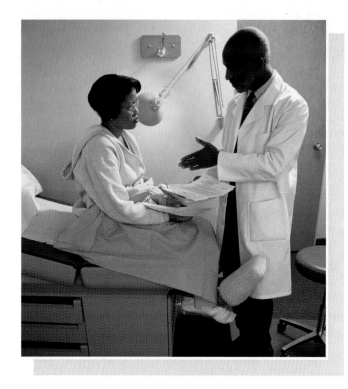

internal medicine, psychiatry, and general practice; the highest-risk specialties are neurosurgery, anesthesiology, and obstetrics (Figure 4.4). As with any insurance policy, the purchaser may set the limits of the coverage and the basic functions of the policy. The limits of professional liability policy usually are stated in two separate dollar amounts, such as $1 to $3 million coverage. The lower figure represents the maximum amount of money available to settle any single incident, and the higher figure represents the maximum amount of money for all incidents that occur within the policy period. A policy period usually is 1 year; therefore policies must be renewed annually.

Professional liability insurance may be purchased to cover the physician for an incident, regardless of when the claim is made, as long as the policy was in effect when the incident took place. This is called an *occurrence policy*. The other type of policy, called a *claims-made policy*, protects the physician only if the policy is in effect when the incident occurs and when the claim is made. Physicians with this type of policy must purchase what is called a tail to provide coverage after they retire.

Common Reasons for Lawsuits

The most frequent grounds cited in medical professional liability suits are negligence, lack of informed consent, abandonment, and missed diagnoses. Professional insurance analysts and medicolegal experts believe that the primary reason patients file professional liability suits against physicians, regardless of the grounds, is a breakdown in the physician-patient relationship caused by a lack of communication. Most of the suits filed are unfounded, but before this is determined the physician and attorneys for the insurance company spend much time and money on the complaint. For this reason, physicians usually strive to prevent lawsuits. By developing and maintaining rapport with patients throughout all aspects of care, physicians can prevent most unfounded lawsuits. This is not to say that communication can take the place of competent, diligent patient care; both these factors are necessary for the best possible practice of medicine. Overall, the important consideration remains the welfare of the patient.

Negligence and Liability

Negligence in the performance of duty constitutes malpractice in any profession. Attorneys, accountants, and clergy are as capable of malpractice as medical professionals. Negligence of a professional duty may be the result of an action or an omission. In other words, physicians are negligent if they perform a service that is not in accordance with the expected standards of care or fail to perform a service necessary for the well-being of a patient. When a patient is injured (physically or mentally) because of the physician's negligence, the patient may sue for financial compensation.

AMA Criteria of Neligence

A physician's liability (responsibility) is determined to exist if four distinct elements—duty, derelict, direct cause, and damages—are present. The AMA's 1963 Committee on Medicolegal Problems produced a report discussing these four elements, known as the *four Ds*. The plaintiff in a negligence suit against a physician must be able to support the claim with evidence of each of these elements.

Duty. Mutual agreement (usually implied) establishes a contract for medical care between the physician and the patient. Once a physician accepts the responsibility for a patient's care, the physician has a duty to provide medical services according to the standards of care.

Derelict. The derelict physician fails in the performance of duty to the patient by either falling short of the expected standards of care or abandoning the patient (Figure 4.5).

Direct Cause. The principle of direct cause means that an explicit act or omission by the physician is directly linked to the injury suffered by the patient. The plaintiff must prove that the physician's actions or lack of action, and no other possible cause, resulted in an injury.

Damages. Damages are the result of actions by a physician that could have been predicted or anticipated. The measure of damages in a professional liability case are classified as compensatory. General compensation is a dollar amount for injury, pain, suffering, and potential loss of earnings; these do not have to be verified. Special compensation might involve actual added costs of medical care, hospital services, rehabilitation, and so on, and these expenses must be documented.

ABCDs of Negligence

For a patient to claim negligence, the physician must have completed the following steps:

- A: Acceptance of a person as a patient
- B: Breach of the physician's duty of skill or care

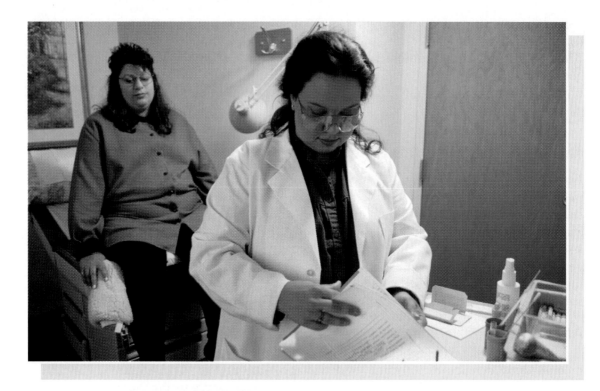

FIGURE 4.5

The physician is derelict if she falls short of expected standards.

- C: Casual connection between the breach by the physician and the damage to the patient
- D: Damage of foreseeable nature

The criteria for negligence is demonstrated in the following example: A board-certified orthopedic surgeon is asked by a pediatrician to treat a 10-year-old boy for a simple displaced fracture of the ulna and radius just about wrist level. The orthopedist examines the child, reviews the x-ray films, and determines the necessary treatment. After discussing the treatment plan and need for anesthesia with the parents and obtaining the parents' written consent, treatment begins. The child is given a general anesthetic, the fracture is reduced, and the proper position of the bones confirmed by x-ray film.. As the physician begins to apply the cast, the administrative medical assistant delivers a message. The message states that the call should be returned as soon as possible. In haste, the physician applies the cast too loosely and without sufficient layers to provide adequate support. About 4 weeks later, a follow-up x-ray film reveals that the bones have changed position and are no longer in alignment. Surgery is necessary to correct the alignment. After the bone has healed completely, it is determined that the child will never have complete range of motion of the arm.

If the parents sue the pediatrician on the child's behalf, the defendant (the pediatrician) should be cleared because the pediatrician fulfilled his duty by recognizing the need for a specialist and referring the patient to a qualified ortho-

PERSPECTIVES ON MEDICAL ASSISTING

Statute of Limitations

A patient has pain in her leg, which began immediately following kidney surgery. For several years following surgery she knew she had phlebitis. She went to another surgeon, who informed her that a vein in her leg had been severed at the time of her first operation. She filed a malpractice suit against the first surgeon. The court determined that the pain in her leg and other symptoms let her know that something was wrong, and that she should have filed a lawsuit immediately. Her failure to do so within the statutory period eliminated her right to sue.

Crawford v. McDonald, 187 SE 2d 542 (Ga. 1972)

pedist. If the parents sue the orthopedist, the judgment should be in favor of the plaintiffs (the parents). Negligence could be demonstrated in each area:

- Duty: the orthopedist did not provide appropriate care for the patient according to acceptable standards of care
- Derelict: the physician was derelict in not applying a proper cast
- Direct cause: direct cause can be demonstrated between the weak cast and the subsequent bone displacement
- Damages: the case involves permanent disability

In a true legal sense, this example is extremely simple and the outcome very obvious. Actual medicolegal cases usually are very complex and require a great deal of research to determine whether the four necessary elements are present.

Statute of Limitations

Each state determines a statute of limitations, the time during which a civil lawsuit may be filed. Filing a claim in court establishes the lawsuit process; this claim does not have to be completed within the statute of limitations. Determination on a claim can take several years. Regardless of the time limit, the typical statute of limitations is worded in such a manner that the claimant may file a claim within a certain period from the time an injury occurs or from the time the injury is discovered.

For example, a state may have a statute of limitations of 1 year. A patient has an annual examination, including a Pap smear, by her gynecologist. A week later the smear is reported by the pathologist as "negative, Class I," and the gynecologist notifies the patient that everything is fine. The patient schedules an appointment 6 months later with the gynecologist because of intermittent vaginal bleeding. A repeat Pap smear reveals a carcinoma in situ (Class IV), and a recheck of the original smear reveals that the slide had been misread. It should have been reported as a Class III, with further study recommended by the pathologist. Although the error occurred 6 months earlier, the patient has 1 year from the date of the second Pap smear to file a claim against the pathologist (see the box above).

TABLE 4-1

Physician's Responsibility for Other Personnel

Associates	Physician's responsibility
Employees	Under the legal doctrine of respondent superior, physicians are responsible for *any* act or omission by their employee in the course of treatment or care.
Borrowed employees (hospital, clinic)	Depends on the physician's control over the selection and direction of the facility's employee; varies by state.
Fellow employees (physicians employed by a facility)	Physicians are responsible for their own actions but *not* for the actions of others not under their direct supervision or control.
Substitute physician	There is no responsibility if the original physician takes reasonable care in selecting a substitute.
Referral physicians	Referred physicians are responsible for their own acts or omissions while treating the patient. The referring physician is *not* responsible if care was taken in selecting the referred physician.
Partners	Each partner is responsible for his or her own actions and the actions or omissions of all legal partners whether or not a partner participated in the care of the patient.
Members of professional corporations	Action may be taken against the responsible physician, direct employee supervisors, and the limited assets of the corporation. Physicians not involved in an incident cannot be held responsible for the actions of other corporate members.
Hospital employees	Physicians are not responsible for employees under the direction and control of the facility. The hospital legally is responsible.

Liability for Others

Physicians are responsible for their own actions and for the well-being of their patients. In the course of protecting patients, physicians are responsible for and potentially liable for the actions of certain associates and employees. Physicians may be held responsible for the personnel listed in Table 4.1.

Administrative Medical Assistant's Role

Physician-employers are responsible for the actions and omissions of each employee listed in Table 4.1. Therefore a basic understanding of the essential

WHAT DO YOU THINK?

Leslie is the administrative medical assistant for Dr. Garfinkle. She works in a very busy family practice office that sees approximately 50 patients a day. Her work area and desk are in the reception area so most of the patients will pass directly in front of her. Today is very busy, with many patients with flu-like symptoms waiting to be seen. She has no work space left on her work area and has stacked some of the medical records, as well as reports to be filed, on the end of the counter temporarily. When Dr. Garfinkle walks by the counter, he gets very upset at seeing the records and reports on the counter and tells Leslie so. She thinks he is angry because the counter is not neat.

Do you think this is the reason for his anger?

legal principles governing the performance of professional duties and limitations under the law will be of great assistance in preventing legal action.

Physicians must be confident that the medical assistants they employ are adequately trained to perform the tasks delegated to them. Medical assistants also must be aware of the legal limits of their role in a practice. The medicolegal risk to the physician can be minimized when assistants have some guidelines about their duties, responsibilities, and limitations. A policy and procedures manual can serve this purpose.

As an administrative medical assistant, you serve as the representative or agent of the physician and must always remember that patients perceive you as the physician's spokesperson. Any comment or directive from the administrative medical assistant can be interpreted as a message relayed from the physician. You are bound legally and morally as a spokesperson of the physician to protect the privacy and confidentiality of physician-patient interactions. The medical assistant must ensure the following:

1. All patient information obtained from or about the patient must only be exchanged with staff members in private.
2. When calling in prescriptions, medical assistants should always take care that they are not in an area where other patients can listen to or observe information regarding other patients and their prescriptions.
3. The patient should always be protected from unnecessary or inappropriate physical exposure.
4. The medical assistant should never discuss a particular patient or case outside the office, even when the patient's name is withheld (Figure 4.6). An exception is made for professional discussions, such as referral of a patient to another office or use of the patient's case (but not the name or facts that may identify the patient) in class.
5. Charts and written documents regarding a patient should be kept out of view of other patients and visitors to the office.

In general, adhering to the guidelines of the physician's and the medical assistant's code of medical ethics, the general statutes covered in this chapter, and the policy of the practice will protect you, the physician, and the patient in medicolegal matters.

FIGURE 4.6

The medical assistant should never discuss a patient or case outside the office—even when the patient's name is withheld.

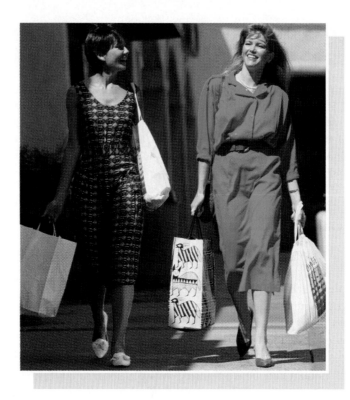

Handling Liability Claims

The best option regarding liability claims is to prevent them altogether.

Communication

As stated in the section on lawsuits, an inadequate or nonexistent physician-patient rapport or a breakdown in communication is the primary reason for most professional liability claims. It therefore follows that communication is the most important element in preventing liability claims. Communication may be spoken or unspoken, and both types are involved in a medical relationship.

Spoken communication deserves a great deal of consideration. Many situations can result in a potential lawsuit. The administrative medical assistant can inadvertently involve the physician in an unwanted contract by giving incorrect instructions or advice and may become liable for suit along with the physician. The physician may omit information necessary for the patient to provide informed consent, in appropriately guarantee results, or withhold important information from the patient regarding his or her condition. Another possible error in spoken communication may result from conversations among members of the health care team. Patients are anxious about their status and keenly aware of the activities and interactions within the facility. When employees speak carelessly, patients can overhear information out of context, learn information about their condition before it is presented properly, or incorrectly apply information about another patient to their own case. Even if such conversations are not misinterpreted by patients, the patient may rightfully question the degree of confidentiality practiced by the facility's personnel.

Unspoken (nonverbal) communication is another important element in patient relations and is the responsibility of all health care team members. Patients are as attuned to nonverbal communication as they are to verbal com-

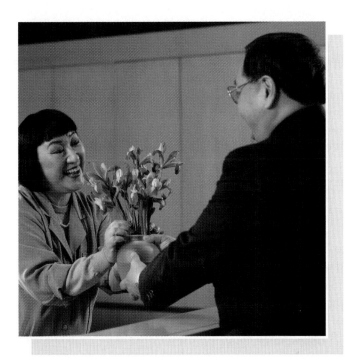

FIGURE 4.7

Unspoken communication is an important element in patient relations and is the responsibility of all health care team members.

munication (Figure 4.7). For example, the administrative medical assistant may inadvertently imply a problem by frowning while reviewing information on the patient information sheet. Or perhaps the administrative medical assistant may neglect to inform the patient making an appointment that the physician is not a member of the insurance plan in which the patient is enrolled. Also, by looking down or turning away while the patient is waiting to be acknowledged, the administrative medical assistant may appear to lack concern for the patient's needs.

In any situation involving communication about or with patients, the medical care team should keep in mind that effective, appropriate communication is the foundation of liability claims prevention.

Records and Documentation

The medical record is the most important tangible element in legal medicine. The patient's record provides documentation (proof) of the care provided, including the time and way it was provided and the consideration of options. The record provides the information necessary to determine whether medical services were given in accordance with the standards of care recognized by law, and it should include the patient's acceptance or refusal of medical advice. The record should clearly indicate the patient's failure to comply with treatment plans or keep necessary appointments for follow-up care and the physician's attempts to inform the patient of the necessity of care.

The physician and other employees responsible for making contributions to the patient's record should be careful to avoid unprofessional comments. Such comments include the following:

- Slang or colloquial terms
- Criticism of the patient's lifestyle, previous physician, or medical care
- Words such as "error," "mistake," and "inadvertently"

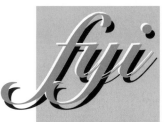

Communication

Communication is defined by Webster as "the process by which we exchange information through a common system of symbols, signs, or behavior." It has always been important for people to communicate verbally and nonverbally to make interaction possible in society.

Verbal communication can be improved if:

1. We develop good listening skills
2. We develop an ability to use the written and spoken word
3. We learn to communicate on different levels
4. We learn to use our voices, words, and phrases well

Nonverbal communication can be improved if:

1. We watch our posture and body movements
2. We are aware of our facial expressions and eye contact
3. We learn to be aware of and respect other people's personal space

Although the medical record is considered the property of the physician (because the physician has acquired, complied, and interpreted the information), other persons have legal access to the record. Patients or their attorneys may acquire copies of the record for review. If a lawsuit is filed, the patient's records become available to the legal representative of the plaintiff, the defendant, and the court. The records also are available to federal or state agencies responsible for payment of the medical care or private insurance (health, life, or disability) companies with the written consent of the patient.

It is in the best interest of both patient and physician if the records are accurate, complete, and legible. If these three criteria are met, the physician can be assured of having an important tool in the prevention of or defense against professional liability claims.

Arbitration

A method of settling a dispute between two individuals or two groups of individuals without resorting to a civil lawsuit is arbitration, a common technique in labor disputes. Arbitration of medical disputes increased in popularity as an alternative to lawsuits during the professional liability insurance crisis of the mid-1970s. An agreement to go to arbitration occurs when a contract for care between the physician and the patient is in threat of lawsuit. A court is involved only in determining the legality of the contract, not the issue or the settlement.

How Does Arbitration Work? Many states have statutes that allow arbitration. Your state medical association can provide information and guidance. Where available, arbitration is viewed as an alternative to large liability insurance premiums. The physician may contribute to a fund for possible settlements. Another option is for a group of physicians to form an arbitration association and pool their funds for this purpose. In either situation, physicians invest much less than they would if they were paying insurance premiums because they avoid the expense of attorneys and the court costs associated with lawsuits. A popular term for doing without professional liability insurance is "going bare."

The Physician's and Administrative Medical Assistant's Roles. In a practice that uses arbitration, each patient should be given an information sheet and an arbitration agreement to read at the time of registration. The administrative medical assistant should tell patients that the agreement is office policy and that the physician will discuss the agreement, answer any questions, and sign the agreement with the patient before the examination.

The administrative medical assistant and the physician should not attempt to legally interpret the agreement to patients. Specific terms such as *tort* and *personal representative* may be defined, but patients should be advised to seek interpretation from their attorneys.

A Typical Agreement. In many respects an arbitration agreement is similar to an informed consent for medical care. The arbitration agreement clearly lists the method of settlement if a dispute arises over the fulfillment of medical care duties or the quality of care. The agreement signed by the physician and the patient usually covers the following:

- Possible issues of dispute
- The voluntary nature of the arbitration contract
- The patient's relinquishment of the right to sue in a court of law
- The binding nature of the agreement

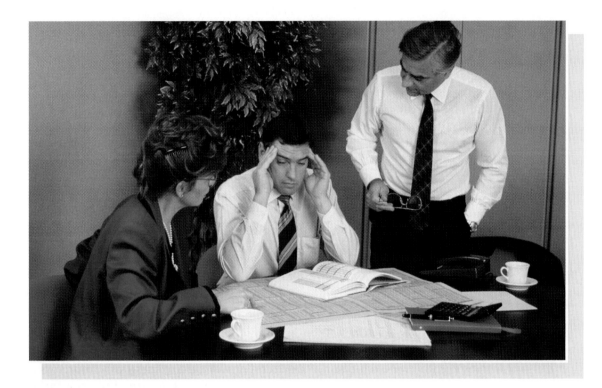

FIGURE 4.8

Arbitrators who are knowledgeable in the field may be used to help settle a dispute between a physician and a patient.

- The method of settlement
- The patient's right to revoke the agreement
- A statement that the agreement is not mandatory for treatment
- A statement of understanding of the agreement

Who Arbitrates a Settlement? A dispute covered by an arbitration agreement is settled by a neutral individual or a panel of three neutral individuals acceptable to both the physician and the patient. Arbitrators are individuals who are knowledgeable in the field in which a decision is required. Professional medical associations or the American Arbitration Association can provide a list of acceptable arbitrators. The latter organization ensures the qualifications of the arbitrators it recommends. One of the requirements to be considered as an arbitrator by the organization is 100 separate endorsements of neutrality (Figure 4.8).

The Results of Arbitration. The binding nature of an arbitration agreement means that the physician and the patient must abide by the decision of the arbitrator. Patients who agree to arbitration may not pursue the dispute in a court of law if they do not agree with the settlement established by the arbitrator. Should either party believe that the arbitrator was not knowledgeable or neutral, an appeal may be made to one of several arbitration associations.

Court Cases

Physicians not using arbitration must settle disputes through the civil court system or with an out-of-court settlement. In either situation, professional liability attorneys are necessary. If the physician has professional liability coverage, the insurance company will provide attorneys. Otherwise the physician must obtain legal counsel.

When a liability claim becomes a legal case and is pursued through the courts, a decision may take several years. During this time the physician will lose practice time to attend legal conferences, depositions, and court proceedings, and the office schedule will be disrupted. More then ever, physicians involved in legal proceedings need the support of their staff.

In some cases, because of the nature of a claim or the anticipated time involved, a physician may be advised to settle out of court. This type of settlement involves negotiations by the attorneys of the defense and plaintiff until a mutually acceptable settlement is determined. An out-of-court settlement may be appealing, but physicians should resist this option if their case is strong. Although some claims settled in court favor the plaintiff and these settlements are steadily rising in dollar amount, most claims are in favor of the defendant (the physician).

Good Samaritan Acts

As the number of lawsuits increased, physicians realized that they must practice defensive medicine. In other words, they had to prevent lawsuits. Physicians even became reluctant to offer emergency care to unknown injured persons at the scene of an accident or during a sudden illness. In 1959, California became the first state to enact a law protecting physicians who volunteer aid when needed. Since then, most states have passed similar statutes, which are known as *Good Samaritan acts.*

Good Samaritan acts encourage voluntary help by protecting physicians from legal liability under civil law. These statutes generally make the physician immune from any suit arising out of emergency care, provided that the help is given with reasonable care under the circumstances and in good faith. In some states the Good Samaritan act extends to registered nurses, but it rarely applies to medical assistants. Medical assistants who wish to offer help at the scene of an accident should be trained in first aid and cardiopulmonary resuscitation (CPR [ideally through a certified program]) and offer help as a private citizen, not as a medical professional.

In general, Good Samaritan acts do not protect the physician in professional settings such as medical offices, clinics, and hospitals. They do not provide immunity if a fee is charged or collected for the service. A physician who provides emergency care as a Good Samaritan should relinquish the patient to emergency medical personnel or an attending physician as soon as possible.

Controlled Substances

A physician who administers, prescribes, or dispenses any drugs listed under the Controlled Substances Act has certain legal restrictions and responsibilities. These restrictions and responsibilities and the role of the medical assistant when drugs are involved are discussed in more detail later in this book.

In general, medical assistants in facilities that dispense controlled substances must be aware of the following:

- Drugs classified as controlled
- Records required by law

WHAT DO YOU THINK?

What Would You Do in This Case?

Tammy and Jody were medical assistants for Ivy Medical Clinic. They both had taken various types of training, including a course in cardiopulmonary resuscitation (CPR [BLS-C]). They had never had to use CPR until one day when they were returning from lunch in the park across from their office. They saw an older man slumped on a park bench and went to see what was wrong. The man was unresponsive so Tammy started CPR while Jody ran to the office to call 911. When she returned, she assisted Tammy with the man. After about 5 minutes, paramedics arrived and took over. The man died. Several months later Tammy and Jody received a letter from the man's family stating that they felt that Tammy and Jody had contributed to the man's death by performing CPR when they were not nurses or physicians.

1. Should they be worried about a lawsuit?

2. Would the Good Samaritan law cover them?

WHAT DO YOU THINK?

Anne worked for Dr. Simson for 4 years in the downtown area. For the first 3 years she was the only medical assistant in the office. Over time the practice seemed to change as more of the new patients seemed to have drug problems. These patients usually were middle-class working persons who paid cash for the visit. The physician would prescribe large amounts of Valium to help these patients try to kick their drug habit, and he would have them come back weekly.

Finally, after several years of this situation, Anne went to her mentor to try to decide what to do. It was suggested that she leave as soon as possible— the mentor even called Anne the next day with some job possibilities. Anne made several appointments for interviews and secured a job almost immediately. She left 2 weeks later; within the next 10 months her former employer was arrested.

1. Would you report your physician to the authorities if you knew he or she was doing something wrong?

2. Should you talk to anyone about the situation or just tolerate it?

- Inventory control procedures
- Required order forms
- Security for drugs and prescription forms
- Reporting responsibilities

Most important, the medical assistant must be aware that only a physician may prescribe drugs and that only a physician or a licensed pharmacist may dispense drugs. Most states have statutes regarding the administration of medication to a patient. A medical assistant should administer medication only under the direct supervision of the physician. The physician bears the responsibility for the act and the outcome (Figure 4.9).

Uniform Anatomical Gift Act

Reason for the Act

Technological advances now permit the transplantation of many organs. Many states have enacted laws allowing individuals to declare their wishes with regard

FIGURE   **4.9**

In general, medical assistants in facilities that dispense controlled substances must be aware of legal requirements regarding records, inventory, ordering, security, and reporting.

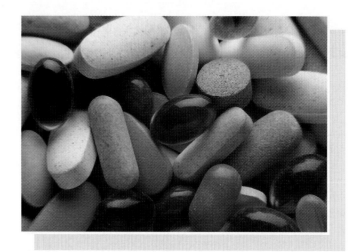

to the disposition of their bodies or specific organs after their death. Previously, state laws varied, and some states had no organ-donor laws; therefore individuals who wished to donate their organs or body could only be assured that their wishes would be carried out in the state in which they legally declared their intentions. To correct this and encourage a valuable service to society, the National Conference of Commissioners on Uniform State Laws approved the Uniform Anatomical Gift Act in 1968. This act serves as the model for state statutes.

Elements of the Act

The basic elements of the Uniform Anatomical Gift Act are as follows:

- The donor must be at least 18 years of age
- The wish to donate should be in writing
- The donor may stipulate specific organs for transplantation, the entire body for research or transplantation, or any acceptable organs or tissues to be used
- The donor's valid statement takes precedence over anyone else's wishes, except when the law requires an autopsy
- An individual's survivors may act on his or her behalf
- If aware of the donor's wishes, the attending physician may dispose of the body under the act
- The physician accepting the donor's organs in good faith is protected from lawsuits
- Death of the donor may not be determined by any physician involved in the transplantation
- The donor may revoke the gift, or the gift may be refused
- No financial arrangements can be made for donated organs

In many states the department that issues driver's licenses also provides Uniform Donor Cards, which have become a part of the license. Law enforcement and emergency medical personnel automatically check the license in the event of an accident. In addition to completing the necessary written documents, potential donors should make their wishes known to their physicians, family, and friends.

Reporting Responsibilities

In the course of doing business, medical practices must fulfill certain reporting responsibilities to various legal agencies. Again, state laws vary.

County, District, or Parish Statistics

Physicians are required to complete and file information on births and deaths that occur within a designated area. Birth certificates must be filed within 5 days after the birth and include information about the child and both parents. Death certificates must be signed by the physician attending the patient at the time of death and include the patient's statistics and place and cause of death.

Public Health

Health departments require that physicians report certain contagious diseases discovered when treating a patient. These diseases include cholera, plague, smallpox, meningitis, scarlet fever, measles, mumps, tuberculosis, and sexually transmitted diseases. Because these diseases have a potential effect on the general public, the patient's consent is not necessary to release information. The physician and the health department do, however, respect the confidentiality of the patient.

When a sexually transmitted disease or tuberculosis is involved, the physician must advise the patient of the need for treatment and of the patient's responsibility to prevent the spread of the disease. Physicians and health department authorities often work together to ensure that the advice is carried out.

Medical Examiner Cases

The medical examiner or the individual serving as coroner must be notified of a death in certain circumstances. Depending on the county, district, or parish, the following circumstances apply:

- Uncertain cause of death
- Death as a result of lack of medical care within a certain time after hospital admission or major surgery
- Death within a certain time after hospital admission or major surgery
- Death as a result of violence or during the commission of a crime
- Death as a result of child abuse

In the past the person reporting a case of suspected child abuse or neglect was subject to a possible lawsuit for libel and slander. In 1967, California passed a statute protecting individuals who honestly and without malice report a possible case, and other states have adopted similar laws. Many states have since gone one step further and now require physicians, nurses, teachers, and other responsible adults to report suspected cases. Suspected cases may be reported to the police or the public welfare department.

Permissive Reports

Physicians may supply information without liability or the patient's consent under statutes that allow permissive reports. The two circumstances that allow permissive reports are as follows:

1. When information is requested by medical organizations, health agencies, or facilities conducting studies to control or cure disease

2. When information is requested by a facility or institution currently treating a patient who formerly was under the care of the physician providing the information

The agency that gathers information by permissive report is responsible for maintaining confidentiality and protecting the patient's privacy.

Consent and Informed Consent

General Considerations

All persons who receive medical care and treatment have the legal right to participate in decisions that affect their well-being. In fact, the final decision regarding care rests solely with the patient or the patient's legal guardian, regardless of whether the physician feels the decision is in the patient's best interest. The physician must respect the patient's right to decide and provide appropriate care based on the limitations of the patient's consent.

There are two types of consent for treatment: permissive consent and informed consent. Either type of consent may be implied (understood or assumed) or expressed orally or in writing. The patient may withdraw consent at any time.

Permissive Consent

During examination and treatment the physician must touch the patient. Permissive consent authorizes the necessary body contact and usually is implied. Touching an individual without consent can result in a charge of assault and battery against the physician. In legal terminology, *assault* is the threat of unauthorized contact and *battery* is the actual unauthorized contact. Even if the services provided have positive results, the patient may sue the physician for damages, pain, and suffering.

If a question or objection should arise during the course of examination, the physician should suspend the examination and answer the patient's questions or provide further explanation. The examination should resume only with the patient's permission. When a female patient is examined by a male physician, a female assistant should be present if possible. The patient might misunderstand a method of examination, and the presence of a female assistant will not only reassure the patient but also guard against inappropriate charges of unauthorized body contact.

Informed Consent

Purpose

Informed consent (Figure 4.10) is a means of involving patients in decisions regarding their medical care and of legally protecting the physician. To make a knowledgeable decision, a patient must understand what is planned, who will provide care, and what the treatment possibilities are.

Situations Requiring Informed Consent

Consent problems are more common in situations involving surgery than in diagnostic procedures or medical care, but informed consent should be

Informed Consent

This information is in regard to your condition and the recommended treatment. This consent form is designed to provide a written confirmation of our discussions by recording some of the more significant medical information given to you. It is intended to make you better informed, so that you may give or withhold your consent to the proposed therapy.

It is explained to me that the following conditions exist:

The potential benefits and risks of the proposed therapy, the likely result without such treatment, and the risk associated therewith, and the available alternatives and risks associated with those have all been explained to me. I understand what has been discussed with me, as well as the contents of this consent form, and have been given the opportunity to ask questions, to which I have received satisfactory answers.

Proposed surgery:

Vaginal hysterectomy (removal of the uterus or womb). **Anterior** and/or posterior colporraphy or repair (a tightening of the vagina done to repair the bladder, rectum and pelvic "floor"). **Partial** or complete vaginectomy (partial always occurs in all "repair" procedures; complete occurs only in certain cancer operations and may or may not occur if you have a completely fallen womb and/or vagina). **Anterior** vesicourethropexy (Marshall Marchetti Krantz procedure) or modified anterior vesicourethropexy (pereyra procedure), one or the other, may be done to elevate the bladder neck. This corrects the anatomical defect that causes you to leak urine when you laugh, cough, lift, or sneeze. **Pelvic** laparotomy (done when the surgeon opens the abdomen for any reason, and may do anything necessary after doing so). **Total** abdominal hysterectomy (removal of the uterus and cervix through an incision or cut in the abdomen). **Unilateral** or bilateral salpingectomy and/or oophorectomy (removal of one or both tubes and/or ovaries). **Enterocele** repair (a hernia of the plevic "floor" that may not be apparent until surgery). **Suprapubic** cystostomy (The insertion of a tube into the bladder through the abdomen. It is removed at a later date after surgery in either the hospital or the office.) **Vaginal** vs. adbodminal: In gynecological surgery the procedure may be done by making an incision in the vagina, the abdomen, or both. Abdominal incisions may be up and down, or across the abdomen transversely. There is very little difference in risk or outcome dependent on method of approach. If the surgeon advises one way over the other, it is his judgment that it is easier and therefore safer for you.

Very rarely, emergency circumstances arise in gynecological surgery that make the removal of the uterus necessary in order to save the patient's life. Examples are vaginal hemorrhage due to many different causes or pregnancy complications (ruptured uterus, ectopic pregnancy), and progression of neglected pelvic inflammatory disease (i.e., ruptured tuboovarian abscess).

Alternatives: Elective hysterectomies have the following alternatives: medical management or living with whatever condition you have, or a combination of both. Examples are chronic inflammation or endometriosis. Pelvic relaxation may sometimes be treated with pessary. This is a mechanical device placed in the vagina to hold the uterus in position. Pessary use may lead to complications. **After surgery:** You may experience discomfort in your lower abdomen or back for a day or so. Medicine will be available for this. You may experience drowsiness from anesthesia. Occasionally, nausea may occur. Very rarely, death may occur as a complication of anesthesia. Any anesthetic may be toxic to kidneys, liver, heart, brain, or other vital organs. Tubes in your bladder (catheters) and arms (IVs) are usually removed in several days. Rarely, tubes down your nose into your stomach may be necessary. Enemas and/or rectal suppositories may be necessary. **Expected results:** Removal of your uterus will render you sterile. You will be unable to become pregnant or have children. You will have no further menses ("monthly," "period"). Preoperative sensations of pelvic pressure, heaviness, engorgement ("fullness") or pain may be relieved, but no guarantee or warranty that this will occur is made or implied. If your ovaries are removed, and you are premenopausal, you will

FIGURE 4.10

Informed consent is a means of involving patients in decisions regarding their medical care and of legally protecting the physician. *Continued*

become instantly menopausal. Estrogen replacement therapy might then follow to replace hormones previously made by the ovaries. If one ovary can be saved, no hormonal replacement would be necessary if premenopausal. If postmenopausal, most gynecologists would recommend ovarian removal. Sex drive and sexual response are the same, and usually are not altered by any gynecological surgical procedure. If you have cancer, you may or may not be cured. Generally speaking, you may feel impoved and your quality of life may be improved. **Hospital stay:** 4 to 10 days. Then, 1 to 2 weeks' home convalescence. Complete recovery usually is by 6 weeks. Return to work may be expected in 6 weeks. If you have radiation therapy before surgery, complete healing of the vaginal vault may take 6 months or longer. **Complications: Death:** Cardiac arrest and unexpected death may occur in any surgical procedure, and may be completely unrelated to anesthesia, blood loss, or surgery itself. **Infection:** Rarely a problem in this antibiotic era. Nevertheless, it can sometimes occur, be resistant to antibiotics, spread throughout the body, and cause prolonged hospitalization, other surgery, further expense, and may rarely cause death. **Hemorrhage:** Similar to infection, this rarely is a problem with elective surgery. If transfusion becomes necessary with whole blood or blood components, rest assured that it has been screened for the absence of the antibodies to the HIV virus. The risk of contracting AIDS via blood bank transfusion is estimated to be one in one million. Contracting hepatitis is a much greater risk and is estimated at 10% to 15% per blood transfusion. **Wound dehiscence:** Wound falls apart—seen in people with poor nourishment or who are debilitated by chronic illness. **Fistula formation:** Tracts or ducts can develop between the bladder, bowel, rectum, and vagina wherein urine or feces drain between them. A rare complication. **Bowel obstruction:** The "locking" of one's bowels resulting in abdominal bloating, cramping, nausea, vomiting, or other gastrointestinal systems. This may necessitate a tube down one's nose, further surgery, and its attendant expense. It may occur shortly after surgery, or may occur years later. **Adhesions:** These may form and lead to bowel obstruction, interference with tubal function, and the ability to become pregnant if no sterilization procedure occurs, or can cause intermittent lower abdominal pain. When vaginal bladder or rectum repair occurs, scarring may lead to vaginal narrowing with subsequent difficulty or painful intercourse. This is very rare. **Damage to surrounding organs:** The bladder, ureter (tube connecting kidney to bladder), small bowel, colon, rectum, and anus are adjacent to the uterus, tubes, and ovaries. If damage occurs, emergency additional surgery may be mandatory without your consent in order to repair the damage. This may lead to prolonged hospitalization, additional expense, and rarely, rehospitalization and additional surgery with associated risks. **Nerve damage:** Cardiac arrest may be reversed, but could lead to brain damage and may not be reversible. Peripheral nerves may be damaged leading to numbness, tingling, foot drop, or "funny feelings" along the course of the nerve. Peripheral nerve damage may be and usually is completely or partially reversible with time, and requires no specific treatment. **Adverse** reaction to medications may lead to an allergic reaction or other damage to heart, brain, lungs, etc. **Blood clots:** These may form in the lower legs or pelvis, jar loose, and go to the lungs (pulmonary embolus) and result in death. **Keloid formation:** An unsightly skin scar caused by cell overgrowth in the healing process. **Lack of expected results:** A realistic understanding of what to expect from surgery is mandatory. A thorough discussion regarding the proposed surgery has been held with me. I understand no guarantee or warranty exists regarding any surgical procedure.

Alternatives to surgery have been discussed with me.

The above has been thoroughly discussed with me by Doctor _____. I understand the risks of the procedure. I understand the alternatives to the procedure. I understand the risks of alternative treatment. I understand second opinions frequently are required. Doctor _____ encouraged and welcomed second opinions whether or not required by my insurance company.

The surgical fee for this procedure will be approximately:

CPT Number: Fee:

FIGURE 4.10, cont'd

For legend see p. 97.

Assistant surgeons fees, anesthesiologist fees, and hospital costs are not included.

Patient's signature   Date:

Patient's printed name:

Witness' signature   Date:

Witness' printed name:

NOTICE: Your decision at any time not to undergo a hysterectomy will not result in the withdrawal or withholding of any benefits provided by programs of projects receiving federal funds, or otherwise affect your right to future care or treatment.

FIGURE 4.10, cont'd

For legend see p. 97.

obtained for any situation that involves risk. When procedures are conducted in the office, informed consent often is oral. In this case, the physician must be careful to note in the patient's record that the necessary information was supplied to the patient and that the patient agreed with the treatment plan.

Providing the Necessary Information

Written informed consent requires the patient's signature on a preprinted form (see Figure 4.10) describing the details of the specific procedure. The patient's signature is witnessed by an employee, such as the medical assistant. Although the patient is expected to read the consent form carefully before signing, the patient often ignores this step because of anxiety, trust, or disinterest. By signing the form, the witness acknowledges that the patient read the form before signing. If there is any doubt, the witness should review each section of the form with the patient before either signs the form.

Avoiding Omissions

Many techniques may be used to ensure that all aspects of the consent are adequately covered. For frequently performed procedures, physicians may develop their own information sheet, purchase one prepared by a commercial medical education organization, or use videotapes. Any educational material from an outside source must be carefully reviewed by the physician for accuracy before it is made available to patients. However, prepared material must never replace oral communication between the patient and the medical care provider.

A prepared checklist of the elements of an informed consent also guarantees that all important information is passed on to the patient. The minimal information to be discussed for an informed consent to exist is as follows:

- The date
- The specific planned procedure
- Any potential risk
- The anticipated benefit or result

- Any alternative treatments or procedures
- Any exclusions (reasons the patient provides that alter the options available, such as allergies to substances or respiratory conditions that will influence the choice of anesthesia)
- Assurance that the patient's questions are always welcome
- The patient's right to withdraw consent at any time
- Any unusual circumstances
- The signature of the patient or the patient's legal guardian or representative
- The signature of the witness to the consent procedure

Who Can Give Informed Consent

Consent for treatment must be obtained from the appropriate individual. As in contracts, the individual providing consent must be of legal age and capable of providing permission. In most instances a minor (a person under the age of 18) may not legally contract for medical care. A legal guardian must be advised of all the information involved in an informed consent. A legal guardian has the power to grant permission. Exceptions to this rule allow minors to provide their own consent in the following circumstances:

- The minor is serving on active duty in the armed services
- The minor is emancipated (self-supporting and at least 16 years old)
- The minor has a communicable disease, including sexually transmitted disease
- The minor is pregnant and not married
- The minor has an illness related to substance (drug) abuse
- The minor desires advice regarding birth control and abortion

Mental capacity is an important criterion for a valid consent. Mental illness, diminished capacity, and mental retardation interfere with the possibility of an individual contracting for care or granting informed consent for treatment. Individuals who are temporarily incapacitated because of medication or shock or who are in a reduced state of consciousness also are incapable of granting informed consent. A legal guardian must be appointed to act on the patient's behalf.

Emergency Care and Consent

In the case of a life-threatening emergency, the survival of the patient is the only consideration. Regardless of the age, capacity, type of health insurance, or religious belief of the patient, treatment cannot be delayed. The physician's judgment prevails in an emergency, and consent is not required.

A Patient's Bill of Rights

The Patient's Bill of Rights, developed and approved by the American Hospital Association in 1973, should also be the credo of the administrative medical assistant. The Bill of Rights appears in the box on the facing page.

PATIENT'S BILL OF RIGHTS

The right to CONSIDERATION AND RESPECT
- The patient is treated as a person and given kind and thoughtful care.
- Personal values, beliefs, cultural practices, and personality are considered when planning and providing care.

The right to INFORMATION
- The patient receives information from the doctor about the diagnosis, treatment, and prognosis in terms the patient can understand.
- Unfamiliar medical terminology is avoided.
- An interpreter is needed if the patient does not understand or speak English.
- The nearest relative or legal representative is informed of the patient's diagnosis, treatment, and prognosis if it is unwise to tell the patient.

The right to INFORMED CONSENT
- The patient receives information and explanations about any treatments or procedures.
- The doctor provides information about a treatment's purpose, risks, alternatives, and the probable length of recovery.
- The patient is told who will perform the treatment or procedure.

The right to REFUSE TREATMENT
- The person can refuse treatment.
- The patient does not have to consent to each treatment or procedure recommended by the doctor.
- The doctor must inform the patient of the risks to life and health involved in refusing the treatment.

The right to PRIVACY
- The patient's body, record, care, and personal affairs are kept private.
- The right to privacy is still protected after death.

The right to CONFIDENTIALITY
- Information is shared with other health workers in a wise and careful manner.
- All health workers must recognize the confidential nature of patient information.

Patients' Bill of Rights, American Hospital Association.

The right to HOSPITAL SERVICES
- The patient has the right to expect that the hospital can provide needed services.
- After immediate needs are met, the patient may be transferred to another agency better equipped to handle the patient's problems and needs.
- The patient is informed of the reason for the transfer and of other alternatives.

The right to INFORMATION ABOUT THE HOSPITAL'S RELATIONSHIP TO OTHER AGENCIES
- The patient is informed of any relationships with schools and other health care agencies.
- Patients have the right to know about these relationships and to know the names of students or other persons providing or involved in their care.

The right to INFORMATION ON RESEARCH AND HUMAN EXPERIMENTATION
- The patient receives information and explanations about research for making an informed decision about participating.
- The patient's consent is obtained before involvement in human experimentation or research.
- The patient may refuse to participate.

The right to CONTINUING CARE
- The patient is informed of the care needed after discharge.
- The patient is given written information about the times and locations of appointments with doctors.

The right to THE PATIENT'S BILL
- The patient has the right to examine bills and receive an explanation of the items in the bill.
- This right exists even if the bill is to be paid by an insurance company or the government.

The right to KNOW HOSPITAL RULES AND REGULATIONS
- The patient is informed of any rules and regulations applying to his or her conduct as a patient.
- The patient and family are given pamphlets that explain the rules and regulations.

Conclusion

Legal medicine is a complex field that requires specialized training and experience. The overview presented in this chapter is intended as a guide for administrative medical assistants in the course of their professional career and is not an absolute statement for legal interpretations. In a doubtful situation, you should seek clarification from the physician-employer, the office procedures manual, or another supervisory source. In every case, the confidentiality of patient information must be protected. The administrative medical assistant also should constantly be aware of the patient's rights.

Review QUESTIONS

1. List six reasons that a physician might lose his or her license to practice.

2. Why is it important to obtain informed consent before treating a patient?

3. What is professional liability?

4. What situations might cause a patient to charge a physician with abandonment?

5. Compose a letter of dismissal to a patient.

6. Name and describe the "four Ds" or the "ABCDs" of negligence.

7. What is the responsibility of medical personnel in a case of suspected child abuse?

8. Explain the need for the Patient's Bill of Rights.

SUGGESTED READINGS

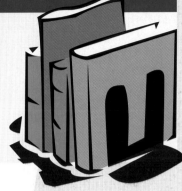

Black HC: *Black's law dictionary,* St Paul, Minn, 1983, West Publishing.

Cowdrey ML: *Basic law for the allied health professions,* Monterey, Calif, 1984, Wadsworth Health Sciences Division.

Kapp MB: *Legal guide for medical office managers,* Chicago, 1985, Pluribus Press.

Tomes JP: *Healthcare records: a practical legal guide,* Dubuque, Iowa, 1990, Kendall/Hund Publishing.

The Role of the Administrative Medical Assistant Receptionist

On completion of Chapter 5 the administrative medical assistant student should be able to:

1 Define the key terms listed in this chapter.

2 Describe reception responsibilities.

3 Discuss the importance of attitude and personal presentation.

4 Discuss the three components of greeting the arriving patient.

5 Instruct the new patient about the necessity of filling out forms completely.

6 List at least two ways that the administrative medical assistant can relieve a patient's stress when the office schedule is backed up.

7 Suggest a way to deal successfully with an angry patient.

K E Y   T E R M S

Patient information brochure	Printed material explaining office policies and procedures.
Patient instruction form	A fill-in sheet summarizing a patient's office visit and outlining follow-up procedures.
Professionalism	Conduct, aims, and qualities characteristic of a profession.
Receptionist	The person responsible for initially greeting patients or visitors in an office or facility.
Stress	A condition composed of an individual's physical and emotional reactions to irritating or stimulating circumstances.

*A*s an administrative medical assistant, you may also serve as the receptionist for the physician's practice. The receptionist usually is the first person to greet the patient, either on the telephone or at the time of the appointment. The receptionist is a very important part of the health care team. In fact, receptionists can make or break the office depending on their attitude and demeanor (Figure 5.1). As a receptionist, you must project a relaxed but interested and concerned attitude. If the office is clean, cheerful, and orderly and the receptionist is friendly and well-groomed, patients are more comfortable and the physician's job is made much easier.

Responsibilities of the Administrative Medical Assistant Receptionist

One of the most important responsibilities of the receptionist is to answer calls, both by telephone and in person. Your work varies depending on the type of call you are handling. As the physician's representative, you are obligated to convey a professional attitude at all times.

FIGURE 5.1

The receptionist's attitude and demeanor can make or break the office.

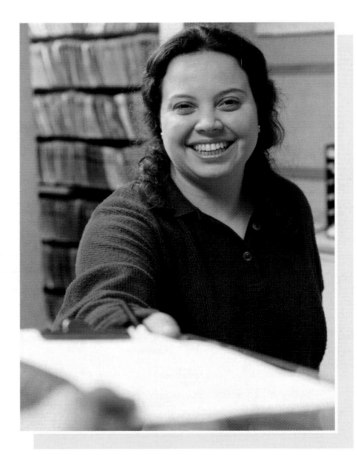

Greeting Visitors

Patients

Patients are the most important visitors to a medical practice. Your role as receptionist usually is linked to your responsibilities for the appointment system. After scheduling the appointment, you are the first person to greet patients as they arrive. The tone of your greeting, as well as your appearance, will set the tone of the visit. The arrival of patients should take precedence over other business of the office.

Other Visitors

Because a medical office or facility is a place of business, you can anticipate a number of visitors during the day. These can include other physicians, pharmaceutical representatives, medical sales representatives, the physician's family or friends, former patients, and relatives of patients. These visitors should be greeted politely and allowed to see the physician according to office policy, which should be written in the policy and procedures manual.

You also may encounter salespeople offering various unsolicited products or services. These callers should be discouraged because they will distract you from your duties and take time away from patient services. You may post a sign that states "No Solicitors"; however, many of these people ignore these signs. Thus you must be polite but firm when you inform the visitor that you and the health care personnel are not interested.

Creating a Positive First Impression

Attitude

All administrative medical assistants should demonstrate pride in themselves and their work. Visitors will notice your attitude as soon as they walk through the door. As the office receptionist, you establish the initial impression of the office and of its personnel. Initial impressions are based on general appearance,

WHAT DO YOU THINK?

Wanted: a receptionist for a busy two-doctor medical office. Should be able to answer incoming calls and make outgoing calls as necessary. Will greet patients and maintain the waiting room. Will schedule appointments and order tests/make referrals as needed. Will order and maintain supplies for both back and front office.

Special attributes:

Must be professional in appearance and able to treat patients in a warm, professional manner.

Must be able to communicate well with people, be able to handle stressful situations, and be able to work in a multitask environment.

Must be reliable, have good health, and have a good attendance record in past employment.

Must be comfortable with multilined phones, have basic computer experience, and be able to adapt to various types of computer software.

1. Does this sound like a job you would like?

2. Would you qualify for this job? Why or why not?

etiquette, and the appearance of the work environment. Remember that as the first person to have contact with the patient, you help determine the visitor's satisfaction and promote good public relations for the office.

Appearance

The basic elements of an employee's professional appearance are appropriate dress, tasteful makeup and accessories, and proper hygiene.

Office policy may include a dress code. Many offices expect administrative medical assistants to wear uniforms; some may allow assistants to choose between a uniform or street clothes (with or without a laboratory coat).

Uniforms may be the easiest option. Uniforms are appropriately styled and attractively designed. Uniforms are available in various styles, including dresses, skirt and blouse combinations, and slacks with a shirt, jacket, or pullover top. The easy-care, durable fabrics used in uniforms allow for daily laundering and retain a crisp appearance. If street clothes are worn at work, they should be tailored in style and subdued in color. A laboratory coat worn over street clothes protects them from excessive wear and helps patients recognize you as a member of the health care team.

Makeup for work should be minimal and conservatively applied. Nails should be subtly manicured and not overly long. Accessories should be limited to a watch, engagement and/or wedding ring, professional pin, and name tag. If you have pierced ears, your earrings should be simple, preferably of the post variety.

Grooming and hygiene should receive as much attention as your wardrobe and makeup (Figure 5.2). Personal hygiene, or cleanliness, means bathing, using deodorant, and caring for your hair, teeth, and breath. *Grooming* refers to the condition of your clothes, the style of your hair, and the appearance of your nails. In other words, grooming is your overall appearance after you have prepared for your day.

Etiquette

The receptionist should be courteous in welcoming people as they arrive at the office. You should greet each person by name and introduce yourself. If the visitor is not a patient, you should determine the reason for the visit, invite the visitor to take a seat in the reception room, and indicate the waiting time.

Dealing with Patients Waiting for Services

Never ignore patients in the reception area. Patients perceive any period of waiting as longer than it actually is; however, a few words from the receptionist will break up the time. You might suggest a magazine you think the patient might enjoy, compliment the patient's outfit, or inquire about a hobby you know the patient enjoys. You may tell the patient the remaining waiting time if you can accurately estimate it. However, you should never underestimate the remaining time in an attempt to pacify the patient. Dishonesty is never acceptable.

Dealing with Others Waiting in the Reception Area
Children

In a pediatric or family practice, you should plan for the presence of children in the reception area (Figure 5.3). Furnishings and recreational materials should be appropriate and safe for small children.

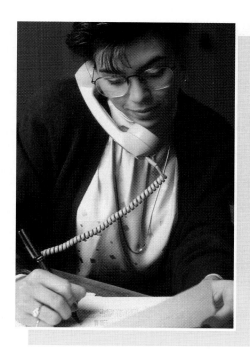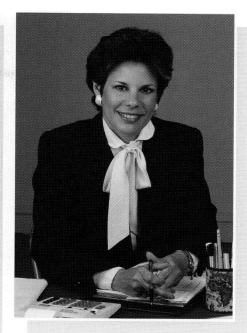

FIGURE 5.2

Grooming and hygiene should receive as much attention as wardrobe, and should be conservative.

MEDICAL ASSISTING STEP-BY-STEP

Etiquette

Etiquette means to act appropriately in social/business situations. It is important that you use courtesy and good taste when you act appropriately. Etiquette encompasses the following:

Considering others—Having a variety of current reading material in the waiting room (possibly safe, noiseless toys in a pediatric or family practice office)

Respecting and encouraging others—Checking to make sure that the patients are comfortable during their stay

Being thoughtful of others—Trying to give the patient the estimated waiting time if the wait is taking longer than 15 minutes

Being democratic in relations—Greeting each patient by name and introducing yourself if they are new; being concerned no matter how you feel that day

Saying "thank you" with sincerity—Always appreciate your patients. They are your "business." Let them know that you care about them.

Using a friendly voice—Your voice lets the patients know if you are empathetic and how you really feel. It should always reflect your care and concern.

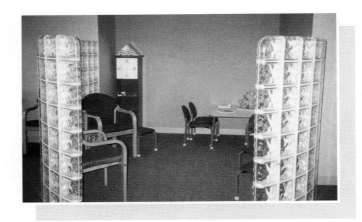

FIGURE 5.3

In a pediatric or family practice you can expect and should plan for children in the reception area.

The reception area should include small chairs and a table with children's magazines and books. Safe, quiet toys also help children pass the time.

Other practices, however, usually are not prepared for children. On occasion, a parent scheduled to see the physician either will arrive with a child (or children) or ask at the time an appointment is made if is all right to bring children. Because children may not be able to be with their parents during the visit with the physician, you may find yourself acting as a baby-sitter. This will create a hardship, especially in a single-employee office. If the child is brought in without advance warning, you can do very little but adapt to the situation. As the parent is leaving the office, however, you can politely explain that the office is not sufficiently staffed to accept responsibility for children and ask that the parent make different arrangements for the next visit. You can offer to schedule an appointment for a time when the child can be cared for at home. If a request to bring children is made in advance, you will have some control over the situation. Again, you should politely explain the staffing situation and the inadequate facilities. To avoid appearing inflexible, you might say, "Yes, you can bring the children, Ms. Adams, as long as you can bring someone with you to watch them while you are with the doctor." The patient usually decides that getting a sitter to watch the child at home is easier than transporting the sitter to and from the office.

Relatives or Friends of the Patient

The people who accompany a patient to an appointment may be anxious about the patient or restless from waiting. You can let them know the approximate time the patient's visit will be completed and perhaps suggest some reading material. You should be careful, however, not to answer questions regarding the patient's condition or treatment. This information is confidential. You should respond to these questions by suggesting they discuss it with the patient.

The Reception Area

The term *reception room* is preferable to waiting room because the latter reminds patients of precisely what they are doing—waiting. A wide variety of popular magazines and educational brochures should be available to patients.

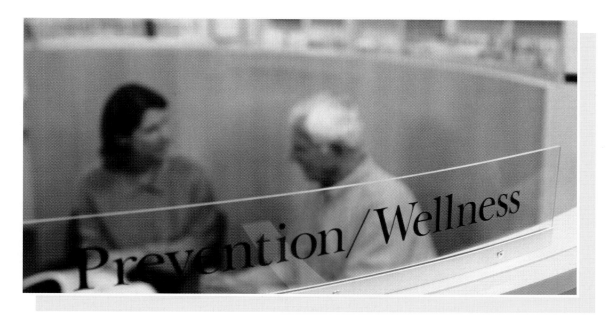

FIGURE 5.4

Try to view the reception area as a patient seeing the room for the first time. What is your reaction?

If a person has been waiting longer than 15 minutes to see the physician, you should speak to him or her and, if possible, give an estimate of the length of waiting time expected. The reception area should be a pleasant, well-lighted area in which patients and visitors can wait comfortably.

The administrative medical assistant's desk is the visitor's focal point on arrival in the office. You should keep the desk neatly arranged. Put unnecessary items into storage and place necessary confidential items where they are not visible.

The counter in front of the receptionist should be the same height as most bank counters. This allows the receptionist some privacy but gives the patient enough space to write a check for payment of services. The areas directly in front of the receptionist should be lined with fabric-covered board or cork to reduce sound from telephone conversations. When working with the patient at the front desk, you should stand or sit in a high chair (as in some banks); eye contact is extremely important when discussing information or payments with the patient.

After arriving at the office each morning, you should immediately check the reception area to see that everything is neat and clean, with all magazines arranged attractively (Figure 5.4). Try to view the reception area as if you are the patient seeing the room for the first time, and judge your reaction. Are the magazines current? Is the room in need of freshening up? Are the chairs clean and the cushions in good condition? Are the pictures attractive? Patients often spend more time in the reception area than they do in the examination room; for this reason a relaxing atmosphere and a clean, cheerful appearance are essential.

Current magazines should be available in an area where they can be replaced easily, preferably in a magazine rack. Patients seem to prefer magazines with many pictures and short stories or articles. Popular choices are *Time, Newsweek, People, National Geographic,* and *Architectural Digest.* Outdated magazines should be discarded and replaced. Attractive, healthy plants or a well-maintained aquarium are interesting additions. Many offices, particularly consulting offices, now provide a corner equipped with a small desk and telephone for local calls. Soft, restful music from a stereo or CD player promotes a relaxed setting. (Do not use a local radio station with advertisements.) The reception area should be well lit, effectively ventilated, and comfortable in temperature (70° to 72° F). A place to hang raincoats and hold umbrellas helps keep the reception area neat.

The seating should be attractively arranged, with a variety of seating options. Most people prefer firm, straight-backed chairs; however, some like soft, lower seating. Many elderly people need sturdy chairs and small sofas or loveseats with firm cushions and arms from which they can push themselves upward.

Artwork in the reception area reflects the taste of the physician-owner but should be relatively conservative in color and design. In many locations the office may be able to rent artwork from a local museum or gallery. Many offices contract with a local florist to deliver a flower arrangement once a week. The office usually can arrange this for under $30 a week; patients also may appreciate fresh flowers. (However, flowers are not good for allergy or dermatology practices because many people may be allergic to certain flowers or scents.)

Check the reception area frequently to see whether patients are still waiting, and straighten the room when you have a free moment. However, do this discreetly: you should be careful not to suggest that you are picking up after the patients.

Patient Registration

Before the patient arrives, the assistant checks the name on the appointment sheet and watches for the patient's arrival. When the patient enters the room, greet him or her by name, making sure that you are pronouncing the name correctly. Sometimes, spelling the name phonetically in the front of the chart is helpful. Ask established patients whether there are any changes in their personal information such as a new address, telephone number, place of employment, and insurance plan. Even if the patient says there are no changes, the assistant must verify the information in the record. Patients often say there are no changes because they have moved, changed jobs, or obtained new insurance 6 months to 1 year ago and the information no longer seems new to them; however, their last appointment may have been 2 years ago. Therefore the receptionist must ask specific questions of each patient who has not been seen in the past 6 months.

Any patient arriving for a first visit requires certain introductory procedures. Most physicians use a preprinted form to gather important information. The administrative medical assistant receptionist may partially complete the form while interviewing the patient over the telephone or ask the patient to complete the form on arrival. If the appointment is made 3 to 6 weeks in advance, the form may be sent to the patient along with directions to the practice and an informational brochure. You should instruct the patient to bring the filled-out forms to the appointment. Otherwise, the forms may be completed in the office. The administrative medical assistant receptionist should review the forms to see that all information has been completed and that all required signatures are in place.

All patient registration forms should include the following information (Figure 5.5):

- Patient's name*
- Address (number, street, city, state, and Zip code)*
- Telephone numbers for both home and work*
- Date of birth
- Sex
- Marital status (particularly when the patient is a child of divorced parents and one parent is responsible for the children's medical bills)
- Social Security number
- Driver's license number
- Referring physician
- Employer
- Responsible party (the parent who brings the child is considered the responsible party even though the other parent is financially responsible for the child's medical care†)

Communicating with Patients and Families

Communication with the patient starts in the reception area. A patient information brochure (see the box about brochures) is an excellent way to begin this process. Ideally, all staff members and the physician should collaborate on the brochure. The patient information brochure should describe office policies and procedures in a pleasant, conversational tone with a minimum of technical terminology. Patients should be referred to as "you" and the staff as "we." The brochure can answer many commonly asked questions and enhance the professional appearance of the practice. It will reduce follow-up telephone calls by introducing the physician and specialty.

As staff members of most practices can attest, interactions with patients and their families can either promote wellness or aggravate a physical or mental

---

*If the patient is a child and the parents are divorced, you must have this information on both parents.
†In some states the parent whose birthday comes first in the year provides the primary coverage and the other parent's carrier is the secondary insurance, provided both parents have health insurance. All information regarding the responsible party—name, address, date of birth, employer, and insurance carrier—is confidential. Insurance information, primary carrier name and address, subscriber's name and address, telephone numbers at both home and work, subscriber's date of birth, relationship to the patient, policy identification, group number, employer, and a signed assignment of benefits to the physician are required. It also is helpful to have information regarding the nearest relative not living with the patient and his or her relationship to the patient.

CLIENT ACCOUNT NUMBER	**PATIENT REGISTRATION FORM**	DATE

PATIENT ACCOUNT NUMBER	CLIENT NAME	☐ NEW ☐ CHANGE

PLEASE TYPE OR PRINT CLEARLY — (DR. CODE — R.D. CODE — CARRIER CODE FOR OFFICE USE ONLY)

PATIENT INFORMATION

PATIENT'S NAME	DATE OF BIRTH	SEX ☐ Male ☐ Female	SOCIAL SECURITY #
ADDRESS — STREET, APT. NO.	REFERRING DOCTOR		
	EMPLOYER		
CITY	STATE	ZIP	TELEPHONE — HOME	TELEPHONE — OTHER

RESPONSIBLE PARTY FOR BILLING

NAME - LAST, FIRST, MIDDLE INITIAL	☐ SAME AS ABOVE	PATIENT RELATIONSHIP TO RESPONSIBLE PARTY ☐ SELF ☐ SPOUSE ☐ CHILD ☐ OTHER
ADDRESS — STREET, APT. NO.		CITY	STATE	ZIP
		TELEPHONE — HOME	TELEPHONE — OTHER

INSURANCE

PRIMARY INSURANCE CARRIER NAME, TELEPHONE	POLICY/ID#	GROUP#
INSUREDS NAME - LAST, FIRST, MIDDLE INITIAL ☐ SAME AS ABOVE	EMPLOYER	EMPLOYER PLAN COVERAGE ☐ YES ☐ NO
ADDRESS OF INSURANCE COMPANY	PATIENT RELATIONSHIP TO INSURED ☐ SELF ☐ SPOUSE ☐ CHILD ☐ OTHER	
	TELEPHONE — HOME	IF CHAMPUS ☐ RETIRED ☐ ACTIVE ☐ DECEASED
CITY STATE ZIP	SOCIAL SECURITY #	BRANCH OF SERVICE:

SECONDARY INSURANCE CARRIER NAME, TELEPHONE	POLICY/ID#	GROUP#
INSUREDS NAME - LAST, FIRST, MIDDLE INITIAL ☐ SAME AS ABOVE	EMPLOYER	EMPLOYER PLAN COVERAGE ☐ YES ☐ NO
ADDRESS OF INSURANCE COMPANY	PATIENT RELATIONSHIP TO INSURED ☐ SELF ☐ SPOUSE ☐ CHILD ☐ OTHER	
	TELEPHONE — HOME	IF CHAMPUS ☐ RETIRED ☐ ACTIVE ☐ DECEASED
CITY STATE ZIP	SOCIAL SECURITY #	BRANCH OF SERVICE:

Please remember that insurance is considered a method of reimbursing the patient for fees paid to the doctor and is not a substitute for payment. Some companies pay fixed allowances for certain procedures, and others pay a percentage of the charge. It is your responsibility to pay any deductible amount, co-insurance, or any other balance not paid for by your insurance.

IN ORDER TO CONTROL YOUR COST OF BILLINGS, WE REQUEST THAT OUR CHARGES FOR OFFICE VISITS BE PAID AT THE CONCLUSION OF EACH VISIT.

To the extent necessary to determine liability for payment and to obtain reimbursement, I authorize disclosure of portions of the patient's records.

I hereby assign all medical and/or surgical benefits, to include major medical benefits to which I am entitled including MediCare, private insurance, and other health plans to:

This assignment will remain in effect until revoked by me in writing. A photocopy of this assignment is to be considered as valid as an original. I understand that I am financially responsible for all charges whether or not paid by said insurance. I hereby authorize said assignee to release all information necessary to secure the payment.

SIGNED _____   DATE _____

FIGURE 5.5

Example of a patient registration form.

FOCUS ON THE WORKPLACE

Sample Patient Brochure

Many offices will use a patient information brochure for their new patients. It describes the basic office policies and procedures of a practice. As an administrative medical assistant, you might be asked to write such a brochure.

John Smith Medical Group, Inc.
347 Oakdale Avenue
Smithfield Heights, MA 13000
Telephone 500-600-8760
Fax 500-600-8761

The staff of John Smith, M.D., would like to welcome you to our family practice, located in the Oaks Plaza medical building. We offer all services, including pharmacy, x-ray, laboratory, and physical therapy.

General Information

Office hours: *The office is open from 9 AM to 5 PM Monday, Tuesday, Wednesday, and Friday. On Thursday the office is open from 8:30 AM to noon.*

Appointments: *Dr. Smith and our nurse practitioner work on a regular appointment schedule. If your appointment is for a special problem, adequate time will be allotted. Routine appointments will be made 1 to 2 weeks in advance. Needs for immediate treatment are taken care of daily, and Dr. Smith is a member of a family practice group that covers emergency care when he is not available. If you cannot keep an appointment, we ask that you cancel 24 hours in advance to open the booking to other patients.*

Payment for Services: *This office accepts most types of basic insurance. Please call our insurance secretary to check coverage on any HMO or other group plan you may have.*

condition. In fact, many experts believe that attending to the patient's mental state is as important as performing expert treatment skills. You should work on your communication skills to communicate a caring attitude toward patients and family members.

Communication, both verbal and nonverbal, is a very important skill. Verbal communication must be clear so it may be interpreted correctly—make an effort not to mumble, slur your words, or speak too quickly. Verbal communication goes beyond the content of what you say. The tone, inflection, and projection of your voice can let others know how you feel at that particular moment—happy, sad, excited, exasperated, impatient, or angry. Nonverbal communication, or body language, also can convey a message. Obviously, communicating a caring attitude toward the patient has a positive effect on the patient and makes your job easier. The following suggestions for good communication will help you in your work:

- Do not interrupt patients or their relatives when they are speaking.
- Take time to listen with patience and kindness to elderly or disabled patients. In an extremely busy practice, waiting and listening to the patient who is slow in speech or thought may be frustrating; however, a kind attitude shows that the patient's concerns and questions are important to you. This projects a positive image, which the clinical staff and the physician—not to mention the patient—appreciates.
- Communicate clearly, without the use of a lot of "uhs" or "you knows."
- Watch out for negative body language. Nonverbal communication can indicate more about a person's feelings than the content of the conversation. Negative body language includes frowning (this implies that you are insensitive to the patient's needs and feelings) and crossing your arms (this indicates that you are closed off to what others have to say).
- Use a positive nonverbal response such as a warm smile and perhaps a brief hug or a gentle pat on the arm or back. (This type of reassurance usually is reserved for long-term patients who are comfortable with physical contact.)
- Treat all patients with kindness and courtesy, no matter what the patient's social or economic status is. Each person who enters the reception area should receive a cordial, friendly greeting.
- Use a personal touch when greeting the patient. Cultivate the habit of greeting each patient in a friendly, self-assured manner. Eye contact and a smile are very important. Even though you are wearing a name tag, introduce yourself to the patient with your name and position title: "Hello, I am De Ann, Dr. Johnson's receptionist."
- Greet established patients by name. Memorize the correct pronunciation of the patient's name. When greeting patients, as a rule of thumb, you may greet most patients your age and under by their first name (if you know them); however, other patients or those older than you should be greeted as Ms., Mrs., or Mr.
- Mention a small piece of personal information regarding a patient, if you can. Appropriate topics include the patient's recent vacation or new grandchild. You may even jot this type of information on the appointment book. Remember, never mention any confidential information.

Consideration for the Patient

After completing the initial forms, the patient expects to see the physician at the appointed time, or very close to it. You do what you can to make this happen or explain to the patient the reason for the delay. Often, if patients understand the reason for the delay (for example, the physician was called to the hospital for an emergency), they are more tolerant and less irritated. This also gives patients the opportunity to decide whether they can wait for the physician or whether they need to make a new appointment. As the medical assistant, you are responsible for conveying both your own and the physician's concern for the patient's convenience. Consideration for the patient's time is extremely important.

Most consultants agree that in a well-managed, busy office, there are never more than three to five patients in the reception area. When surveyed, patients complain most often about the amount of time they spend waiting before the doctor can see them. In fact, frequently when patients object to the amount of the fee or the quality of their care, they are really complaining about the amount of time spent waiting in the reception area. Remember that patients' time is as valuable to them as your time is to you. For example, business people, who are in the habit of making the most of their time, are particularly upset by the appearance of inefficient scheduling of appointments. Any delay of more than 15 minutes should be explained to the person waiting. Many physicians simply can never be on time, which leads to major frustration in the front office. In this situation, you may want to suggest that working patients call ahead and confirm whether the physician is running on time. If the physician has fallen behind, for any reason, you can reschedule the appointment for later in the day. This practice shows busy patients that their time is a consideration for you.

If the patient is already in the reception area and the wait becomes excessive, you must explain the delay to the patient. You may be able to spend a little extra time, perhaps offering a cup of coffee or making brief conversation with the patient who is becoming visibly upset at waiting. Some patients are fearful and tense, and an extended waiting period may worsen the problem. You can frequently put them in a better frame of mind with just a friendly smile or a show of concern.

If you are the only member of the front-office staff, you can help keep appointments on schedule by tidying up each examination room and moving the next patient in (Figure 5.6). This will save time for the physician. However, once the patient has been gowned, draped, and positioned on the examination table, waiting for an extended period of time is unacceptable. If a short delay is unavoidable, current magazines in the examination room will help patients pass the time.

Consideration for Elderly and Disabled Patients

When the family accompanies the patient to the office, it usually is because the patient is a child or an adult who needs assistance. In many instances, the patient is elderly or disabled. When you are aware that the patient is elderly or disabled, consider certain additional practices to make the patient's visit more comfortable (Figure 5.7). Some techniques you may use are as follows:

1. Reserve time for the first appointment after lunch, particularly if the family member is employed; this may allow the family member to take time off from work. Early-morning appointments tend to be difficult for elderly and disabled people.

2. Speak clearly and slowly, particularly if the patient has difficulty understanding, either because of age, a related hearing impairment, or a language barrier. If you are aware that the patient needs an interpreter, ask if the family can assist the patient or bring an interpreter with them. Simply because a patient has difficulty understanding what you are saying is not a reason to shout or speak loudly to the patient. Speaking loudly or shouting does not enhance or clarify what you are trying to say, and only succeeds in embarrassing you and the patient.

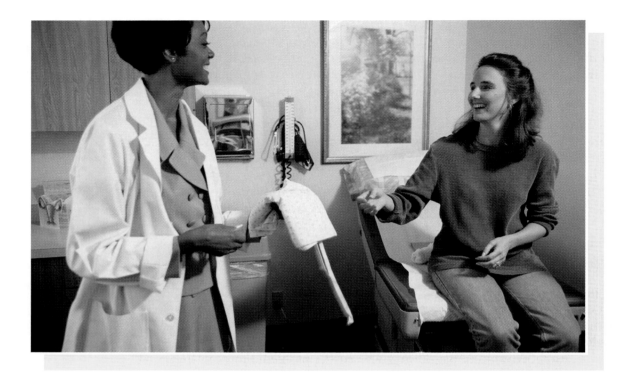

FIGURE 5.6

If you are working solo in an office, you will assist in keeping patients on
schedule by preparing and moving the next patient into each examination room.

FIGURE 5.7

When you are aware that
a patient is disabled, consider additional practices
to make the patient visit
more comfortable and
easily managed.

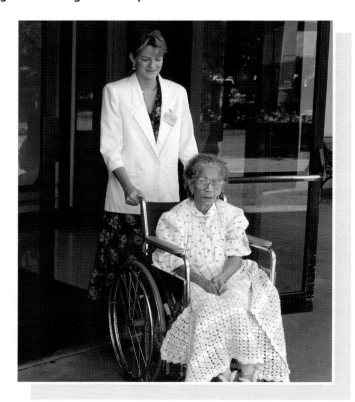

3. Provide assistance in filling out patient information and patient registration forms in a well-lighted area.

4. Be knowledgeable about which insurance plans the physician has joined, as well as supplemental insurance for Medicare patients.

5. Provide surgical instructions in large, bold type; many older patients have visual impairments.

6. Provide information sheets on special subjects related to geriatric patients, such as cardiovascular disease, arthritis, and osteoporosis.

7. Provide refrigerator magnets that include the physician's name and telephone number. You might also provide the same type of stickers to place on the telephone.

8. Maintain a warm temperature in the examination rooms.

9. Add the name and telephone number of the patient's nearest relative, close friend, attorney, or clergy to the patient's chart.

Sometimes, patients are accompanied by relatives. If the patient requires assistance, a relative may (if the patient so desires) come to the examination room and participate in further discussion with the physician and the patient regarding the patient's medical care and treatment plan.

Patient Complaints

In every practice there comes a time when a patient will complain about something. The administrative medical assistant must learn to listen and project a feeling of sympathy. Many times the patient is only reacting to fears or problems within his or her own life. However, you must be aware that no complaint, no matter how small or big, is to be ignored. Everyone must remember that the services provided to the patient produces the income that pays the health care team's salary and the office overhead. Take the complaint seriously, and make every attempt, within your area of responsibility, to resolve the problem. Express your concern, explain that you will make every attempt to solve the problem, and then report back to the patient your findings and the final determination for solution. Every patient deserves the right to understand the process that you used and the steps you took to solve the problem. Many times this will ease the tension and relieve the situation. Do not get excited or yell at the patient; always remain calm and under control. If you cannot solve the problem, report it to the supervisor and ask him or her to let you know how it was resolved.

Upset Patients and Excessive Talkers

At one time or another you will be confronted with the upset or angry patient. The anger may simply be a reaction to an unexpected wait in the reception area. This problem can be prevented by remaining calm, sure of yourself, and low key. Sometimes patients are angry because of events over which you have no control, or fearful of what they are going to hear from the physician. It is most important that you do not display anger or become argumentative.

Other patients are lonely or isolated and enjoy talking to the receptionist. These people also may take up large amounts of the physician's time. Although

FOCUS ON THE WORKPLACE

The Receptionist and the Angry Patient

1. Mr. Lyons: "Where is Dr. Kyle? My appointment was at 2:00 and it's 2:30—and no doctor yet!"
   A. Bad response—"Mr. Lyons, you'll just have to wait like all the other patients. You're not special, you know."
   B. Good response—"Mr. Lyons, the doctor was delayed at the hospital during his lunch break. He has called and should be in anytime. Can I do anything to make you more comfortable?"
2. Mr. Sanchez: "My time is valuable as I have a business to run. I should charge your doctor for my time."
   A. Bad response—"Mr. Sanchez, go right ahead and do that. Doctor doesn't like threats and usually discharges patients who threaten him."
   B. Good response—"Mr. Sanchez, I'm sorry that you feel that way, but our doctor is very conscientious and would always take the necessary time with you if you were hospitalized. It certainly is not his intention to make you wait."

they mean no harm, they can be very disruptive to the practice with their constant telephone calls or need for attention. Experienced receptionists usually can spot this type of personality at the first meeting. A prearranged signal to alert the physician that the next patient has arrived should be established, thus allowing the physician to exit gracefully. Such a signal could be just a knock on the examination room door to let the physician know how many other patients are waiting, with fingers extended to represent the number of waiting patients. Once you have learned which patients take additional time, you can schedule their appointments for the end of the day so other patients are not inconvenienced.

Interoffice Communication

Co-Workers

Medical assistants are hired because they have knowledge and specific skills that are needed to complete the job. Their interests, personalities, or backgrounds may not be compatible with those of the other health care professionals in the practice. Establishing a good working team is essential, but it is not easy. No two people are alike. Co-workers may view things differently than you do. Their values, habits, and personalities may conflict with yours.

Patients usually are very sensitive to the degree of harmony that exists in the medical practice or facility, and their well-being depends on their being treated in a caring atmosphere. If personality problems exist among the staff members, these conflicts should be openly discussed and resolved at staff meetings. You must take care to avoid criticism of others or to participate in office gossip. Inevitably, some co-workers enjoy gossiping, back-stabbing, and petty quibbling. This behavior not only is unpleasant for those around you but also is extremely detrimental to the practice and almost always destructive to the initiator.

Cooperation is the ability to work with others. You must extend yourself to be helpful to others. You learn cooperation by not thinking of yourself and your own immediate concerns but thinking of the total welfare of all the health care professionals and patients in the facility. Cooperation usually is an expression of unselfishness. You are expected to work cooperatively as a member of the health care team. Occasionally, you may observe that a co-worker is behind in his or her work, and you should offer to step in and assist the co-worker. You should do this without complaint; however, you must recognize if and when a co-worker is taking advantage of your good spirit of cooperation. If a co-worker attempts to place more and more work on you that is not within your job description, you should first let the co-worker know in a dignified, quiet manner that you cannot continue to process the work because it will jeopardize your own position and that if the co-worker needs assistance he or she should talk to the office manager. You should never say, "That is not my job." The qualified administrative medical assistant should be able to step in and handle any portion of the front office positions.

Teamwork also is based on the ability of one staff member to count on another staff member. Every person on the team is important and must complete a share of the workload. When you think of yourself as a team member, you need to keep in mind the following rules:

1. Think before you speak.
2. Do not take advantage of your co-workers, and do not allow them to take advantage of you.
3. Never let your emotions overrule your brain.
4. Always remain reserved about making judgments of others; put yourself in the other person's shoes.
5. Often, little comments such as "please," "thank you," "good morning," and "good night" are extremely powerful in the work environment; politeness simply lets others know that you appreciate them.

Patience is a virtue; not every person can catch on to new ideas and routines at the same time. You should remain calm when helping a new co-worker learn a new routine. Be patient when answering questions. Simply remember that someone took the time to teach you, and now it is your turn to teach the newcomer. You should always do the best job that you can do. Working in a medical practice is one of the most stressful occupations that you can pursue, but a little humor goes a long way toward relieving stress.

Supervisors

Supervisors sometimes appear extremely successful, but they may feel totally unappreciated. Remember the old saying: "The higher you climb on the ladder of success, the more lonely it is at the top." Like everyone, supervisors have personality quirks, strengths, and weaknesses; good days and bad days; and hopes and fears. You should respond to your supervisor as a professional and a real person. You will get along better with your supervisor when you remain calm, positive, and respectful.

Most supervisors have a definite style of managing people. You should become acquainted with the various styles of management; you can then develop a good working relationship with your supervisor. There are three basic

FIGURE 5.8

The democratic supervisor encourages employee participation in management, making use of committees of staff members to make decisions and suggest policies.

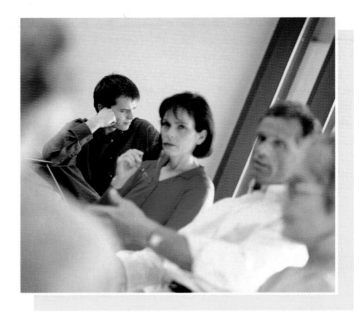

styles of management: autocratic, democratic, and laissez-faire. Each style has its own rules and characteristics.

The autocratic supervisor is a leader who dictates policy, procedure, and tasks. This type of person tells you not only how to do a task but also when and where. An autocratic person may feel uncomfortable delegating authority and rarely accepts employees who demonstrate initiative, creativity, and assertiveness. Autocratic supervisors may not wish to accept your positive recommendation. These individuals would like to think that only their ideas are the best; however, this type of thinking is the result of the individual's own insecurities. When working for such a supervisor, be sure that you follow all directions and adhere strictly to the rules of the practice or facility.

The democratic supervisor encourages employee participation in the management process (Figure 5.8). This type of individual exercises a moderate degree of control over the employees and frequently seeks input from them. Sometimes referred to as a "born teacher," this supervisor always seems to have time to explain policies and procedures to employees. This type of supervisor encourages you to see yourself as a part of the management team by asking for your ideas and considering them. In the office with a democratic supervisor, committees of staff members often make decisions and suggest changes to current office policies.

The supervisor with a laissez-faire management style exercises little or no control over the employees. This person usually provides minimal guidance and allows the staff to work independently. Such a supervisor encourages initiative and creativity. You have the freedom to complete your work using your best judgment and creative talents and relying on your past experiences. If you are assertive and creative, you will work well in this environment and with this type of supervisor.

Because of a difference in education and training, the physician may treat the administrative medical assistant as a subordinate. The physician may have a poor "bedside manner" not only in interactions with patients but also with other staff members. You can improve interactions with the physician by using your human relations skills. Be patient. It may take time, but even the gruffest

WHAT DO YOU THINK?

What type of management style do you prefer? (Answer the following true/false questions.)

1. In a large office or clinic, there should be an effective work structure. T F

2. The "chain of command" is the direction that authority and information are sent. T F

3. Respect for your superiors is necessary for you to work efficiently. T F

4. You should "go around" your immediate supervisor when there is a case of sexual harassment. T F

   A. Do you prefer to have the people at the top make the decisions?

   B. Do you feel strongly that you should be able to make important decisions?

physician eventually responds to a compliment, some light-hearted humor, or reassurance. Many physicians deal with emotionally draining situations every day: the death of a terminally ill patient, the stress of life-threatening emergencies, and the medical complaints of a full caseload of patients. Understandably, such a routine can harden even the most dedicated physician. Be sure not to let a doctor's complaints and frustrations affect you personally. Use your social skills and human sympathy to break through barriers and get in touch with the vulnerable human being inside the physician's coat.

Your supervisor's basic personality and style of management probably will not change. As the employee, you must learn to adapt to the style of the practice. When you discover which management style best suits you (see the box about preferred management style), you should direct your efforts toward securing employment in a health care facility where the management style suits your style.

Discrimination

Discrimination is a word used to describe unfair treatment of a person because of race, sex, religious affiliation, or disability. This behavior often is based on an attitude that has no place in the medical practice or facility. This attitude might be the belief that people of a particular race tend to be lazy. If you refuse to work with a person of a particular race or will not assist a person with a particular disability, you are guilty of discrimination.

The first step in handling discrimination in the practice or facility is to recognize it. When prejudice becomes a part of your personality or when you learn to accept unfair treatment based on prejudice, you begin to experience a form of personal decay. Work is not satisfying, and conflicts occur daily. Prejudice is difficult to overcome, but you must learn to recognize and refuse to accept discrimination in the workplace (see the box on p. 124).

AT WORK TODAY

Discrimination

Discrimination is unfavorable treatment based on prejudice. Related words are: bigotry, bias, intolerance, favoritism, one-sidedness, and inequity.

Following are examples of ways we might act that would show discrimination:

1. Race
   A. Mimicking someone's style of speech to "communicate better"
   B. Staring at a patient when he or she has an unusual hair or dress style
2. Age
   A. Talking loudly to the patient, assuming that he or she does not hear well
   B. Showing impatience when directing the patient to the examination room or having him or her prepare for an examination
3. Sex
   A. Acting cool and stilted when dealing with the opposite sex

   B. Discussing your opinions of "rights," either with your patients or where they can hear you
4. Religion
   A. Questioning something someone is wearing, whether it is clothing or a symbolic item
   B. Criticizing someone's diet when it is related to his or her religious beliefs
5. Disabled
   A. Trying to help the patient without asking first if he or she wants you to, for example, assisting a patient into the examination room or filling out forms for him or her
   B. Acting self-conscious around the patient; talking too much and not treating him or her normally

Office Emergencies

Sometimes patients brought into the office during office hours require emergency care. You must maintain a flexible attitude so that you can adjust on a moment's notice to any type of emergency. React calmly in a situation that demands immediate attention. This includes following planned procedures, particularly if the reception area is crowded with patients waiting for their own appointment. If a patient stops breathing, you should be prepared to perform cardiopulmonary resuscitation (CPR). Classes in this technique are given in most localities. First-aid training also can make it easier to cope with office emergencies. Because a medical emergency can occur when a physician or nurse is not available, these situations should be discussed and understood, with written directives placed in the procedures manual.

Normally, patients who have had an accident or who have suddenly become very ill are brought to the office by a very worried member of the family or close friend. The patient should immediately be moved into an inner examination room, away from patients in the reception area. While waiting for the physician or nurse, you must remain calm yet show concern. You should not give medical advice or discuss the situation at length; conversation should be limited to emotional support. If the patient mentions a relevant medical detail, pass this information on to the physician before the physician enters the treatment area.

Conclusion

The role of the administrative medical assistant receptionist is vital in the successful management of a practice. The medical assistant receptionist must have intuition, finesse, and a variety of skills to work successfully in this position. Whereas the clinical personnel are significant in their role of working with patients on a physical level, the receptionist must work on a psychological level and should present and maintain an image that the office is efficient and well managed.

Review QUESTIONS

1. List four types of visitors to the medical office.

2. Explain the way attitude affects the patent's overall impression of the office.

3. Describe the four basic elements of an employee's professional appearance.

4. Describe the type of desk that should be in a reception area.

5. Discuss the two types of communication—verbal and nonverbal— in the front office

6. Explain the importance of eye contact.

7. List at least four ways you can make keeping an appointment easier for an elderly or disabled patient.

8. Describe a situation in which you should assist a patient in filling out forms.

9. Why is it important to cooperate with other members of the health care team, and what can you do to achieve this goal?

SUGGESTED READINGS

American Medical Association: *The business side of medical practice,* Chicago, 1989, The Association.

Manning FF: *Medical group practice management,* Cambridge, Mass, 1977, Ballinger Publishing.

Medical office management Institute, San Francisco, 1991, Conomikes Associates.

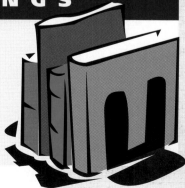

Telephone Skills

OUTLINE

On completion of Chapter 6 the administrative medical assistant student should be able to:

1. Define the key terms listed in this chapter.
2. Discuss the importance of telephone communication.
3. Communicate effectively over the telephone.
4. Handle incoming calls in a courteous and efficient manner.
5. Place various types of calls for the practice and the physician.
6. Use the telephone message pad effectively.
7. Coordinate calls for all health care professionals in the facility.
8. Handle and direct emergency calls.
9. Set up conference calls.
10. Respond appropriately to callers who have specific questions.

K E Y   T E R M S

Answering service	A business that specializes in taking and relaying telephone messages for offices that are closed.
Cellular telephone	A portable telephone (either in the automobile or a handheld set) that uses a satellite computer-controlled communication system to connect the telephone system to a network of cells that provide service through satellites for mobile radiotelephones.
Communication	The exchange of thoughts or opinions between persons or business firms; any means of conveying ideas or information in person or with auxiliary equipment.
Conference call	A prearranged telephone call that allows several people in different locations to hear and speak to one another at the same time.
Directory	An alphabetical list of names with addresses and telephone numbers or telephone extension numbers.
Electronic transmission	An electronic means of sending information via the telephone lines.
Enunciate	To declare or state; to pronounce clearly when speaking.
Etiquette	The rules of conduct observed in social or business interactions; polite behavior.
Handset	The portion of the telephone that is held in one hand and allows the user to hear and speak with others.

Continued

KEY TERMS

(Continued)

Hold (on the telephone)
The ability to keep a telephone call in an inactive state.

Telephone recording device
An instrument attached to the telephone that mechanically intercepts calls and preserves the caller's message; also called an *answering machine*.

ral communication is a vital part of the medical practice. It is important in any business, but it is even more important in patient care (Figure 6.1). The administrative medical assistant has a responsibility to patients and physicians to develop effective techniques of oral communication. Each member of the health care team also has a responsibility to maintain good communication with other members of the team. Oral communication occurs through face-to-face encounters and through the use of the telephone and its auxiliary services.

Types of Equipment and Services
Telephone Systems

After the deregulation of the telephone industry in the late 1980s, many companies introduced various types of business telephone equipment, along with a multitude of services. Messages can be held on voice mail or sent from computer to computer with E-mail (electronic mail). Some systems have direct chat capabilities. The systems can hold up to 300 preprogrammed numbers in a telephone directory and can automate calling with one-touch dialing. The physician and the administrative medical assistant may make entries up to 60 days in advance on a daily calendar. Electronic messages can be displayed on a screen. A search engine and automatic speed dialing of any number stored for the name on the message can be activated. A common feature is the ability to prerecord frequently called telephone numbers; these numbers can be changed at any time. If the physician is on a line and the receptionist receives another call, the receptionist can direct the call either to the physician (who may choose to place the person on hold) or to the physician's voice mail.

Several types of telephone systems are available. Many are very popular and can support from one to more than 30 lines, with the ability to overlay incoming 800 numbers over existing numbers. Many of the new telephones have two-digit codes that can be programmed easily to dial the numbers of those businesses or people that you call most frequently. Conference calls, privacy buttons (the option to prevent anyone from listening to the call), intercom, hold, call waiting, and voice mail are just some of the features today.

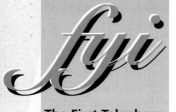

The First Telephone

Alexander Graham Bell was not trying to invent the telephone per se when the telephone became a reality. He had always been interested in the education of hearing-impaired people. He invented the microphone and then in 1876, his "electrical speech machine" (the telephone). He set up the first telephone exchange in 1878 and by 1884, long-distance connections were made between Boston and New York City. Today, many people with hearing impairments use a special display telephone to communicate, and fiber optics have improved the quality and speed of data transmission.

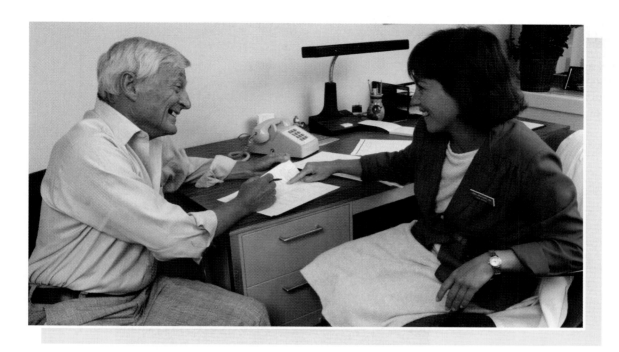

FIGURE 6.1

Oral communication, whether in face-to-face encounters or over the telephone, is vital in business, but especially in patient care.

We now are able to send data electronically over the telephone lines using computer modems and faxes.

Cellular Telephones

The cellular telephone has become very popular, especially among physicians. Car phones (either installed or portable) and pocket-size cellular phones allow busy physicians to respond to emergency situations and return nonemergency calls at their leisure (Figure 6.2). Cellular phones may receive interference when used near mountains, airports, radiology centers, and military facilities. Moreover, the call must be received within the region of a cellular station.

Telephone Features

The most common source of telephone equipment is the Bell telephone system; however, many manufacturers supply all types of telephone systems. The necessary equipment may be leased or purchased from most of these companies, although a local service company will have to be contracted for hookup of the equipment to the local system. If there is an equipment fee, it will be separate from the monthly service charge. Some services, such as long-distance calling, may be supplied by private companies. Private telephone companies commonly are referred to as *interconnective systems.*

The type of equipment chosen for the medical office depends on the present and future needs of the practice. Telephone specialists can assist with the

FIGURE 6.2

Car phones and pocket-size cell phones have allowed much greater flexibility for the physician.

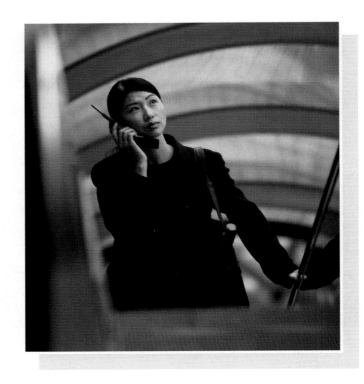

selection of appropriate equipment when setting up or making changes in a practice. Some of the options available on telephone equipment are described below.

Six-Button Key Set

The six-button key set is one of the most common types of telephone equipment used in a solo-practice office. One of the buttons is red and is used to put a call on hold. This allows the person answering the phone to retrieve information or transfer the call. The remaining buttons are clear plastic and may be delegated to incoming lines or intercom lines. (Figure 6.3). The term *incoming lines* does not indicate that the lines are limited to calls received by the office; it simply refers to the number of lines available for use by the office. An intercom line is used exclusively in the office suite. Personnel are able to communicate with each other via intercom and thereby save time and unnecessary movement about the office.

When a line is in use, a steady light is visible through the clear button. An intermittent flashing light indicates an incoming call, and a rapidly blinking light means that the call is on hold. The six-button set may have an old-fashioned rotary dial, but push-button dials are by far the most common. The latter is more efficient, usually requiring only 3 seconds to dial a seven-digit number.

Ten-Button Key Set

Increased telephone activity in a practice may require a set with additional lines. The 10-button set provides one hold button and nine lines for external or internal communication.

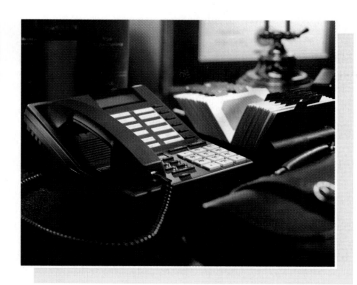

FIGURE 6.3

Increased telephone activity in a practice may require a set with more than one line.

Communications Key

An office with a large amount of floor space may select a communications key (com key) version of the 10-button set. It provides seven incoming lines and allows users to communicate by intercom from multiple sites at one time, make announcements over a loudspeaker, and select the time and place that various phones in the facility will ring.

Desk Sets

A facility with several physicians, many patients, and a busy telephone system may require an 11- to 30-button telephone set. Some models serve as a desktop switchboard, allowing the operator to place another call without breaking the original caller's connection, or establish conference calls by simultaneous depression of the necessary buttons.

Touch Tone

The touch-tone phone usually allows storage of 31 frequently called numbers in a memory. The face of the telephone instrument has a column on which to write the name or number stored in the memory next to a small button. You may place a call to any number in the memory by lifting the receiver and pressing the button for the person or place you wish to call. The number is dialed automatically. If you need to call back to a number just dialed, you may use the last-number-dialed button. This button automatically redials the most recently dialed number.

Speakerphone

An attachment inside the telephone instrument, the speakerphone allows the user to speak to and hear the person on the line without holding the receiver. This leaves the hands free to handle papers or make notes regarding the conversation. Users of speakerphones must be careful, however, to maintain privacy if confidential information is discussed where it might be overheard by others nearby.

WHAT DO YOU THINK?

Match each item on the left with its description on the right.

Item	Description
1. Six-button key set	a. Allows storage of 31 frequently called numbers on a memory
2. Ten-button key set	b. Allows individuals to speak and hear without holding the receiver
3. Com key	c. One of the common types of telephones used in a solo-practice office
4. Desk sets	d. This feature clips over the head or ear to provide more freedom of movement
5. Touch tone	e. A set with more lines for a busy practice
6. Speakerphone	f. Used in offices with larger floor areas
7. Headset	g. Has 11 to 30 buttons for a facility with several physicians

Headset

Many telephone systems feature headsets, which either clip over the head to glasses or over the ear. A small tubelike device is inserted into the person's ear, and a small rotatable, wirelike device is positioned in front of the person's mouth. This device has a very powerful but tiny microphone in the tip. A connecting wire usually clips to the user's clothing, allowing freedom of movement. Receptionists can take advantage of this feature to do paperwork or make notes regarding the conversation.

Telephones should be located with consideration given to efficient use and privacy. Appropriate location is as important as the type of equipment. Telephones should not be placed where they are easily available to patients or visitors to the office. Pay telephones usually are available in medical buildings or facilities; people requesting a telephone should be referred to them. You may, however, have one telephone in the reception area that is restricted to local calls and is available for patient use.

Other Useful Tools

Telephone service companies charge for directory assistance (411) to locate local telephone numbers. In addition, waiting for a prerecorded message to play before you can speak to an information operator wastes valuable time. Therefore you should develop a personal system to quickly locate the numbers you need to conduct business.

Local Telephone Directories

The local telephone company automatically provides customers with a local directory. Directories for other cities also can be supplied and should be requested for cities in which you conduct business. Local telephone books are divided into two major sections, commonly called the *White Pages* and the

Yellow Pages. These references may be combined or in separate volumes, depending on the size of the metropolitan area.

The White Pages may contain the following:

- An introductory section describing available telephone services, including emergency police, fire, and ambulance numbers; area codes; long-distance calling instructions; time zones; and instructions on handling obscene or harassing calls
- Emergency first aid and disaster-survival guides
- A government section listing the offices of local, state, and federal agencies
- Alphabetically listed names, most addresses, and telephone numbers of individuals (except those who request unlisted numbers)

The Yellow Pages lists the names, addresses, telephone numbers, and advertisements of businesses according to the service or product provided. Physicians are listed alphabetically and also have the option of a second listing according to specialty. Any listing in the Yellow Pages results in an additional monthly charge based on the number of lines and the size of the print or advertisement requested.

Medical Society Directories

County medical societies publish an annual directory of all members of the organization. Usually a photograph of each physician is included with his or her name, office address and telephone number, medical school, and year of graduation. This directory is a convenient alphabetical reference source of many local physicians. For the offices you call frequently, you may wish to note the name of the assistant responsible for answering the phone under the physician's entry. People appreciate being recognized by name, and the practice establishes a positive tone for subsequent conversations.

Hospital Directories

Local hospitals may print a directory of hospital services and departments, listing the corresponding extensions or the direct-dial numbers. Knowing the extension number reduces the time you spend waiting for the hospital operator to look up this information. If direct dialing to service areas is available, you can bypass the hospital operator altogether.

Personalized Directories

You also should develop a system for quick access to numbers that you use frequently. A rotary file or a desktop box containing 3 x 5 index cards is most commonly used for this purpose (Figure 6.4). Each is supplied with alphabetical dividers. Emergency numbers can be highlighted by using colored cards or a colored tab or by edging the card with colored tape. A separate card should be used for each business or person in the file and should include the following information:

- Name, spelled correctly
- Complete address, including Zip code
- Telephone number, with area code when appropriate
- Pertinent information such as services, equipment, or supplies provided

FIGURE 6.4

A rotary file is most commonly used in developing a system for quick access to frequently used numbers.

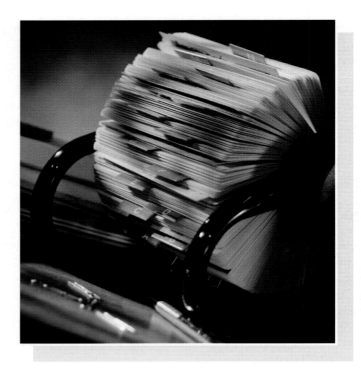

You can create a cross-index for your personal directory with your office procedures manual. In the section on telephone procedure, you should prepare the following lists:

- Physicians, by specialty, to whom your employer commonly refers patients
- Professional agencies or services such as hospitals, ambulance companies, pharmacies, home health agencies, visiting nurses associations, laboratories, and specialty practices
- Business suppliers or services such as medical-surgical suppliers, bankers, stationers, equipment maintenance companies, instrument repair services, and linen suppliers
- Employer's personal and private numbers, such as for family, friends, insurance broker, accountant, and attorney

Incoming Calls

Incoming calls (see the box about answering a call) make up approximately 80% of the daily telephone activity in an office or agency. Up to 50% of this activity involves patients or potential patients. Because the telephone is considered a valuable public relations tool, you must develop effective telephone techniques.

General Courtesy

The telephone should be answered as quickly as possible, preferably on the first or second ring. This gives the caller an impression of efficiency and considera-

MEDICAL ASSISTING STEP-BY-STEP

Answering a Call
- Answer promptly
- Hold the instrument properly
- Identify the office and yourself

MEDICAL ASSISTING STEP-BY-STEP

Answering a Call When You Are Unable to Complete the Conversation
- Answer promptly
- Hold the instrument properly
- Identify the office and yourself
- Allow the caller to identify himself or herself
- Restate the caller's name
- Ask the caller if he or she can hold for a moment
- Wait for the caller's reply
- Thank the caller, and depress the hold button
- When you return to the call, thank the caller again and continue with the conversation.

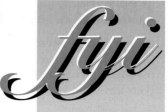

Communications/ Telephone

The first ingredient essential for good telephone skills is communication. Remember the four Cs:
- **Complete**
- **Concise**
- **Correct**
- **Clear**

tion. Answering quickly does not mean hastily. If you are rushing and sound breathless, the caller will notice. If you must rush to the telephone, pause briefly, take a deep breath, and then pick up the receiver. If you must answer but are unable to complete the conversation, be courteous. You would not appreciate placing a call that was answered, "Doctor's office, please hold," and placed on hold before you could respond. The box above lists the steps of a more considerate technique to use for answering a call when you are unable to complete the conversation.

Hold the instrument properly. Remove the telephone receiver gently from the cradle with your nondominant hand at the center of the handset. This leaves your dominant hand (the one with which you write) free to write notes or take messages. Place the receiver to your ear with the mouthpiece approximately 1 inch away from your lips. This position transmits your voice most effectively (Figure 6.5). The position can be checked by looking in a mirror or by passing the width of two fingers between the mouthpiece and your lips. Your fingers should just barely pass through. Never prop the handset between your ear and shoulder. This causes the mouthpiece to be pressed against your chin and distorts your voice, interfering with your ability to enunciate. Should you accidentally drop the receiver, retrieve it, apologize to the caller, and continue the conversation.

Identify the office and yourself. Office procedure should guide all personnel in the preferred manner of identifying the office and the person answering. Most telephone specialists suggest some variation of the following: "Dr. Smith's office, Ms. Jones speaking." In a multiphysician office, each physician's name

FIGURE 6.5

On the phone, speak with the receiver approximately 1 inch away from your lips.

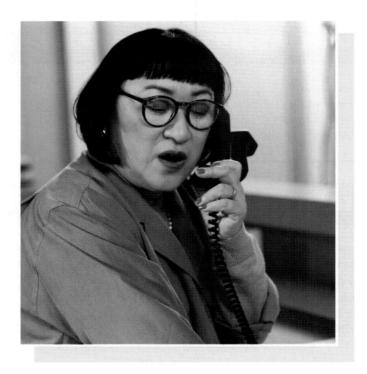

can be stated (for example, "Drs. Smith, Adams, and Caldwell, Ms. Jones speaking."). With more than three physicians, you may consider answering, "Doctor's office." Some multiphysician offices are incorporated or have adopted a group name. In that case you can answer, for example, "Valley Medical Group, Ms. Jones speaking."

If time permits, you may include a greeting such as "Good morning" or "Good afternoon" or ask, "May I help you?" after stating your name. The caller will appreciate the pleasant greeting.

Some states have regulations regarding the telephone identification of an incorporated medical practice. The physician's attorney and the office procedures manual should guide you in this matter. Some attorneys have linked the incorporation rules to the need for identifying the office by merely stating the telephone number. This procedure should be avoided. It is bewildering to the caller, who usually replies, "Is this Dr. Adam's office?" By the time the identification is made, time has been wasted and callers feel that they are dealing with an impersonal medical office.

Use the hold button properly. The hold button should be used any time you are not speaking with the caller. This includes brief interruptions to retrieve information or bring another person to the telephone. Placing the receiver on the desk without using the hold button allows the caller to overhear office conversations. This is extremely unprofessional. Placing a hand over the mouthpiece is an inadequate substitute for using the hold button and may even magnify what is being said.

The hold function also must be used when directing a call (that is, transferring it to the person for whom it is intended). After the caller is put on hold, you may use the intercom line to identify the caller and the line on which the call can be picked up.

MEDICAL ASSISTING STEP-BY-STEP

Interrupting a Call to Answer Another Call

1 Excuse yourself from the person on the line. Explain that you have another call coming in and that you will be right back.

Rationale
The caller will appreciate the courtesy, and understanding the reason will generate cooperation.

2 Answer the second call, and put the second caller on hold as previously suggested.

Rationale
The caller will be reassured that he or she has reached the office and will be more willing to wait.

3 Return to the first caller, thank him or her for waiting, and mention that the other line is on hold.

Rationale
Knowing that another caller is waiting may encourage the individual to be concise.

AT WORK TODAY

Telephone Etiquette

Just remember that the first 15 seconds of a phone call are crucial. Telephone skills can "make or break" the practice. Some good advice is:
- Use your natural voice
- Sit up straight
- Answer calls with "a smile"

- Address your patients appropriately
- Notice the response of your callers (that is, can they understand you?)
- Listen actively
- Obtain needed information

When you are speaking to one caller and another line rings, you must respond to the new call. An appropriate procedure to follow is listed in the box about interrupting a call to answer another.

A caller should not be allowed to wait on hold indefinitely. You should speak with the person on hold at 2-minute intervals and inform him or her of the status of the call. For example, you may have a caller waiting to speak to a physician who is on another line. When you check back with the caller, you might say, "Dr. Smith is still on the other line. Would you like to continue to hold, or can the doctor call you back?" This lets the caller know that you have not forgotten him or her, and your courtesy shows your understanding of the caller's needs.

WHAT DO YOU THINK?

"Hello, doctor's office. What do you need?"

What is wrong with this greeting? What is missing?

"This is Mrs. Green. Can you please give me the results of my daughter's pregnancy test?"

How would you take care of this question? What would you say?

"This is Smith Brothers Pharmacy, Joe speaking. Mr. Gaines has called for a refill of his Vicodin, which was filled 2 weeks ago."

To whom does this call go? What do you tell the pharmacist?

"Dr. Ander's office? I'm Mary Harkins, and I want to know why you overcharged me on the bill!"

The patient seems angry. What would you say?

MEDICAL ASSISTING STEP-BY-STEP

Handling Calls

1. Be prepared.
2. Get the information you need.
3. Control the call.
4. Log the call.

Telephone Call Records

You must always be ready to take a message when you lift the handset from the cradle (see the box about handling calls). Being prepared to note information is the first step in handling messages. A message or notepad should be near the telephone at all times, and you should have a pen or pencil in your hand. A notepad, such as a stenographer's spiral book, may be appropriate aid for initially answering the telephone because it also can be used to make notes to yourself. You may even want to note who is on which telephone line when you are dealing with several calls at once.

To minimize the amount of time you spend on each call, develop techniques for controlling calls and procedures for classifying and disposing of calls. Callers may forget that you must handle numerous duties and respond to many telephone calls each day. In addition, if they are anxious, they may include a great deal of unnecessary information in their conversation.

All telephone calls should be logged. The best method is to use a two-part NCR form because it provides a copy for the patient's chart and a permanent copy for the office. These logs should be kept a minimum of 7 years. If the physician treats children, the logs should be kept until the child is 21 years old. The importance of documentation cannot be overstressed. At no time should scraps of paper be used for patient information or documentation of phone calls. Many pharmaceutical companies provide scratch pads as a method of advertising product. These pads should not be used for message taking; however, if they are, the information should be transferred to the NCR log as quickly as possible.

When screening a call, first acquire the basic information. If the caller has not volunteered a name, you should ask, "Who is calling, please?" If necessary, ask for the correct spelling of the name, which saves time if you need to locate records. You also should obtain the caller's telephone number and the reason for the call.

Retain control of the call by asking specific questions rather than allowing the caller to give a lengthy account of the reason for calling. You should not be rude or sound rushed, but you can learn to conserve time with each caller. For example, a patient calling for an appointment because of an upper respiratory infection may mention the illness and then attempt to tell you what he or she thinks happened last week to cause it. At the first opportunity, you might interject, "This type of infection is common in this area now. Dr. Smith can see you this afternoon at 2:00 or at 3:30. Which time would you prefer?" With this technique you can curtail potentially lengthy conversation while demonstrating that you understand the caller's needs and are offering assistance. You can learn additional telephone techniques from articles in *The Professional Medical Assistant* and by observing experienced co-workers.

Troublesome Callers

On occasion, you will receive calls that are considered troublesome. These callers may fit into the following categories:

- The angry caller
- The repeat caller
- The appointment juggler
- The caller seeking aid beyond your duties
- The caller requesting confidential information
- The unidentified caller

You will need to deal with these callers in a tactful manner but also in a way that indicates you are in control of the situation.

The Angry Caller
With the angry caller, it is in your best interest to remain calm, determine the issue, and assure the caller that you are interested in helping (Figure 6.6). You may be able to reduce the caller's anger by saying, for example, "I understand you are upset, Ms. Jones. I may be able to help if you will answer a few questions for me." You may then ask the questions necessary to determine the issue.

The Repeat Caller
You occasionally will deal with people who repeatedly call the office for clarification of the doctor's instructions, for reassurance, or perhaps to discuss information from the media that concerns them. Many calls may be eliminated by providing patients with printed instructions or diet slips that have been prepared for routine situations in your office. The instructions may be reviewed by patients before they leave the office. This provides them with an opportunity

FIGURE 6.6

With the angry caller, it is in your best interest to remain calm, determine the issue, and assure the caller that you are interested in helping.

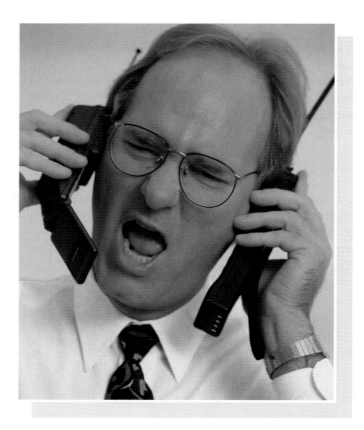

to ask questions. Individuals making repeated calls about items covered in the information sheet may be referred to the guide they were given. This will reduce the time spent on the call and will subtly suggest that the call was unnecessary. A statement such as "I believe that is covered in the instruction sheet you received during your last visit" may be all that is needed. If the caller persists, you may suggest scheduling an appointment to discuss the concerns with the doctor. Often the prospect of spending additional time and money on another office visit separates true concerns from insecurity.

The Appointment Juggler

Patients occasionally may need to change a scheduled appointment. This certainly is understandable, and the change usually is for a valid reason such as an unplanned business trip, a change in work or school schedule, or car trouble. However, some patients constantly change appointments, often at the last minute. If you notice this pattern developing, you should speak to the patient. At the time an appointment change is requested, you might say, "Mr. Smith, I will try to help you with your requested change, but I think you should know that it helps to have more notice when you cannot keep an appointment. Another patient could be scheduled."

The Caller Seeking Aid Beyond Your Duties

Occasionally, patients ask for help with matters that are beyond the scope of your duties and would require time away from your responsibilities. Many times, this involves a request to check with the patient's insurance company about the status of a claim. Patients should be told that the insurance company can provide the information directly to them if they call the company. A diplomatic way to do this is to mention that insurance companies prefer to speak to the patient directly because they wish to protect the patient's privacy. This call also may be directed to the billing person. Other requests, such as to change appointments with laboratories or other offices, also should be tactfully declined by saying, "I can give you the office's number, and you can speak with the appointment secretary directly. That way you can select a time that will best fit with your schedule."

The Caller Requesting Confidential Information

Callers may seek information of a confidential nature for many reasons. Some of these individuals are interested friends, insurance companies, the media (if the patient is newsworthy), or employers. You know that the patient's written consent is necessary to release the information and should state this to the caller. If you receive a call from an institution stating that they admitted your patient and need information from the patient's record, you should be sure to do the following:

- Request some identifying data on the patient, such as date of birth or Social Security number.

- Request the caller's name and telephone number, stating that you will call back immediately after pulling the patient's chart for the physician. By returning the call, you can verify the institution and person to whom you are speaking.

The Unidentified Caller

You may occasionally receive calls from individuals who refuse to identify themselves or who misrepresent their identity or the nature of their business. This technique for gaining access to the physician is increasingly common among salespersons, particularly those selling financial investments. Some of the statements you may hear in response to your request for information include the following:

- "This is Ms. Jones, regarding the doctor's financial statement."

- "This is Mr. Smith, regarding the doctor's stock portfolio."

- "This is Simpson from the Human Aid Society to see if the doctor will be matching last year's donation." (In truth the physician may not have made a donation last year.)

Office policy will direct you on how to deal with calls of this type. Some possibilities are as follows:

- For callers who refuse to identify themselves, advise them that you may not transfer a call without the information you have requested, but they may state their business in a letter to the physician.

- For callers who imply that they are the physician's established representative (and you know they are not), you might reply, "The doctor's broker handles the portfolio. Thank you for calling. Goodbye."

- If you are in doubt about the validity of the representative, check with the physician.

WHAT DO YOU THINK?

1. Mrs. Salez says, "May I speak to the doctor? I saw the doctor for a kidney infection last week, and I'm still having problems." What would you do?
2. Jan Greenwich calls and says, "I've been sick for 2 days with a sore throat and aches and pains." Can I be seen today?
3. Joan Collins begins, "I need to speak to the doctor immediately. My husband, Fred, is having chest pains and I don't know what to do."
4. Mrs. Hale calls and asks for a well-baby checkup at the end of the current week. She says she forgot to make an appointment when she was in 6 weeks ago.

What is the urgency of these calls? (Rate these calls in order of importance.)

For contributions, say, "The doctor reviews contribution requests submitted in writing. If you care to send your literature, the doctor can make a decision. Thank you for calling."

Classification of Calls

Establishing a policy defining the various classifications of calls is important. Classifying calls is necessary to determine how and by whom calls will be handled. The common groupings for calls received in a medical office or agency are detailed in the following sections.

Emergency Calls

Emergency calls require the immediate attention of the physician. In emergency situations, symptoms are as follows:

- Loss of consciousness
- Heavy bleeding
- Severe pain
- Severe vomiting or diarrhea, particularly in children
- Fever greater than 102° F (38.9° C)

If the physician is not in the office, you should locate him or her immediately. On average, 2% to 3% of calls to the office are true emergencies.

Routine Patient Calls

The majority of calls from patients concern routine matters. Most of them are handled by the medical office personnel. Routine patient calls include the following:

- Requests for appointments
- Clarification of instructions
- Inquiries about statements
- Inquiries about routine laboratory results
- Status reports

In most offices the first four types of routine calls are handled by the administrative medical assistant; the physician usually prefers to speak to the patient about status reports and abnormal laboratory results. You should tell the patient when the physician typically returns nonemergency calls. This is a valuable service not only to the patient but also to the practice in general. It eliminates many additional calls from patients wanting to know when the physician will return their calls.

Medical Business Calls

Medical personnel from other offices or facilities call the physician's office through the course of the day. Medical business calls can be expected from the following people and institutions:

- Other physicians
- Hospitals
- Pharmacies
- Laboratories
- Ancillary services (physical therapy, visiting nurses)
- Professional associations

You should take a message with the pertinent information from each caller. Preprinted forms are available for recording laboratory data. These forms save time because you will not have to write out each element before writing the value found. The laboratory technician also will appreciate this time-saving technique.

The use of a recording device is extremely helpful in offices that receive numerous prescription refill calls. This allows the recorder to log as many as five or six calls regarding prescriptions. Then all charts may be pulled and documented at the same time and sent back for refiling. This type of system usually results in fewer telephone calls on the part of the staff. Information regarding this service should be preprinted in the practice's brochure.

Other Business Calls

Maintaining an office requires contact with many individuals who represent various services, including the following:

- The office accountant
- The physician's attorney
- The physician's insurance broker
- Medical-surgical supply sales representative
- Pharmaceutical company representatives seeking an appointment to talk with the physician

Most physicians do not usually interrupt patient care to speak with business callers but return their calls when possible (Figure 6.7).

Personal Calls

Physicians usually receive some personal calls from family or friends during business hours. Friends tend to call because it is easier to reach the physician at the office, or they may not want to interfere with the physician's limited free

FIGURE 6.7

Maintaining an office requires contact with many individuals who represent various services, including accountants, attorneys, insurance firms, and sales representatives.

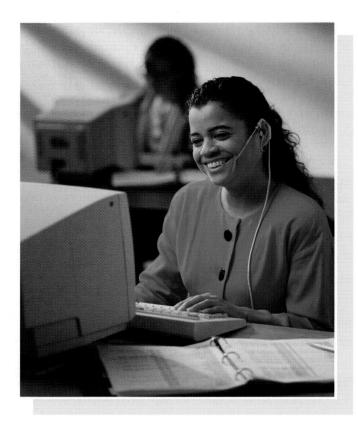

time at home. Family members may wish to confirm tentative plans or remind the physician of a personal appointment. On rare occasions, you may be asked to perform a service or do an errand for the physician's spouse or children. You must be tactful, but you should not allow a habit to develop. You may reply, "I would be happy to help if time is available after completing my office duties," or, "I will check with Dr. Smith to see if our schedule will permit the time you request." Physicians usually prefer to reserve office personnel for business and will support your stand.

You and other members of the staff cannot expect the privilege of receiving or making personal telephone calls at work. Office policy usually states that staff members should discourage personal calls; if they receive a personal call, employees should advise the caller that they will return the call from home that evening. Sometimes personnel need to accept very important calls from their spouses, family, or babysitter. These calls should be kept as brief as possible.

Disposition of Calls

Once a call has been received and classified, you can determine the disposition, or appropriate management, of the call. Making the proper choice in handling incoming calls saves time for the caller, the physician, and the office personnel.

Referred to the Physician

Calls that typically are referred to the physician include the following:

- Emergencies
- Patient status reports

- Reports of laboratory results to patients
- Calls from other physicians
- Calls from hospitals
- Calls from professional associations
- Calls on nonmedical business other than from medical suppliers, such as attorney, accountant, and so on
- Personal calls

Handled by the Medical Assistant

The medical assistant usually is responsible for resolving the needs of most callers contacting the office. These needs include the following:

- Scheduling appointments
- Clarification of instructions (may be referred to nurse or physician)
- Inquiries about fees and bills (may be referred to the billing person)
- Requests from pharmacies (may be referred to back office staff)
- Laboratories calling with reports (may be referred to nurse or physician)
- Scheduling meetings with hospital and professional association committees
- Calls from medical-surgical suppliers
- Laboratory results to patients (with physician's approval)

Your policy manual should have a chart to use for quick reference regarding the appropriate handling of a call. See Table 6.1 for a sample disposition chart.

Outgoing Calls

General Guidelines

Telephone Etiquette

When you place a telephone call, you should remember that you may be interrupting another person's activities. Your calls should be designed to save time and respect the other person's needs. Above all, they should be conducted in a courteous manner. Business etiquette suggests that it is most appropriate for individuals to place their own calls. Physicians who wish to speak with a colleague, business associate, or medical facility should dial the call, identify themselves, and state the name of the person with whom they wish to speak. Because of experience with being placed on hold for a lengthy period, some physicians ask the medical assistant to place their calls for them. This may evolve into a game of protocol, in which neither physician wants to be put on the line first and have to wait for the other physician to be put on the phone. If you work with physicians who insist that you place their calls, you can reduce the waiting and interoffice manipulation by placing the call when you know your employer is readily available. If the receiving medical assistant demands that the calling physician be put on the line, you may put the call on hold and inform your employer that the call will be put through as soon as he or she is on the line. The colleague's subtle message may be received. If the receiving assistant puts the call

TABLE 6-1

Guide for Disposition of Incoming Calls

Disposition	Patient Emergency	Patient reporting back on treatment	Patient seeking Reinstruction on Treatment plan	Other Physicians	Hospital, Urgent	Hospital, Nonurgent	Pharmacies	Laboratories Reporting Results	Nonmedical Business	Personal	Patient: Appointment Scheduling	Patient: Administrative Inquiries
Calls Requiring Physician												
Physician in office												
Interrupt immediately	X			X	X							
Return as soon as possible		X				X						
Return at fixed, routine time (medical assistant to advise caller of approximate time)		X					X		X			
Return when convenient									X	X		
Physician out of office												
Contact physician immediately for handling or instructions	X			X	X							
Hold messages until physician calls for them		X				X	X	X	X	X		
Calls Processed by Medical Assistant												
Administrative								X			X	X
Clinical			X					X				

From Zakus SM et al, editors: *Mosby's fundamentals of medical assisting: administrative and clinical theory and technique,* ed 2, St. Louis, 1990, Mosby.

through directly, and you are greeted by the physician being called, you will be able to thank the physician and put your employer on the line immediately.

Planning Your Calls

Thinking about a telephone call that you need to make and preparing for it will, in the long run, save time for you and the person answering the call. Planning calls also demonstrates your efficiency. Your preparation in planning a call includes the following measures:

- Locating the correct telephone number
- Compiling the information needed during the call
- Keeping a notepad and writing instruments nearby

The information needed varies depending on the purpose of the call. If you need to set up or change a patient's appointment, you will need the appointment book to know the days and times available. To order supplies, you will need a list of the items needed, including a description of the items, catalog numbers, and the quantity desired. To discuss a patient's account, you will need the billing record and filed insurance claims. The experience of practicing and placing business calls will help you plan for these calls. Over time, the preparation will become automatic. The person receiving the call will appreciate your efforts and will feel confident about your ability to conduct business.

Dialing Errors

If you make a dialing error when placing a call, you should always apologize to the person you disturbed. If the call involves an additional charge (such as a long distance call), you should attempt to learn the number you have reached. Many people are understandably uncomfortable about giving their phone number to an unknown caller, and their rights must be respected. In this case, state the number you were calling and ask if it is the number you reached. If it is the number you dialed, you will know your file was wrong. If it is not the number you intended to call (and you are certain you dialed the number correctly), dial the operator, state the number you were attempting to reach, and request credit for the error. The misdialed call will not be charged on the monthly statement.

Use of Directories

Directories should be readily available to all personnel who place outgoing calls. The office should acquire as many directories as necessary to avoid frequently moving them from one site to another. Most practices require a set of directories at the desks of the office manager, the administrative medical assistant, and the physician.

Directory Assistance

Local Assistance

To locate a number within your area code, dial "411." As noted, the local telephone company may charge for use of the 411 service. This is another reason for acquiring the directories of nearby cities or counties if they are included in your area code. Dialing "0" for directory assistance instead of "411" also results in an extra charge.

Long-Distance and International Assistance

Help in locating long-distance numbers may be obtained by dialing the area code of the business or person and then dialing "555-1212." Your telephone directory lists most area codes. International calls also may be dialed directly if you know the local telephone number. To complete an international call, you must dial the following, in order:

- 011 (the international access code)
- The country code (available in your directory White Pages)
- The city code (from the directory White Pages)
- The local number

FIGURE **6.8**

Dialing 911 connects the
caller in most communities
with a public safety
answering point, from
which the dispatcher can
provide the appropriate
services.

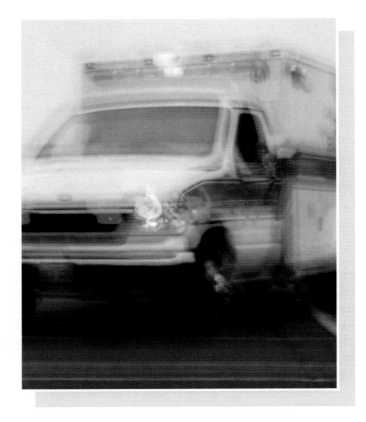

A sample international direct dial might look like the following:

011	+	61	+	12	+	218-362
(international access code)		(country)		(city)		(local + # number)

Local numbers in other countries can have more or fewer digits than numbers in the United States. You can expect approximately a 45-second wait after dialing before the connection is complete and the telephone rings.

800 Numbers

Many companies throughout the country provide toll-free (800) numbers so that callers may conduct business or place orders at no charge. If you want to determine whether a business provides a toll-free number, call 800 information by dialing 1-800-555-1212.

Emergency Assistance

Some cities have instituted a means of summoning emergency aid by dialing "911." Where the system is in effect, you can even dial the number from a pay telephone without inserting a coin. Dialing "911" connects the caller with a public safety answering point from which the dispatcher can provide the following services:

- Fire rescue
- Police or highway patrol
- Ambulance
- Paramedics (Figure 6.8)

This number must be used only in a true emergency. When you use the 911 access number, the number from which you are calling is automatically displayed on the dispatcher's message screen, even if the number is unlisted. This aids the dispatcher in case you are cut off before completing the call. If it is not a true emergency, you must locate and dial the individual number of the service you need.

Types of Calls

Local

The majority of calls you place from the office will be local—that is, within your area code. Most local calls are covered by the basic monthly service charge. Some calls within an area code but beyond a predetermined distance are still considered local but are billed based on the distance, the time spent on the telephone, and the time of day that the call was placed.

Long Distance

Long-distance calling is increasing in popularity because it reduces the amount of paperwork necessary to conduct business. The cost of long-distance calls depends on the company supplying the service, the method used in placing the call, the distance between the caller and the recipient, the time spent on the call, and the time of day the call takes place.

Various companies have different rates for long-distance service. In general, the cost of long distance has been greatly reduced in recent years. If your office or agency uses long distance often, you should investigate the many options available for saving money.

The cost of long distance also is influenced by the method you choose in placing the call. Direct dialing is the least expensive method of placing a call and is termed *station-to-station calling*. To place a station-to-station call, you simply dial the area code and the seven-digit number you want. In most areas you must dial "1" before the area code to gain access. Your direct dial number would be, for example, "1-361-123-4567."

Operator-assisted long-distance calls involve the services of a telephone operator, which increases the cost of the call. The operator is necessary for collect calls, some credit card calls, and person-to-person calls. A person-to-person call is used when you want to reach a specific person who may not be in the office when you call. An operator-assisted call is placed by dialing "0," the area code, and the seven-digit number. The operator intercepts the call, obtains the necessary information, and then allows the call to proceed.

The time of day must be considered when placing a call. The least expensive times for placing calls do not usually coincide with business hours, but time must be considered for another reason. The world is divided into various time zones. The continental United States is divided into four time zones. From the West Coast to the East Coast, these time zones are titled *Pacific, Mountain, Central,* and *Eastern.* Each time zone involves a 1-hour difference from the zone on either side of it. For example, when it is 9:00 AM Pacific time, it is 10:00 AM Mountain time. See your telephone directory for the geographical areas included in each time zone. You must consider these time zones when placing calls to reach a business during working hours. A call placed from New York at 10:00 AM Eastern time to an office in San Francisco will be too early, since it

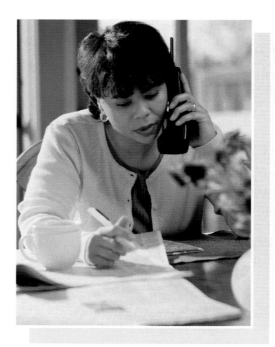
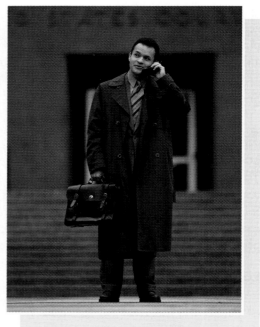
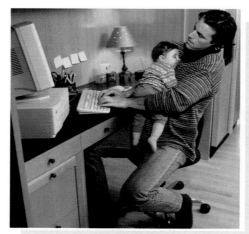
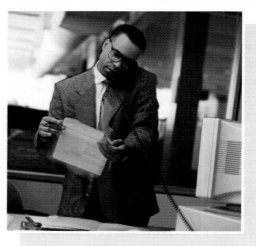

FIGURE 6.9

Conference calls allow between 3 and 14 different geographic points to be connected at one time, all involved in one call.

will be 7:00 AM Pacific time. A call placed to North Carolina from Colorado at 4:30 PM will be too late, since it will be 6:30 PM Eastern time. Your local telephone directory includes a time zone chart to assist you in planning long-distance calls.

Conference Calls

Conference calls allow between 3 and 14 different geographical points to be connected at one time. Each person at each geographical point can speak to and be heard by all other persons involved in the call (Figure 6.9). Conference calls

PERSPECTIVES ON MEDICAL ASSISTING

The Physician's Outside Life

Amy was a medical administrative assistant who worked for Simeon French, M.D. Dr. French's wife, Samantha, resented her husband's obligations to his patients. At times, she would not answer the phone at home when the answering service was trying to reach the doctor. Amy would come into the office the next morning to be greeted by the service telling her that they could not reach Dr. French the night before when they needed him. Amy talked to Dr. French regarding her concerns, and he agreed he would talk to his wife to resolve the situation.

are of great value in sharing information among several physicians or among the physician and members of a patient's family in different geographical areas. Being able to discuss an issue with several people at once saves valuable time.

Conference calls are billed at the person-to-person rate applicable to the two farthest points involved in the call, with each additional line charged at a reduced rate. You can establish a conference call by contacting the local operator and requesting a connection to the conference operator. The conference operator will need the name, area code, and number of each person participating in the call and the time the call will take place. The conference operator will contact the parties in advance and ask each person to hold. Once all connections are made, the operator will open the lines to all participants. Some of the newer systems allow an in-house switchboard operator to handle this operation within the facility.

Telephone Services

Answering Services

Physicians or their associates must be available to patients 24 hours a day, 7 days a week. Because a medical office may be open only 8 eight hours a day, some arrangement must be made for patients to reach the physician after business hours. Ethically and legally, physicians are bound to fulfill this duty to their patients. If patients are unable to reach their physician or the physician's on-call colleague in a time of need, they may sue the physician for abandonment.

Recording Devices

Telephone answering devices are becoming more common in our society. People are used to listening to the recorded message and leaving their name, telephone number, and the reason they wish to speak with the physician. There are positive and negative aspects to using recording devices to monitor after-hours telephone calls. These are presented in Table 6.2.

TABLE 6-2

Pros and Cons of Electronic Recording Devices

Pros	Cons
Less expensive than operator-assisted services	Viewed by some as impersonal
Valuable in areas where answering services are not available	Requires a back-up number or instructions if call is an emergency
Medical assistant does not have to call answering service when arriving at or leaving the office	Systems subject to interruption if there is a failure of electricity or telephone service
Can be equipped with a remote control device, allowing physician to collect messages from any telephone outside of office	Systems that page physician via beeper in the event of mechanical difficulty are expensive

From Zakus SM et al, editors: *Mosby's fundamentals of medical assisting: administrative and clinical theory and technique*, ed 2, St. Louis, 1990, Mosby.

Operator-Assisted Services

Answering services are available with operators who will assist patients in contacting the physician after office hours. The patient can be connected with the answering service in one of two ways. First, the number of the service can be listed in the telephone directory immediately below the private number for the office. The directory entry may read as follows:

```
Jones, James
6 Main Street       123-4567 Office
24 hours call       765-4321
                    or if no answer, call 765-4320 Services
```

The second option is to arrange with the telephone company and the answering service for an automatic relay of calls from the office to the service. With this arrangement, the patient places only one call. As the office is closing, the medical assistant calls the answering service and notifies it to begin intercepting the calls. The answering service operators are trained to make decisions regarding the classification and disposition of calls.

There are two types of operator-assisted answering services: general and specialty. General answering services accept clients from a variety of businesses and individuals who require 24-hour telephone coverage, such as attorneys, plumbers, and consultants. Specialty services limit their clients to members of a particular field. Some county medical societies have developed physician-only answering services with operators trained in handling medical situations. If available, specialty answering services are the best choice for a medical practice.

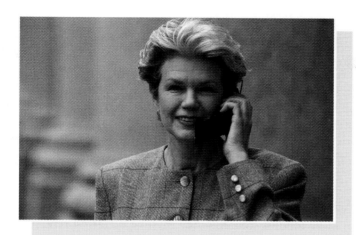

FIGURE 6.10

When a pager is used, the physician can be reached almost anywhere and receive important messages.

Coordinating After-Hours Telephone Services

The medical assistant is responsible for coordinating the after-hours telephone services. If a recording device is used, it must be on and working before the office is closed. The medical assistant should periodically check the recorded message for clarity and quality of sound. If an operator-assisted service is used, the medical assistant should notify the service, sometimes referred to as the *exchange,* when the office closes. When signing out, you should be prepared to inform the service how to reach the physician and supply necessary telephone numbers.

In addition, the efficient medical assistant periodically checks on the manner in which the office telephones are answered when the office is closed. This can be done by calling the office number when the office is closed and evaluating the efficiency and effectiveness of the recording device or answering service. Another method of checking is to ask patients who had to reach the physician after hours if everything was satisfactory.

Pagers

Pagers, commonly called *beepers,* are small, pocket-sized devices that the physician can carry. If the medical assistant or answering service needs to speak with the physician, a telephone code can be dialed and the pager will signal the physician. The physician can then call the office to obtain the message (Figure 6.10). Some pagers have a button that allows the physician to hear the message without calling in. The one drawback to pagers is that the medical assistant cannot be assured that the message was received.

Pagers are valuable because they save time for the physician and the medical assistant. Pagers eliminate the need for multiple calls to locate physicians who are ahead of or behind the schedule they left with the medical assistant. After office hours the answering service can hold the patient's call, page the physician, and connect the patient directly with the physician. This is reassuring to the patient and eliminates the need for the physician to place two calls.

Call Forwarding

Telephones can be adapted to forward telephone calls from the physician's offices to any number programmed into the system. This system is an advantage to practices with more than one office and more than one telephone number. Patients calling one office are automatically transferred to the site where the physician and staff are. This reduces confusion for the patient and eliminates the need for redialing.

If call forwarding is used for after-hours calls, physicians may find it a disadvantage because unwanted callers may easily trace them.

Dictation Services

The need for clear medical records may involve dictating reports for the office files or for the records of hospitalized patients. Private transcription services and hospital medical record departments often provide special telephone dictating equipment. You will be provided with special telephone numbers that the physician can dial for direct, immediate access to the equipment. The dictation is recorded and transcribed by personnel at the facility.

Some physicians prefer to dictate information regarding patients for clear and concise records for the patient's chart. Today's requirements for clear and legible documentation of medical records make dictation advantageous. The physician can select from several types of recording devices; one of the most popular is the voice-activated tape recorder. The data may be typed on plain white sheets or on what are called "sticky sheets" with a self-adhering backing (which may be cut, pulled apart, and placed in the medical record after typing). This data may be transcribed by office staff or sent out to a transcription service.

Telegraph Services

The telephone is used for access to telegraph services. These services include regular and overnight telegrams and mailgrams. Telegrams are sent through Western Union and Mailgrams through the U.S. Postal Service. If you wish to send a telegraph message, contact the appropriate agency and dictate the message to the operator. The message is transmitted by telephone or computer to the point of delivery, where it is printed and delivered to the proper person. Either service can be charged to your telephone number.

Conclusion

Oral communication is one of the most vital systems in a medical facility. Establishing rapport with patients provides the foundation for the subsequent relationship between the patient and the physician. The importance of telephone services cannot be overemphasized, and the medical assistant is the key to efficiency and effectiveness of the system. Keep in mind that the telephone provides the primary link between the patient and necessary medical services. You will need to monitor the operating efficiency of the office telephone equipment, the auxiliary services, and, particularly, your communication techniques and skills.

Review QUESTIONS

1. List the four basic factors that influence oral communication, and explain the way they influence it.

2. Describe how you will apply the standard techniques of effective communication when working with an angry patient.

3. Why is the telephone considered so vital to the medical practice?

4. List and describe six possible types of medical office telephone equipment.

5. Write a sample dialogue between you and a caller, keeping in mind the four elements of general courtesy. Produce an accurate message from the call.

6. List the five major categories of incoming calls, and describe the appropriate disposition of each type.

7. Explain how you would handle the following:
   a. An angry patient
   b. A repeat caller
   c. An appointment juggler
   d. A request for help beyond your capability
   e. A request for confidential information
   f. An unidentified caller

8. What auxiliary services can you expect to encounter in a complete telephone system?

SUGGESTED READINGS

American Medical Association: *The business side of medical practice,* Chicago, 1989, The Association.
Southwestern Bell: *Your voice is you,* Oklahoma City, 1985, Bell Telephone Systems.

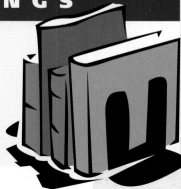

Appointment Scheduling

OUTLINE

OBJECTIVES

On completion of Chapter 7 the administrative medical student should be able to:

1 Define the key terms listed in this chapter.

2 List and discuss the three reasons for time management.

3 List and discuss the various types of appointment systems.

4 Describe the equipment necessary for an appointment system.

5 State the patient information needed to schedule an appointment; state the information given to the patient about the appointment.

6 List and discuss at least five major guidelines for scheduling office appointments.

7 Discuss the steps that should be taken to protect the physician legally when a patient fails to keep or cancels an appointment.

8 Describe what to do and say to visitors who are not patients (for example, other physicians, pharmaceutical representatives, salespeople, family members, friends, and former patients).

KEY TERMS

Appointment management	A systematic method of using the time available to the best possible advantage.
Medical emergency	A state or condition that could result in the loss of the patient's life if not treated.
No-show	A failure to keep an appointment without notification to the office.
Receptionist	The person responsible for initially greeting visitors in an office or facility.
Scheduling system	A preplanned method of dividing available time to provide services efficiently to the greatest possible number of patients.

*M*anaging the appointment scheduling system for the patients in your office or facility is one of the most important responsibilities you will have as an administrative medical assistant (Figure 7.1). Properly managed, the scheduling systems will control the time available in each working day and allow each member of the health care team to plan for patient care. The efficiency of a scheduling system depends on the ability of the person who develops and manages it and the cooperation of the health care team and patients.

Appointment Scheduling Systems

There are three basic types of appointment systems: open office hours, scheduled appointments, and flex hours. Regardless of the system chosen for an office or facility, the method should be used consistently and meet the needs of the patients, physician, and staff. Choosing a system requires evaluation of the

FIGURE 7.1

Managing the appointment scheduling system for patients is one of the most important responsibilities you will have as an administrative medical assistant.

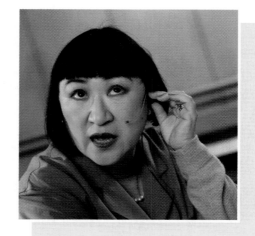

type of practice, the preference of the physician-owner, the number of patients seen, and the available facilities.

Open Office Hours

The least structured and least commonly used method of scheduling patients is the open-hours system. Drop-in or walk-in clinics fall into this category. Patients are advised that the office is open during a certain block of time, such as from noon to 4:00 PM, and they may come in anytime between those hours. Patients know in advance that they will have to wait varying lengths of time before seeing the physician. Although this method may at first seem less stressful than making appointments, it prevents planning for the various duties associated with a practice. You may be faced with the problem of several patients arriving at the same time—possibly at the end of the day. Such unforeseen events can keep you from attending to your regular duties. For the medical office, this is an inefficient method of time management and should be avoided if possible. However, this system is perfectly suited for urgent-care settings.

Scheduled Appointments

Physicians are able to see more patients with less pressure on patients, staff, and themselves when appointments are scheduled. If appointments are made by telephone, the patient's impression of the practice or facility begins with that initial call. Few people, including the physician, rarely appreciate the skill required for proper scheduling of appointments. Many times this task is delegated to the least-qualified medical assistant. Although the skill and attitude of the assistant who manages the appointment desk is very important, the ultimate success of the system lies in the cooperation of the physician(s).

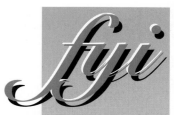

Formula for Effective Appointments

The doctor—who arrives on time and sees patients in a timely manner

+

The patient—who schedules in advance as much as possible, and who is on time for appointments or who calls in advance when an appointment cannot be kept

+

The administrative medical assistant—who schedules the patient to meet with the doctor (the appointment) and looks at the time, length, and necessity of appointment to make these arrangements

PERSPECTIVES ON MEDICAL ASSISTING

The First Appointment Schedules

Early physicians in America only saw patients as the need arose, usually at the patients' homes or the site of an accident. Later, when physicians kept an office first at home and then in a professional office building, they posted hours on the door to inform people when they would be there. People came on a first come–first serve basis. Physicians still only saw patients with problems who needed to see them. There were no "did not keep" appointment problems.

Although some medical offices still have open hours, most physicians use regular scheduled appointments to improve patient waiting time and also to practice preventive medicine (that is, healthy people for examinations and rechecks).

Clinics and urgent-care centers usually are the only offices that use open appointments routinely.

Scheduling appointments appropriately requires an understanding of the following factors:

- The type of practice (pediatrics, family practice, surgery, neurology, cardiology, and so on)
- The physician's personality and habits
- The amount of time needed for each patient

By planning appointments carefully and ensuring to the best of your abilities that the physician starts on time and stays on schedule, you will please the patients, make the practice more successful, and promote a calmer atmosphere for the physician, staff, and patients.

Flex Hours

Most methods of scheduling are relics from the days when the father was the wage earner and the mother stayed at home. Today, both parents usually work. Consequently, many primary care practices (for example, general practitioners, pediatricians, gynecologists) offer extended or flexible office hours. Staff hours must then be staggered to meet the demand. For example, once a week, the office hours might begin at 6:00 AM and end at 3:00 PM; on another day, they might begin at noon and end at 8:00 PM. The remaining days may be scheduled for the traditional hours of 9:00 AM to 5:00 PM. This practice gives the patient numerous options. Flex scheduling is best suited to group practices or partnerships consisting of four or more physicians because more physicians are available for time rotation.

Scheduling Tools

Appointment Books

Appointment books or scheduling systems are the foundation of all practices. The practice has its beginning from the voice on the phone to the availability of the first appointment that can be scheduled. Appointment books and/or scheduling systems are available in many styles. One might consider the traditional appointment book (Figure 7.2) for the new practice. Some basic features should be considered when selecting an appointment book. The book or scheduling system should include space for scheduling at least one calendar year. Most books or systems come with preprinted or preset time slots, usually at 10- to 15-minute intervals. Most appointment books are either spiral bound or loose leaf and will lie flat on the writing surface. Most will fit the desk space available, and will have sufficient space to accommodate the practice's needs. An efficiently designed appointment book should provide space for the date, time, patient's full name, reason for appointment, and telephone number.

At the beginning of each year, the administrative medical assistant should block off those periods when the physician(s) will not be available to see patients. These times include committee meetings, days off, hospital rounds, hospital meetings, and holidays. The administrative medical assistant also should maintain information regarding other family or social commitments.

AT WORK TODAY

The Matrix

The appointment book is the matrix.
Matrix: The basic structure from which something develops

Before appointments can be made, it must be established when the doctor will be available. Most offices mark off the periods when there will be no doctor by using X's or slanted lines (see the example below).

A brief statement explaining why the doctor will not be available also should be recorded in the appointment book. Also, some doctors like to use the book to remind them of their personal obligations after hours. Examples of these statements include "Hospital rounds," "Surgery," "Days (or hours) off," "Meeting," "Vacation," or "Holiday."

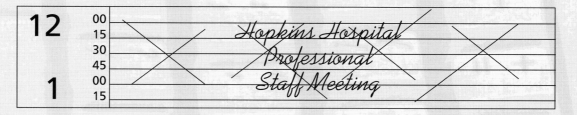

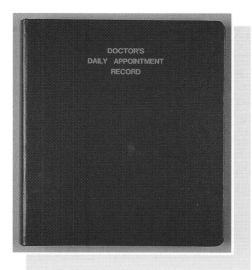

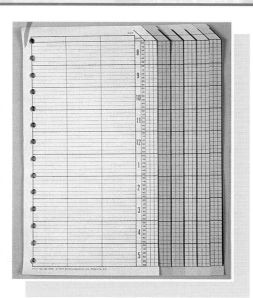

A

B

FIGURE 7.2

A, Cover of a traditional appointment book. B, Preprinted appointment-setting grid typically found in a traditional appointment book.

Although it has long been taught that a pen is the only appropriate writing instrument, many employers realize it can be impractical to use. Although a pen provides a permanent record, using it to record information in the appointment book becomes impractical when schedule changes require crossing out a patient's name to insert another. In recent years the appointment book, although written in pencil, has remained a legal document. The appointment book also can be used to verify some information noted in the chart.

If your employer requires you to use ink, one color (either blue or black) should be selected and used consistently in the appointment book. The neatness and consistency of notations in the book lend credibility to the document. Some offices select one alternate color to record the name of a first-time patient. Red is an excellent contrast to the blue or black ink used to record established patients. The alternate color entry will alert the staff at a quick glance whether new patients are to be seen each day. This will help with appointment management, since new patients require extra time for registration, chart preparation, and discussions of office policy.

Computer Appointment Systems

Computer systems allow for a great deal of flexibility. Most systems will allow the practice to set the time frames for physician appointments. Most systems also allow for working days as well as nonworking days and for location of appointment. The majority of the appointment systems will search a physician's schedule to find available appointment times that are acceptable to the patient. The system should allow space for appointment time, patient name, telephone number, reason for the appointment, and any appropriate notes regarding the patient. The schedule then can be printed out daily. This system also may be able to print out a schedule for the complete month. Most systems will show on the screen all appointments scheduled for the day, with overlays for each physician or department. For example, a patient may be scheduled for a consultation, an electrocardiogram (ECG), and a thallium treadmill. If the scheduled physician is delayed at the hospital because of an emergency, this type of system allows for the patient and all additional scheduled services to be moved as a group to the on-call physician. This allows the patient to be seen in a timely fashion, particularly when he or she has come to the office or facility from a significant distance and cannot be reached in time to reschedule with the previously scheduled physician.

Computerized appointment systems usually will allow the user to review the patient's scheduled visits for a selected period, block out meeting times for the physician, and list both primary physician and secondary physician, as well as offer other customized features.

Appointment Cards

The appointment card is an important reminder for patients, since patients have numerous things on their minds by the end of their visit. The appointment cards should be kept in a convenient holder near the appointment book. They will be used each time a patient schedules an appointment while in the office. You also may send an appointment card, along with a patient information pamphlet, to a new (nonemergency) patient who schedules advance appointments or to patients who made advance appointments by telephone.

The standard appointment card is imprinted with the physician's name, address, and telephone number and a line on which to write the patient's name, usually preceded by the letter "M" (Figure 7.3). This allows the person filling out the card to follow the "M" with an "r" or "s" to indicate Mr. or Ms. and

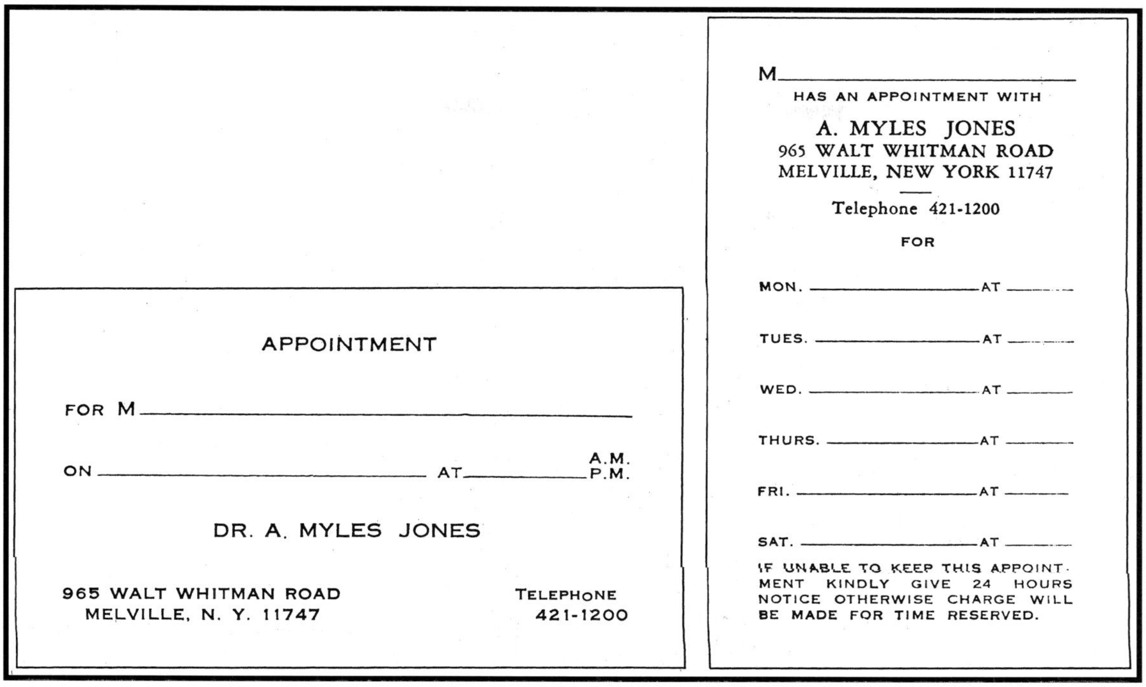

APPOINTMENT

FOR M_____

ON _____ AT_____ A.M.
                                              P.M.

DR. A. MYLES JONES

965 WALT WHITMAN ROAD   TELEPHONE
MELVILLE, N. Y. 11747   421-1200

M_____
HAS AN APPOINTMENT WITH

A. MYLES JONES
965 WALT WHITMAN ROAD
MELVILLE, NEW YORK 11747
—
Telephone 421-1200

FOR

MON. _____AT _____

TUES. _____AT _____

WED. _____AT _____

THURS. _____AT _____

FRI. _____AT _____

SAT. _____AT _____

IF UNABLE TO KEEP THIS APPOINT-
MENT KINDLY GIVE 24 HOURS
NOTICE OTHERWISE CHARGE WILL
BE MADE FOR TIME RESERVED.

FIGURE 7.3

Appointment cards. (From Zakus SM et al, editors: *Mosby's fundamentals of medical assisting: administrative and clinical theory and technique*, ed 2, St. Louis, 1990, Mosby.)

then to insert the patient's name. This may take a few extra seconds of your time, but it personalizes the interaction and indicates to the patient that you see him or her as an individual. Below the line for the name are spaces to enter the day, date, and time of the scheduled appointment. You may choose a card with a preprinted line that states, "If unable to keep appointment, kindly give 24 hours' notice." If the office intends to charge for missed appointments, this must be stated either on the appointment card, in the statement of services, or in the patient information pamphlet.

Some appointment cards are designed to serve a second purpose. The back of the card may serve as a business card or provide a map with the location of the office. A dual business/appointment card may serve a purpose in the office but does not look professional when physicians exchange business cards with colleagues. If the office location requires directions they should be provided in the patient information pamphlet. The patient will not require this information for every visit.

Considerations in Scheduling

The method of scheduling appointments should be individualized for the specialty or practice. One of the most important considerations in determining office hours and appointment times is the specifics of the area served. Is this an agricultural, industrial, or retirement community? Who are the patients? Is it appropriate to utilize flex hours or even Saturday appointments? However, when making an appointment in any practice, you should keep in mind the following considerations:

- The patient's problem and needs
- The physician's habits and preferences
- The available facilities and equipment

Patient Needs

Time must be specifically allotted to the patients with respect given to the patients' particular needs. After asking the patient a few questions, the medical assistant receptionist will be able to ascertain the patient's needs and considerations, which will help in scheduling the appointment.

A medical office or facility exists to fulfill the needs of patients. Because a patient often is under stress in a medical environment, it is important to develop an appointment system that reduces confusion and tension. You should keep in mind that the patients also have schedules that they must keep, and an effective appointment system will provide some flexibility to respond to their needs.

Work or School Schedules

Work or school schedules are important to patients, and patients hesitate to disrupt them unnecessarily. Every attempt should be made to accommodate the patient's schedule. You might be able to schedule these patients for the first or last appointment of the day, so they will be able to limit the time away from their duties.

Travel Time

Some patients will be concerned about appointments if they must travel some distance and wish to avoid commuter times. Older patients traveling by public transportation also may wish to avoid being on the bus or train when schoolchildren or business commuters are using the system. You and the patients will be aware of these commuter periods, and you can schedule appointments nearer midday to avoid them.

Childcare Needs

The potential problems of having children unsupervised in the reception area means you will want to make every effort to accommodate patients who want to work around childcare schedules (Figure 7.4).

Special Needs

When scheduling appointments for patients with disabilities, you must consider their transportation needs and the possible extra time required during the visit to accommodate any mobility difficulties. These patients may have to adapt their schedules to those of the people who assist them in getting to the physician's office. You should be as flexible as possible when scheduling appointments under the circumstances. You also should include in the planned

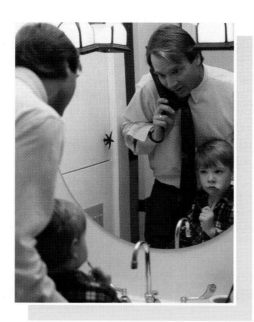

FIGURE 7.4

It is in everyone's best interest to make every effort to accommodate patients who call in trying to work around childcare schedules.

WHAT DO YOU THINK?

Susan has been working with Drs. Fife and Smith for 2 months, and her new job is to handle the appointments and referrals. She has glanced at the appointment book and thinks the job will be easy. Her first experience is to schedule Ms. Flowers for a complete history and physical at 4:00 PM on Friday.

Is this a good scheduling procedure? If not, why not? How much time should be allowed?

Betty is in charge of computer operations in Dr. Liu's office. She takes care of appointment scheduling and electronic insurance billing. The practice is a very busy one, and it includes a nurse practitioner to assist the physician. Betty usually is very efficient,

but she did not back up the work she had done on her computer before going home the previous evening and lost some of her files, including the next week's appointment files.

What should she do to avoid this problem again?

Tom is working at the appointment desk today. Mr. Long came to see the doctor today and, since he is hearing impaired, communication between the doctor and Mr. Long was difficult.

What would you suggest Tom communicate to Mr. Long in writing to prevent this problem from happening again?

appointment any extra time you anticipate needing once the patient arrives at the office. Making the patient aware of the extra planning done for his or her benefit is not necessary; your actions will be recognized and appreciated.

Communication Problems

Occasionally you will encounter patients with special communication problems. Hearing impairment is one type of problem; another may involve non-English–speaking patients. If you or your co-workers are not fluent in the patient's language, you should request that a translator accompany the patient.

Physicians' Habits and Preferences

Developing and implementing an appointment scheduling system will depend on the attitude and preference of the physician. Some physicians like a very orderly workday, and others prefer not to be restricted by the clock. These examples represent extreme perspectives, and reality will fall somewhere in between. In most practices, absolute structure is impossible because you must allow for emergencies. In contrast, complete lack of structure creates long waits and unhappy patients. You should discuss the physician's preferences and evaluate them in relation to the needs of the patients and the staff. The system that you devise will have to consider all of these factors to work effectively.

Some physicians will worry if patients are kept waiting, while others will become upset if the reception area is not packed with waiting patients. These habits and preferences become an important part of appointment scheduling.

Appointment Scheduling Guidelines

One of the elements necessary for efficient management of the appointment system is knowing, in advance if possible, whom you will be seeing each day and for what reasons you will be seeing them. Advance appointment scheduling is ideal, because it also allows you to save some time each day for unexpected events, such as emergency patients or friends of the physician who drop in. Often, one 15- or 30-minute segment in the morning and one in the afternoon provides enough cushion to end the day on time.

Necessary Information from the Patient

In making advance appointments, you need a minimum amount of information from each patient.

Patient's Full Name

The correctly spelled name allows you to locate the patient's chart quickly or label the chart cover, registration form, and account card for new patients in advance.

Daytime Telephone Number

Noting the daytime telephone number in the appointment book or computer file allows for quick reference if you need to change or remind a patient of an appointment.

Reason for the Visit

Determining the reason for the visit will allow you to determine the amount of time to reserve for the visit. There will be times when this is a delicate situation that will require perception, tact, and diplomacy. Patients may hesitate to provide the reason because, for example, they are calling from work and lack privacy. If you suspect this is the situation, simply ask the patient. You then can suggest that he or she calls you from a private telephone during a break. Patients also may hesitate because they are shy or embarrassed about the condition or about speaking to a member of the opposite sex regarding the condition. Your diplomacy and professional manner of speaking usually will relieve the situa-

MEDICAL ASSISTING STEP-BY-STEP

New Patient Appointment Guidelines

1. New patients need to feel comfortable with the office when making their first appointments.
2. You will need to get their full names, daytime phone numbers, and reason for the visit. In addition, you will need the referral source and insurance information.
3. Be sure to explain any office policies that the new patient should know before coming to your office. Tell them how to get to the office (give specific directions and if there is time, mail an office map).
4. Try to give them some idea of how long their visit may take. Many practices devote at least 30 to 45 minutes for the first visit.
5. Ask if there are any questions and, before you end the call, be sure to confirm the time and date of the appointment with them.

tion. You might say, "Mr. Sims, having a general idea of why you wish to see the doctor will allow me to reserve the correct amount of time for you." With this type of statement, you demonstrate consideration of patients and their needs and assure them that you are not pressing for details.

Referral Source

For new patients, the referral source should be noted in the appointment book or computer log, on the medical record information sheet, and possibly on the financial record. If the source was a physician, established patient, or professional group, the physician will want to acknowledge the referral. Also, a referral source may be needed to locate the patient at a future time.

Insurance/Payment Information for New Patients

Information about insurance or financial responsibility should be acquired without implying that obtaining services is based on finances.

Necessary Information for the Patient

When making an appointment for a patient, either in person or over the telephone, you must be sure the patient has the correct information. State the appointment day, date, and time as you note the patient's name in the appointment book or computer listing, and state them again before you complete the call. An appropriate closure to the call might be, "Thank you for calling, Ms. Adams. I will see you on Friday, March 4th at 3:00 PM." This demonstrates courtesy and individualized attention and reconfirms the appointment information. Also, make certain that new patients have directions to your office.

Follow-Up Appointments

At the end of an office visit, the physician will advise patients regarding whether they need a follow-up appointment. If a subsequent appointment is necessary, try to schedule it while the patient is still in the office. This eliminates the patient needing to call back to make the appointment (and possibly forgetting to call) and allows you to give the patient an appointment reminder card.

Scheduling Appointments by Telephone

Patients also may telephone for an advance appointment. After the date and time have been agreed on, you may send the patient a written appointment card and, for new patients, a patient information brochure.

Appointment Management Techniques
Time-Specified

In a time-specified system, each patient is given an appointment for a definite time. This method provides time for advance planning to prepare for the patient's needs. The interval between appointments depends on the type of medical practice and the service to be provided during the visit. A complete physician examination may require 1 $\frac{1}{2}$ hours, whereas a blood pressure recheck will take only a few moments. Therefore the medical assistant responsible for scheduling appointments will need to determine the reason for each visit.

Because time-specified systems also provide structure to each day, this method actually allows physicians to see more patients during office hours without the stress of having a backlog of people in the reception area (Figure 7.5).

A patient visit most commonly includes a preliminary question-and-answer period, a physical evaluation, and a postexamination discussion period between the physician and the patient. Although you never want to interrupt a necessary discussion and you should understand that some social conversation often occurs before the visit ends, you and the physician will recognize that some patients engage in lengthy, unnecessary conversations. Planning can prevent these conversations from interfering with another patient's time. For example, several minutes before the scheduled end of a visit, you might contact the doctor on the intercom and simply mention the time left until the next appointment. The physician then can gracefully direct the conversation toward closure.

FIGURE 7.5

Time-specified systems allow physicians to see more patients during office hours without the stress of having a backlog of people in the reception area.

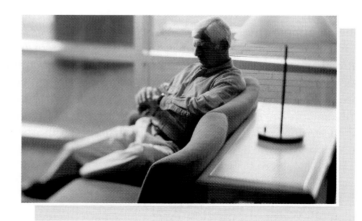

Wave

Some physicians and medical assistants feel that the time-specified system is too structured and prefer a method that provides flexibility. The wave method of scheduling is designed to self-adjust to the unpredictable variances caused by patients. These variances include patients who arrive late, require more or less time than estimated, fail to keep their appointment, or arrive without an appointment.

The wave system is based on the average time spent with each patient on a routine visit. An hour is divided by the average appointment time to determine the number of patients that can be seen in an hour. A certain number of patients are then told to arrive at the beginning of each hour. Patients are seen in the order of their arrival. For example, an office staff may determine that an average visit requires 15 minutes; some will be shorter and some longer. Therefore four patients can be seen each hour. Table 7.1 demonstrates the possible outcome of a 1-hour period when four patients are instructed to arrive at 2:00 PM. Many other outcomes are possible, but in general, you can expect that patient waiting periods will vary while the office remains relatively on schedule. However, you should know that patients eventually become aware that the 2:00 PM appointment is not exclusively theirs. When patients are waiting in the reception area, they speak to one another, and the topic is often the office. Patients soon learn that others also were scheduled for the same time. Explaining the

TABLE 7-1

The Wave Appointment System and the Effects of Double Booking

Patient	Time of arrival	Time required for visit	Time visit begins	Waiting period (from time of arrival)	Time visit ends
1	2:00	15 min	2:00	0 min	2:15
2	2:00	25 min	2:15	15 min	2:40
3	2:05	15 min	2:40	35 min	2:55
4	2:25	10 min	2:55	35 min	3:05

Patient	Appointment time	Time required for visit	Time visit should be finished if on time	Patient's time waiting	Time visit finished	Cumulative time office is "behind schedule"
1	2:00	15	2:15	0 min	2:15	0 min
2	2:00	15	2:15	15 min	2:30	15 min
3	2:15	20	2:30	15 min	2:50	20 min
4	2:15	10	2:30	35 min	3:00	30 min
5	2:30	15	2:45	30 min	3:15	30 min
6	2:30	10	2:45	45 min	3:25	40 min

From Zakus SM et al, editors: *Mosby's fundamentals of medical assisting: administrative and clinical theory and technique,* ed 2, St. Louis, 1990, Mosby.

reason that four people were scheduled for one time is difficult without causing the patients to feel manipulated.

Modified Wave

A modified wave system is similar to the wave system in that an hour is the basic block of time. The modification involves prespacing the arrival times of the patients planned for a given hour. Using the previous example, you may schedule two patients for 2:00 PM and two for 2:30 PM, or you might schedule the four patients at 10-minute intervals between 2:00 and 2:30 PM, reserving the second half of the hour to complete the visits. The modified wave technique will reduce the possibility of having to answer questions from patients concerned about the scheduling system, but this system may still result in varying waiting periods.

Double Booking

Double booking actually is a form of wave scheduling and occurs when two patients, both requiring the physician's attention for the total appointment slot, are scheduled for the same time. Consider an office that schedules patients at 15-minute intervals and also double books. Table 7.1 demonstrates the waiting periods that can occur for patients and the cumulative time the office will be off schedule with double booking. As in the wave system, patients may compare scheduling and feel manipulated.

In general, you can see that open office hours, the wave system, the modified wave system, and double booking result in waiting time for patients. More often than not, these methods will put an office behind schedule rather than on schedule. Time-specific systems are the most efficient if they are respected and provide time for unplanned events.

Grouping Procedures

Booking similar examinations or procedures within specific blocks of time is another method of appointment management. For example, a pediatrician might decide to reserve three mornings a week and divide them into 1-hour appointment intervals during August to accommodate demands for preschool physicals. A cardiologist might schedule patients requiring diet counseling in one afternoon so that the nutritionist can assist several individuals in one day. Grouping may be in response to an anticipated special situation or may be a routine occurrence. You may need to test a grouping system several different ways until you find an acceptable schedule.

Types of Appointments

When developing an appointment system for the office, you need to consider the needs of the patients, the preferences of the physician, and the personnel, facilities, and equipment available. You also will need to plan for advance scheduling and scheduling exceptions, including emergencies, patients in acute need, and other potential disruptions.

MEDICAL ASSISTING STEP-BY-STEP

Compare Regular Appointments and Wave System

Regular System

Advantages

1. Each patient has a definite appointment time.
2. The time allotted is planned for the patient's need.
3. This method allows for the physician to see more patients more efficiently.

Disadvantages

1. Some patients take too much time, which puts the schedule out of balance.
2. When the physician is delayed starting the schedule, the entire day's schedule is delayed.

Wave System

Advantages

1. Because 2 to 3 patients may be scheduled at the same time, usually a patient is waiting, although one patient may be late and the other early.
2. It provides more flexibility because it accounts for no-shows and people without appointments.

Disadvantages

1. When all of the patients arrive at the same time and become aware that they all have the same appointment time, they might become frustrated.
2. When the schedule fails, the patients have to wait longer.

Routine Appointments

Staff members can plan on most patients being scheduled for appointments that are considered routine. Routine visits will vary depending on the type of practice and the specialty of the physician. In general, routine visits require a limited time period (15 to 20 minutes), necessitate only basic equipment, and are easily handled by the administrative medical assistant. The staff can anticipate a predictable transition between routine visits.

Specialized Services

Some offices or facilities offer specialized services or counseling that requires individuals with training in the specialty. Often the specialty personnel are not full-time members of the staff but come to the office on a limited schedule or on an on-call basis (Figure 7.6). If they are in the office on a limited schedule, you will need to incorporate some grouping techniques in the appointment

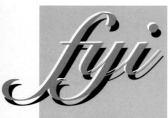

FIGURE 7.6

Specialty personnel, such as this physical therapist, usually come to the office on request or on a limited schedule to see specific patients.

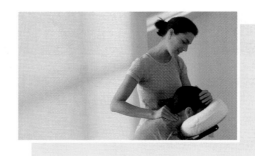

Advance Scheduling

Preplanned advance appointments can and should be scheduled for routine follow-up visits, physical examinations, and special diagnostic or treatment procedures. The advance planning is to the patient's advantage, because the appropriate amount of time can be reserved to avoid a rushed atmosphere. Occasionally, patients will request an appointment on the day they call. You should inquire about the reason for the appointment before making a firm statement about the need for advance planning to fulfill their request. You may be misunderstanding the patient's terminology. Consider the following example. A patient requests a same-day appointment, stating that he needs a physical examination. You take the patient literally and explain that physical examinations must be scheduled at least 2 weeks in advance. The easily intimidated patient does not disagree but instead accepts your restriction even though he is in need of care on the day of the call. In reality, the patient was trying to request an appointment to the physician to examine him for a painful physical problem.

system so the specialty therapist and the patients who need the service are in the office at the same time. On-call personnel will come to the office on request to see a specific patient. However, even these visits must be preplanned. The term *on-call* does not imply immediate availability in all situations; it implies "as needed." Some of the specialty personnel you may be planning for your office schedule include:

- ECG (electrocardiogram) technician
- EEG (electroencephalogram) technician
- Nutritionist
- Occupational therapist
- Physical therapist
- Respiratory therapist

In managing a scheduling system that involves specialty personnel, you will need to keep in mind that you must coordinate time for both the provider and the patient. The additional temporary staff person also may require your attention to assist him or her regarding the necessary facilities and equipment to provide the services.

Scheduling by Exception

Scheduling by exception refers to unplanned situations that require an immediate appointment. These situations can include emergency patients, acute-need patients, and physician referrals.

Emergency Patients

Criteria. Determining what constitutes an emergency in relation to the classification of incoming telephone calls is discussed in Chapter 6. Briefly, emergencies are serious situations in which the patient may have a temporary or continued loss of consciousness, heavy bleeding, severe pain, severe vomiting or diarrhea, or fever.

Screening. An experienced administrative medical assistant will be able to determine an emergency call and proceed as necessary. If there is any doubt about the situation, the physician or other supervisory medical staff, if readily available, should be given the call to make a decision. If the physician is out of the office, he or she should be contacted immediately for instructions. When in doubt, it is better to treat the situation as an emergency than underestimate its severity.

Scheduling Emergency Patients. Many emergencies are first evaluated in the medical office or facility. Emergency patients have priority in scheduling and, on arrival at the office, are seen before previously scheduled and waiting patients. The situation may be obvious to the patients who are waiting, but you should briefly explain to them that it is an emergency and they will be seen as soon as possible.

Acute-Need Patients

Criteria and Screening. Patients in acute need of care should be seen on the same day that they call. Acute conditions include infections, moderately elevated temperature, newly discovered masses (such as a breast lump), or moderate pain of recent onset. Some symptoms, such as slight vaginal bleeding, may seem acute to the patient when actually they may not be. However, you cannot disregard the patient's anxiety and need for reassurance.

Scheduling Acute-Need Patients. Patients in acute need should be given the first possible appointment on the day that they call. If all appointment times are filled, you will have to resort to double booking. Patients should be advised of the scheduling situation and made to understand that they may have a limited wait when they arrive. They should be reassured that they will be cared for as soon as possible.

Referrals

Physicians frequently refer patients to one another for specialized care or consultation. The referring physician's medical assistant might make the appointment for the patient, or the patient may be given the new physician's name and telephone number to make his or her own appointment. Because referring physicians are a valuable source of patients for a practice, every effort must be made to accommodate the patient as quickly as possible.

Your responsibilities will include assisting patients who are referred from your office to another office or facility for consultation, diagnostic studies, or hospitalization. Patients feel protected in their own physician's care and will feel somewhat insecure when referral is necessary. They will ask questions such as, "What is the other doctor like?" "Will the procedure hurt?" and "Will the treatment work?" You should be able to reassure patients requiring referral as well as assist with the arrangements.

You must be careful, however, that your reassurance is based on accurate information. When patients ask what the other physician is like, they are asking for a comparison with their primary physician. You should be discreet and nonjudgmental and focus on the patient's benefit. You might say, "Dr. Smith is less talkative than Dr. Adams but just as conscientious." If you know a procedure is painful say, "Yes, there is some discomfort involved, but the procedure is important and the staff will help you stay as comfortable as possible." Patients will appreciate your honesty, and it builds their trust in you. You must be extremely careful with questions about the outcome of treatment. Patients with questions seeking a promise of cure should be redirected to the physician. You might respond with a question such as, "Did Dr. Adams talk with you about the treatment? If you still have questions, the doctor will be glad to speak to you again before you leave." Various types of referrals involve certain scheduling responsibilities and options.

Scheduling Physician Consultations

Patient Schedules Appointment. Patients who wish to schedule their own appointment with the consultant should be given, in writing, the name, address, and telephone number of the consulting physician. A preprinted patient referral slip can be given to the patient with this information and other data the consultant might desire. You also can give the name of the administrative assistant in the consultant's office, if you know it. This helps the patient feel that the transition is more personal. You might also place a brief call to the consultant's office so that the patient's call will be expected. With managed care, if your physician is the primary care physician you may need to provide a written referral slip (Figure 7.7).

Assistant Schedules Appointment. If you make the appointment for the patient, you may be able to expedite the process and reduce the patient's stress. The medical assistant in the consultant's office might be persuaded to supply an earlier appointment when speaking to another medical assistant rather than the patient. Showing preference to a medical assistant over a patient is not appropriate behavior, but it can exist. Rather than reacting negatively, remember that the patient's well-being is the important issue. You should develop and maintain rapport with the other office personnel, because it will be to your patient's benefit. Once the appointment is scheduled, you can note the information on a patient referral slip.

Physician Schedules Appointment. Occasionally the patient may need to be seen by the consultant as soon as possible, perhaps even the same day. If the medical assistant is unsuccessful in obtaining an appointment, another approach may be necessary. This option involves the referring physician speaking directly with the consulting physician, and it should be reserved for special situations. The referring physician usually is very effective in acquiring the necessary patient service.

Diagnostic Studies (Outpatient)

Appointment Scheduling. Diagnostic studies frequently are scheduled for patients at other offices or facilities. You usually will be responsible for scheduling these studies because of the medical terminology involved.

Scheduling Information. When calling an office to schedule a diagnostic study, you should first identify yourself and the physician's office you represent and state the name of the study you would like to schedule. The diagnostic office assistant may need to retrieve a special appointment schedule. Next, you will need to supply certain information that you have gathered before placing the call, including the following information about the patient:

- Name
- Age or date of birth
- Insurance carrier
- Suspected diagnosis or reason for study

The patient will need a referral slip. You may keep blank slips on hand (see Figure 7.7), or the diagnostic office may provide you with preprinted forms with their name, address, and telephone number. You fill in the date and time of the appointment and the study to be performed.

Patient Instructions. Many diagnostic studies require preparations of the patient in advance of the examination. Preparations might include a special

MARIN IPA

REFERRAL REQUEST
For HPR Member

Referral
Number **607242**

125 East Sir Francis Drake Blvd. Suite 400 Larkspur, Ca 94939

TEL (415) 925-6555   FAX (415) 925-6560

Patient's Name (Last)	(First)	(M. Intial)
1 40410		

Address

I.D.#	Date of Birth	Telephone No.
		--

Referring PCP Name (Print)	Telephone No.
2	

Specialists/Facility Name	Telephone No.
3	

Address

Reason for Referral   **PAINFUL BUNIONS**

5 PRE-AUTHORIZATION REQUEST

MANDATORY PRIOR TO ALL SERVICES LISTED BELOW

☐ OUT OF PLAN (NON MARIN IPA) PROVIDER
☐ PHYSICAL/OCCUPATIONAL/SPEECH THERAPY
☐ PSYCHOTHERAPY/PSYCHIATRY/MENTAL HEALTH
☐ COST OF SERVICE EXCEEDS $450.00
☐ MRI/CT
☐ BENEFIT REVIEW REQUESTED
☐ RETROACTIVE REFERRAL
☐ EXTENDED SERVICE (exceeds 3 mo.)
    NOTIFICATION OF APPROVAL/DENIAL SENT TO
    PATIENT AND REFERRING M.D.
☐ INFERTILITY STUDIES / TREATMENT
☐ WORKERS COMPENSATION
☐ THIRD PARTY LIABILITY (IE: MVA) Date of Injury
☐ OTHER:

HEALTH PLAN USE ONLY

☒ Approved   ☐ Denied   01/22/97
☐ Urgent / Verbal Approval
PCP AUTH'D

Number of Visits Requested	☐ Single/Consult Only	☒ 2

Single Visit Expires 45 Days After Issue Date.
Multiple Visits Expire 90 Days After Issue Date.

4 **If Pre-Authorization Required-Complete Section 5 And Submit
Entire Form To Marin IPA.**
If Pre-Authorization Is Not Required-Retain Yellow Copy For
PCP Records. Patient Carries All Other Copies To Specialist.

DR. HUNTER/ CFR 132254/ MFC	01/22/97		
SIGNATURE - REFERRING PHYSICIAN / PCP	DATE	SIGNATURE - MEDICAL DIRECTOR	DATE

**REFERRAL TO NON MARIN IPA PROVIDER VALID ONLY IF PRE-AUTHORIZED (Section 5).
ALL ANCILLARY SERVICES MUST BE PRE-AUTHORIZED (Section 5).
SPECIALISTS REPORT, DIAGNOSIS and TREATMENT (must complete and return to Marin IPA)**

SEE BELOW

VISIT REQUEST BY SPECIALIST	REASON FOR EXTENSION:
☐ 1 ADDITIONAL VISIT REQUESTED	3/5/97 AUTH 2 ADD'L VISITS FOR CASTING & ORTHOTICS./PC URC.
More than 1 additional visit requested:	4-22-97 REQ 2 ADDTL VISITS./JHM URC
☐ 2 ☐ 3 ☐ 4 ☐ 5 ☐ 6	4/24/97 AUTH 2 ADD'L VISITS./PC UR COORDINATOR.
More than 6 additional visits requested:	
specify number of visits:	
Date requested:	

SIGNATURE OF SPECIALIST	DATE

**NON MARIN IPA PHYSICIAN EXTENSION
VALID ONLY IF PRE-AUTHORIZED BY
MEDICAL DIRECTOR.**

MEDICAL DIRECTOR	DATE

A COPY OF THIS REFERRAL MUST ACCOMPANY ALL BILLINGS
This authorization certifies medical necessity only. This guarantees payment only if the member proves to be eligible at the time services were rendered.

Specialist   Patient   IPA   Attending

48 MFC

FIGURE 7.7

Referral request. (Courtesy Marin IPA, Larkspur, Calif.)

diet, fasting, or medication. Most diagnostic offices will provide you with preprinted forms that you can give to and review with the patient. If the diagnostic office is in your building or nearby, the patient can be directed to stop at the office for instructions and, if needed, preparatory substances. The latter option will save you time and provide an opportunity for the patient to meet the diagnostic office assistant.

Hospitalization

Elective and Emergency Admissions. *Elective hospitalization* refers to an admission process that is preplanned and may be necessary for certain diagnostic studies, treatment, or surgery. An emergency admission is based on the criteria discussed in scheduling emergency office appointments. Either you or the physician will schedule an emergency admission. If the patient is first examined in the office, you generally will make the hospital arrangements. As in any scheduling situation, certain information must be available before the call is placed, and you must be prepared to supply information to the patient.

Information Needed by the Admissions Office. The admissions office personnel often will be your first contact with the hospital. The information needed to schedule a hospital admission usually includes the following:

- Admitting physician's name and the names of any other physicians involved in the patient's care
- Patient's name and date of birth
- Admitting diagnosis
- Patient's Social Security number
- Patient's insurance carrier
- Subscriber's ID number for insurance
- Room preference, such as private, semiprivate, smoking, nonsmoking
- Prior admission and date of last admission
- Possible prior authorization requirement
- Insurance carrier's telephone number

The patient's medical record should provide you with all of the necessary information.

Surgical Cases. When a patient is being admitted for elective surgical treatment, you will need to contact the operating room secretary first. You cannot determine the date of admission before you know the date that the surgery can be scheduled. In some instances, the patient can be admitted to the hospital the morning of the surgery; in other cases, the patient is admitted the day before the surgery. The operating room secretary will need to have the following information:

- Surgeon's name
- Procedure planned
- Time the procedure is expected to take
- Anesthesia requested
- Name of assistant surgeon for major cases
- Patient's name, age, and sex

Once the surgery is scheduled, you may call the admissions office. However, in an emergency situation, the patient is admitted first, and the operation is scheduled as soon as possible. Operating rooms are prepared to handle emergency cases 24 hours a day.

Instructions to Patients. Patients to be admitted to the hospital are naturally anxious and will need your help during the process. Your calm and organized manner will reassure the patient. First you should provide the patient with written or preprinted referral slips (see Figure 7.7), which should include the following information about the hospital:

- Name
- Address
- Telephone number
- Check-in time

Patients also will ask you questions regarding various hospital policies. It will be helpful if you familiarize yourself with some basic information about the hospitals frequently used in your practice. You can anticipate inquiries about billing, insurance deductibles, prepayments needed for the uninsured, and visiting hours.

Patients may need to be advised about what they should bring with them to the hospital. Few items actually are needed. These include robe, slippers, personal hygiene items, and some diversionary materials (for example, books and writing materials). If the patient is scheduled for surgery, you should be prepared to tell them that before admission, certain routine procedures may be performed, including the following:

- Chest x-ray
- Laboratory tests
- ECG
- Visit from the anesthesiologist
- Special skin preparations

If the patient knows that these procedures are routine, anxiety can be greatly reduced. In all referral procedures the importance of communication cannot be overstressed. Taking time to explain an activity to patients will make them feel more comfortable and make the process smoother for everyone.

Disruption of the Appointment System

A schedule can be disrupted for various reasons, and you must be prepared to adapt to unplanned events. The common causes of scheduling disruptions are as follows:

- Patient failure to keep appointments
- Patient cancellations
- Delayed arrival of the physician
- Physician absence as a result of an emergency

Each disruption requires different handling, but all have two things in common: the disruption should be kept to a minimum and the patient's needs and comfort should be foremost in your mind.

Patient Failure to Keep Appointments

Should a patient fail to keep an appointment or cancel an appointment with or without rescheduling, this information must be noted in the appointment book. In either of these situations, a single line should be drawn through the name and the reason for the cancellation noted. The single line indicates the appointment was not kept, and the name can still be read and verified. You might note N/S (for no-show) or F/S (failed to show) for the patient who does not arrive. "C" or "canc" should be noted after the name of an individual who cancels an appointment. If an appointment is cancelled, you also should note the date of the new appointment if one is made or note "w/c" (will call) if the patient states he or she will reschedule at another time.

Without Notification

Handling Technique.   Occasionally, patients will fail to keep an appointment without notifying the office. This patient action is termed *no-show.* Anyone can inadvertently miss an appointment. If you contact the patient or the patient calls the office, you should be courteous and understanding and schedule another appointment. If the situation occurs repeatedly, you will have to explain diplomatically the problems that result. It may be effective to explain that when you do not know that the reserved time will be free, you cannot offer the time to another patient. When repeated failure to keep appointments interferes with proper care of a patient, the physician may choose to dismiss him or her. Be aware of the legal implications of dismissing a patient (see Chapter 4).

Recording.   Any failure to keep an appointment without notification should be recorded in the appointment book and in the patient's chart. Each document verifies the other.

With Notification

Rescheduling.   When a patient cancels an appointment, you should attempt to reschedule it during the same telephone call. This will allow you to maintain continuity of care for the patient and maintain your scheduling system. Rescheduling at the time of the cancellation gives you immediate access to the time required and the reason for the appointment. This will reduce the time spent on the call.

Notations.   Cancelled appointments should be noted in the appointment book and the patient's chart along with the date of the rescheduled appointment. These notations help you in documenting a patient's cooperation or lack of cooperation in participating in his or her own care.

Use of Time.   If the appointment is cancelled with sufficient notice, the appointment time can be offered to another patient. If it is a late cancellation, the time may serve as a buffer against unplanned patient appointments or used to accomplish other duties.

Delayed Arrival of the Physician

Reasons and Staff Notification

Physicians can be delayed in arriving at the office for various work-related reasons. An operation may begin and end late because of scheduling difficulties at the hospital, the physician may remain with an emergency patient until an ambulance arrives, or a medical society meeting may run overtime. These delays are understandable and relatively infrequent. The important issue is that the physician notify the office staff of the delay as soon as it is evident and estimate the time of arrival so that the staff can make adjustments. You may have to remind the physician occasionally of the importance of staff notification.

Notifying Patients

Given a valid reason for the delay, patients usually respond with understanding, especially if it is not a common occurrence. They realize that the situation was beyond your control.

You will need first to explain the situation to the patients who have already arrived. Some medical assistants find this an uncomfortable duty. Remember that patients respond well to a frank explanation; it is highly preferable to sitting in the reception area guessing at the cause of the delay. Your next step is to attempt to reach patients by telephone in the order that they are scheduled to arrive at the office. Patients in transit to the office will have to receive an explanation of the situation when they arrive. The remaining patients can be notified at home or work before leaving for the appointment. Each patient should be offered the option of either waiting for the physician to arrive or rescheduling the appointment. Because of your experience, you will be able to help the patient decide. In any case, patients should be aware that the remainder of the day is likely to run behind schedule.

Physicians also may be delayed in arriving at the office because of personal delays or habitual lateness. As previously suggested, you may be able to schedule patients who may see other members of the clinical staff for early-morning appointments.

It also may be possible at staff meetings to include a training program for the physician and staff in discussions about the appointment system (Figure 7.8). Rather than pointing out the physician's part in disrupting the schedules, the subject can be introduced as an office problem and suggestions for remedies requested. You might state during a staff meeting, "We seem to be getting further and further behind schedule each day. Can we discuss what we can do to remedy the situation, either by changing our habits or by altering the system?" Such an introduction to the subject is diplomatic and nonaccusatory and allows each staff member to make suggestions.

If you identify a specific problem that you are unable to correct with behavior modification, your alternative is to adjust the system. For example, if patient-care hours begin at 1:00 PM and the physician routinely arrives between 1:15 and 1:25, you could schedule the first patient for 1:30 PM. You also may encounter a patient who is chronically late. The ideal option would be to explain the importance of arriving on time (provided your office functions on schedule) and securing the patient's cooperation. If this approach does not alter the behavior, you will simply have to accept it and adjust. Perhaps the late patient can be scheduled next to a patient who typically arrives early. In effect

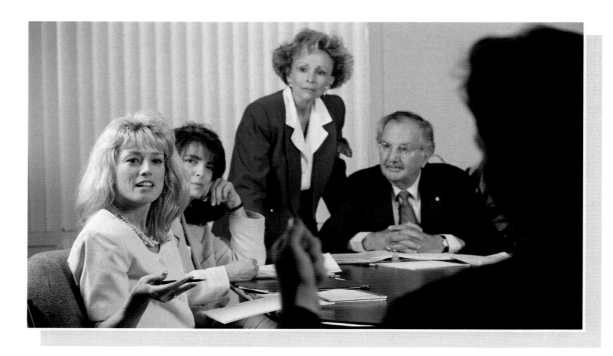

FIGURE 7.8

It may be possible, at staff meetings, to train the physician and staff in using the appointment system.

WHAT DO YOU THINK?

A physician's arrival at the office may be delayed for many reasons. The fact remains, however, that patients and their medical problems cannot be cared for without the physician.

Ideally the physician will notify you if he or she will be delayed and give you an anticipated time of arrival. You then will need to explain the delay to waiting patients and also try to reach patients who may still be at home or work regarding whether they want to wait or change their appointment.

Because it is crucial for the physician to see patients, what do you do and say if he or she is habitually late, regularly causing delays in the schedule? Do you invent reasons as to why the physician is late? Should you insist on a meeting to discuss this with the physician? Can you make some suggestions as to what might help the situation?

the patients cans switch their appointments for you, and your schedule can continue uninterrupted.

Physician Called Away from the Office

Physicians can be called out of the office after office hours have begun. This might be for a medical emergency or perhaps to deliver a baby. Whatever the reason, it will disrupt the office schedule. The same procedure is followed in this situation as when the physician is delayed in arriving at the office.

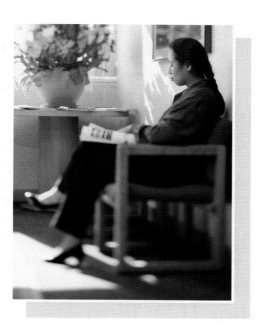

FIGURE 7.9

The most common complaint of patients surveyed about medical care is the time spent in the office reception area.

Importance of Effective Appointment Management

Patients' Most Frequent Complaint

The most common complaint of patients surveyed about medical care is the time spent in the office reception area (Figure 7.9). Most patients make every effort to arrive on time or even early for a scheduled appointment. Unfortunately, some patients have experienced waiting periods as long as an hour before being taken to the treatment area, where they have another wait before seeing the doctor.

You should not be surprised if the result of this waiting is angry patients, and it is not uncommon for patients to express their anger to the medical assistant rather than to the physician. If the delay is unusual, keeping patients informed about the reason for the delay and the anticipated time involved usually will offset the anger. If delays are common, you will need to reevaluate the system and observe the staff members' effects on the efficiency of the system.

Acceptable Wait

Surveys and evaluation of patient questionnaires both show that the maximum acceptable wait in an office before seeing the physician is 20 minutes. Most people recognize that the nature of the business requires some flexibility on the part of everyone involved. However, patients who notice a constant pattern of lengthy waits might ignore the appointment time they are given and arrive at their convenience. They also might begin calling the office in advance to check on the schedule or waiting time, creating more telephone calls for you to answer. The final step a patient might take because of repeated scheduling difficulties is to change physicians.

Stress Reduction

Effective appointment management reduces stress for patients and the health care team. Patients always feel more comfortable when they know what to expect and when to expect it. The comfortable patient is a cooperative patient. Reduced stress in the medical environment means less time dealing with the stressful situation and more time available for patient care. The stress of a disorderly appointment system also influences the health care team and is disruptive to the working relationships among the staff and the physician. Eliminating staff tension will have a good effect on patients and on staff relationships and will enhance a pleasant working environment.

Visitors Other Than Patients

From time to time you can expect visitors other than patients to arrive at the office requesting to see the physician. Predetermined office policy will dictate the manner in which each visitor will be handled. Protocol for certain types of visitors follows.

Physicians

When another physician arrives at the office, the visitor should be announced and escorted immediately to the physician's private office. If the physician is in an examining room with a patient, the visitor should be seated in the private office. The physician in the treatment room should be notified of the guest's arrival. The physician either will leave the treatment room to speak with the visitor or tell you how soon he or she can see the visitor. You then can tell the visitor the waiting period.

Pharmaceutical Representatives

Representatives from pharmaceutical companies are frequent visitors to medical offices and facilities. Many will simply drop in; some will call in advance to see what the best time is to see the physician. Physicians usually have an established policy about seeing pharmaceutical representatives. Some never see them; if this is the case, you must politely inform the representatives of the policy. Physicians who see pharmaceutical representatives usually prefer to limit the visit to a brief call, perhaps 5 minutes. The representatives are aware of this and will respond to your cue. The well-run office will recognize the need for the physician to know and understand about new medications. In many offices, the physician and staff will set aside perhaps one lunch hour per month to see pharmaceutical representatives. Usually the pharmaceutical representative will provide the lunch and have it delivered to the office. Because the "reps" want to be able to call again, they will respect this opportunity and respect the office policy.

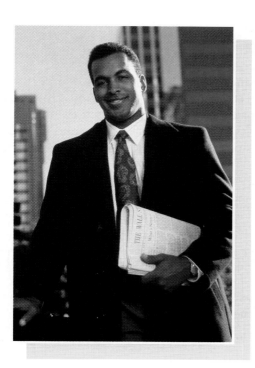

FIGURE **7.10**

Sales representatives are seen by the person responsible for routine purchases, but they must be screened by you before approaching the physician.

Sales Representatives

Sales representatives can be seen by the person responsible for routine purchases. Major purchases usually are decided by the physician, but the representative usually is greeted by the medical assistant, who will gather the basic information to be passed on to the physician. Your responsibility at this point is to know that the representative must be screened by you before approaching the physician (Figure 7.10).

Family Members and Friends

Although physicians often discourage the habit of family or friends dropping into their office, it still will occur occasionally. When it does, the person should be greeted politely and the physician notified. If the physician's office is available, the caller may be seated there to wait for the physician.

Former Patients

It is a source of pleasure to a physician when a former patient drops in to say hello and share some news. The visitor usually is very aware of the physician's schedule and does not wish to interrupt. This former patient should be asked to wait in the reception area while you check to see if the physician is available. If at all possible, the physician usually will try to see the visitor. If it is impossible to interrupt the physician or if the physician is away from the office, the visitor will understand. You should tell the visitor that you will make certain that the physician knows of the visit, and you should offer to take a message.

Conclusion

The administrative medical assistant is the pivotal person in developing and maintaining an effective appointment system. This administrative system involves planning for expected and unexpected events and, most importantly, tactfully dealing with many people in the office and in outside facilities. Managing appointment systems is a challenging and rewarding experience.

Review QUESTIONS

1. At the most, how long should a patient have to wait in the reception area before seeing the physician?

2. What are your responsibilities to the waiting patient?

3. What should appointment management accomplish?

4. What callers can you expect to a medical office, and how should they be handled?

5. What role does the administrative medical assistant play in a caller's first impression of the medical office?

6. What are the administrative medical assistant's responsibilities in creating a good first impression?

7. Describe the basic equipment for the appointment system and for scheduling referral appointments for patients needing consultation with another physician, diagnostic studies, or hospitalization.

8. Describe the methods of handling visitors other than patients to the medical office, including other physicians, pharmaceutical representatives, sales representatives, family or friends, and former patients.

S U G G E S T E D   R E A D I N G S

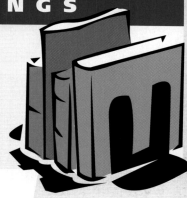

American Medical Association: *The business side of medical practice,* Chicago, 1989, The
    Association.
American Medical Association: *Winning ways with patients,* Chicago, 1981, The Association.
Medical office management institute, Atlanta, 1991, Conomikes Associates, Inc.

Correspondence and Mail Management

OUTLINE

OBJECTIVES

On completion of Chapter 8 the administrative medical assistant student should be able to:

1 Define the key terms listed in this chapter.

2 Discuss the importance of written communication.

3 List and describe the equipment necessary to produce outgoing correspondence.

4 Discuss four basic communication skills.

5 List and describe the three acceptable styles for letters and the 12 possible parts of a letter.

6 List five Postal Service suggestions for preparing envelopes, and describe the folds used for three different envelopes.

Continued

OBJECTIVES

(continued)

7 Describe the five special services provided by the Postal Service.

8 Contrast the four classes of mail.

9 Discuss the four elements that should be included in office policy regarding incoming mail.

10 Describe the types of incoming mail, the proper sequence for stacking items, and the equipment needed to accomplish the task.

11 Discuss the medical assistant's role in annotating or responding to correspondence.

12 Describe the method of handling incoming mail when the physician is absent from the office.

KEY TERMS

Affidavit A written statement signed, as under oath, to affirm the truth of the document.

Affix To attach.

Annotate To reduce a written communication to a limited explanatory statement.

Bond paper A superior quality paper with a firm surface used for correspondence.

Confidential Private or secret.

Consultation report The decision and plan determined necessary for the care of an individual.

Narrative An account of an observation or event in writing.

Organizational title The official position of an individual within the structure of a business or company.

Proofread To review a written work for errors.

Stationery The paper and envelopes required for correspondence.

Transcription The act or process of converting notes or dictation to a complete, typed form.

*W*ritten communication is the unspoken exchange of ideas between individuals, who in many instances have never met one another. The manner in which you handle communication responsibilities will affect the efficiency of the office. Many aspects of written communication and mail handling will be addressed in this chapter.

Mail Processing Equipment

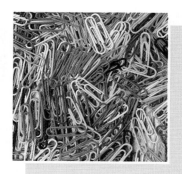

Good equipment for processing mail can save many hours of work. You will need the following equipment: a letter opener, paper clips, date stamp, stapler, postage machine, and weight scale. In larger offices, which receive a great deal of mail daily, you will need an automatic mail opener. These machines may be purchased separately, or the automatic opener may be an additional function of your postage machine. If using a hand opener, you will want a firm and narrow one, with a handle that provides for a good, solid grip and a blade that is sharp enough to slide under the sealing flap of an envelope and separate it without leaving ragged edges. Paper clips, which are used to group pieces of correspondence that arrive in the same envelope, should be clean and have no rough edges.

Some offices use a date stamp to indicate on the item the date and time that it arrived in the office. This will help you evaluate the efficiency of the methods you use in responding to items that require an answer.

A stapler is needed for securing small items enclosed in a letter or similar items that will be stored together, such as a series of laboratory reports made on the same day.

A postage machine (also called a postage meter) for automatic stamping of mail is absolutely necessary when the practice routinely sends large amounts of mail, such as statements, claims, and reports. Most postage machines not only stamp the mail but will also seal the envelopes. These machines save hours of time in hand-processing. You can easily change the amount of postage according to the weight of your letters or class of mail. When using a postage machine, the medical assistant must remember each day to do the procedure described in the box about postage machine techniques.

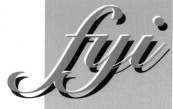

The Postage Meter

Advantages of the postage meter are that it addresses a large amount of mail, the amount of postage needed can be selected easily, and a meter can be selected that also seals the envelopes.

Disadvantages of the postage meter are that it requires daily care, that is, the date must be changed and specific postage amounts set; a weight scale is needed to determine postage amounts; and additional postage must be added or electronically credited by the post office; it will "lock up" when it gets low on postage.

Writing Equipment

The following equipment is necessary for preparing correspondence:

- A word processor or typewriter
- Dictation equipment
- Dictionaries (standard and medical)

Word Processors

A word processor is a computer program that handles various typing and editing functions (Figure 8.1). There are two basic sets of equipment that can

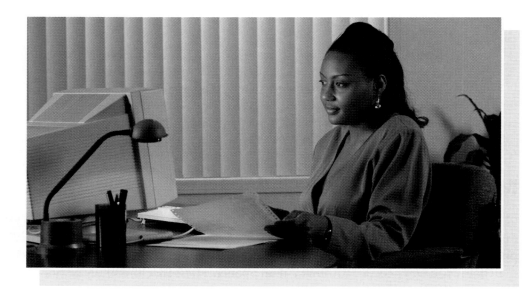

FIGURE   8.1

Computers with word processing programs are fast increasing in offices that generate a large amount of correspondence and reports.

MEDICAL ASSISTING STEP-BY-STEP

Postage Machine Techniques

1. Change the date each day.
2. Check and set the amount of postage on the machine before stamping the envelope.
3. Make certain the postage is imprinted on the upper right-hand corner of the envelope.
4. Deposit mail on the date shown on the envelope.
5. Save all unused or incorrectly stamped envelopes and tapes and apply periodically (usually every 6 months) for a refund from the Post Office. The post office supplies the refund form for you to complete.
6. Stamp or mark envelopes for bulky items before placing data inside, and write "Hand Stamp" in large letters on the front and back of the envelope.

Note: Every practice requires a weight scale to determine the amount of postage required for packages, heavy envelopes, and special classes of mail.

be purchased or leased for word processing functions. One type includes an electronic typewriter and a television-type screen, or monitor. The typewriter allows an operator to enter information into the word processor via a keyboard. The information is stored on a computer disk and displayed on the monitor for you to proofread before printing the permanent copy. When you are satisfied with the material, you can print it out. This type of equipment has the advantage of allowing you to use the typewriter independently or in conjunction with a computer. The other equipment option includes a keyboard that is similar to a typewriter keyboard, a monitor, and a separate printer. This type of word processor functions the same as the other one except that it cannot be used independently for typing.

Computers with word processing programs are fast increasing in popularity, particularly in offices that generate larger amounts of correspondence and reports. Because many reports are redundant, with only minor wording changes, a word processor significantly reduces the amount of typing that is required. The basic letter or report is stored in the computer or on disks and can be displayed on the screen as needed. The variable information can be inserted before printing. After the document has been printed, the variable information can be removed so that the basic format is ready for the next use.

Other advantageous features of word processors include the following:

- Personalization of multiple letters
- Rapid drafting or revision of lengthy documents
- Capacity for adding, deleting, and moving words, phrases, sentences, and paragraphs without retyping the entire page or document
- Automatic realignment of margins
- Automatic alignment of figures, tables, and graphs for statistical reports
- Spell check
- Thesaurus
- Change of fonts

Word processing equipment can be purchased or leased for use in the office or facility. Should the employer not wish to acquire the equipment, word processing services are available, some limited to medical services. These services often return the finished report within 24 hours and guarantee complete confidentiality. Because you may be involved with word processors, either through direct use or through a service, you should familiarize yourself with their basic functions and applications.

Typewriters

The typewriter is another type of basic writing equipment used in preparing correspondence. Your typewriter should be kept in good condition. Many offices have a service maintenance contract that keeps their typewriters in the best working order. Typewriters are available with a variety of styles of type. Many newer typewriters are single-element machines, which means they print using a movable ball or wheel rather than individual characters. This element eliminates the need for a movable carriage, allowing the typewriter to rest in a more compact space. Elements also are available with a dual-pitch option, which allows an easy change from pica to elite type.

Some typewriters have regular keyboards and no built-in correction capabilities; with these you must use white correcting sheets or liquid. Other models have a self-correcting key that uses lift-off tape. Some incorporate a feature called *word spell or spell check,* which allows for the verification of correct spelling. Many typewriters now incorporate a limited amount of memory for letters or reports that are frequently produced with minor changes.

Typewriter or Printer Ribbons

Most modern typewriters use correctable film ribbon that passes through the spool only one time and therefore does not deteriorate gradually. However, if your typewriter or printer uses a cotton or silk ribbon that becomes lighter with use, be sure to change it regularly.

Dictation Equipment

The vast majority of physicians prefer electronic dictating equipment. A large variety of equipment is available. Many physicians use the very small handheld voice-activated recorders that use microcassettes. This allows physicians to carry the microrecorders with them, using them to record patient and hospital information by dictating notes as they move from patient to patient or travel to and from facilities.

Dictionaries (Standard and Medical)

All practices need to have available both standard and medical dictionaries. Although they may not be used regularly, they are certainly helpful to have when needed. Although most word processing programs include dictionaries, they are rarely complete.

Supplies

Office supplies are necessary in every office. Numerous discount office product suppliers are available from which to order supplies. Most vying for your business will offer free delivery for orders totalling more than $50, or they will match another supplier's reduced charge for items if it is called to their attention.

It is important to keep an inventory of supplies and order items regularly.

Stationery

Quality

The stationery selected for formal correspondence should be of high quality that reflects positively on the practice. The quality of paper is measured by grade or weight. The materials used in making paper (wood pulp or cotton fiber) also affect its appearance. Business stationery usually is within the 16- to 24-pound range and contains at least 25% cotton fiber.

Size

Most offices purchase stationery in two sizes. Standard-size letterhead ($8 \frac{1}{2} \times 11$ inches) is the basic stationery for business letters and formal reports, with envelopes matching in size, weight, and fiber content. Brief, informal letters usually are sent on $7 \frac{1}{4} \times 10 \frac{1}{2}$-inch letterhead called *monarch or executive-size stationery,* also with corresponding envelopes. Informal stationery should match the standard-size stationery in weight and fiber.

Embossed vs. Engraved Letterhead

The letterhead can be applied to the stationery in three ways. Engraving impresses each letter and number into the stationery—if you pass your fingertips over the engraved letterhead, it will feel flat. Embossing raises the letters and numbers above the surface—an embossed letterhead will feel "bumpy" to the touch. Embossing is considered more elegant and is more expensive. Printing has become an acceptable alternative to engraving or embossing of letterhead.

Second Sheets and Copies

Lengthy correspondence that requires a second page is continued on a plain sheet that matches the letterhead in quality. A copy of each letter is retained for the office files, and additional copies are sometimes required for other persons interested or involved in the subjects of the correspondence. "Copy sheets" also are available; they are much lighter in weight than the originals, and one margin is marked vertically in red letters with the word *copy.* The use of copy sheets has been greatly reduced in favor of the use of photocopy equipment.

General Processing of Incoming Mail

Each medical office should have an established policy regarding the processing of incoming mail. This should include a statement about who is to process the mail, what may or may not be opened, how mail is routed within the office, and what mail should be left for the physician to open.

Usually the administrative medical assistant is responsible for processing all incoming correspondence. If the assistant is away from the office, a predetermined alternate employee will fulfill the responsibility. The alternate employee should be trained and prepared before he or she is needed.

Opening the Mail

Office policy should be established regarding what mail can and cannot be opened and examined by the medical assistant. Usually items marked "Personal" or "Confidential" are left sealed and opened only by the individual to whom the mail is addressed. The physician may also indicate specific items, such as bank statements or attorney correspondence, that are to remain sealed.

Routing Incoming Mail

Routing mail means separating it by addressee. Once this is accomplished, the items are either paced in a predetermined spot for pickup or delivered to the appropriate person. The larger the office or facility, the more formal the routing system will be.

Physician's Mail

Each physician will have a preference about where the mail should be placed until it can be reviewed. The primary consideration is privacy, and the mail (opened or closed) should be placed out of the line of vision of callers to the office. Most physicians will want the mail placed on their desk.

Sorting Mail

Types of Incoming Mail

Mail usually is sorted and stacked according to class, with special delivery, mailgrams, electronic mail (E-mail), facsimile (fax), and first-class mail on top. Note that E-mail and faxes do not come in the regular mail, and equipment sources for these items may need to be checked periodically during the day. Following this sorting technique, you or the physician will encounter the most important items first. If the mail has been properly sorted and stacked, the items you can expect to see, from top to bottom, will be:

- Telegrams; faxes; express, certified, registered, and priority mail
- E-mail, personal letters, business correspondence from other professionals
- Payments from patients, insurance forms, invoices, letters regarding accounts
- Medical reports, laboratory and x-ray reports
- Professional materials, meeting announcements, medical bulletins
- Medical journals, journal reprints
- Magazines, newspapers
- Pharmaceutical literature or samples
- Advertisements

Mail-Opening Process

The process of opening the mail will be completed more efficiently if there is adequate working space and the necessary equipment close at hand (Figure 8.2).

AT WORK TODAY

Sort the Mail

Mail in a one-doctor medical office is sorted according to the following general categories:

1. Urgent or emergency—telegrams, faxes, express mail
2. Personal/confidential mail—E-mail, personal letters
3. Routine correspondence—patient payments, letters
4. Medical reports—laboratory, x-ray reports
5. Medical journals—research magazines, reprints
6. Miscellaneous magazines, newspapers—for doctor, waiting room
7. Advertisements—pharmaceutical literature, other ads

Annotation

Some physicians prefer that the medical assistant thoroughly review each piece of correspondence, highlighting the key points by underlining them in a highly visible color or briefly summarizing them in the margin. This process is called *annotation,* and it saves the physician a great deal of time. If the correspondence relates to a patient or previous communication, the necessary documents should be retrieved and attached to the current letter.

MEDICAL ASSISTING STEP-BY-STEP

Processing Mail

1. Presort the mail into separate stacks by class (first class, second class, and so on) to determine which pieces of mail you may or may not open.
2. All envelopes to be opened then can be placed face down with the seals pointing in the same direction so that each piece is ready for insertion of the letter opener.
3. After each item has been opened, place it face up for the next step.
4. Set aside mail for other employees in the envelope for routing to the addressee.
5. Remove each item of correspondence for the physician, except for personal mail.
6. Clip the envelope to the correspondence, if the sender's address is not on the correspondence.
7. Review each letter for necessary action and to be sure that indicated enclosures are included.
8. Note missing enclosures on the correspondence, and notify the sender.
9. Stamp and date each item, if this is the office policy, and route.

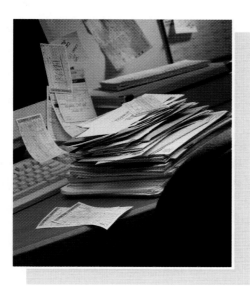

FIGURE 8.2

Every medical office should have an established policy regarding the processing of incoming mail.

Mail Processed by the Administrative Medical Assistant

Beginning early in your career, you will be expected to handle certain items and inquiries that arrive in the mail. These responsibilities may include handling insurance forms and inquiries, payments from patients, and pharmaceutical samples; and ordering supplies. The details of handling these items are discussed in various appropriate chapters.

When the physician is away from the office for meetings or vacations, you will need to adjust your technique of handling the mail. First, you will need to know precisely where the physician is and now to get in touch with him or her. Second, each piece of mail must be evaluated for the urgency of the requested response. The physician will need to be contacted regarding correspondence that cannot await his or her return, unless it is a routine matter that the office staff can handle.

You will handle items that require an immediate response. If the mail includes a notification of a meeting that will take place before the physician's return, you should notify the organization or meeting chairman to obtain an excused absence. Requests for reports, conferences, or records may be deferred, but the requester should be notified that the physician is away and will fulfill the request on his or her return. All mail needing the physician's attention should be stored in a safe and private location until the physician can review it.

Responding to Inquiries

As you gain experience with correspondence, you may be delegated the responsibility of responding to some inquiries without the physician's direction. This too will save time for the physician, and accepting the responsibility will enhance your value to the health care team.

Special Mail Processing

Certain types of incoming mail are to be protected and therefore will need special processing. With the increasing ability to transmit data quickly via mailgrams, E-mail, and fax machines, the administrative medical assistant must be aware of this incoming mail. Many times this mail is urgent or sensitive in nature and must be processed or given to the physician immediately.

Mailgrams

Mailgrams are a special service offered jointly by the U.S. Postal Service and Western Union. Messages charged by 100-word units may be dictated by telephone to Western Union, which transmits them to the destination city for next-day delivery by the postal service.

Electronic Mail

Electronic mail, also called *E-mail,* is the process of sending, receiving, storing, and forwarding messages and data over computer telecommunications equipment. The great advantages to this type of mail are the speed by which it is transmitted and the cost savings. The sender leaves a message in the electronic mail box via a computer, where it remains until the receiver retrieves it. Any message stored can be seen on the screen, then printed or saved to disk. In large offices the E-mail also may be used to send memos throughout the office. Several on-line information services incorporate E-mail within their services. If the E-mail is of a sensitive nature, it should be delivered immediately to the office administrator or physician. Many offices have only one personal computer (PC), and this equipment is used primarily by the receptionist or the only medical assistant in the office.

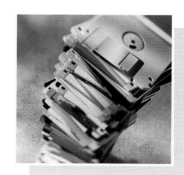

Facsimile (Fax) Communication

Facsimile communication is more commonly termed *fax communication*. It is a wonderful communication tool for sending and receiving information in a fast, reliable, and inexpensive manner. Today physician offices use the machines to transmit medical records, insurance information, laboratory and x-ray reports, prescriptions, and sometimes other very sensitive information. You must protect the patient's confidentiality at all times. If the information that you are going to transmit or receive is sensitive, those faxes should be sent and received only to and from machines located in areas of restricted access. The medical assistant should fax health information only when absolutely necessary, and then usually at the direction of the physician or administrator.

Outgoing Correspondence

Spelling

Correct spelling is vital to the impression transmitted by written communication. If you know you have difficulty with spelling or are occasionally in doubt

WHAT DO YOU THINK?

Two new types of mail are becoming more common so you will need to know how to deal with them.

Electronic mail (E-mail) has become popular with the advance of the computer age. Certain legal problems have arisen with E-mail because it is considered company property. You should be careful what you say in E-mail correspondence and how you say it—do not use words that someone can misinterpret. The advantages of E-mail are that it saves time and can eliminate having to immediately contact a person with the telephone. Messages sent can be stored, brought up on the computer screen, and saved to a disk or printed.

Fax (facsimile) communication has become an important tool for sending and receiving copies over the telephone lines. The copies are instant and inexpensive, and can be used to obtain preautho-

rizations, send prescriptions to the pharmacy, resubmit insurance forms, and send medical information anywhere in the country. The main concern is faxing records, which should only be done when it is critical to save time. Do not fax records to open areas such as mail rooms and lobbies. Have properly completed authorizations from the patients. Check to make sure that documents requiring signatures are legal, if faxed. Because patient confidentiality is an issue, always verify the telephone number and make prior arrangements for the receipt of the fax.

How can you as an administrative medical assistant maintain confidentiality with these methods? Can you prevent someone from reading E-mail on the computer? Can you send signed documents using the term signature on file?

about a word, use the appropriate dictionary. If you are using a word processor, always verify your correspondence through the spell checker. Even if you use spell check, you must proofread your correspondence. Spell check will only verify that the words are spelled correctly; it will not correct inappropriate words. For example, if you have used "he" rather than "the," spell check will not correct your error because "he" is a correctly spelled word. Extreme care should be taken to spell all names correctly. The addressee's title should be verified if you are in doubt.

Punctuation

Standard methods of punctuation should be used throughout all correspondence. If the salutation of the letter is formal, stating the addressee's title or courtesy title (Mr. or Ms.) and last name only, it is followed by a colon. If the salutation is informal, using the addressee's first name, it is followed with a comma.

Transcription

To do transcription, one must have taken courses in medical terminology and use of dictation equipment, and be fully familiar with medical procedures handled within the practice. Skill in transcription is developed primarily through practice and concentration. The quality of transcription may be influenced by the quality of dictation, but experience usually compensates for halting dictation.

Editing and Proofreading

For important communication or communication that is still in the developmental stages, you may want to make a rough draft. This first draft is typed on inexpensive quality paper. A good recycling tip is to save and use the clean side of previously typed or printed items that are to be normally discarded. Form may be ignored, and the draft is double-spaced throughout to allow room for comments or changes. Comments and changes at this stage are referred to as *editing*. Once the draft is acceptable, the material can be prepared in final form. With the use of word processors and computer-based word-processing programs, these type of changes may be made much easier. Therefore the first draft may often appear very close in format to the final correspondence.

Letter Styles

Physician's Preference
The choice of which style to use in office correspondence usually is based on the physician's preference. If the physician does not show a preference, you may choose the style best suited to the practice and most convenient for the volume of correspondence.

Acceptable Styles
Blocked. In the blocked letter style, the dateline, subject line, complimentary close, and typed signature begin at the center point from left to right of the page. All other parts of the letter begin at the left-hand margin (left justified).

For an example of this style, see Figure 8.3.

Semi-Blocked. The semi-blocked style is similar to the blocked style except that the beginning line of each paragraph in the body of the letter is indented five spaces. For an example of this style, see Figure 8.4.

Full-Blocked. In the full-blocked style, all lines or all parts of the letter begin at the left-hand margin. For an example of this style, see Figure 8.5.

RICHARD C. OSWALD, M.D.
2385 Bayor Road
Brookline, MA 02146

May 10, 1999

Robert C. Parsons, M.D.
Women's Clinic
240 Woodside Road
Boston, MA 02134

Re: Mary O'Malley

Dear Doctor Parsons:

I saw our mutual patient, Mary O'Malley, in my office today for a follow-up examination. As you are aware, she has been taking Dyazide, one tablet daily.

On physical examination: Weight 106 pounds. Blood pressure supine 120/80 in the right arm, pulse 86; standing 108/72 in the right arm, pulse 90. Lungs were clear to auscultation and percussion. Carotids were normal. There was no jugular venous distention present. Peripheral pulses were full, equal, and symmetric. Extremities revealed no edema, cyanosis, or clubbing.

An electrocardiogram, a copy of which is enclosed, was within normal limits.

I will be seeing Ms. O'Malley again in 3 months. If you have questions, please call me.

Sincerely,

Richard C. Oswald, M.D.

RCO:ep

Enclosure

FIGURE 8.3

Example of blocked letter style. (From Zakus SM et al, editors: *Mosby's fundamentals of medical assisting: administrative and clinical theory and technique,* ed 2, St. Louis, 1990, Mosby.)

RICHARD C. OSWALD, M.D.
2385 Bayor Road
Brookline, MA 02146

May 10, 1999

Robert C. Parsons, M.D.
Women's Clinic
240 Woodside Road
Boston, MA 02134

Dear Doctor Parsons:

Mary O'Malley

I saw our mutual patient, Mary O'Malley, in my office today for a follow-up examination. As you are aware, she has been taking Dyazide, one tablet daily.

On physical examination: Weight 106 pounds. Blood pressure supine 120/80 in the right arm, pulse 86; standing 108/72 in the right arm, pulse 90. Lungs were clear to auscultation and percussion. Carotids were normal. There was no jugular venous distention present. Peripheral pulses were full, equal, and symmetric. Extremities revealed no edema, cyanosis, or clubbing.

An electrocardiogram, a copy of which is enclosed, was within normal limits.

I will be seeing Ms. O'Malley again in 3 months. If you have questions, please call me.

Sincerely,

Richard C. Oswald, M.D.

RCO:ep

Enclosure

FIGURE 8.4

Example of semi-blocked letter style. (From Zakus SM et al, editors: *Mosby's fundamentals of medical assisting: administrative and clinical theory and technique,* ed 2, St. Louis, 1990, Mosby.)

Parts of a Letter

Letterhead

The embossed, engraved, or printed letterhead normally is centered near the upper edge of the page and usually includes the name of the physician, practice, or facility and the address of the practice or facility. Often the telephone number and practice specialty also are included.

RICHARD C. OSWALD, M.D.
2385 Bayor Road
Brookline, MA 02146

May 10, 1999

Robert C. Parsons, M.D.
Women's Clinic
240 Woodside Road
Boston, MA 02134

Re: Mary O'Malley

Dear Doctor Parsons:

I saw our mutual patient, Mary O'Malley, in my office today for a follow-up examination. As you are aware, she has been taking Dyazide, one tablet daily.

On physical examination: Weight 106 pounds. Blood pressure supine 120/80 in the right arm, pulse 86; standing 108/72 in the right arm, pulse 90. Lungs were clear to auscultation and percussion. Carotids were normal. There was no jugular venous distention present. Peripheral pulses were full, equal, and symmetric. Extremities revealed no edema, cyanosis, or clubbing.

An electrocardiogram, a copy of which is enclosed, was within normal limits.

I will be seeing Ms. O'Malley again in 3 months. If you have questions, please call me.

Sincerely,

Richard C. Oswald, M.D.

RCO:ep

Enclosure

FIGURE 8.5

Example of full-blocked letter style. (From Zakus SM et al, editors: *Mosby's fundamentals of medical assisting: administrative and clinical theory and technique,* ed 2, St. Louis, 1990, Mosby.)

Dateline

The dateline indicates the date that the correspondence was transcribed and is placed two line spaces below the letterhead. The month should be spelled out in full, not abbreviated, followed by the day, a comma, and the year in four digits. The international order of writing day first, then the month, and finally the year is not considered appropriate in American correspondence.

Inside Address

The inside address contains three, and possibly more lines, all of which are flush with the left margin. It is placed a minimum of four single-spaced lines below the dateline; more space if appropriate if needed to center the letter attractively. The following information should be listed in this order:

- Addressee's name
- Organizational title, if appropriate
- Company name, if appropriate
- Street address or post office box number
- City, state, and Zip code

The addressee's name is preceded by a courtesy title such as Ms., Mr., Dr., or Prof. If the addressee is a physician, the courtesy title is omitted and the initials M.D., D.O., PhD and so on follow the name.

Subject Line

Placed two line spaces below the inside address, the subject line usually is centered regardless of the letter style to be used. This line is intended to alert the reader to the reason for the letter; centering it commands attention. The subject (frequently a patient) is preceded by "Re:" which means regarding. The subject line may be underlined for further emphasis.

Salutation

The salutation is a greeting to the addressee. It is placed two lines below the inside address or the subject line, whichever is lower. The greeting may be formal or informal. Each begins with the word "Dear," followed either formally by a courtesy title and the addressee's last name or informally by the addressee's first name. If a physician is greeted formally, the courtesy title is not abbreviated (Dr.) but spelled out (Doctor). Occasionally, your employer will strike out a formally typed salutation to a colleague and write in the addressee's first name. This is a recognized technique of personalizing the correspondence.

Body of the Letter

The body of the letter is begun two lines below the salutation, according to the style you have chosen. The body of the letter is the message conveyed to the recipient.

Second-Page Heading

If a second page is necessary to complete a communication, it should have a heading for identification in case it is separated from the first page. The heading should include the addressee's name, the date, the page number, and the subject (if it was used on page 1). The heading for page 2 of a letter might read as follows:

<pre>
Robert C. Parsons, M.D.   May 10, 1999
Re: Mary O'Malley   Page 2
</pre>

Complimentary Close

The complimentary close is the method of ending a communication, and the closure selected should be in keeping with the tone of the salutation. A formal letter should be closed "Very truly yours" and an informal one "Sincerely," "Warm regards," or "Best wishes." The closure is placed two lines below the last line of the body of the letter, in the position appropriate to the style.

Typed Signature

The typed signature is a courtesy to the reader, especially if the sender's name does not appear on the printed letterhead. The typed signature is placed four lines below and flush with the complimentary close.

Reference Initials

The reference initials are placed two lines below the typed signature. The physician's initials are capitalized, and the transcriber's are lowercased. The initials are separated by a diagonal slash or a colon.

Enclosure or Carbon Copy Notation

If the letter is accompanied by additional materials you will indicate this by stating "Enclosure:" two lines below the reference initials. You then can indicate the number of enclosures being sent with the correspondence. You also may indicate what those enclosures are. The following are examples of enclosure notations:

> Enclosure
> Enclosures: 2
> Enclosures: Lab results for Mary Smith and patient chart

If others are to receive a copy of the letter, the initials "cc" (for xerox copy) or "pc" (for personal computer copy) are noted two lines below the reference initials or the enclosure line, whichever is last. The notation "pc:" is followed by the name or names of those receiving a copy. If multiple copies are sent, the names are listed one below the other in alphabetical order or order of rank.

Signature of the Sender

The physician will sign the letter after reviewing it for content and accuracy. If for some reason the physician is not available to sign the communication but instructs the transcriber to send it on completion, the transcriber can sign the physician's name and follow it with a slash and the transcriber's initials. The transcriber also may insert a line two spaces below the typed signature stating: "dictated but not read." This relieves the physician of complete responsibility for communication errors.

Correspondence Generated by the Administrative Medical Assistant

Much outgoing office communication is the responsibility of the medical assistant. The skill and timeliness with which this communication is handled will reflect on the assistant and ultimately on the physician. Each letter that leaves a medical office reveals subtle information about the intelligence, ability, and efficiency of the writer.

Some of the administrative medical assistant's correspondence responsibilities might include:

- Responses to patient inquiries on administrative procedures
- Exchanges with suppliers and business associates
- Account collections
- Exchanges with insurance companies
- Notification to patients of surgery or hospital arrangements
- Letters of solicitation

Because of the importance of written communication, planning should be an integral part of each letter.

Preparing a Letter

Preparing a letter or any communication involves the following four basic steps:

- Organizing the information
- Drafting a reply
- Editing the rough draft
- Preparing the final letter

A natural inclination is to attempt to save time by bypassing some of these steps, but doing so rarely saves time and often results in lost time. The most important step is organizing the information. Organizing a letter means to prepare the information in a logical manner that can be easily followed by the reader.

Having the necessary information in the proper order will allow the other steps to be accomplished easily. A rough draft allows you to see your statements more clearly. If you are working with a word processor, the third and fourth steps of editing and final letter are almost completed. Always review your work critically, as if you were the recipient rather than the writer.

Preparing the Envelope

The proper preparation of the envelope is important so that the correspondence reaches the addressee quickly. A business envelope is prepared with the sender's name and address printed in the upper left-hand corner. The addressee's name, company name, street address or post office box number, and city, state, and Zip code should be typed on the face of the envelope (Figure 8.6).

Special notations, such as "Attention: Ms. Adams" or "Personal" should be placed in the lower left-hand corner on the face of the envelope.

In an effort to speed mail processing with the use of automated envelope readers, the postal service offers some suggestions for preparing the envelope. A sample of these guidelines follows:

1. When using the No. 10 envelope (business letter size), you should begin typing the address 12 lines from the top and four inches from the left edge of the envelope. On smaller, standard-size envelopes (No. 6 $^3/_4$), begin the address 12 lines down from the top and 2 $^1/_2$ inches from the left edge.

De A. Eggers & Associates
Medical Accounts Management
and Consulting

565 First Street West
Sonoma, CA 95476

AirTech Corporation
P. O. Box 6666
Everytown, CA 99999

FIGURE 8.6

A properly addressed business envelope.

2. Use capital letters to begin words throughout the address.

3. Eliminate all punctuation.

4. Identify the state, district, or territory according to its standard two-letter abbreviation (see the box on p. 206).

5. The last line of the address must contain the city, state, and Zip code in 22 total spaces, including blanks between words. Because the state abbreviation, the Zip code, and the spaces between the city and state and the state and Zip code total 9 digit spaces, the letters of the city must not exceed 13 digits. Approved abbreviations have been developed for cities with lengthy names.

Contact your local post office for guidelines on abbreviations to use when preparing correspondence.

Folding Letters

Tri-fold for No. 10 Envelope

Letters on standard business-size (8 ½ × 11) stationery are folded in thirds beginning at the bottom. The top then is folded down over the rest of the letter. When completed, there will be three sections, or two creases. The crease made by folding the top down is the edge inserted first into a No. 10 envelope.

Tri-fold for No. 6 3/4 Envelope

Letters or forms on standard-size sheets that must be inserted into No. 6 3/4 envelopes are folded in three motions that will produce the creases. The lower

AT WORK TODAY

Two-Letter State/District/Territory Abbreviations

Alabama	AL	Illinois	IL	Montana	MT	Puerto Rico	PR
Alaska	AK	Indiana	IN	Nebraska	NE	Rhode Island	RI
Arizona	AZ	Iowa	IA	Nevada	NV	South Carolina	SC
Arkansas	AR	Kansas	KS	New Hampshire	NH	South Dakota	SD
California	CA	Kentucky	KY	New Jersey	NJ	Tennessee	TN
Colorado	CO	Louisiana	LA	New Mexico	NM	Texas	TX
Delaware	DE	Maine	ME	New York	NY	Utah	UT
District of Columbia	DC	Maryland	MD	North Carolina	NC	Vermont	VT
Florida	FL	Massachusetts	MA	North Dakota	ND	Virgin Islands	VI
Georgia	GA	Michigan	MI	Ohio	OH	Washington	WA
Guam	GU	Minnesota	MN	Oklahoma	OK	West Virginia	WV
Hawaii	HI	Mississippi	MS	Oregon	OR	Wisconsin	WI
Idaho	ID	Missouri	MO	Pennsylvania	PA	Wyoming	WY

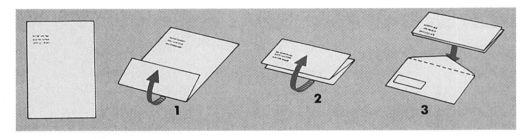

FIGURE 8.7

Letters on standard business-size stationery are folded in thirds, beginning at the bottom. (From Cooper MG et al, editors: *The medical assistant,* ed 6, St. Louis, 1993, Mosby.)

edge of the paper is lifted up and toward the top until the edges and corners match. The crease you make will produce a sheet folded in half. Next, lift the right-hand edge and fold one third of the way across the page. Then lift the left-hand edge and fold over the previous one-third segment. The last crease made is the first inserted into the envelope.

Folding for Window Envelopes

The fold required for envelopes with windows is a tri-fold that resembles pleating (Figure 8.7). It is used for most statements that you receive in the mail.

The first fold is made by lifting the bottom edge and creasing at one third the length of the sheet. The correspondence then is placed face down, and the free edge is lifted up and back so that the inside address is facing you. The sheet then is placed in the envelope with the inside address facing the window. Before sealing the envelope, turn it over and be sure the entire name and address are visible through the window.

Outgoing Mail

Affixing Appropriate Postage

Using a postage scale, determine the weight of the item to be mailed. For first-class mail the first ounce is charged one fee; each subsequent ounce costs less. Do not incorrectly calculate the total postage by multiplying the total ounces by the cost of the first ounce. Instead, determine the total weight in ounces, subtract 1 ounce, and multiply the remainder by the lesser fee for subsequent ounces. Add this amount to the fee for the first ounce to determine the total postage due. Affix the postage by meter or in stamps to the upper right-hand corner on the face of the envelope.

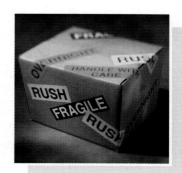

The administrative medical assistant can control the expense of outgoing mail and postage expenses in numerous ways. Letters and packages that need to be quickly received by a person or facility should be taken directly to the post office. The following are some cost-saving steps the administrative medical assistant can take:

1. Encourage patients to pay for services at the time of their office visit, particularly their co-pays. You also may hand them their statement with an envelope.
2. Avoid additional postage fees by using only standard-sized envelopes.
3. If mail is not metered through a postage machine, purchase a postage scale and keep it accurately adjusted.
4. Use the proper mailing class to avoid being charged first-class rates when you don't need the first-class services.
5. Preprint "address correction requested" on mailing envelopes for statements.

Classes of Mail

First Class

First-class mail includes rapidly processed correspondence such as handwritten or typed letters, postcards and business mail. The majority of mail sent out is first-class mail.

Second Class

Newspapers and periodicals (magazines, journals) are mailed at second-class (reduced) rates under a special permit issued to publishers of printed materials that come out at least four times a year. The public can mail single copies of books or other printed materials at second-class rates if the item weighs less than 16 ounces. Items over this weight are mailed at fourth-class rates.

Third Class

Third-class mail consists of unsealed or marked and sealed matter that weighs less than 16 ounces. This category includes circulars, booklets, catalogs, and so forth. Third-class mail is commonly called *advertising mail.*

Fourth Class

Fourth-class mail is commonly referred to as *parcel post* and consists of all mailable matter that weighs 16 ounces or more and is not considered first-class or second-class mail. The upper limits of parcel post are 70 pounds or a total of 100 inches in combined length and circumference. Fourth-class mail must be packed and wrapped carefully because of the rough handling it receives.

Remember that any package must be sealed with regular or reinforced packing tape approved by the postal service. Packages sealed with twine, string, masking tape, or cellophane tape will be rejected.

If in doubt about the proper class or most efficient way to send an item, call the local postal service information number. A postal employee will assist you.

International Mail

International mail is divided into two categories: postal union, which includes letters, cards, and packages; and parcel post, which is governed by agreements with foreign countries that place restrictions on materials that enter their borders. Most letters sent to various foreign geographical regions will be sent airmail at international rates determined by the U.S. Postal Service based on half mail weight. First-class mail to Canada and Mexico is sent the same as U.S. rates. Window envelopes cannot be used for international mail.

Combination Mail

Combination mail may be used when a letter is sent with a parcel. First-class postage is placed on the letter, which is attached to the parcel. Postage for the parcel is paid separately, and both items must be addressed exactly the same. This package travels with mail of the class in which the bulky item falls. If a letter is placed inside the package, the notation "Letter Enclosed" must be placed on the outside of the package, unless the package is sent priority mail. This classification is used frequently by medical offices for mailing x-ray films with a letter.

Special Mail Services

Certified Mail

For a fee in addition to the regular postage, certified mail provides a record of delivery that is retained at the addressee's post office for 2 years. A return receipt, signed by the addressee or addressee's agent, can be acquired and returned to the sender to verify that the item was received. An additional fee is charged for this service.

Express Mail

Express mail is a fast, intercity delivery system geared to the special needs of business and industry. It offers reliable transfer of time-sensitive documents and products. Overnight delivery is guaranteed, with about a 95% reliability record (Figure 8.8).

The five service options for express mail are:

- Door to door—item is picked up at sender's office and delivered to addressee's office
- Door to destination airport—item is picked up at sender's office and delivered to airport in addressee's city, where it is picked up

MEDICAL ASSISTING STEP-BY-STEP

Mailing Notations for Envelopes

If you have special instructions for the postal service, they should be noted on the envelope. These notations specify special mailing instructions and should be written using all capital letters—on line nine from the top edge of the envelope, below the postage stamp. Examples are "REGISTERED," "SPECIAL DELIVERY," or "RETURN RECEIPT."

If you have special instructions for people delivering mail in the office, these also should be noted on the envelope. These notations are to the addressee and are written using all capital letters—four spaces from the left edge and four spaces below the return address. Examples would be "CONFIDENTIAL," "PERSONAL," or "PLEASE FORWARD."

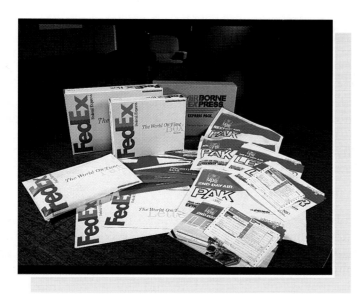

FIGURE 8.8

Express mail is a fast, intercity delivery system geared to the special needs of business and industry. Overnight delivery is guaranteed, with about a 95% reliability record.

- Sender's airport to addressee—item is taken by sender to nearest airport for direct dispatch to addressee
- Airport to airport—item is dispatched to and retrieved from respective airports
- Regular express mail service—mail taken to designated postal facilities by 5:00 PM may be picked up at addressee's designated postal facility at 10:00 AM or delivered to addressee's office by 3:00 PM the next day

AT WORK TODAY

Speedy Mail

In a world in which it has become increasingly important for transactions to occur in a minimal amount of time, it has become critical that mail travel faster.

1. The U.S. Postal Service offers express mail, which is used when an item needs to arrive at its destination the next day. If an item is deposited in a special box or turned in at the window by 5:00 pm, guaranteed delivery is by noon the next day.

2. United Parcel Service is available in most larger cities and towns and also will deliver overseas. It also provides overnight service. In some cities, UPS will pick up articles at your office if they have been properly weighed and payment is ready at pickup.

3. Federal Express (FEDEX) is similar to UPS. It has overnight service and may be preferred by some people. Items to send by FEDEX include manuscripts, reports, or medical specimens.

Insured Mail

Third-class and fourth-class mail may be insured against loss and damage up to $400. The insurance fee is based on the stated value of the item.

Mailgrams

Mailgrams are a special service offered jointly by the U.S. Postal Service and Western Union. Messages charged at 100-word units may be dictated by telephone to Western Union, which transmits them to the destination city for next-day delivery by the postal service.

Priority Mail

Priority mail is the special service for first-class mail that weighs more than 11 ounces but not more than 70 pounds. It is the fastest way to get heavier mail to its destination, with a 2- or 3-day delivery assured. Using the special red, white, and blue envelopes provided by the postal service assures first-class handling. You also may get special red, white, and blue stickers from the post office to place on packages.

Registered Mail

First-class and priority mail may be registered if the contents are valuable. The value of the item is declared by the sender. The fee for this service is based on the declared value of the item, and the sender is given a receipt that must be retained until the item is received by the addressee. A return receipt also may be included with this service for an additional fee. If registered mail is lost or damaged in transit, the postal service will pay the declared value up to $10,000 if the item is not also insured by another source. If commercial insurance is carried on the item, the postal service can pay up to $2,000 in a coordinated effort with the insurance carrier to pay for the total value of the item.

Special Problems
Change of Address

If the office or facility site is to be changed, the postal service should be notified at least 1 month in advance. This will ensure that mail is forwarded without delay. If the office is moved to another city, you must sign a form accepting responsibility for the cost of forwarding all mail other than first-class items.

If you wish to locate an addressee who has moved without notifying the office, you should note "address correction requested" on the envelope. It is a good idea to have this message preprinted on the office statement envelopes. If the post office can forward the mail, the new address is noted on a card and returned to the sender with postage due for the service. This is money well spent if you are attempting to collect a large outstanding account.

Nonstandard Mail

Extra postage will be required for items deemed nonstandard in size by the postal service. Because the criteria for determining nonstandard size involve minute and confusing measurements, many manufacturers of odd-sized envelopes place a notice in the spot where postage is to be placed stating extra postage required. The fee schedule can be obtained from the postal service.

Tracing Lost Mail

If you believe that a piece of first-class, registered, certified, or insured mail is lost, you should notify the post office and complete the required forms. When reporting the loss, you should bring along any receipts associated with the item.

Recalling Mail

If you wish to intercept a mailed item before it is delivered to the addressee, you may make a written request, accompanied by an identically addressed envelope, to the local post office. If the letter is already in transit, the postmaster will attempt to intercept the item at the destination post office. Any expenses incurred, such as for long-distance telephone calls or telegrams, are the sender's responsibility.

Nonmail Items Dropped into a Mailbox

Should you inadvertently drop a nonmail item into a mailbox and you wish to retrieve it because of its value, a special procedure is required. Notify the postal service immediately, using the emergency number if it is after business hours. The postal service will take the location of the mailbox, your name, and the type of item lost. A "special pickup" then will be ordered. The person handling your call will advise you to wait at the mailbox and give you the approximate waiting time. When the driver arrives, the entire contents of the box will be collected, and the driver will advise you where to retrieve the item. Do not ask the driver for it; it is temporarily the property of the postal service. Be prepared to provide a detailed description of the item and sign affidavits before recovering the item.

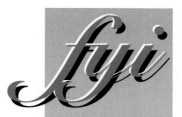

What About Mail Size?

Because the U.S. Postal Service uses machines to sort mail, standards have been developed so the machines will work properly. Domestic mail must be at least 0.007 inch thick. Mail that is $1/4$ inch or less in thickness must be $3^1/2$ inches in height and at least 5 inches long.

Mail that does not meet this standard is considered nonstandard. The post office places a surcharge on any nonstandard mail. It also will place a surcharge on first- and third-class mail weighing 1 ounce or less if the length exceeds $11^1/2$ inches, the height exceeds $6^1/2$ inches, and the thickness exceeds $1/4$ inch.

Conclusion

Developing skill in handling the various aspects of written communication will help you as an individual and project a positive image of you and your employer to patients and business contacts. Written communication requires constant attention, because it provides permanent documentation of events and transactions on details that you could not possibly remember. Constant monitoring of the system will ensure its efficiency and effectiveness.

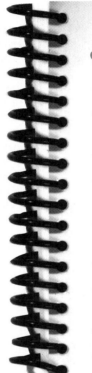

Review QUESTIONS

1. Explain the key terms listed in this chapter.

2. What equipment is needed to prepare correspondence and process it for mailing?

3. What skills will help you in preparing correspondence?

4. Prepare a letter in full-blocked style, and label the 12 parts of the letter.

5. How will you determine which class of mail is correct for an item you are preparing to send?

6. What special services does the postal service provide?

7. Name and describe four problems you might encounter with outgoing mail.

8. Develop an office policy for handling incoming mail.

9. List in order the sequence in which you would stack incoming mail, beginning at the top of the stack.

SUGGESTED READINGS

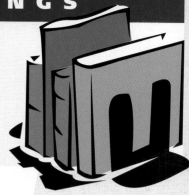

Sabin W: *The Gregg reference manual,* ed 6, New York, 1991, Gregg Division/McGraw-Hill.

Schwager E: *Medical English usage and abusage,* Phoenix, 1991, Oryx Press.

The postal manual, Superintendent of Documents, Washington, DC, 1991, US Government Printing Office.

Patient/Medical Records Management

OUTLINE

OUTLINE

OBJECTIVES

On completion of Chapter 9 the administrative medical assistant student should be able to:

1 Define the key terms listed in this chapter.

2 Define and state the purpose of a medical records management system.

3 Describe at least four organizational divisions of a medical record.

4 List the subjective and objective patient data contained in the medical record.

5 Describe the process of making deletions from a medical record; state the reasons for and techniques of making corrections in a medical record.

6 Describe the techniques for protecting medical records.

7 Discuss opinions on the retention of medical records.

8 Explain how color coding of medical record files can be advantageous to the facility.

9 Discuss the method of destruction of medical records.

K E Y   T E R M S

Chronological	Arranged in the order of time.
Confidential	Information to which a person may be privy and cannot be shared without the express authorization of the person to which it pertains.
Cumulative	Growing in number by repeated additions.
Derogatory	Tending to discredit or belittle.
Diplomatic	Skillful in the conduct of affairs.
Microfilming	Photographing records in a reduced size on film for retention.
Retention	The act of keeping in one's power or possession.
Scrutiny	Close inspection or examination.
Subpoena	A written court order commanding a person to appear in court.

*R*eceiving, processing, and gathering papers in an orderly manner for storage are necessary functions in every business. Records management is the development and maintenance of a systematic method of fulfilling these functions. The management of medical records is a responsibility that should be orderly and systematic. The main purpose of keeping accurate and complete medical records is to assist in giving the best possible care and treatment to the patient. Therefore, attention to the details of records management requires the special attention of the administrative medical assistant.

Purpose of Records Management

Single Location of Data

One factor in providing the best possible medical care is having all of the information regarding a patient in one place. That place is the patient's individual medical chart. Every patient's chart is stored ideally in a single location, either the filing cabinet or record-storage area (Figure 9.1). If patient information is systematically stored in a known, single location, it will be readily available to the physician and personnel when needed.

Continuum of Information

The medical record provides the medical staff with a chronological history of a patient's care, illnesses, injuries, responses to treatment, and general condition at all stages throughout the relationship with the physician. Patients frequently forget various events and responses to particular medications, and the physician cannot possibly remember the details of care given to each individual because

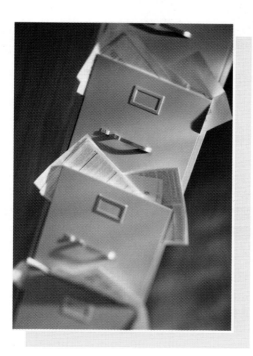

FIGURE 9.1

Every patient's chart is stored ideally in a single location, either the filing cabinet or record-storage area.

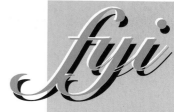

The Medical Record

The medical record is the "storehouse" for a patient's medical information. It needs to contain all past and current information related to patient history, diagnosis and treatment, test results, reports, and letters.

The medical record also is a permanent legal record and should contain anything that has happened to or transpired with the patient, such as office visits, telephone conversations, and prescription refills. All entries should be accurate and legible with no blatant or unnecessary comments.

Remember, the physician is accountable for anything in the record.

The physician also is accountable for putting secondhand information into the record. An example of secondhand information might be: "Sister states that a friend of the patient has indicated that he (the patient) might be a secret alcoholic." The physician should include this statement in the record if laboratory results have ever shown that alcoholism might be a factor with the patient.

of the great number of patients for whom he or she cares over the course of a career. The well-maintained medical record provides a detailed and logical sequence of events to the benefit of both the patient and the physician.

Comprehensive Record of Data From Various Sources

The office medical record is developed around the observations and notations of the physician based on conversations with and examinations of the patients. In addition, the record serves as a storage unit for information from a variety of sources. This outside medical information includes reports from laboratory and diagnostic facilities of examinations requested by the physician, detailed information gathered if the patient is hospitalized, consultations requested of other physicians, and records from other health care providers who have treated the patient. This cumulative information assists the current physician in the continuing care of the patient.

Rapid Retrieval of Information

Proper development, maintenance, and storage of patients' medical records allows for rapid retrieval of information. The speed at which patient data can be located and transmitted can affect a positive outcome for a patient in need. Consider the situation of a child brought to an emergency room after ingesting a parent's prescription medication. The parent, concerned about getting care for the child, leaves for the emergency room without the medication bottle and cannot remember the name of the medication. When your office is contacted, the speed with which you can provide the information could be vital to the child survival.

Legal Protection of the Patient

Confidentiality

The proper maintenance and storage of patient's medical records will provide for the confidentiality of the information contained in them. You should think of the record as the person, and the same privacy you would provide for the patient should be provided for the record. This will create an atmosphere in which the patient can feel confident in being totally frank with the physician.

Protecting Patients' Identities

The protection of your patients and their records should always be your first thought when any inquiries are made about them. Some requests will be perfectly innocent and should be handled diplomatically. For example, one patient may notice another person leaving the doctor's office and inquire, "Was that Sam Johnson? I haven't seen him in years. Do you have his number? I'd really like to call him." Because you may not confirm the patient's name or release his telephone number, you might reply, "I am sorry, Mr. Simpson, I cannot give out anyone's phone number, just as I would not give out yours to anyone without your permission." With this type of statement, you have not confirmed or denied the departing patient's identity and have subtly educated the patient on confidentiality.

When a subpoena for a medical record is delivered in person, the server must present it to the medical assistant along with a check to cover the cost of processing the chart. If it turns out that the person is not a present or former patient, the check is retained and the subpoena is returned after the assistant signs a form stating that no records are available. In an effort to cut costs, some subpoena firms call an office in advance to inquire if the records are available. This is a method of determining if an individual is under the physician's care. If you respond that you have a record for that patient, you are breaching confidentiality. The appropriate response would be, "If you will forward the subpoena, I can check our files."

Release of Records

There is to be no release of patient records without signed consent of the patient or the patient's representative. In all instances for which consent is required, the permission should be obtained in writing and placed on file. Most offices keep a supply of preprinted forms with blanks for the appropriate information (Figure 9.2).

Protection of the Physician

Documentation of Care Provided

The patient's medical records provide the primary documentation of the evaluation, examination, treatments, and conclusions determined by the physician. Entries in medical records should be written clearly and legibly. Physicians

CLIENT ACCOUNT NUMBER	PATIENT REGISTRATION FORM	DATE

PATIENT ACCOUNT NUMBER	CLIENT NAME	☐ NEW ☐ CHANGE

PLEASE TYPE OR PRINT CLEARLY — (DR. CODE — R.D. CODE — CARRIER CODE FOR OFFICE USE ONLY)

PATIENT INFORMATION

PATIENT'S NAME	DATE OF BIRTH	SEX ☐ Male ☐ Female	SOCIAL SECURITY #

ADDRESS — STREET, APT. NO.	REFERRING DOCTOR		
	EMPLOYER		

CITY	STATE	ZIP	TELEPHONE — HOME	TELEPHONE — OTHER

RESPONSIBLE PARTY FOR BILLING

NAME - LAST, FIRST, MIDDLE INITIAL	☐ SAME AS ABOVE	PATIENT RELATIONSHIP TO RESPONSIBLE PARTY ☐ SELF ☐ SPOUSE ☐ CHILD ☐ OTHER		

ADDRESS — STREET, APT. NO.	CITY	STATE	ZIP
	TELEPHONE — HOME	TELEPHONE — OTHER	

INSURANCE

PRIMARY INSURANCE CARRIER NAME, TELEPHONE	POLICY/ID#	GROUP#

INSUREDS NAME - LAST, FIRST, MIDDLE INITIAL	☐ SAME AS ABOVE	EMPLOYER	EMPLOYER PLAN COVERAGE ☐ YES ☐ NO

ADDRESS OF INSURANCE COMPANY	PATIENT RELATIONSHIP TO INSURED ☐ SELF ☐ SPOUSE ☐ CHILD ☐ OTHER	
	TELEPHONE — HOME	IF CHAMPUS ☐ RETIRED ☐ ACTIVE ☐ DECEASED

CITY	STATE	ZIP	SOCIAL SECURITY #	BRANCH OF SERVICE:

SECONDARY INSURANCE CARRIER NAME, TELEPHONE	POLICY/ID#	GROUP#

INSUREDS NAME - LAST, FIRST, MIDDLE INITIAL	☐ SAME AS ABOVE	EMPLOYER	EMPLOYER PLAN COVERAGE ☐ YES ☐ NO

ADDRESS OF INSURANCE COMPANY	PATIENT RELATIONSHIP TO INSURED ☐ SELF ☐ SPOUSE ☐ CHILD ☐ OTHER	
	TELEPHONE — HOME	IF CHAMPUS ☐ RETIRED ☐ ACTIVE ☐ DECEASED

CITY	STATE	ZIP	SOCIAL SECURITY #	BRANCH OF SERVICE:

Please remember that insurance is considered a method of reimbursing the patient for fees paid to the doctor and is not a substitute for payment. Some companies pay fixed allowances for certain procedures, and others pay a percentage of the charge. It is your responsibility to pay any deductible amount, co-insurance, or any other balance not paid for by your insurance.

IN ORDER TO CONTROL YOUR COST OF BILLINGS, WE REQUEST THAT OUR CHARGES FOR OFFICE VISITS BE PAID AT THE CONCLUSION OF EACH VISIT.

To the extent necessary to determine liability for payment and to obtain reimbursement, I authorize disclosure of portions of the patient's records.

I hereby assign all medical and/or surgical benefits, to include major medical benefits to which I am entitled including MediCare, private insurance, and other health plans to:

This assignment will remain in effect until revoked by me in writing. A photocopy of this assignment is to be considered as valid as an original. I understand that I am financially responsible for all charges whether or not paid by said insurance. I hereby authorize said assignee to release all information necessary to secure the payment.

SIGNED _____ DATE _____

FIGURE 9.2

Example of a patient registration form with blanks in which to record information.
(Designed and provided by De A. Eggers & Associates, Sonoma, Calif.)

AT WORK TODAY

The Medical Record: a Legal "Safe"

At a time when people commonly sue others and companies for as much compensation as possible, the medical record has become an increasingly important document.

It is vital that the record be an accurate, complete document so that the physician can:

1. Protect himself or herself in court by being able to prove that he or she gave adequate treatment, that is, "the standard of care"

2. Support insurance company billings with the correct coding justification

3. Use the information recorded to complete the reports required by law in the case of child abuse, communicable diseases, and criminal actions such as gunshot wounds and stabbings

---

cannot be expected to remember previous impressions of the patient's health or treatments prescribed and must depend on the accuracy of the record. Should a legal issue be raised regarding the care or condition of a patient, the medical record usually is the first source of information evaluated.

Permanent Protection

A medical record is a lasting proof of care and is credible regardless of the time elapsed since an entry was made. Because a lawsuit may be filed years after an event, the record is considered more reliable than the physician's memory. For the record to provide protection, it must be carefully prepared and maintained.

Statistical Information

Physicians may wish to gather and evaluate data on the effectiveness of a treatment plan or follow the course of several patients with the same diagnosis. Medical records can provide this information, which can be abstracted and maintained in a separate file. The increasing use of computers to store records and abstract data is a great help with statistical information. You should remember, however, that this information, whether abstracted by you or a computer, still is confidential and must be protected.

Medical Record Content

Patient Data

The first step in developing the patient's record is to gather demographic data from the patient on his or her first visit to the office. This information will be used initially to introduce the patient to the physician. It also is used to contact the patient if necessary, to establish the account records, and to assist with insurance billing. The information most often requested includes the following:

- Full name
- Date of birth

AT WORK TODAY

Patient Information—Why Is It So Important?

Current patient information is retrieved from the patient registration form and gives all the basic information about the patient, including complete name, address, telephone number, and date of birth. Other information found on the patient registration form includes the following:

- If the patient is working: the company address and telephone number
- If the patient is married: the spouse's name and other pertinent information
- Insurance information: company and policy information; type of policy, whether group or individual
- Referral/emergency information: who referred the patient or a reference name, address, and telephone number

This information is used to contact the patient, bill the insurance company for payment of charges, and trace the patient if he or she needs to be reached and has moved without leaving a forwarding address. The patient registration form also is used to contact someone in case of an emergency involving the patient.

- Health questionnaire: this form either is completed by the patient or accomplished through an oral interview by the administrative medical assistant. It gives the doctor past and current information regarding the patient's prior health problems and current condition. This information is used by the doctor to evaluate a patient and will guide him or her in the future care and treatment of the patient.
- Release of information/assignment of benefits: this may be included in the data section so that the data in the record may be released to other physicians, insurance companies, or hospitals.

The patient may or may not sign these documents. Having the patient's signature on these documents allows the office to release the information to various agencies or doctors as needed. Always remember that the medical record is privileged information.

- Sex (name may not be indicative)
- Complete home address
- Home telephone number (or number where messages can be left)
- Marital status
- If married, spouse's name or if unmarried, the next of kin
- Occupation, employer, work address, and telephone number
- If married, spouse's work information
- Insurance carrier and identification numbers
- Insurance carrier's address
- Referral source
- Social Security number
- Driver's license number
- Name of individual to contact in an emergency (someone who does not live with the patient)

Changes in social attitudes regarding independent identity may cause a married patient to decline to provide information about a spouse. This wish must be respected, but you could explain that the information is for notification purposes, particularly in the event of an emergency, and not an assumption of dependence. Some patients may refuse to give their Social Security number or driver's license number. This too must be respected, since it will be difficult to explain that the information is requested so that the patient may be traced in the event an account is not paid. Fortunately, the majority of insurance carriers use a patient's Social Security number as a policy identification number.

Methods of Patient Registration

The demographical information may be obtained by two methods: a patient-completed form or an oral interview.

A patient-completed registration form may be one of your own design or may be selected from those offered by office-supply companies. The form, secured to a hard writing surface such as a clipboard, is handed along with a pen or pencil to the patient on his or her arrival in the office. The patient is asked to complete the form and return it to the receptionist. If the practice has a significant number of elderly patients, a small desk in the reception area for filling out the form is very handy. If the appointment is made far enough ahead of time, patients will appreciate your sending them the forms to fill out and bring with them to the appointment. This also allows time for the patient to complete the form more accurately. The form usually is put into the record as is, although you may wish also to have the information typed onto a patient-history form.

Gathering demographical information by interview is a more personal technique, but you must be careful to provide privacy during the interview. The data may be handwritten or typed directly into a computer system as the information is acquired. Each method has advantages and disadvantages.

Personal and Medical History

The personal history, including social habits and family history, and medical history are necessary to prepare a foundation for the physical examination and subsequent treatment. This information also can be gathered by patient-completed forms or by interview (Figure 9.3).

Reason for Visit

The patient may have given the reason for the visit at the time the appointment was made, but he or she usually is asked again at the beginning of the visit. Normally the receptionist might ask, "Are you here for your injection or flu shot?" This information is recorded in the patient's own words, in the patient's chart, before the patient is escorted by the back office staff to an examination room.

Objective Data

The objective entries in a medical record are based on observations made during the course of examining the patient and through reviews, diagnostic studies, and subsequent care. Objective findings and conclusions include:

- Physical measurements
- Physical examination findings
- Diagnostic study reports
- Diagnosis and prognosis
- Treatment plan
- Outcome of treatment

Text continued on p. 231.

Andrus/Clini-Rec®
General Health History Questionnaire
&
Physical Examination
Male or Female

C
O
N
F
I
D
E
N
T
I
A
L

INSTRUCTIONS TO MY PATIENT

One of the most important parts of the medical record your doctor keeps for you is a health history concerning your past and present health problems, and any personal information which might affect the state of your health.

Your answers will be treated confidentially as are all parts of your visit. Please return this questionnaire to your doctor or to the doctor's nurse or assistant after you complete it.

Take all the time you need to complete this questionnaire. Answer each question as best you can by filling in the information asked for or by putting an "X" in the appropriate space. Choose the answer to each question which in your mind comes closest to applying to you.

If there is any question you have difficulty answering, just circle the question. You can discuss it with the doctor when you return the questionnaire.

If you have completed this questionnaire at home, be sure to bring it with you so that you and the doctor can go over your answers during your appointment within a confidential setting.

If this is a RE-EXAMINATION and you have previously filled out one of these "Patient Administered Comprehensive Health History Questionnaires", fill in PART A - Present Health History, sections I & II. *You do not* have to redo sections III & IV, or PART B - Past History.

Any changes which have occurred since you last filled out the questionnaire should be noted.

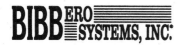

Created and Developed by
"Medical Economics" Professional Systems

BIBBERO SYSTEMS, INC.
1300 N. McDOWELL BLVD.
PETALUMA, CA 94954

Copyright © 1979, 1983 Bibbero Systems International, Inc.

STOCK NO. 19-742-4 8/95

FIGURE 9.3

Andrus/Clini-Rec General Health History Questionnaire and Physical Examination Male or Female. (Courtesy Bibbero Systems, Inc., Petaluma, Calif.)

Continued

ANDRUS/CLINI-REC® HEALTH HISTORY QUESTIONNAIRE

Chart No. _____

Identification Information

Today's Date _____

Name _____ Date of Birth _____

Occupation _____ Marital Status _____

PART A – PRESENT HEALTH HISTORY

I. CURRENT MEDICAL PROBLEMS
Please list the medical problems for which you came to see the doctor. About when did they begin?

Problems

Date Began

_____ _____

_____ _____

_____ _____

What concerns you most about these problems?

_____

_____

If you are being treated for any other illness or medical problems by another physician, please describe the problems and write the name of the physician or medical facility treating you.

Illness or Medical Problem | Physician or Medical Facility | City

_____ _____ _____

_____ _____ _____

II. MEDICATIONS
Please list all medications you are now taking, including those you buy without a doctor's prescription (such as aspirin, cold tablets or vitamin supplements).

_____ _____ _____

_____ _____ _____

III. ALLERGIES AND SENSITIVITIES
List anything that you are allergic to such as certain foods, medications, dust, chemicals or soaps, household items, pollens, bee stings, etc., and indicate how each affects you.

Allergic To: | Effect | Allergic To: | Effect

_____ _____ _____ _____

_____ _____ _____ _____

IV. GENERAL HEALTH, ATTITUDE AND HABITS

How is your overall health now?	Health now:	Poor _____ Fair _____ Good _____ Excellent _____
How has it been most of your life?	Health has been:	Poor _____ Fair _____ Good _____ Excellent _____
In the past year:		
Has your appetite changed?	Appetite:	Decreased _____ Increased _____ Stayed same _____
Has your weight changed?	Weight:	Lost _____ lbs. Gained _____ lbs. No change _____
Are you thirsty much of the time?	Thirsty:	No _____ Yes _____
Has your overall 'pep' changed?	Pep:	Decreased _____ Increased _____ Stayed same _____
Do you usually have trouble sleeping?	Trouble sleeping:	No _____ Yes _____
How much do you exercise?	Exercise:	Little or none _____ Less than I need _____ All I need _____
Do you smoke?	Smokes:	No _____ Yes _____ If yes, how many years? _____
How many each day?		_____ Cigarettes _____ Cigars _____ Pipesfull
Have you ever smoked?	Smoked:	No _____ Yes _____ If yes, how many years? _____
How many each day?		_____ Cigarettes _____ Cigars _____ Pipesfull
Do you drink alcoholic beverages?	Alcohol:	No _____ Yes _____ I drink _____ Beers _____ Glasses of wine _____ Drinks of hard liquor - per day
Have you ever had a problem with alcohol?	Prior problem:	No _____ Yes _____
How much coffee or tea do you usually drink?	Coffee/Tea:	_____ cups of coffee or tea a day
Do you regularly wear seatbelts?	Seatbelts:	No _____ Yes _____

DO YOU:	Rarely/Never	Occasionally	Frequently	DO YOU:	Rarely/Never	Occasionally	Frequently
Feel nervous?	_____	_____	_____	Ever feel like committing suicide?	_____	_____	_____
Feel depressed?	_____	_____	_____				
Find it hard to make decisions?	_____	_____	_____	Feel bored with your life?	_____	_____	_____
Lose your temper?	_____	_____	_____	Use marijuana?	_____	_____	_____
Worry a lot?	_____	_____	_____	Use "hard drugs"?	_____	_____	_____
Tire easily?	_____	_____	_____	Do you want to talk to the doctor about a personal matter? No _____ Yes _____			
Have trouble relaxing?	_____	_____	_____				
Have any sexual problems?	_____	_____	_____				

CONFIDENTIAL

STOCK NO. 19-742-4   8/95   Page 1

FIGURE 9.3, cont'd

For legend see p. 223.

PART A – PRESENT HEALTH HISTORY (continued)

IV. GENERAL HEALTH, ATTITUDE AND HABITS (continued)

Have you recently had any changes in your: If yes, please explain:

Marital status?   No_____ Yes_____   _____

Job or work?   No_____ Yes_____   _____

Residence?   No_____ Yes_____   _____

Financial status?   No_____ Yes_____   _____

Are you having any legal problems
  or trouble with the law?   No_____ Yes_____   _____

PART B – PAST HISTORY

I. FAMILY HEALTH

Please give the following information about your immediate family:

Relationship	Age, if Living	Age At Death	State of Health Or Cause of Death
Father	_____	_____	_____
Mother	_____	_____	_____
Brothers and Sisters	_____	_____	_____
	_____	_____	_____
	_____	_____	_____
Spouse	_____	_____	_____
Children	_____	_____	_____
	_____	_____	_____
	_____	_____	_____
	_____	_____	_____

Have any **blood relatives** had any of the following illnesses?
If so, indicate relationship (mother, brother, etc.)

Illness	Family Members
Asthma	_____
Diabetes	_____
Cancer.	_____
Blood Disease	_____
Glaucoma	_____
Epilepsy.	_____
Rheumatoid Arthritis.	_____
Tuberculosis	_____
Gout	_____
High Blood Pressure	_____
Heart Disease	_____
Mental Problems	_____
Suicide.	_____
Stroke	_____
Alcoholism.	_____
Rheumatic Fever	_____

II. HOSPITALIZATIONS, SURGERIES, INJURIES

Please list all times you have been hospitalized, operated on, or seriously injured.

Year	Operation, Illness, Injury	Hospital and City
_____	_____	_____
_____	_____	_____
_____	_____	_____

III. ILLNESS AND MEDICAL PROBLEMS

Please mark with an (X) any of the following illnesses and medical problems <u>you</u> have or have had and indicate the year when each started. If you are not certain when an illness started, write down an approximate year.

Illness	(x)	(Year)	Illness	(x)	(Year)
Eye or eye lid infection	____	_____	Hernia	____	_____
Glaucoma	____	_____	Hemorrhoids	____	_____
Other eye problems	____	_____	Kidney or bladder disease	____	_____
Ear trouble	____	_____	Prostate problem (male only)	____	_____
Deafness or decreased hearing	____	_____	Mental problems	____	_____
Thyroid trouble	____	_____	Headaches	____	_____
Strep throat	____	_____	Head injury	____	_____
Bronchitis	____	_____	Stroke	____	_____
Emphysema	____	_____	Convulsions, seizures	____	_____
Pneumonia	____	_____	Arthritis	____	_____
Allergies, asthma or hay fever	____	_____	Gout	____	_____
Tuberculosis	____	_____	Cancer or tumor	____	_____
Other lung problems	____	_____	Bleeding tendency	____	_____
High blood pressure	____	_____	Diabetes	____	_____
Heart attack	____	_____	Measles/Rubeola	____	_____
High cholesterol	____	_____	German measles/Rubella	____	_____
Arteriosclerosis			Polio	____	_____
(Hardening of arteries)	____	_____	Mumps	____	_____
Heart murmur	____	_____	Scarlet fever	____	_____
Other heart condition	____	_____	Chicken pox	____	_____
Stomach/duodenal ulcer	____	_____	Mononucleosis	____	_____
Diverticulosis	____	_____	Eczema	____	_____
Colitis	____	_____	Psoriasis	____	_____
Other bowel problems	____	_____	Venereal disease	____	_____
Hepatitis	____	_____	Genital herpes	____	_____
Liver trouble	____	_____	HIV test	____	_____
Gallbladder trouble	____	_____	AIDS	____	_____

CONFIDENTIAL

FIGURE 9.3, cont'd

For legend see p. 223.

PART C – BODY SYSTEMS REVIEW

Please answer all of the following questions.

Circle any questions you find difficult to answer.

__MEN:__ Please answer questions 1 through 12, then skip to question 18.

__WOMEN:__ Please start on question 6.

MEN ONLY

1. Have you had or do you have prostate trouble? . . . . No _____ Yes _____
2. Do you have any sexual problems or a problem with impotency? . . . . No _____ Yes _____
3. Have you ever had sores or lesions on your penis? . . . . No _____ Yes _____
4. Have you ever had any discharge from your penis? . . . . No _____ Yes _____
5. Do you ever have pain, lumps or swelling in your testicles? . . . . No _____ Yes _____

Check here if you wish to discuss any special problems with the doctor . . . . □

MEN & WOMEN

		Rarely/ Never	Occasionally	Frequently
6.	Is it sometimes hard to start your urine flow?	_____	_____	_____
7.	Is urination ever painful?	_____	_____	_____
8.	Do you have to urinate more than 5 times a day?	_____	_____	_____
9.	Do you get up at night to urinate?	_____	_____	_____
10.	Has your urine ever been bloody or dark colored?	_____	_____	_____
11.	Do you ever lose urine when you strain, laugh, cough or sneeze?	_____	_____	_____
12.	Do you ever lose urine during sleep?	_____	_____	_____

WOMEN ONLY

Do you:

		Rarely/ Never	Occasionally	Frequently
13. a.	Have any menstrual problems?	_____	_____	_____
b.	Feel rather tense just before your period?	_____	_____	_____
c.	Have heavy menstrual bleeding?	_____	_____	_____
d.	Have painful menstrual periods?	_____	_____	_____
e.	Have any bleeding between periods?	_____	_____	_____
f.	Have any unusual vaginal discharge or itching?	_____	_____	_____
g.	Ever have tender breasts?	_____	_____	_____
h.	Have any discharge from your nipples?	_____	_____	_____
i.	Have any hot flashes?	_____	_____	_____

14. How many times, if any, have you been pregnant? . . . . _____
15. How many children born alive? . . . . _____
16. Are you taking birth control pills? . . . . No _____ Yes _____
17. Do you examine your breasts monthly for lumps? . . . . No _____ Yes _____
17a. What was the date of your last menstrual period? . . . . Date _____

Check here if you wish to discuss any special problem with the doctor . . . . □

MEN & WOMEN

		Rarely/ Never	Occasionally	Frequently
18.	In the past year have you had any:			
a.	Severe shoulder pain?	_____	_____	_____
b.	Severe back pain?	_____	_____	_____
c.	Muscle or joint stiffness or pain due to sports, exercise or injury?	_____	_____	_____
d.	Pain or swelling in any joints not due to sports, exercise or injury?	_____	_____	_____

19. Do you have dry skin or brittle fingernails? . . . . No _____ Yes _____
20. Do you bruise easily? . . . . No _____ Yes _____
21. Do you have any moles that have changed in color or in size? . . . . No _____ Yes _____
22. Do you have any other skin problems? . . . . No _____ Yes _____

23. In the last 3 months have you had:
   a. A fever that lasted more than one day? . . . . No _____ Yes _____
   b. Sores or cuts that were hard to heal? . . . . No _____ Yes _____
   c. Any cold sores (fever blisters)? . . . . No _____ Yes _____
   d. Any lumps in your neck, armpits or groin? . . . . No _____ Yes _____
   e. Do you ever have chills or sweat at night? . . . . No _____ Yes _____

24. Have you traveled out of the country in the last 2 years? . . . . No _____ Yes, Traveled in: _____

25. Write in the dates for the shots you have had: . . . .
   Measles _____ Smallpox _____
   Mumps _____ Tetanus _____
   Polio _____ Typhoid _____

26. Have you had a tuberculin (TB) skin test? . . . . No _____ Yes _____ Date _____
   If so, was it negative or positive? . . . . Neg _____ Pos _____
27. Have you had an HIV test for AIDS? . . . . No _____ Yes _____ Date _____
   If so, was it negative or positive? . . . . Neg _____ Pos _____

© 1979, 1983 Bibbero Systems International, Inc.   __PLEASE TURN THIS PAGE__   STOCK NO. 19-742-4 __8/95__   __Page 3__

FIGURE 9.3, cont'd

For legend see p. 223.

REMOVE THIS PAGE AFTER COMPLETING QUESTIONNAIRE

CONFIDENTIAL

VISION / HEARING

28.	Do you wear eyeglasses?	No_____	Yes_____	Wears eyeglasses
29.	Do you wear contact lenses?	No_____	Yes_____	Wears contacts
30.	Has your vision changed in the last year?	No_____	Yes_____	Vision changes in last year

		Rarely/ Never	Occasionally	Frequently	
31.	How often do you have:				
a.	Double vision?	_____	_____	_____	Double vision
b.	Blurry vision?	_____	_____	_____	Blurred vision
c.	Watery or itchy eyes?	_____	_____	_____	Watery/itchy eyes
32.	Do you ever see colored rings around lights?	_____	_____	_____	Sees halos
33.	Do others tell you you have a hearing problem?	_____	_____	_____	Hearing problem
34.	Do you have trouble keeping your balance?	_____	_____	_____	Loses balance
35.	Do you have any discharge from your ears?	_____	_____	_____	Discharge from ears
36.	Do you ever feel dizzy or have motion sickness?	_____	_____	_____	Dizzy / motion sickness
37.	Do you have any problems with your hearing?	No_____	Yes_____ Hearing Problems		
38.	Do you ever have ringing in your ears?	No_____	Yes_____ Ringing in ears		

NOSE / THROAT / RESPIRATORY

		Rarely/ Never	Occasionally	Frequently	
39.	How often do you have:				
a.	Head colds?	_____	_____	_____	Head colds
b.	Chest colds?	_____	_____	_____	Chest colds
c.	Runny nose?	_____	_____	_____	Runny nose
d.	Stuffed up nose?	_____	_____	_____	Head congestion
e.	Sore/hoarse throat?	_____	_____	_____	Sore / hoarse throat
f.	Bad coughing spells?	_____	_____	_____	Coughing spells
g.	Sneezing spells?	_____	_____	_____	Sneezing spells
h.	Trouble breathing?	_____	_____	_____	Trouble breathing
i.	Nose bleeds?	_____	_____	_____	Nose bleeds
j.	Cough blood?	_____	_____	_____	Cough blood
40.	Have you ever worked or spent time:				
a.	On a farm?	No_____	Yes_____	Worked on a farm	
b.	In a mine?	No_____	Yes_____	Worked in a mine	
c.	In a laundry or mill?	No_____	Yes_____	Worked in a laundry/mill	
d.	In very dusty places?	No_____	Yes_____	Worked in high dust concentrations	
e.	With or near toxic chemicals?	No_____	Yes_____	Exposed to toxic chemicals	
f.	With or near radioactive materials?	No_____	Yes_____	Exposed to radioactive materials	
g.	With or near asbestos?	No_____	Yes_____	Exposed to asbestos	

CARDIOVASCULAR

		Rarely/ Never	Occasionally	Frequently	
41.	Do you get out of breath easily when you are active (like climbing stairs)?	_____	_____	_____	Out of breath quickly when exercising
42.	Do you ever feel light-headed or dizzy?	_____	_____	_____	Dizziness
43.	Have you ever fainted or passed out?	_____	_____	_____	Fainted
44.	Do you sometimes feel your heart is racing or beating too fast?	_____	_____	_____	Rapid heartbeat
45.	When you exercise do you ever get pains in your chest or shoulders?	_____	_____	_____	Chest/shoulder pains in exercise
46.	Do you have any leg cramps or pain in your thighs or legs when walking?	_____	_____	_____	Pain in thighs or legs when walking
47.	Do you ever have to sit up at night to breathe easier?	_____	_____	_____	Sits up at night to breathe easier
48.	Do you use two pillows at night to help you breathe easier?	_____	_____	_____	Breathing problems during sleep
49.	Would you say you are a restless sleeper?	_____	_____	_____	Restless sleeper
50.	Are you bothered by leg cramps at night?	_____	_____	_____	Leg cramps at night
51.	Do you sometimes have swollen ankles or feet?	_____	_____	_____	Swollen ankles/feet

DIGESTIVE

		Rarely/ Never	Occasionally	Frequently	
52.	How often, if ever:				
a.	Are you nauseated (sick to your stomach)?	_____	_____	_____	Nauseated
b.	Do you have stomach pains?	_____	_____	_____	Stomach pains
c.	Do you burp a lot after eating?	_____	_____	_____	Burps after eating
d.	Do you have heartburn?	_____	_____	_____	Heartburn
e.	Do you have trouble swallowing your food?	_____	_____	_____	Trouble swallowing food
f.	Have you vomited blood?	_____	_____	_____	Vomited blood
g.	Are you constipated?	_____	_____	_____	Constipated
h.	Do you have diarrhea (watery stools)?	_____	_____	_____	Diarrhea
i.	Are your bowel movements painful?	_____	_____	_____	Painful bowel movements
j.	Are your bowel movements bloody?	_____	_____	_____	Bloody bowel movements
k.	Are your bowel movements dark or black?	_____	_____	_____	Dark bowel movements
53.	Have you ever had a sigmoidoscopy?	No_____	Yes_____ Date_____		Date of last sigmoidoscopy?

PLEASE TURN TO BACK PAGE AND COMPLETE QUESTIONS ON NUTRITION.

© 1979, 1983 Bibbero Systems International, Inc.

FIGURE 9.3, cont'd

For legend see p. 223.

Andrus/Clini-Rec®

BIBBERO SYSTEMS, INC.

COMPREHENSIVE PHYSICAL EXAMINATION
MALE OR FEMALE
NEW OR ESTABLISHED PATIENT
CPT # 99201 - 99215

(For Office Use Only)

	TODAY'S DATE _____
NAME _____ AGE _____ YRS. OLD	DATE OF BIRTH _____

Key: [O] Neg. Findings [+] Positive Findings [X] Omitted [✔] See Notes/CIRCLE WORDS OF IMPORTANCE & EXPLAIN

C O N F I D E N T I A L

#			
1	GEN. APPEARANCE	[ ]	Apparent Age/Nutrition/Development/Mental & Emotional Status/Gait/Posture/Distress/Speech –
2	HEAD / SCALP	[ ]	Size/Shape/Tender over Sinuses/Hair/Alopecia/Eruption/Masses/Bruit –
3	EYES	[ ]	Conjunct/Sclerae/Cornea/Pupils/EOM'S/Arcus/Ptosis/Fundi/Tension/Eyelids/Pallor/Light/Bruit –
4	EARS	[ ]	Ext. Canal/TM's/Perforation/Discharge/Tophi/Hearing Problem/Weber/Rinne –
5	NOSE / SINUSES	[ ]	Septum/Obstruction/Turbinates/Discharge –
6	MOUTH / THROAT	[ ]	Odor/Lips/Tongue/Tonsils/Teeth/Dentures/Gums/Pharynx –
7	NECK	[ ]	Adenopathy/Thyroid/Carotids/Trachea/Veins/Masses/Spine/Motion/Bruit –
8	BACK	[ ]	Kyphosis/Scoliosis/Lordosis/Mobility/CVA/Bone/Tenderness –
9	THORAX	[ ]	Symmetry/Movement/Contour/Tender –
10	BREASTS	[ ]	Size/Size-Consistency/Nipples/Areolar/Palpable Mass/Discharge/Tenderness/Nodes/Scars –
11	HEART	[ ]	Rate/Rhythm/Apical Impulse/Thrills/Quality of Sound/Intensity/Splitting/Extra Sounds/Murmurs –
12	CHEST / LUNGS	[ ]	Excursion/Dullness or Hyperresonance to Percussion/Quality of Breath Sounds/Rales/Wheezing/Rhonchi/Diaphragm/Rubs/Bruit –
13	ABDOMEN	[ ]	Bowel Sounds/Appearance/Liver/Spleen/Masses/Hernias/Murmurs/Contour/Tenderness/Bruit/ING Nodes –
14	GROIN	[ ]	Hernia/Inguinal Nodes/Femoral Pulses –
15	MALE GENITALIA	[ ]	Penis/Testes/Scrotum Epididymis/Varicocele/Scars/Discharge –
16	FEMALE GENITALIA	[ ]	Vuvla/Vagina/Cervix/Uterus/Adnexae/Rectocele/Cystocele/Bartholin Gland/Urethra/Discharge – Pap Smear (if done ✔) ☐
17	EXTREMITIES	[ ]	Deformity/Clubbing/Cyanosis/Edema/Nails/Peripheral Pulses/Calf Tenderness/Joints for Swelling/ROM –
18	SKIN	[ ]	Color/Birthmarks/Scars/Texture/Rash/Eczema/Ulcers –
19	NEUROLOGICAL	[ ]	DTR's/Babinski/Cranial Nerves/Motor Abnormalities/Tremor/Paralysis/Sensory Exam – (touch, pin prick, vibration)/Coordination/Romberg –
20	MUSCULAR SYSTEM	[ ]	Strength/Wasting/Development –
21	RECTAL EXAM	[ ]	Sphincter Tone/Hemorrhoids/Fissures/Masses/Prostate/Stool Guaiac (if done ✔) ☐ Pos ☐ Neg –

Impression: ☐ Check If Normal Physical Examination

Summary: _____

_____

Signature _____ Date _____

Page 4   © 1979, 1983 Bibbero Systems International, Inc.

FIGURE   9.3, cont'd

For legend see p. 223.

Body Area Number	REMARKS:	PHYSICIAN'S NOTES:

C O N F I D E N T I A L

R   L   L   R

R   L

HEIGHT_____	**VISION**	**AUDIOMETRIC TESTING**	**BLOOD PRESSURE**

VISION

Without Glasses

Far   R ^{20}/   L ^{20}/

Near   R ^{20}/   L ^{20}/

HEIGHT_____

WEIGHT_____

With Glasses

R ^{20}/   L ^{20}/

R ^{20}/   L ^{20}/

BUILD_____

PULSE_____

Tonometry R_____ L_____

RESP._____

Colorvision_____

TEMP._____

Peripheral Fields R_____ L_____

AUDIOMETRIC TESTING

	250	500	1000
R	____	____	____
L	____	____	____
	2000	4000	8000
R	____	____	____
L	____	____	____

Gross Hearing _____

BLOOD PRESSURE

Sitting

R   /   L   /

Standing

R   /   L   /

Lying

R   /   L   /

Diagnostic Test:	Results:

The space below is provided for additional information when these data are being forwarded to a hospital, insurance company, a referral physician, etc.

Significant Comments/Recommendations:

_____

_____

_____

Physician's Name _____

Address _____

_____

Telephone (area code) _____

FIGURE 9.3, cont'd

For legend see p. 223.

NUTRITION AND DIET

1. How many meals do you eat each day? .... _____ <u>Meals each day</u>
2. Do you usually eat breakfast? .... ☐ No ☐ Yes <u>Breakfast</u>
3. Do you diet frequently and/or are you now dieting? .... ☐ No ☐ Yes <u>Diets</u>
4. Do you consider yourself .... ☐ Underweight ☐ Overweight ☐ Just right? <u>Weight</u>
5. Do you snack? .... ☐ More than once a day ☐ Usually daily ☐ Rarely? <u>Snacks</u>
6. Do you add salt to your food at the table? ..... ☐ Almost always ☐ Sometimes ☐ Rarely <u>Salts food</u>
7. Check the frequency you eat the following types of foods:

	More than once daily	Daily	3 times weekly	Once weekly	Twice monthly	Less or never
a. Whole grain or enriched bread or cereal						
b. Milk, cheese, or other dairy products						
c. Eggs						
d. Meat, Poultry, Fish						
e. Beans, Peas, or other legumes						
f. Citrus						
g. Dark green or deep yellow vegetables						

List any food supplements or vitamins you take regularly: _____

Additional Patient Comments: _____

_____

_____

_____

_____

_____

_____

Thanks for completing this questionnaire. Please review for skipped questions, sign your name on the space to the right and return it to the physician or assistant. If you wish to add any information, please write it in the spaces provided above.

Patient's Signature _____

Physician's Notes: _____

_____

_____

_____

_____

_____

CONFIDENTIAL

To order, call or write:
Bibbero Systems, Inc.
1300 N. McDowell Blvd., Petaluma, CA 94954-1180
Toll Free: 800-BIBBERO (800 242-2376)
  Or Fax: 800-242-9330
STOCK NO. 19-742-4   8/95

FIGURE 9.3, cont'd

For legend see p. 223.

WHAT DO YOU THINK?

John Ames was a regular patient of Joseph Burkes, M.D. He had several medical problems, including severe asthma and congestive heart failure with hypertension. He had an appointment with the doctor on Wednesday to have his blood pressure checked, but he missed his appointment and did not call. On Friday he called to say he was on his way to the emergency room because he could not breathe and needed immediate care. Mr. Ames died shortly after arriving at the emergency room. Several months later Dr. Burkes received a subpoena for a court hearing regarding Mr. Ames' medical care. When reviewing the medical record, the doctor found no reference to the Wednesday appointment or the Friday telephone call.

What charting problems have occurred here?

Is there anything that can be done to correct this?

Legal Considerations Regarding Entries

Unalterable

The entries in a medical record are unalterable. In other words, notes written in a patient's medical record cannot be changed or removed. If records are handwritten, all notations should be made in a neat and legible manner. If an error is found, a special technique should be used to correct it. This technique will be discussed later in this chapter.

Authorized Personnel

Because of the importance of the medical record, office policy should be established indicating which personnel are authorized to make entries in a patient's record. As an administrative medical assistant you undoubtedly will be responsible for medical records, including entry making. You must always keep in mind the importance of the medical record for patient care and for legal purposes.

Entries to be Avoided

A thoughtless comment in a patient's chart could give the impression that the physician is uninterested in the care or prejudiced in his or her opinion of the patient. This impression can influence the credibility of the physician and the quality of care provided, and cause legal problems for the physician. Humorous or sarcastic remarks should never be written in a patient's record.

Physicians and assistants also should take care not to attempt to describe another physician's findings or treatments. Information provided by the patient can be enclosed in quotation marks to indicate the source. If more information is required, the patient can sign a records release so that the other physician's records can be acquired.

Organization of the Medical Record

Each office will develop a procedure for the organization of a medical record that suits the needs of the personnel working with the record and the personal preference of the physician. Many prefer to divide the chart into subsections: physician's notes, diagnostic and hospital records, correspondence, and insur-

MEDICAL CHART ORGANIZATION

Left Side
- List of medications
- Prescriptions and renewals
- Telephone messages and disposition

Right Side
- Progress notes
- X-ray reports
- Laboratory results
- EKGs, EEGs, and so on

MEDICAL ASSISTING STEP-BY-STEP

Styles of Progress Notes

Physicians have different preferences for writing style in the patient records (charts). The two most common are as follows:
1. Narrative—is the oldest method. After the administrative medical assistant writes in the date, chief complaint, and vital signs, the physician notes what was wrong with the patient, his or her examination findings, and what treatment he or she is using.
2. SOAP—is used with a problem-oriented medical record and means Subjective, Objective, Assessment, and Plan. Subjective is what the patient says is wrong; objective is what is seen in the examination of the patient, including vital signs and tests. Assessment is the physician's impression of what is wrong with the patient, and plan is what is going to be done for the patient, that is, medication, special tests, referrals, return in 10 days, and so on.

ance forms (see the box about medical chart organization). Each subsection is maintained in chronological order and secured with metal clips attached to the chart. Staples should be avoided because of the damage they cause to individual sheets when they are removed or replaced to add new information.

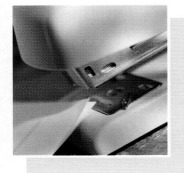

Physician's Notes

The physician's notes begin with the information history and initial evaluation. Subsequent visits are noted on sheets called *progress notes*. The notes are stamped with the date of each visit. Most physicians prefer that progress notes, the first section encountered when the chart cover is opened, be maintained in reverse chronological order, with the sheet describing the most recent visit on top and the oldest entry on the bottom. This avoids having to turn multiple sheets to locate the space to begin notations for the present visit. Usually the cover for this section will have space for a record of current medications.

Diagnostic and Hospital Records

The next section in the medical record contains diagnostic studies. This section frequently is referred to by the physician for monitoring the patient's condition or progress and in discussions with patients regarding their care. Diagnostic reports usually are stored in reverse chronological order, with the most recently dated report on top. Some common subsections are as follows:

- Progress notes
- Consultations
- Laboratory reports
- X-ray reports
- Operative reports
- Correspondence
- Prescriptions and medications

Correspondence

The correspondence section contains letters and narrative reports from physicians or facilities that previously have provided care for the patient. Correspondence from the patient also can be included in this section. Patients often send the physician cards from vacation spots or announcements of special events in their lives. Retaining these items in the record will serve as a reminder for the physician to mention the greeting or event during the patient's next visit.

Insurance Forms

The fourth section of the patient's record contains copies of insurance forms prepared by the administrative medical assistant. It is particularly important to retain copies of Medicare and Medicaid forms (if you do not have a computer), which might be subject to inspection and are necessary for documentation of services. Some offices store insurance forms in separate chronological files, by date of service. If you need to compare the patient's record with the insurance form, you will have to retrieve information from two sources.

Medical Record Applications and Personal Computers

Technology to maintain medical records has leapt forward dramatically since 1992. The federal government, through the Health Care Financing Administration (HCFA), has indicated that medical offices and facilities must be able to transmit medical records electronically by the year 2000, with every practice having that availability by the year 2005. In 1995 the Committee of XII was appointed to set the standards for medical record transmission under federal guidelines of the American National Standards Institute (ANSI). In light of the ANSI directive, a significant number of programs are available and will make the necessary program changes to comply with ANSI guidelines. Almost every system designed for medical billing either is developing a program or is purchasing a program that will be compatible with the billing programs in order to adhere to government guidelines. One of the ANSI guidelines currently in place is the directive that the chart must be legible. If the chart is not legible and the physician's accounts are audited by Medicare, Medicaid, or any other

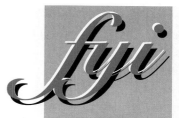

Separate Information/Charts

The following types of information should not be filed in a patient's regular medical record:

1. **Worker's Compensation cases** —should have a separate record since they will be billed and handled differently.

2. **Patient's records from another source**—these records may come from another physician or hospital/urgent care office. They may be added if the physician reviews them and decides to add them to the patient's regular medical record.

3. **Consulting physician's reports**—should not be included unless they have been reviewed and are consistent with the regular chart or differences are justified.

4. **HIV/drug or alcohol reports**—some state laws mandate that such information be kept separate.

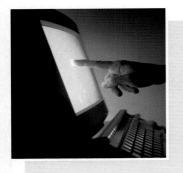

government-subsidized health care program, the auditors can demand that the reimbursement made to the physician for that patient must be returned to the government program from which it came.

Touch Programs

One highly developed computer program uses a touch screen. The patient is placed in front of the computer; the program then asks the patient a series of questions pertaining to patient history, family history, a particular surgery, or a procedure that the patient is about to have performed. The patient has only to press his or her finger to the screen and choose from among a variety of answers the one the best fits him or her. When the patient has completed all questions (in some instances the patient may press, "I don't know" or "I don't understand"), the program then produces a printed report of the questionnaire and the answers for the patient to review. The program also enters this information into the patient's medical record. At the same time, the program produces for the physician a list of questions or indicates areas in which the patient needs further explanation regarding the information requested. The physician then may use the visit time to the greatest advantage. The physician also may dictate directly into the computer for further charting.

Voice-Activated Systems

With the voice-activated system, the monitor (CRT) is placed in an examination room, and the clinical medical assistant then brings up on the screen the record of the patient's last visit. The patient's complete chart is available to the physician on the computer. As he or she examines the patient, spoken information is transmitted directly into the computer and added immediately to the record. The chart therefore is kept completely up to date, without the need for later dictation by the physician. The physician can turn off the voice controller and instead make notes for later dictation, although doing so can cause a delay in charting.

Direct Input Systems

Direct input systems have been developed by specialty and are customized toward the physician's dictation patterns. These systems usually review with the physician their previous methods of charting, their normal speech patterns, phrases they frequently use, and then customize the program around those areas and by specialty. When the physician finishes examining a patient, he or she has only to step into the consultation room, select the patient by name or account number from the fee slip (Superbill), select the phrases that best suit the patient, and fill in the blanks with that patient's information. This allows for immediate update of the chart without delay of dictation. The physician also may request a printed record to review for accuracy.

Scanning Systems

The scanner system is able to scan typed records into a file for electronic transmission. Many of these systems also attempt to scan the physician's handwritten notes from previous records for inclusion in the complete patient chart stored in the computer system. Because the handwriting of physicians often is

FOCUS ON THE WORKPLACE

Altered Records?

The plaintiff was seen by a physician for a blocked tear duct. During treatment, an instrument brushed her cornea and caused abrasions. After the incident, the plaintiff's daughter (a nurse), requested permission to review the patient's medical records. After seeing the records, the plaintiff filed a suit against the physician. At the trial, the daughter testified that her mother's records, which she had reviewed at the physician's office, had been altered by the time they were admitted for evidence. It also was noted that an office visit after the accident was not recorded in the record.

The court ruled that altered records create a presumption of negligence.

James v. Spear, 338 P. 2d 22, (Cal. 1959).

difficult to read, a number of problems with this type of record review and transfer to the electronic chart have occurred.

Deletions and Corrections of Medical Records

Deletions

Deletions are sometimes made in medical records at the direction of the physician in an effort to keep the chart as concise and orderly as possible and to reduce the overall storage space required for medical records.

Only the physician should decide what specific material may be deleted from an office medical record. Medical assistants should never take it upon themselves to make such a decision, even if an exact duplicate of a report already is in the record. The physician should always be consulted for items not discussed in the policy manual.

It is recommended by most medical associations that documents removed from patient charts either be microfilmed or retained in a permanent storage area.

Delegated Staff Actions

Once a decision has been made on what material may be deleted, the physician may designate certain staff members to complete the procedure. Usually this will be the administrative medical assistant. Should the physician decide to complete the task personally, the assistant should not take it negatively. Most physicians are rightfully very cautious with records because of their legal importance and because the physician is ultimately responsible for the contents and condition of the record.

Typical Material Deleted

The material that may be safely deleted with the physician's approval from the medical record includes the following:

- Duplicates of diagnostic studies
- Hospital studies over 3 years old (the hospital will have the originals if needed) that show normal findings; retain any report of abnormal findings
- Insurance forms over 7 years old

Individual progress notes or pages of notes should never be deleted from a medical record. Entry errors may be corrected as described later in this chapter.

Protecting Confidentiality

Extreme care must be taken to make sure that material removed from the patient's chart is disposed of properly. No one should be able to discern the patient's name or connect the name with a report when it is discarded. The best method is to destroy the document by burning or shredding. The other option is to tear the document carefully into very small pieces. For the correct procedure for discarding data from a chart, refer to the office procedures manual.

Corrections

Reasons For Corrections

Occasionally it is necessary to make a correction in the progress notes of a patient's record. This occurs when incorrect data are recorded in the patient's record or an entry is made in the wrong chart. Incorrect data might be discovered while, for example, recording a patient's weight as 103 pounds and noting that it was recorded as 156 pounds on a previous visit. One of the notations probably is incorrect. The fact should be rechecked, and the entry corrected. Data can be recorded in the wrong chart if, for example, you have several charts in your hands at one time and inadvertently make an entry intended for the chart of one patient in the progress notes of another. Again, a correction is in order.

Correction Technique

Information noted in the chart, whether factual or not, becomes part of the permanent record. You must never attempt to obliterate a chart entry. If an error in charting is discovered you should:

1. Strike a single line through the error.
2. Date and initial the strikeout.
3. If the problem is incorrect data, enter the corrected information directly below the strikeout.
4. If the entry is made in the wrong chart, follow step 1 and note, "Recorded in chart by error. Information transferred to chart of John C. Adams."
5. Date and sign the strikeout and explanation. Step 4 is vital for legal purposes, because it can be verified. It is not considered a breach of confidentiality.

Maintenance of Medical Records

One of the greatest problems in medical offices is keeping the records up to date. Medical records must be constantly and methodically kept current. It is the responsibility of the administrative medical assistant to see that this is done.

Reports, case histories, consultations, and laboratory results may accumulate on the physician's or medical assistant's desk during each day (Figure 9.4). After the last patient has left, check each record to ascertain that all necessary

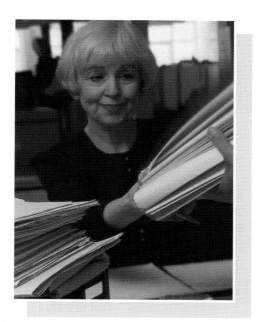

FIGURE 9.4

Reports, case histories, consultations, and laboratory results may accumulate on the physician's or medical assistant's desk during each day.

information has been recorded for that visit and that each entry is sufficiently clear for future understanding. Give the physician all extra reports, such as laboratory and x-ray, to be reviewed and initialed. After the physician's review, the reports will be filed in the patients' charts.

While the physician is reviewing these reports, you should pull the charts of those patients the physician has seen outside of the office that day (such as nursing home or hospital patients). You also should pull the charts of patients who were provided with telephone instructions or prescriptions; however, it is to your advantage to pull the charts while the patients are on the telephone and record the information immediately rather than waiting until the evening. This may be handled by either front office or back office personnel.

After all records have been reviewed, they should be placed in a file tray and locked away for overnight, if you do not have time for filing on the same day. Do not leave medical information of any sort on the desks overnight.

The physician may prefer to dictate all progress notes, rather than write in longhand. Many offices have an outside service for transcription. As soon as the dictation has been returned to the practice, have the information reviewed by the physician before filing in the chart.

The medical assistant should continually attempt to maintain and improve medical records management. One should evaluate the efficiency of the filing system annually. Many times inactive charts remain in the active section too long when they should be purged to increase filing space. One easy way to spot charts that need to be purged is to use special tabs that are placed on the chart the year the patient first comes to the office. Once a year you can review your charts and immediately identify the charts of patients who have not been to the practice for 2 or 3 years. These charts should be pulled, a notice for a checkup sent to the patient, and the charts boxed and held in the office for approximately 2 weeks. If the patient has forgotten to come in for a checkup, this may remind him or her to make an appointment before the chart is sent to storage.

Transfer and Retention of Medical Records

Each office must establish a policy regarding when a record should be considered inactive and transferred to storage. In most situations this will depend on:

- Age of the chart (date since last visit)
- Type of practice
- Space available in the "active" filing cabinets

Many offices find that 2 to 3 years since the last visit is an appropriate time span for considering a record for storage. The other two factors are strictly individual. Closed charts should be transferred within 6 months. Closed charts include those of:

- Patients who have died
- Patients who have moved away and did not request their chart
- Patients who have otherwise terminated their relationship with the physician

When a chart is transferred to inactive status, it may be stored on the premises or at some other location. In either case a list of inactive charts should be retained in the office to avoid unnecessary searching. A small file box containing 3 × 5 cards is an easy technique of noting inactive charts, since the cards can be easily alphabetized when new names are added. Another method is to set up a file in the word processor. In this manner you may add patient names, and show the storage unit in which the chart is filed. This is a particularly nice system when the practice must utilize more than one storage unit.

Period of Records Retention

Debates continue about the amount of time records should be retained after certain events. These events include the following:

- Treatment of a minor
- Closure of a case
- Death of a patient
- Retirement of the physician
- Death of the physician

Opinions vary from one state to another. Attorneys, medical associations, and management consultants also have varied opinions regarding the period of retention.

When care involves a minor, the record should always be kept at least until the patient is 21 years old, and thereafter until the local statute of limitations runs out.

Closure of a case, as in a specialist's care, may warrant destroying a chart after a given time period. Most agree that the chart should be retained for at least 10 years.

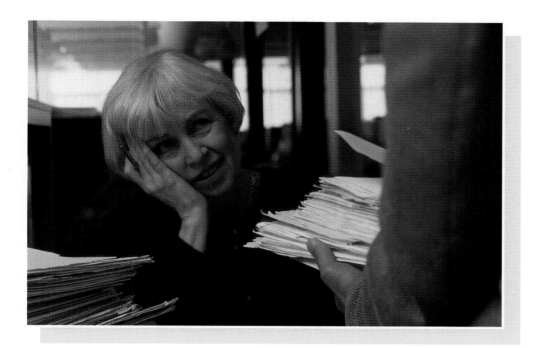

FIGURE 9.5

Because of the frequency of professional liability suits and variations in state statutes, the only safe option for records retention is to retain them forever.

After the uncomplicated death of a patient, some professionals suggest that the chart be retained through the statute of limitations and then destroyed.

In the event of a physician's retirement, the charts of deceased patients may be destroyed after a selected time period following the death and following appropriate notification of the next of kin. The records of living patients may be transferred to the physician continuing the practice or to a physician of the patient's choice on receipt of written authorization.

On the death of a physician, the patient's records are put under the care of a custodian of records, who often is the physician's spouse or a former employee who is willing to perform the duties involved. The disposition of the records is similar to the method that follows a physician's retirement.

General Advice

Because of the increasing frequency of professional liability suits and the variations in statutes, many authorities are beginning to agree that the only safe option for records retention is to retain them forever (Figure 9.5). In other words, medical records should never be destroyed. If the physician retires or dies, the requested records should be forwarded to the physician of the patient's designation, and the others retained by the physician or his or her estate. Sometimes the practice will be sold; in this instance, the charts stay with the practice or are transferred to the physician of the patient's choice.

Storage Sites

Inactive records may be stored in specifically designed file boxes in a storage area on the office premises, with a professional storage company, or on microfilm. Storage on the premises is the ideal option for an active practice, because inactive records may be needed from time to time. Professional storage facilities are appropriate if the physician has retired or died, but this option causes retrieval problems for an active practice. Microfilm is an ideal option from the perspective of saving space, but it is relatively expensive.

Medical Record Protection

Records Temporarily Out of File

The common reasons for taking a record out of the filing cabinet and the methods of monitoring its whereabouts using OUTguides are discussed in Chapter 10. However, you must protect and pay particular attention to medical records that are out of the office because they were subpoenaed. If you must send a record out, be certain to photocopy at least the doctor's notes, since they can never be replaced.

Most subpoena services are prepared to microfilm a record in your medical office, although they may not volunteer the option. You should ask if it is possible, particularly for a sizable record. You then avoid the possibility of losing the record in the mail and the additional cost of photocopying.

Keep a record of charts that must be sent out, the date they are sent, and to whom they are sent. If the chart has not been returned within 10 days, contact the subpoena service and ask them to locate the record and notify you regarding when it will be returned.

After-Office Hours

At the end of each day all possible records should be returned to the filing cabinet for security purposes. As you leave the office, the cabinets should be closed and, if possible, locked. This will prevent scrutiny by maintenance-service personnel and may preserve them in case of fire.

Records Removed by Physician

When the physician removes a group of records from the file to take them home to work on, the resulting problems can be disastrous (Figure 9.6). The physician runs the risk of having the records stolen from his or her vehicle; accidently dropping them, resulting in papers being scattered or destroyed (particularly if it is a windy or rainy day); or leaving them at home when the patient is due into the office. All malpractice carriers advise physicians to never remove medical records from the office.

Destruction of Medical Records

As previously discussed, each state has a statute of limitations regarding how long to keep medical records. You may destroy records as stated earlier after checking with the physician's malpractice carrier and attorney.

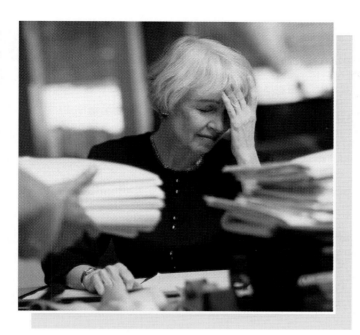

FIGURE 9.6

When the physician removes a group of records from the office, the resulting problems can be disastrous.

Informal Record Systems

Medical assistants usually develop informal record systems to help them efficiently accomplish their varied responsibilities.

Master Calendars

A master calendar, usually one that displays a month at a glance, allows you to list well in advance items and events that recur annually or on the same date every month. You may then preplan the time necessary to deal with the events and assist the physician with notification of upcoming financial needs. The categories and the items included in master calendars are presented in Table 9.1. This list demonstrates the integration of various duties.

Tickler Files

The common term for a file system designed to remind you of patients or events that require follow-up is a *tickler file.* The tickler file may take various forms, but it is always organized in chronological order.

Many times the office will maintain a small file box containing 3 x 5 cards and dividers for each month. At the beginning of each month, the cards in that section are pulled out, and the necessary action is taken. Each card will contain a separate activity or patient's name and the reason the card is in the file. Most often the cards are used to recall patients for routine examinations, such as physical examinations or annual Pap smears. You can notify the patient by telephone or mail. Once the appointment is made, the card may be inserted behind the divider for the same month next year.

TABLE 9-1

Common Items on a Master Calendar

Insurance premiums due	Routine payments	Renewal dates	Tax dates	Meetings	Holidays
Property	Salaries	Medical licenses	Federal tax deposits	Annual conventions	Traditional holidays
Life/health	Rent Janitorial services	Narcotics licenses	State & federal quarter taxes	Committees	Religious holidays
Professional liability	Leased equipment	Association membership	Annual state and federal taxes (4/15)		Legal holidays
Disability	Laundry service Medical-surgical supplies	Subscriptions			

FIGURE 9.7

A small file box or desk calendar may be used to recall and notify patients of examinations.

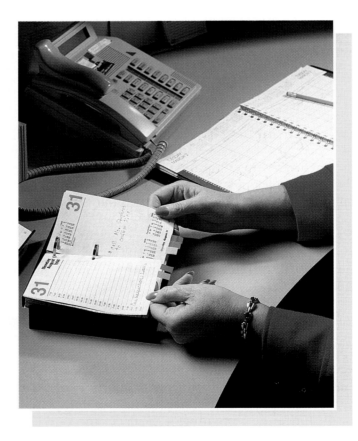

Some administrative medical assistants prefer to maintain this information on their computer or with the computerized date book. This allows them to access the event files, and have the dates of the events, contact person, and telephone numbers available. Most medical billing systems also will maintain the tickler file for recalls to patients. They will print a message to the patient regarding the need and reason, such as an annual examination or Pap smear, for a visit. The computerized system will provide the assistant with a top sheet that is not mailed but can be used to call the patient and remind him or her of the appointment.

A desk calendar (Figure 9.7) also may be used as a tickler file. This can work quite well if you are able to accomplish all the items noted on a given day. If not, you must take time to rewrite them on a subsequent day.

Medical Correspondence Not Related to Patients

Every office receives a certain amount of correspondence that is medical in nature but unrelated to individual patients. This correspondence can be stored by subject in separate folders for ready access. Materials that you will receive could be classified under the following headings:

- Professional associations
- Physician's personal file (correspondence with friends and colleagues)
- General medical information such as U.S. Food and Drug Administration bulletins, drug company bulletins, and statistics on communicable disease
- Business correspondence

Correspondence regarding the business operations of the office also needs to be retained in subject folders for future reference. These files might have the following titles:

- Rental agreements
- Leased equipment
- Maintenance contracts
- Individual folders for each major supplier

The permanent financial records must be stored in a secure and safe location, preferably a fireproof cabinet. These records include the following:

- Checks
- Bank statements
- Accounting ledgers
- Bank deposit receipts
- Patient account records

If these items have been used during the course of the day, they should be returned to their storage site before the office is closed.

Physician's Personal Records

Monitoring the physician's personal records generally is not your responsibility, but you may be asked to maintain a master list of the storage location of certain items such as the following:

- Wills
- Property deeds
- Insurance policies
- Contracts

Most commonly these are stored in bank safety-deposit boxes.

Conclusion

The importance of a systematic approach to records management cannot be overly stressed. Records provide documentation for all medical care provided and for all business transactions. Your role is fundamental to the development and maintenance of an effective and efficient records management system.

Review QUESTIONS

1. What are the five major purposes for maintaining an organized records management system?

2. What options do you have when registering a new patient? What information do you collect?

3. How would you organize the physician's notes in the medical record? How would you organize the diagnostic and hospital reports, correspondence, and insurance forms?

4. Who may decide what material to delete from a record? What material usually can be deleted?

5. What actions would you take to protect medical records temporarily out of the filing cabinet, after hours, and when transferring files to inactive status?

6. How long should a medical record be retained? How can it be stored?

SUGGESTED READINGS

Anderson BH: *Review for medical records administration,* 1996, Delmar.
Chute J: *Electronic medical records,* Brooklyn, NY, 1998, Springer-Verlag.
McMiller K: *Being a medical records clerk,* New York, 1992, Prentice-Hall.
Roach W: *Medical records and the law,* Englewood Cliffs, NJ, 1993, Aspen.

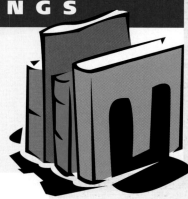

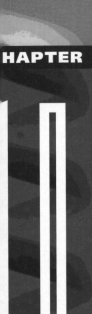

CHAPTER

11

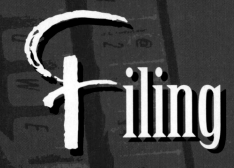

Filing

On completion of Chapter 10 the administrative medical assistant student should be able to:

1 Define the key terms listed in this chapter.

2 Assemble equipment and supplies to establish or update a filing system.

3 Prepare data for filing

4 Understand the advantages of an alphabetical filing system.

5 Establish a color-coded filing system.

6 Understand the rules for indexing.

K E Y   T E R M S

Alphabetical filing	An arrangement of names or documents in order according to the alphabet.
Chart	A specific type of file folder designed for use in the medical office.
Divider guide	Guides that divide the file cabinets into designated areas.
Label	Placed on the outside of each folder or chart for identification purposes.
OUTguides	A heavy guide that is used to replace a medical record that has been temporarily removed.

orrect filing is a must for every medical office. When information is filed incorrectly, data or charts cannot be found and the office practically comes to a standstill while everyone searches for the chart or information. It is essential in every office that the file clerk be interested in keeping the office organized and on schedule. Therefore the file clerk is one of the major team players.

Equipment and Supplies

Equipment

To maintain charts and files in an orderly manner, they must be properly identified and storage equipment must be sturdy, easily accessed, and secure. Medical records may be stored in various cabinet styles and types designed to protect them. Considerations that must be made in selecting filing equipment for the office are as follows:

- Available space
- Expense of space and equipment
- Size, type, and amount of records to be filed
- Confidential requirements
- Structural requirements
- Retrieval speed
- Fire protection

Although expense is a factor when considering which type or style of cabinets to use, the best quality will be the most economical in the long run.

Drawer Files

Drawer files within large, traditional filing cabinets are best used for filing personnel, personal, accounts payable, and other files that require a fireproof, secure system (Figure 10.1). This type of file should have full suspension; the file drawers should roll easily, close tightly, and have a locking device. These files require more space to allow the drawer to be pulled out to its full extension. Filing is slower because only one person can work in front of the file at a time.

Shelf Files

Shelf files need doors to protect the files. A common type of shelf file has doors that slide up and back into the cabinet; the door to the shelf below the drawer in which you are filing can be pulled out and used as a work space, increasing the amount of usable space by 100%. The shelf units hold files sideways and may be much taller, allowing for additional filing space because there are no drawers to pull out (Figure 10.2). Because several persons can work at the same time, file retrieval is much faster. You also may purchase open shelf files without doors; however, these files provide no protection or confidentiality for the records. Nor do they protect the files from fire or water damage. Shelf files

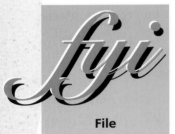

File

1. It is a folder for holding loose papers.
2. It is a set of papers kept in a folder.
3. In computing, it is a collection of data stored under one name.
4. It means to place something (for example, papers) in a file.
5. It means to classify or arrange (for example, papers).
6. It means a portfolio, a folder, a box, or a case.
7. It means to classify, organize, systematize, categorize, alphabetize, put in order, or arrange.

To the medical office, many of these words apply, but it is most important to learn to file accurately. Lost (misfiled) records can cause major problems in an office routine and ultimately an unhappy physician!

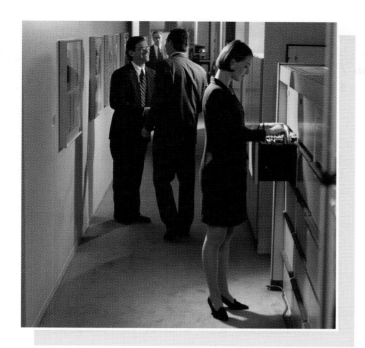

Drawer files within large traditional filing cabinets are best used for filing personnel, personal, accounts payable, and other files that require a fireproof, secure system.

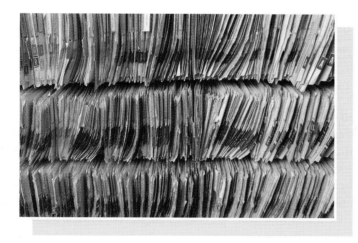

Shelf units hold files sideways; they allow for additional filing space because there are no drawers to pull out.

come in many attractive colors, and some have doors that are covered with fabric to complement the office decor.

Compactible Files

Compactible files are good for very small offices that require a significant amount of filing space. These files are a variation of the shelf files. The files are mounted on tracks in the floor, and the units slide along the tracks so that access is gained to the needed files. These types of cabinets may either be automated or manual. The only inconvenience is that the charts are not all available at the same time.

Lateral Files

Lateral files often are good for the physician's personal office since they provide lockable filing space and can be made of high-quality wood to match the physi-

AT WORK TODAY

File Cabinets

Most common
  Lateral files—with 2 to 3 drawers
  Floor-to-ceiling, open shelf files—with sliding doors that resemble bookcases. These types of files hold more material.
  Vertical files—upright with four or five drawers; a traditional file cabinet

Used in a larger setting (hospital/large clinic)
  Automated files—expensive but retrieve files for individual operators
  Rotary (circular) files—files are stored in units that spin or stack behind each other; offer maximum space utilization; are used in a large office or clinic

cian's office furniture and decor. They occupy more wall space than the vertical drawer but do not extend into the room as far. Files are positioned sideways in this type of file, left to right, instead of front to back as in a vertical or drawer file.

Rotary Circular Files

Rotary circular files will hold large volumes of records. They save space and revolve easily, usually with push-button controls. Another advantage is that several persons can file and use records at the same time. However, they afford less privacy and protection than files that can be closed and locked.

Automated Files

Automated files are extremely expensive and normally require more maintenance than do the other types of file cabinets. You usually will find this type of system in very large facilities or clinics. Automated files bring the files to the operator; when the operator presses a button indicating the proper shelf, the shelf automatically moves into position in front of the operator for file removal. The automated file is fast and can store many records in a small space. A disadvantage is that only one person may use the unit at a time.

Sorting Files

A sorting file can save a significant amount of time. Items that need to be filed, such as insurance forms, charts, and laboratory reports, are placed in the proper section of a portable file cart. This is a very handy tool to presort the filing for later.

Supplies

Guides/Dividers

Guides or dividers are available to assist you with rapid location and retrieval of records. They are available for alphabetical, numerical, geographical, and subject filing systems. Dividers allow you to subdivide major headings into segments of your choice. Dividers should be of good quality pressboard so that they may be used longer.

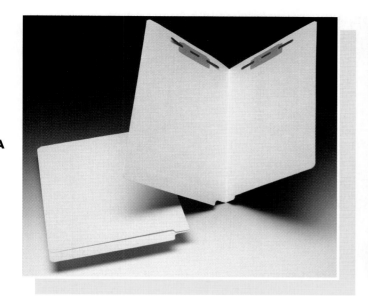

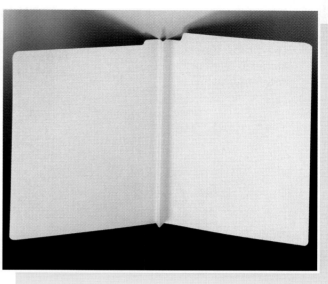

A

FIGURE 10.3

A, Chart folders. B, Manila folder. (Courtesy Bibberro Systems, Inc., Petaluma, Calif.)

OUTguides

An office with several employees and physicians find that time is lost each day attempting to locate charts that are being used in various areas within the office. Although the practice should be discouraged, it also is possible that a physician may take a chart out of the office to dictate a report or compare it with hospital records. OUTguides should be made of very firm paper in the shape of a chart cover or an actual folder and left in place of the record that was removed from the files. There are several types of OUTguides to choose from; some have pre-lined spaces to note the file name, date removed, name of person who removed file, and location to which the file was taken. OUTguides may be made of very firm pressboard and may have a plastic pocket for inserting an information card. They also may be made of plastic and have a plastic pocket. OUTguides should have a distinctive color so that the assistant can quickly spot which files are out. The chart then is easily located, saving the staff time and frustration.

Folders

Chart Folders. Chart folders come in various types (Figure 10.3, *A* and *B*). These folders can be customized to the type of practice, with inserts that separate the chart into sections for progress notes, X-ray reports, laboratory reports, history/physical, medication, insurance and correspondence, ECG strips, or whatever is most useful to the practice. They are designed with inside fasteners embedded or heat bonded to the chart in various places. They may have inside pockets for small notes from patients; some are designed so the entire chart does not have to be taken apart to file something in a particular area of the chart. These charts can be used in any number of ways. They also may be color

FIGURE **10.4**

Chart tabs. (Courtesy
Bibberro Systems, Inc.,
Petaluma, Calif.)

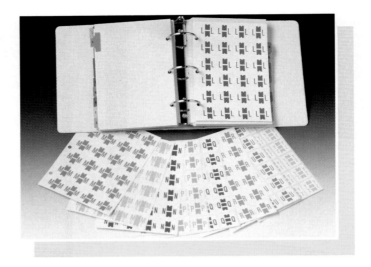

coded; for example, blue for patients with retinal problems and red for patients with cataracts.

Manila Folders. Manila folders are designed to store and protect the forms and documents of an individual's medical record. Each record is stored in a separate folder.

Folders are available in two basic styles: top-tab (used most conveniently in drawer-type filing) and side-tab (for the shelf-type cabinet). Either style folder is available with color-coded tabs (Figure 10.4). Color coding is discussed under alphabetical filing systems later in this chapter. There are many variations of folder styles available for special purposes.

Classification folders normally are used to file accounts payable and have headings such as "American Express (Corporate)," "Auto–Payments," "Auto–DMV," and "Auto–Repairs." These folders will designate those accounts for which regular payments are made.

OUTfolders. OUTfolders are used like the OUTguides and provide space for temporary filing of data. Hanging or suspension folders are used in drawer or lateral files. These folders are made from heavy paper, with tabs at the top, and hang on metal rods on the sides of the drawer. They may only be used with drawers equipped with suspension rods.

Labels

The label is a necessary tool for filing and finding data. Use labels to identify each shelf, drawer, divider, and folder.

Cabinet Labels. The doors of drawer and shelf-type filing cabinets have holders for cards that identify the contents. The card should indicate the range (alphabetical, numerical, or chronological) of the data filed in that drawer or shelf, for example, "Patient charts A–F," or "General Correspondence 1995–1997."

Folder Labels. A label must be affixed to the tab of each file folder. The label on the folder identifies only the items in that folder or that individual's name. You will need a label for each patient seen, business correspondence, or anything that needs to be filed.

Pregummed or self-adhesive labels may be purchased in almost any size, shape, or color to meet the needs of individual offices (Figure 10.4). Many

AT WORK TODAY

Paper Files vs. Computer Files

A paper file usually is a manila folder with side or top tabs (depending on lateral or vertical file system). In a medical office, it usually is letter-sized, and the outside cover often is used to inform the staff of drug reactions, allergies, and so on. Some offices color code their files to separate special problems such as those in the areas of ophthalmology or dermatology, or in a group practice to identify the physician who attends the patient.

A computer file is an electronic file containing all of the patient's information and would be part of an electronic management system. The file can be retrieved to the computer screen as needed, and information requests can be done quickly by requesting automatic printouts. Passwords can be used for security purposes. Computer files need to be backed up to a tape daily to preserve them in case of power or computer failure.

office supply companies are happy to send you a catalog to review the products that you will need for filing.

Chart labels are available on rolls or on sheets and may be self adhesive or pregummed. The name, with last name first, should be typed accurately on both sides of the label (typing the name on both sides of the label enables it to be read from either side of the file folder) before it is affixed to the tab.

Filing Systems

There are four basic filing systems:

- Alphabetical by name
- Numerical
- Geographical
- Subject

A fifth system of filing, chronological, is seldom used in the physician office. You may find that you will primarily use the alphabetical and numerical systems; however, physicians who serve in several cities or communities may wish to have records of patients located in those areas filed by location.

Alphabetical

The alphabetical filing system is the easiest and most commonly used system for organizing patients' records. Labeled folders are arranged in the same sequence as the letters of the alphabet. The filing cabinet is divided to accommodate each letter, and the divider guides also supply subdivisions for letters that typically include more charts than others. For example, you will notice that many charts appear in section A. Divider guides may be positioned for both the first and second letter of the last name at various intervals, for example, A, Ad, Al, and Ap. Other letters, such as I, O, and Z, usually do not hold many charts and are therefore not subdivided.

The alphabetical system of filing is the easiest to use in medical practice, because it is the most common and for many people the easiest method to learn. The one drawback to this system is in rapidly growing practices, in which many charts are added to each section, and space for each alphabetical section must be expanded periodically. This usually involves shifting all of the charts in the system to redistribute the space.

Color coding is the technique of using predetermined colors to assist in the rapid location of files and the avoidance of misfiling records. The selected colors may be incorporated into the folder tabs or, for reasons of economy, may be added by attaching labels edged in various colors to the tabs. The greatest advantage to color coding is the ease with which a misfiled chart can be located.

To initiate a color-coding system, first select the colors to be used and then determine the letters of the alphabet that will be represented by the various colors. Then apply your color-coding system to the second letter of the last name of each patient. Do not use the first letter because otherwise large sections of the cabinet would display the same color. By using the second letter you reduce the number of charts displaying each color in each section, and all the colors are repeated in each alphabetical segment.

Your color code reference card may read as follows:

If the second letter of the last name is:	The folder or label color is:	As in:
A, B, C, D	Blue	Kane Oben Eckhart Idor
E, F, G, H,	Red	Benson Ufus Agerman Chan
I, J, K, L, M	Green	Hines Bjorn Akerman Clayborn Emerson
N, O, P, Q	Yellow	Inorson Borden Epson Aquinas
R, S, T, U, V, W, X, Y, Z	Purple	Braverman Esterly Otter Pulver Aver Ewell Oxley Ayers Izuno

You can see that if you misfiled Inorson as Imorson, the chart with the yellow tab for the N would stand out against the green tabs, which represent M.

Color coding also can be used to indicate type of insurance, the patient's primary physician in a multiple-physician practice, or patients with certain diagnoses under study. The primary alphabetical color system remains unchanged, but the additional identification may be added with color-coded tabs for the

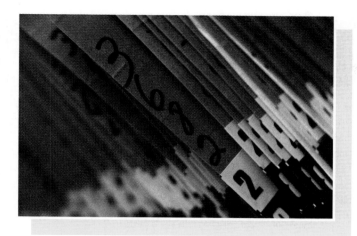

FIGURE 10.5

In numerical filing, materials are categorized first by number and second by an alphabetical cross-reference.

first two to three letters of the last name. Usually the color-coded tabs are reserved for use with the manila folder.

Any number of ready-made alphabetical filing systems are available (for example, Acme, Ames, Bibbero, Colwell, Remington Rand, TAB, and VisiRecord). Self-adhesive, color letter blocks with either two or three letters are supplied in rolls. The color blocks with the appropriate letter are placed on the index tab of the folder, along with the patient's full name. The letters are in pairs so they may be seen from either side of the chart. Using the different colors creates a band of color in the files, making it easy to spot a misfiled folder (Figure 10.4).

Numerical

In numerical filing, materials are categorized first by number and second by an alphabetical cross-reference (Figure 10.5). Each new patient is assigned a number in sequence; this may be the account number assigned by the computer billing system. A cross-reference is established after the number has been assigned. Either an index card or ledger card is arranged alphabetically and followed by the previously assigned numerical code. Office computers also can store and arrange this information for you. The advantages of the numerical system are its capacity for expansion without rearrangement of the cabinets (as in alphabetical filing) and clear identification of individuals with similar or identical names. You usually encounter this system in hospitals, large clinics, or group-practice.

Geographical

Filing according to the patient's place of residence is a technique normally used in major clinics or medical centers and must be cross-referenced by an alphabetical system. This system may be used in facilities wishing to gather statistical data or trying to locate a disease process within a geographical area. In recent years as more physicians have become "circuit riders," that is, seeing patients in as many as five to six locations per month, this system has proved helpful in quickly identifying the location for those patients. It is, in fact, a method more

AT WORK TODAY

Numerical Filing

Several filing systems are used to manage medical records. The alphabetical system is the most commonly used in smaller to middle-size offices. Numerical filing is an indirect system that becomes more practical when there are 10,000 to 15,000 charts as can be found in a multiphysician office or clinic.

Numerical filing require an alphabetical cross-reference (usually a 3 × 5 card filed alphabetically in a smaller vertical file box). It allows unlimited expansion of files without having to shift them continually, and it maintains privacy.

There are two types of numerical filing systems. In the consecutive system, individuals are assigned numbers as they become patients of the practice. The numbers are assigned consecutively. This is the simplest numerical system, but it does not work well after 10,000 files. In the terminal digit system, patients also are given consecutive numbers but the digits are separated into groups of twos or threes and are read in groups from right to left. Records are filed backward in groups.

Examples: 02 88 00
            00 70 01
            04 44 11
            01 65 20
            89 33 22
            90 33 22

You also can use middle-digit filing, in which you start with the middle digits, followed by the first digit, and finally by the terminal digit (the digit on the far right).

Numeric filing probably is harder to learn but if it is learned well, there will be fewer errors than with the alphabetical system and the errors can be found more easily.

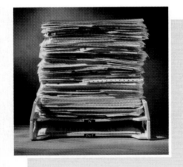

commonly used in business than in medicine. You will rarely encounter this system in medical practice.

Subject

Subject filing may be used for patient records as a cross-index if the physician is interested in gathering statistics on various disease processes. You will use subject filing in the business aspect of the practice for keeping information and correspondence in appropriate categories. Folders are prepared and labeled to store information on subjects such as equipment maintenance contracts, office policies, office procedures, worker's compensation injury reports, and so forth. These folders may be kept in a file drawer in the administrative assistant's desk for easy access.

Filing Procedures

Every item arriving in the office that pertains to a patient or to business must eventually be processed for filing. Approach this task in an orderly and systematic manner to limit the time involved and to ensure accurate disposition of the material.

A filing procedure usually includes the following steps:

• Examination
• Indexing

- Coding
- Sorting
- Storing

These steps should be carefully developed and then outlined in the office procedures manual.

Examining

When an item arrives at your desk for filing, you must first check for a predetermined indicator that it has been reviewed by the physician. This is particularly important for diagnostic reports and consultations that will require patient follow-up. The indicator to file often is the physician's initials in an agreed-upon location, such as the upper right-hand corner of the document.

You also will be reviewing business correspondence for filing. This may be initialed by the physician with instructions to follow before the document is stored, such as "check the cost of maintenance contract last year." You then will check for the information requested, attach it to the correspondence, and return the document to the physician. You will eventually receive it back with further instructions.

Any item ready for filing should be checked for unnecessary clips, staples, or tears in the document. Before processing, the clips and staples should be removed and the tears mended with tape to prevent further damage to the document.

Indexing

Indexing is a method of determining the destination of each document to be filed. Diagnostic studies usually arrive with the patient's name near the top of the record. Some correspondence may have a subject line (RE:) that will tell you the person or subject, but other correspondence may have information buried in the body of the document.

Coding

After determining the name or subject of a document, it must be highlighted in some manner. This activity is called *coding*. One method of coding is to write the indexing factor in the upper right-hand corner of the page; another is to circle or underline it where it appears in the document. Whatever method you choose you must use it consistently, since others responsible for sorting and storing the documents will depend on the code for guidance.

Sorting

The fourth step in a filing procedure is sorting, a method of subdividing the documents. Because most filing is associated with patients' records, which are typically filed alphabetically, the alphabetical method will be discussed here.

Sorting By Major Headings

The documents to be filed each day are first sorted by the first letter of the last name. This provides you with a crude series of major subheadings. If you have

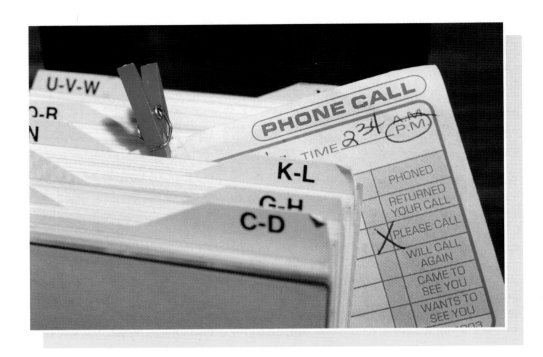

FIGURE 10.6

Commercial desk sorters have a series of sturdy dividers attached at one end and open at the other end, and are deep enough to hold many standard-size sheets of paper without obstructing the sorting tabs.

a large, private work area on which the documents can be placed in separate stacks alphabetically, you can accomplish your sorting in this manner. If space is limited, you may use a sorting aid (Figure 10.6). Commercial desk sorters are instruments that have a series of sturdy dividers attached at one end and that are open at the other end to allow you to insert your documents. The dividers are staggered, so that when the instrument is flat on the desk, each tab with the individual letter of the alphabet is visible. The effect is similar to the one you would see if you spread a deck of cards horizontally so that the number or letter would be visible along one edge of each card. Each divider is deep enough to hold many standard-size sheets of paper without obstructing the sorting tabs.

Once you have completed sorting by major headings, all items in each letter of the alphabet must be indexed.

Alphabetical Indexing

Alphabetical indexing is a method of organizing documents in the order in which the folders are placed in the filing cabinet. Standard indexing rules like the ones developed and maintained by the American Records Management Association are used in most businesses, including medical practices.

Rules of Indexing. Indexing is based on dividing a name into units. Units are numbered beginning with 1. Three units usually are sufficient for the average medical practice (see Table 10-A on p. 263). A detailed description of the rules of indexing is presented here.

1. Persons' names are indexed with the last name as Unit 1, the given (first) name as Unit 2, and the middle name or initial as Unit 3. For example, John C. Jones is indexed as:

Unit 1	Unit 2	Unit 3
Jones	John	C.

2. Once in units, the names are read from left to right, compared, and then placed in alphabetical order according to the first letter that differs. Thus Jones, Jane A. will be filed before Jones, John C. because the "a" in Jane is the first letter that differs alphabetically from the "o" in John.

3. Initials used in place of a first name are considered a unit and placed before a spelled-out name. Thomas Jones, J. or Jones, J. Charles is placed before Jones, John C.

4. Any hyphenated name is considered a single unit; the hyphen in disregarded. Thus Clayton-Moore, Sylvia is indexed as:

Unit 1	Unit 2
Claytonmoore	Sylvia

5. Apostrophes are disregarded in indexing. Thus Morton's Pharmacy is read as Mortons Pharmacy.

6. Names with foreign prepositions or articles are filed as one unit, and the space between the preposition or article and the name is ignored. Thus Claude de Mason is read and indexed as:

Unit 1	Unit 2
Demason	Claude

7. Abbreviated portions of names are read and indexed as if written in full. Thus Mary St. John is indexed as:

Unit 1	Unit 2	Unit 3
Saint	John	Mary

and Wm C. Cosgrove is indexed as:

Unit 1	Unit 2	Unit 3
Cosgrove	William	C.

8. The prefixes Mac and Mc may be filed in one of two ways: (1) You may use individual dividers to establish a separate section for all Mc's and another for all Mac's. These would become a subsystem within the files in which the name following the prefix becomes the first indexing unit. Following the Mac divider, the names MacDonald, MacAndrew, MacHenry in proper order would be indexed as:

Unit 1	Unit 2	Unit 3
Andrew	Elizabeth	D.
Donald	Joseph	
Henry	Sharon	L.

Mc would be the next divider and include names organized in the same way as those under Mac. The dividers would then resume the normal alphabetical order. (2) You may disregard the prefix and treat it the same as indicated in Rule 4. Thus MacDonald, MacHenry, and MacAndrew would be read, indexed, and filed as follows:

Unit 1	Unit 2	Unit 3
MacAndrew	Elizabeth	D.
MacDonald	Joseph	
MacHenry	Sharon	L.

9. Titles and seniority indicators either preceding or following a name should be disregarded. These are noted on the record only so that you can address the person properly. Thus Dr. Mary A. Smith and Henry R. Adams, Jr. are indexed as:

Unit 1	Unit 2	Unit 3
Smith	Mary	A. (Dr.)
Adams	Henry	R. (Jr.)

10. Married women who have adopted their husband's surname are indexed using the woman's given name. For example, put the file under Mrs. Helen J. Smith, not Mrs. John C. Smith (Helen J.).

11. Government offices are indexed by level of government. This first is stated by nationality, followed by department, bureau, and division, requiring additional units. This knowledge is used more often in locating information in a telephone directory. Thus the United States Justice Department, Bureau of Narcotics and Dangerous Drugs is indexed as:

Unit 1	Unit 2	Unit 3	Unit 4
United	States	Justice	Narcotics

12. Banks are indexed by city, bank name, and state. Thus First Interstate of Tulsa is indexed as:

Unit 1	Unit 2	Unit 3
Tulsa	First Interstate	Oklahoma

13. Persons' surnames that can be mistaken for given names should be cross-indexed by placing an OUTguide or blank folder in the correct site. For example, John R. James should be properly indexed as follows:

Unit 1	Unit 2	Unit 3
James	John	R.

The mistaken site marker for this patient should read:

Unit 1	Unit 2	Unit 3	
John	James	R.	SEE
James	John	R.	

Storing

The final step in the filing procedure is the storing of the documents. Your responsibility is to see that the items are placed in the proper folder, the proper section within the folder, and in proper chronological order within the section. You must also see that the folder is replaced in the proper position in the filing cabinet.

File Organization

Patient Charts

It is very important that all patient records be organized systematically. The correct method for placing information in the patient chart is discussed in Chapter 9. It should be emphasized that when a patient chart is not in actual use, there is only one place it should be, and that is in the medical records files. Many hours can be lost looking for a misplaced chart or records that were carelessly left lying around and not filed. The patient chart should be filed immediately after the patient has been seen, new information has been added to the chart, or new reports have been filed in the chart.

Medical Correspondence

If medical correspondence pertains to a patient, it should be filed in the patient's chart. However, if the medical information pertains to matters such as a new drug study that the physician is participating in, then it should be filed in a manner that relates to the particular pharmaceutical company and the medication being studied.

General Correspondence

Because the physician's office is a business, there will be general correspondence pertaining to the operation of the office. You should have a file drawer specified for other correspondence. The correspondence should be indexed according to the subject matter or names of correspondents. The guides in a subject file may appear in several positions depending on the number of headings, subheadings, and subdivisions.

fyi

Record Safety

1. **Do not leave files unattended on desks or counters. Patients are always curious about information laying out. Remember that records are confidential.**
2. **Be sure that file drawers are closed when not in use. Someone could see names on files in the drawers.**
3. **When the office is closed, files should be locked to maintain confidentiality.**
4. **If your files are on computer, be sure that the computer is positioned so that only the operator may view the screen.**
5. **For security use passwords to access individual files.**

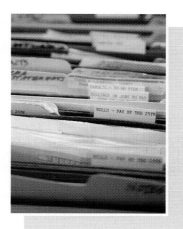

Conclusion

Maintaining an effective filing system is very important in the medical office. Proper filing of records makes retrieval time shorter and less frustrating. Your role is fundamental to the development of effective and efficient records control.

Review QUESTIONS

1. What is the basic equipment needed to set up a filing system?
2. State the seven sequential steps to follow in filing a document.
3. List the advantages of color coding files.
4. List types of filing systems.
5. Type a list of names in indexing order and arrange them alphabetically for filing.
6. What is indexing?
7. What is coding?
8. Describe one way to use geographical filing.

SUGGESTED READINGS

Diamond SZ: *Records management: policies, practices, technologies,* ed 2, New York, 1991, Anacom book division, American Management Association.

Krevolin N: *Filing and records management,* Englewood Cliffs, NJ, 1986, Prentice-Hall.

Sabin WA: *The Gregg reference manual,* ed 6, Westerville, Ohio, 1991, Glencoe Division, Macmillan/McGraw-Hill.

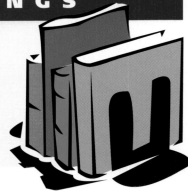

TABLE 10-A

Summary of Indexing Rules

Rule on	Name	Unit 1	Unit 2	Unit 3
Proper names	John C. Jones	Jones	John	C.

Proper names given in:
  Initials in place of a
    given name
	J. Jones	Jones	J.	

Initial as first name with middle name provided	J. Charles Jones	Jones	J.	Charles
Hyphenated names	Sylvia Clayton-Moore	Claytonmoore	Sylvia	
Apostrophes	Morton's Pharmacy	Mortons	Pharmacy	
Prefixes	Claude de Mason	Demason	Claude	
	Elizabeth D. MacAdams	Macadams	Elizabeth	D.
Abbreviations	Mary St. John	Saint	John	Mary
	Wm. C. Cosgrove	Cosgrove	William	C.
Titles	Dr. Mary A. Smith	Smith	Mary	A. (Dr.)
Seniority	Henry R. Adams, Jr.	Adams	Henry	J. (Jr.)
Married women using husband's name	Mrs. John C. Smith (Helen J.)	Smith	Helen	J.
Government offices	Federal Justice Department	United	States	Justice
Banks	First Interstate of Tulsa	Tulsa	First Interstate	Okla.

Medical Office Management

OUTLINE

On completion of Chapter 11 the administrative medical assistant student should be able to:

1. Define the key terms listed in this chapter.

2. Discuss the concept of medical office management and its primary purpose.

3. List the six types of management systems.

4. List the six basic qualities an office manager should possess.

5. Discuss the duties and responsibilities of the office manager.

6. List and discuss the seven possible recruiting sources for new employees.

7. Discuss the steps to be followed when selecting a new employee.

8. List and discuss eight general topics that should be covered in a procedures manual.

9. Describe a facility procedures manual.

10. Explain the purpose of OSHA.

KEY TERMS

Consumer An individual who takes advantage of the services of a facility. In a medical facility the consumer is the patient.

Cost containment An effort to provide high-quality services by the most economical method.

Dynamic process The progressive, adaptive quality of a management system, allowing for changes in the internal and external environment of a medical practice.

Facility The site at which medical care is provided.

Integrated Various components of an organization joined or brought together to function cooperatively and produce a positive effect.

Level of care A determination of the degree of care required to assist the patient's return to optimal well-being. An acute-care hospital is the highest level of care because it can provide all necessary specialized personnel and equipment. The cost of care is proportional to the level of care; an acute-care hospital is the most expensive care.

Management The process of directing or controlling the functions of an organization.

Management system Based on the goals and objectives of the physician-owner, an organized approach to the elements that make up the business portion of a medical practice.

Continued

KEY TERMS

(continued)

Manual A book developed as a reference source of the policies or procedures of an organization.

Outpatient setting A level of care provided to individuals able to reside at home and able to report to a facility for a specific examination or treatment; the most cost-efficient level of care.

Patient recall A method of notifying individuals that a return visit is necessary for examination or treatment.

Policy An established course of conduct based on the goals and objectives of an organization or medical practice.

Private sector Any business providing goods or services, including health care, provided with funds from nongovernment sources.

Procedure A detailed course of action; a step-by-step method of accomplishing an activity.

Provider An individual who supplies a service for others within the health care system. Health care providers include physicians, technicians, medical assistants, nurses, and therapists.

Provider services Professional functions performed by individuals for the well-being of others.

Public sector Any goods or service provided or supported by a government agency.

System A combination of parts that function together in an orderly manner to accomplish a predetermined task.

Administrative medical assistants today increasingly are in demand for their skills. The growing complexity of medical services and the trend toward specialization require greater numbers of well-trained administrative medical assistants (Figure 11.1). In addition, both public (government) and private (for example, insurance carriers, independent physicians associations) agencies responsible for paying for medical services are encouraging and in some cases demanding an emphasis on care in outpatient settings. This shift will likewise create positions for administrative medical assistants and expand their roles through increased contact with the patient-consumer. The purposes of this shift toward treatment in outpatient settings are to ensure consumer use of the appropriate level of care and encourage cost containment. Because patients may not understand the restriction to outpatient services, the medical assistant as educator will, whenever possible, be responsible for explaining these requirements and reassuring the patient that the staff will coordinate other necessary outpatient services to minimize inconvenience.

As payers place more emphasis on outpatient care and the complexity of provider services increases, the need for careful organization emerges. The professional medical assistant is the key to an effective, efficiently managed medical practice. The physician and staff are concerned chiefly with the care and treatment of patients, but there are many other details that must be attended to in maintaining a successful practice.

Principles of Medical Office Management

Management is based on the planning and organization of the various components that make up the administrative (business) portion of a medical practice. The primary purpose of systems management is to achieve patient care and comfort by maintaining an efficient and effective medical practice.

In the management of administrative systems, the administrative medical assistant must be aware of the following principles:

- Each system is used in every medical practice or agency in varying degrees of complexity
- The various systems are integrated and function simultaneously
- The efficiency of each system depends on and affects all of the other systems

After each system has been planned, developed, and instituted, the medical assistant observes, monitors, and evaluates the process for efficiency and effec-

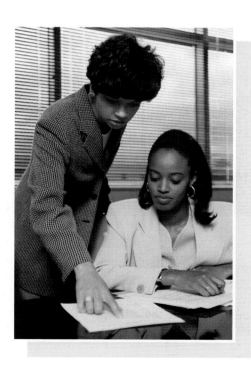

FIGURE 11.1

The growing complexity of medical services and the trend toward specialization have resulted in a greater demand for well-trained administrative medical assistants.

tiveness. As long as a system supports the goals of a medical practice, it may continue unchanged; when a system is not functioning optimally it must be revised.

To prepare for work in a medical office, the medical assistant student will need to develop an understanding of the elements of the following administrative systems:

- Personnel management
- Communications (oral and written)
- Appointment systems
- Records management
- Financial management
- Facility and equipment management

Personnel management and facility and equipment management are discussed in detail in this chapter. The remaining four systems are detailed in other chapters.

Personnel Management
Solo Assistant Office

All administrative systems are equally important, and the employee is the foundation on which all systems are based. In a limited medical practice employing a single medical assistant, the physician-owner takes the role of manager and decision maker. The medical assistant is responsible for carrying out directives and maintaining all systems necessary for the efficient operation of the facility. The medical assistant in this position must be an especially organized and self-directed individual. The assistant will be responsible for the duties of both front and back office.

Multiple-Employee Office
The Office Manager

As a practice grows, increased clinical responsibilities require more personnel, and the management time available to the physician is reduced. To allow the

---

MEDICAL ASSISTING STEP-BY-STEP

Decision-Making Steps

- Define the problem or purpose
- Establish the criteria
- Generate possible solutions
- Test the solutions and make the decision
- Evaluate the decision

physician the freedom to concentrate on the primary goal of providing patient care, an office manager is hired. The office manager, in turn, coordinates the clinical and administrative staff duties necessary to promote total patient care.

Selecting the Office Manager. After the need for an office manager has been established and a job description has been written, the employer has two options for filling the position: he or she may select a current employee or hire a new employee. Each option has advantages and disadvantages that must be recognized and evaluated (Table 11.1). Each office or facility is different, and the employer should select an office manager to fulfill the responsibilities unique to the practice.

Qualifications of the Office Manager. Each office or facility will establish its own qualifications for the office manager. However, some general qualities that are basic requirements for any manager include the following:

- Objectivity
- Organizational skills
- Creativity
- Effective communication skills (written and oral)
- Diplomacy

Duties of the Manager. The office manager is responsible to both the physician and the other staff members, and he or she serves as the information link between the two (Figure 11.2). The administrative medical assistant must see to it that information relating to all six administrative systems flows in both directions between physician-employer and the staff. Just as the office staff is the foundation of the medical practice, the office manager sets the tone for the effective and efficient management of all systems. The manager will either work with the physician-owner or be delegated total responsibility for the various functions of personnel management.

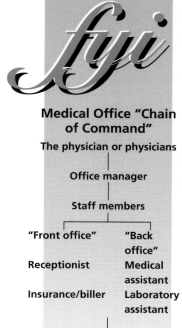

fyi

Medical Office "Chain of Command"

The physician or physicians
|
Office manager
|
Staff members

"Front office"	"Back office"
Receptionist	Medical assistant
Insurance/biller	Laboratory assistant

Appointments

All of these positions may or may not be used in each setting, depending on the size of the practice and the number of employees needed.

WHAT DO YOU THINK?

A medical office manager is a "person who wears many hats." She or he needs to be able to perform all types of duties and train personnel to perform the duties that can be delegated to them. Here is a list of skills and flaws to evaluate:

Management Skills
- Possesses self-awareness
- Manages personal stress
- Solves problems creatively

Management Flaws
- Insensitive to others
- Cold, aloof, arrogant
- Betrays trust
- Performance problems

Management Skills
- Establishes good communication
- Motivates employees
- Can delegate/make decisions
- Manages conflict

Management Flaws
- Unable to delegate
- Too ambitious for self
- Cannot think logically

How would you rate these lists as to their importance? Which is the worst or the best in each list? Which flaws do you think someone can overcome with effort?

TABLE 11-1

Selection Options for Office Managers

	Advantages	Disadvantages
Current employee	Acquainted with staff	May create friction with nonselected employees
	Knows existing systems	Will have preexisting opinions
	Established trust and rapport	Inexperienced as manager
	Known skills and loyalty	Disruption of routine during transition
New employee	Offers a fresh perspective	Orientation time
	Offers objectivity	May not be accepted by current employees
	Able to select individual with proven managerial experience	Will probably command a higher salary
	No established interoffice relationships	Unknown loyalty

FOCUS ON THE WORKPLACE

Employee Motivation

Ted, an administrative medical assistant, is coming in 10 to 15 minutes late periodically. Yours is a busy pediatrics office, and the phones start ringing at 8:30 AM for appointments. Today Ted is 30 minutes late, and the phones are busier than usual. The doctor has just come through the door, and patients are already waiting for their 9:15 appointments. When Ted comes in, you are very upset and think, "Maybe I should just threaten to fire him, and maybe he'll get the hint. He is a very good worker when he is here, and I really don't want to lose him. How can I motivate him to be on time every day and not make him angry?"

Motivation refers to the employee's desire and commitment, and shows as effort. To resolve the problem, you, as the office manager, will need to discuss it with Ted, suggest solutions, and provide positive reinforcement. Documentation of the discussion should be placed in Ted's employee file, after he has signed it.

The larger the facility, the more experience and education the office manager or administrator will need. Many facilities that have 50 or more physicians will need a manager who has studied business exclusively and perhaps has at least a bachelor's degree in business administration or even a master's degree in this field. Many managers in smaller offices simply come up through the ranks.

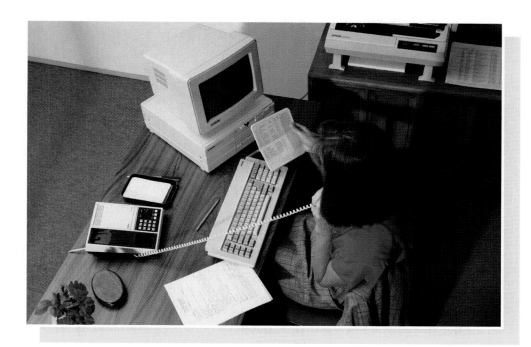

FIGURE 11.2

The office manager is responsible to both the physician and other staff members and serves as the information link between the two.

AT WORK TODAY

Impact of the Information Age

The changes brought about in the medical office by the "age of information" has made management a greater challenge. Sophisticated new technology includes desktop computers, telephones with voice mail, fax machines, and electronic mail (E-mail), which can send or receive messages by computer using a modem or network. Offices have moved from the traditional forms of medical insurance plans to the HMOs, IPAs, and PPOs of the managed care systems, which control most of the "new" world. The administrative medical assistant should have advanced training and be able to move into management when time and experience dictate.

It is predicted that soon the educational level of the labor force in general will need to be higher and that service industries, especially in health care and business, will grow the most rapidly. The position of office manager will continue to be a challenge as technology advances and as the job requires more effort to stay current, but it will be rewarding also.

Recruiting and Selecting Employees

Recruiting Sources. A medical practice or agency that needs to replace personnel or add personnel should approach the process in a logical manner. The first concern is how to recruit enough applicants to make an intelligent choice. The person responsible for hiring new employees may want to use one or more

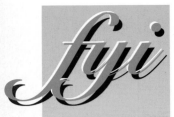

Ways to Change People Without Being Offensive

1. Always begin with praise and honest appreciation.
2. Call attention to people's mistakes indirectly.
3. Talk about your own mistakes before criticizing others.
4. Ask questions instead of giving orders.
5. Praise any improvement, no matter how slight.
6. Give the other person a good example to follow.
7. Use encouragement.
8. Make the other person happy about doing what you suggest.

TABLE 11-2

Recruiting Sources

Resource	Advantages	Disadvantages
Newspapers Post office box given Newspaper box number	Reach vast audience Least expensive Quickest results Initial screening simplified Demands sample of writing skills	Heavy influx of calls May disrupt routine No personal contact Discourages applicants
Private employment agency	Prescreening done by a professional Specialized medical agencies available	Expensive Fee paid by employer
Professional association placement	Applicants generally rated good to excellent Fees less than private employment agencies	Screening for specific skills may be weak
State employment offices	Good for paraprofessional employees No fees	Inadequate screening
Local formal training program	Candidate graduate of accredited program No fees	Availability based on program completion dates
Friends or relatives of current employees	Quick, convenient contact New employee begins with a positive attitude toward practice	Feeling of favoritism among other employees Ill will if referral is not selected
Walk in/write in	Approach demonstrates the applicant has initiative and is self-directed	May arrive at a time when no positions are available

of the many possible recruiting sources. The common recruiting sources and the advantages and disadvantages of each are noted in Table 11.2. One relatively common method used to recruit potential employees is called *pirating*. This method involves seeking out and hiring qualified employees away from other medical offices or facilities in the community. Pirating was not included in Table 11.2 because it is not openly acknowledged and is not considered professional. However, it does exist. Personnel managers must be aware of this practice to prevent the loss of valuable employees to others who use this method.

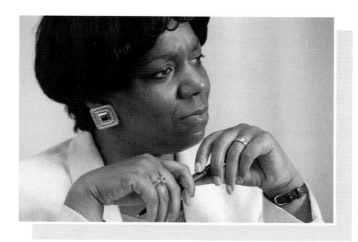

FIGURE 11.3

All interviews should be conducted by the same person; this allows the interviewer to make appropriate, firsthand comparisons of the applicants.

Selection Process. Once candidates are recruited for the position, the selection process begins. The tendency at this point may be to rush the selection in an effort to fill the vacant position quickly. This should be avoided, regardless of the urgency. Hasty selection may result in hiring an individual who is not qualified for the position or does not work well with the other employees. The appropriate selection process is an orderly one that should follow these steps:

- Accept employment applications
- Conduct interviews
- Contact references
- Rank applicants
- Select the most qualified applicant

The application form can be designed specifically for your facility or you may use one that has been tested and proved appropriate by others. The latter form may be the best to avoid legal problems that may arise from requesting inappropriate information, such as age, marital status, or ethnic origin. The application should include an authorization to contact the applicant's current employer.

Once the applications have been completed, each potential employee is scheduled for an interview. The office manager may have the authority to make the final hiring decision or may only do the screening interview after the initial interview, in which case the next step is to schedule appropriate applicants for a second interview with the physician-employer. If the physician-employer conducts the second interview, the office manager usually works cooperatively with that person throughout the remainder of the selection process. Regardless of who conducts the interviews, the following basic rules apply:

- All interviews should be conducted by the same person. This allows the interviewer to make appropriate, firsthand comparisons of the various applicants (Figure 11.3)

- Following a brief, precise description of the specific job by the interviewer, the applicant should do most of the talking. This provides a means to evaluate the applicant's oral communication skill
- The interviewer should use the written application as the foundation for questions asked during the interview
- An application file should be kept with notes on each applicant recorded immediately after the interview
- The interviewer should avoid making any verbal commitment or offering an opinion of the applicant's possibility of obtaining the position

After the interviews the three or four most acceptable candidates for the position should be selected. These applicants then will be considered until the final selection is made.

The third step in the selection process is checking references. The person responsible for hiring the new employee may wish to trust his or her own intuition about the applicant. However, although impressions are important, they should never replace direct contact with former employers, personal references, or both.

References may be checked formally by writing either on a preprinted form or in a letter to the reference source to request a written reply. Although this method will provide a permanent record, it has limitations. These limitations can be overcome by checking references by telephone when possible. Speaking directly with the reference sources offers the advantage of hearing the respondents' vocal inflections and detecting their reactions to questions or omissions of answers. The respondents also may be more candid during a conversation than they might be in a written response for a permanent record. However, there is an increasing reluctance by employers to provide telephone references, as legally they must have the written consent of the applicant to provide such information. In this instance, they may choose to say that the applicant was employed from this date to this date, and give no further information. At this point it may be helpful to ask if the applicant would be rehired for the current position if the opportunity presented itself. The answer to that question alone will be very telling.

The final step in the selection process involves choosing the three best candidates and ranking them as first, second, and third. The position then is offered to the first-choice applicant. If he or she declines, the job then is offered to the second-choice applicant.

Employment Process

The Employment Offer. A position should be offered in writing; however, the offer may be made orally with a follow-up written confirmation. At the time the offer of employment is made, the minimum information supplied to the job candidate should include the following:

- Starting salary
- Salary payment schedule
- Benefits
- Job description or list of major duties and responsibilities

- Employment status
- Work hours
- Dress code
- Office policies and procedures

When the job offer had been accepted, the office manager is responsible for notifying the candidates who were not accepted; this should be done in writing.

Employment Status. Employment status relates to a condition of the employee's position. The employee will be categorized as one of the following types:

- Temporary
- Part-time
- Probationary
- Permanent

The temporary employee works in the facility for a short time to provide interim services. A temporary employee may be necessary to substitute for permanent staff members who are absent for reasons such as vacations, illness, or jury duty. The temporary employee usually is paid hourly and is not eligible for benefits.

Part-time employees usually work half-time or less on a predetermined schedule and at a fixed, prorated salary. Generally, benefits such as health insurance are not available to part-time employees.

When an employee is hired with the intention of making him or her a permanent member of the health care team, a trial period of employment usually is established. This probationary period ranges from 30 to 90 days, and the employee usually is not eligible for benefits such as sick leave, vacations, or insurance during this time. The length of the probationary period must be clearly established. At the end of the probationary period, the employer and employee with meet to determine whether the employee will remain as a permanent staff member (Figure 11.4). The option to terminate without prejudice may be made at this time by either the employer or employee.

Permanent employees have established positions and functions in the medical facility. They receive full salaries and are eligible for all benefits.

Terminations

Ending an employer-employee relationship is called a *termination*. A termination may be classified as voluntary or involuntary.

Voluntary. Voluntary terminations are initiated by the employee, who might wish to leave a position to return to school, work in a different type of facility, or move to another area. The possibility also exists that an employee may wish to terminate because of interpersonal difficulties within the facility or because of an inability to adapt to particular methods of operation. The voluntary termination process should include the following:

- A letter of resignation from the employee, giving appropriate notice (2 weeks to 1 month)
- An exit interview. This will give the employer the opportunity to determine the possible reasons for the resignation. There may be

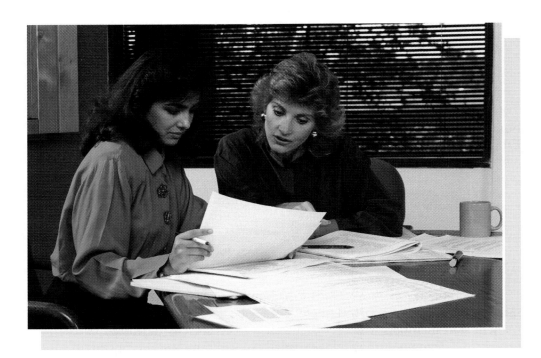

FIGURE 11.4

At the end of the probationary period, employer and employee meet to determine whether the employee will remain as a permanent staff member.

internal problems of which the employer is unaware and about which the existing employee can elaborate. However, the employee should be careful to relay significant information accurately and diplomatically; petty information will diminish credibility.

- A forwarding address for the employee so that documents such as W-2 forms and retirement fund information can be sent

Involuntary. Involuntary terminations are initiated by the employer or office manager and usually are unpleasant experiences. They must be conducted in the most professional and diplomatic manner possible.

One type of involuntary termination is a layoff. Layoffs occur in circumstances such as reduced workload, the relocation of a practice or facility to another area, or the retirement of the physician-owner. Although a layoff may be easier for the employee to understand than a firing, it still is an unsettling experience.

Firing an employee usually follows an accepted protocol that includes the following steps:

- Verbally warning the employee of unacceptable performance
- Warning the employee in writing if the behavior continues
- Terminating the employment, verbally and in writing, if the employee's performance fails to meet established standards

Usually the person responsible for hiring must also conduct the dismissal process. The terminated employee should be given notice as predetermined by office policy. Because it may be uncomfortable for all concerned to have the dismissed employee work through the notice period, the employer should pay all salary, vacation benefits, sick leave benefits, and/or retirement benefits (if possible) through the notice period and so allow the employee to leave immediately. Experience has demonstrated that dismissals should be given privately, preferably at the end of a workday, and on a Friday if possible.

The only situation that precludes the warning process and notice period occurs when the employee is found guilty of a gross breach of ethics, such as betraying a patient's confidentiality or if a legal issue, such as embezzlement, is involved.

In any involuntary termination, it is absolutely necessary for the employer-office manager to have clear, well-documented records detailing the warning process and the circumstances that led to the termination.

Employee Compensation

Salaries. Employee compensation includes salary and selected benefits. Salaries vary depending on the part of the country, the setting (urban or rural), the medical assistant's experience and length of service, and the duties of the position. The trend is toward improved salaries for medical assistants. This trend may be influenced by recognition of the profession, improved training programs, standardized certification examinations, and professional associations.

Salary advances should be scheduled and based on the cost of living as well as considerations of merit. Cost-of-living increases are based on a set percentage for all employees; merit raises are based on individual performance evaluations. Raises usually occur after the probationary period, at which time the employee becomes a permanent staff member. Raises continue according to the established schedule. Annual salary increases may occur on a fixed date for all employees, on the employee's birthday, after a job performance evaluation, or on the anniversary of the employee's attainment of permanent status.

Benefits. Benefits will vary depending on the employment site and whether a practice is incorporated. However, most employees can anticipate basic benefits such as the following:

- Health insurance
- Sick leave
- Vacations and holidays
- Retirement plan

As previously noted, information on salary and benefits should be discussed with the employee at the time the job offer is made.

Records And Forms

Personnel files should be complete and well organized. Each employee's file includes the employee's job application, job description, references, salary and performance reviews, and necessary records and forms. The office manager keeps attendance records, W-4 forms, payroll deduction information, and enrollment forms such as benefit insurance applications.

The information in each employee's personnel file and the tax reports generated from the employee's payroll records must be treated as strictly confidential. The personnel file is a matter between the employer or his or her authorized representative and the employee.

Orientation and Training

Orientation for a new employee involves introducing her or him to co-workers, the work environment, and the guidelines for operations and relationships within the practice.

Because much of a medical assistant's preparation today takes place in formal training programs as described in Chapter 1, on-the-job training requirements have been greatly reduced but not eliminated. Each employer or agency and its employees are unique, with their own variations of office policies and procedures. Although formal training provides a theoretical foundation for a medical assisting career and an externship or other experience enhances that formal training, the new employee still needs a training period to learn and adapt to these variations. This preliminary orientation and training period also helps the new employee to understand fully what is expected of her or him and to develop to her or his full potential. This period coincides with the probationary period.

On accepting a position, the new employee should not be surprised if the departing employee is not available to train her or him. Although it is not a desirable situation, often the position cannot be filled in time for the departing employee to provide adequate orientation and training to the new employee. Thus the new employee will need to ask the office manager, employer, or another medical assistant any questions regarding the position. It is common for the new employee to be placed in a position of self-training. This is particularly true for receptionists and insurance billers.

Foundation of a Training Program. The orientation and training plan is based on information outlined in the office or agency policy and procedures manual. All practices, regardless of size, should develop and maintain these manuals. They are necessary as a foundation for all services. The office manager will work with the employer to develop the policy manual and with the health care team to develop the procedures manual. Once the manuals have been developed, follow-up duties include monitoring and evaluating the effectiveness and efficiency of each system and maintaining or revising the procedures manual as needed (Figure 11.5).

Staff Meetings

Staff meetings are preplanned gatherings attended by the employer and employees at which issues relevant to staff relations and office management are discussed. Some decisions are by their nature reserved for the employer, and others are decided by the majority. Staff meetings provide a continuing-training technique within the office that contributes to maintaining the cooperative spirit among the employees and between the employees and the employer.

Many offices find that it is easiest to set aside a lunch hour, order in lunch, and have a regular structured meeting. These meetings need not be long or overly formal, but someone should be appointed to take notes. The office manager should have an organized agenda or a simple outline of the issues to be dis-

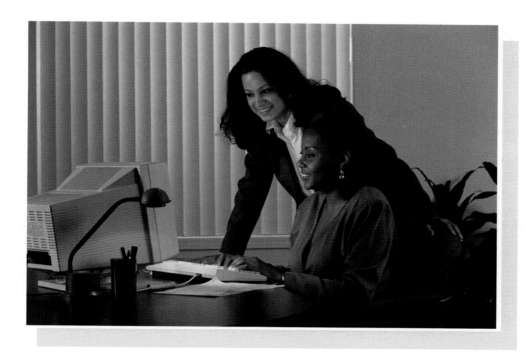

FIGURE 11.5

Even after formal training and a possible externship, the new employee still needs a training period to learn and adapt to office variations.

cussed and any supporting information needed for the meeting. Staff members should be encouraged to submit ideas or information for discussion.

Staff meetings vary in purpose. Some are simply informational; others are for brainstorming to solve an office problem. They may be work sessions to update manuals or discuss information that may pertain to one particular function of the practice, such as billing, but that will affect the entire staff. The staff should discuss new ideas or cost-cutting measures, but under no circumstances should the staff meeting be allowed to become a gripe session. The staff meeting is not a place to air gripes and should a staff member attempt to do so, he or she should be asked by the office manager to meet later. It is to the advantage of all if the physician(s) attend these meetings. Some of the best ideas for the practice come from the staff members working in a particular position, such as billing or the front desk.

Policy Manual

A policy is a general statement that serves as a guideline for operating a business and that governs the employee-employer relationship. Policies are based on the goals and objectives of the facility. A policy manual is a binder, preferably a loose-leaf one, in which statements of policy can be organized and stored. The policy manual in a medical practice serves as a reference source for all employees. It is used to orient and train new employees, and it enables the staff to make changes with minimal disruption of routine. Some of the topics that should be discussed in a policy manual are presented in Table 11.3 and the box

AT WORK TODAY

Effective Staff Meetings

To hold effective staff meetings in the medical office, four important considerations should be made. They are as follows:

1. Deciding when to have the meeting—arranging a time when your staff can be there. Check the appointment book and mark meeting times in it.
2. Deciding who to invite—if staff meetings are hard to arrange so that all staff members are able to attend or if not all staff members need to attend a particular meeting, then decide in advance whom to invite. You also must decide if the physicians should be there and, if so, then let them know.
3. Making preparations for the meeting—be sure to have an agenda and any needed handouts or equipment. You must have a room or space set up with seating for all expected.
4. Managing the meeting—make sure everyone feels comfortable with one another. Avoid confrontations, and manage the discussions to include all.

TABLE 11-3

Policy Manual Topic Areas

Employment	Attendance and timekeeping	Salary	Employee benefits
Confidential information	Absences	Payroll	Health insurance
Employee status	Work breaks	Employee progress review	Pension plan
Employment procedure	Time off (medical/dental appointments)	Overtime	Vacations
Probationary period	Work schedules	Salary advances	Holidays
Recruiting and selection	Timekeeping		Life insurance
Retirement			Sick leave
Terminations			
Unemployment insurance			
Job description and duties			

From Zakus SM et al, editors: *Mosby's fundamentals of medical assisting: administrative and clinical theory and technique,* ed 2, St. Louis, 1990, Mosby.

about office policies. Sound management principles indicate that an office policy manual should be well thought out and well designed. Once in use it also must be periodically reviewed and updated.

Procedures Manual

The procedures manual provides a more detailed aid in personnel and systems management (Figure 11.6). The manual should be a loose-leaf binder with a

OFFICE POLICIES

1. Requirements for payment from patients
2. Forms of payment accepted
3. Policy relating to private insurance
    Full fee due?
    When?
    Accepting assignment?
    Bill insurance for patient?
    Fee for rebilling insurance?
4. MediCare/Medicaid
    Does the practice participate?
    Does the practice accept new patients with this coverage?
        By referral only?
        By emergency only?
        By family member reference only?
5. Practice policies for payment plans
6. Policy for other fees that may be charged to the patient
    Broken appointment
    Interest/finance charge
    Laboratory handling fee
    Rebilling charge

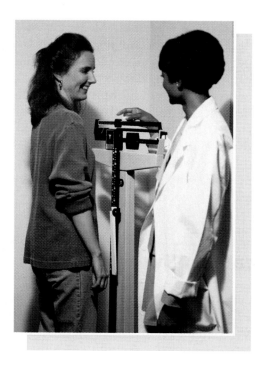

FIGURE 11.6

The procedures manual provides guidance in both administrative and clinical duties, including gathering physical measurements and vital signs.

separate sheet devoted to each staff position and procedure. The manual can be divided in several ways, including the following:

- By clinical and administrative duties
- By employee position and job description
- By job title

The first method is the most definitive and can be subdivided easily. The administrative section can be arranged according to the six administrative systems listed in this chapter. The clinical section can be organized according to the following areas:

- Physical measurements, vital signs, temperature, pulse, respiration, weight and height
- Health history and physical examinations
- Infection control, asepsis, and sterilization
- Surgical asepsis and minor surgery
- Collecting and handling specimens
- Pharmacology and drug administration
- Laboratory orientation
- Diagnostic radiology
- ECGs
- Common emergencies and first aid

Once the format for the manual has been selected, specific procedures are detailed in the appropriate sections. Each procedure is a step-by-step outline or a list of tasks. Having defined procedures serves as an educational tool, because it reduces confusion regarding work distribution. It also provides a guide for new employees, the employee who must fill in for another, and temporary employees who are brought into the facility. As the manual is developed and revised, the various personnel involved should have a chance to offer their ideas about procedures that affect them. Each procedure includes the date it was established. As procedures are revised, the outmoded procedure sheet should be discarded, and the new procedure sheet should be substituted and dated as a revision (for example, Rev. 12/00/97).

Complete procedures manuals are kept by the physician(s) and the office manager and should be accessible to all employees. Copies of individual sections should be given to the employee responsible for the duties as detailed. A sample procedure sheet is shown in Table 11.4.

Communication Systems

An effective communication system is another vital component of medical office management. Communication systems include both oral and written communication. These systems should be thought of as a key link between the physician and the patients. Effective communication also is a form of public relations that links the physician with colleagues and office personnel with pro-

TABLE 11-4

Sample Procedure
Answering Service Sign In/Sign Out

Procedure	Rationale
Call the answering service on arrival at the desk.	Answering service (exchange) is relieved of the responsibility of answering the telephone. Patients can make direct contact with facility personnel.
Obtain any messages left with the service.	
Receive a report from the service on the physician's whereabouts.	Reduces time involved if the physician is needed by office personnel.
Distribute messages to the appropriate personnel for processing.	
If the office closes for lunch, notify the service (1) of where and how the physician can be contacted and (2) the time you will reopen.	
Call the service on return from lunch.	
Sign out at the end of the workday, supplying the same information as at the lunch-hour sign out.	

fessionals in other offices and health care agencies. The impression made through communication reflects on all personnel and on the medical practice in general. Two important means of communication for health care facilities are the telephone (see Chapter 6) and written correspondence (see Chapter 8).

Scheduling Systems

An effective method of scheduling appointments is necessary for the efficient organization of the work involved in a health care facility. These appointment systems (discussed in Chapter 7) must be well developed, since they affect all personnel and, most importantly, the patients who will be using the services provided by the health care facility.

Records Management

An efficient system of managing patients' medical records (discussed in Chapter 9) is essential for a well-run medical office. This includes structured systems for patient registration, preparing records, and handling and storing charts. In addition, informational reminder systems help ensure the smooth operation of a medical office.

Responsibility for the patient's medical record usually involves many, if not all, of the office personnel. Techniques in the development, handling, and storage of these documents are presented in Chapter 9.

Financial Management

The management of financial systems in a facility involves the following three areas of responsibility:

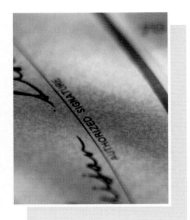

- Billing systems
- Insurance
- Banking and Bookkeeping

Good financial management systems are essential to run a medical office. The income generated by billing (discussed in Chapter 13) and insurance (discussed in Chapter 14) provides the funds with which the practice or agency conducts business. One employee may be responsible for all financial records management, or the responsibility may be distributed among various staff members with specific skills who specialize in one or more aspects of the responsibility. The practice's income is accounted for by banking and bookkeeping techniques (discussed in Chapter 19).

Facilities and Equipment Management

The facilities and equipment of the office provide the structural support for the services provided. Facilities must be organized and maintained for maximum efficiency, and the equipment required to fulfill the various assisting responsibilities must be acquired and monitored.

Facilities Management

The general responsibility for the management of facilities and equipment usually is assigned to the administrative medical assistant or office manager. Specific duties should be detailed in the office policy manual. In small and moderate-sized practices, the job description for one employee may include the entire responsibility for this management system. Managers of large practices or facilities may find that the responsibility for facilities and equipment must be divided, usually by administrative and clinical areas, and that job descriptions must be written to reflect the division of duties.

Areas of Consideration

As a system for managing the facilities and equipment is developed, four basic factors must always be considered:

- Patient comfort
- Accessibility of equipment and supplies
- Safety
- Security

The comfort of patients while they are in the facility is of primary concern for all personnel and involves both psychological and physical comfort. You will need to develop methods of conveying a sense of privacy and dignity that will be reassuring to patients.

Accessibility to equipment and supplies is important to personnel both for their sake and for that of the patients. Maintaining adequate supplies in convenient locations saves time that can otherwise be spent addressing the patients' needs. It also eliminates unnecessary, fatiguing movement expended while searching for items to accomplish assigned tasks.

Monitoring the premises and equipment for safety is the responsibility of all personnel and is for the benefit of both patients and employees. Areas of concern include the unsafe placement of furniture, ripples in carpets, slippery floors caused by excess wax or spills, frayed or improperly grounded electrical cords, overloading of electrical outlets, and improperly labeled or stored fluids and chemicals. These potential problem areas and others unique to your facility require constant monitoring, and you should develop the habit of periodically evaluating the premises from the perspective of someone entering for the first time. Another important safety consideration involves the predetermined course of action to be taken in the event of an emergency. An evacuation plan should be developed and practiced in the event that a fire occurs. A fire extinguisher should be easily accessible. Each employee should be assigned specific areas of responsibility, with notification of the fire department and attention to patients having the highest priority. If time allows, you also will want to consider closing all filing cabinets to protect records, removing financial records, and notifying the answering service from an off-premise telephone to monitor incoming calls. Plans also should be developed for events common in your geographical area, such as earthquakes, floods, hurricanes, and tornadoes. These plans should be detailed in the office procedures manual and reviewed by all staff members periodically.

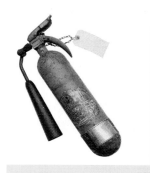

A security system is the final area that must be developed to protect the office and contents during and after work hours. While the office is open, a signaling method to indicate when someone enters the reception room is needed. This most commonly is a bell that is activated when the door is opened or when an individual passes through a light beam. Special attention is required for the protection of medications, especially narcotics, kept on the premises. After hours, the office can be protected by checking all windows and doors to be sure they are securely locked. Office buildings usually have a burglar alarm for additional security. Freestanding private offices should have their own alarm systems.

Physical Resources

Facilities management begins with the physical layout of the office, the choices made regarding furnishings and colors, evaluation of traffic patterns, and general maintenance.

WHAT DO YOU THINK?

The physical environment of the medical office includes lighting, space, furniture, health, safety, and security.

1. Color influences the way people think and feel.

What colors do you think might influence patients to feel better while waiting?

2. Lighting can be too bright from direct sunlight.

What type of lighting do you think might be effective in the waiting room, examination rooms, and work stations?

3. The temperature of the waiting room, as well as the work areas in the back office, is important.

What do you think the temperature range should be from waiting room to back office?

4. Space and furniture are important and should be arranged in a practical manner to accommodate patients comfortably but safely.

What type of furniture should be used?

5. Safety is very important in any setting The Occupational Safety and Health Administration provides guidelines for regulation of the workplace. The waiting room/office setting should have no loose wire, floor coverings should be secure (not loose), and office furniture should be safe, with no sharp edges.

What suggestions would you add to this list?

6. A secure environment is important not only for the contents of the office but also for the safety of the patients and staff.

How can a secure environment be set up? What type of services could be used?

Delineation of Space
The internal office space can be thought of as four distinct areas, which are designated as follows:

- Public area
- Control area
- Medical area
- Storage area

Activity in and maintenance of one area affects the others, but each area will be discussed separately.

Public area
The public area of an office or agency is the reception area and the entrances to it. Most offices have a single reception area, and it should be evaluated and planned to meet the needs of many individuals. Seating should be adequate, with a minimum of three to four chairs provided per physician in the practice. Some large practices with available space (Figure 11.7) can accommodate special needs such as a play area for children or an isolation room for infectious cases.

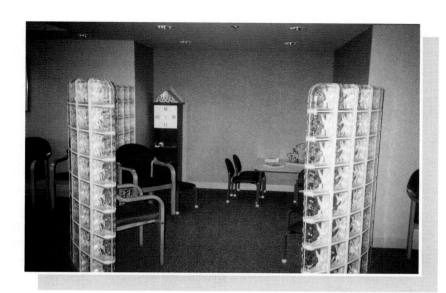

FIGURE 11.7

Some large practices with available space can accommodate special needs such as a play area for children.

Control area

The space from which personnel can monitor activity to and from all other areas is the control area, generally known as the administrative offices. When working in this area, you will be responsible for reception, registration, appointments, medical records, and telephone activity.

Because all patients and visitors must pass through and stop at this area between the reception and medical areas, it must be organized for efficiency and security. The control area is a very active space, and access to records, funds, and prescription pads requires particular attention.

Medical area

The medical area includes the rooms reserved and furnished for the examination and treatment of patients and the physician's office or consultation room for patient interviews and postexamination discussions (Figure 11.8). In the examination-treatment room, particular attention must be paid to privacy for patients. Windows should be appropriately covered, and examining tables should not be placed opposite the door, in case it must be opened after an examination has begun. Sound control should be checked to ensure confidentiality. Light sources and equipment should be placed for easy access to save time during the course of an examination or treatment.

Storage area

Extra supplies and equipment require storage space that does not intrude on the other areas of the office. Supplies and equipment also must remain readily available to personnel who need to replace items used in the course of daily activities. This area should be spacious enough to receive supplies as they arrive and hold them until invoices can be checked against the items delivered. Visitors and sales personnel should not be permitted in this area.

Arrangement of Furnishings. Furnishings, particularly in the public area and consultation room, should be selected and arranged for utility and aesthetics. Chairs of varying height and firmness should be provided to accom-

A 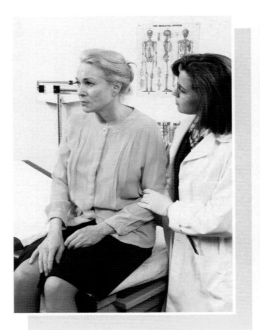   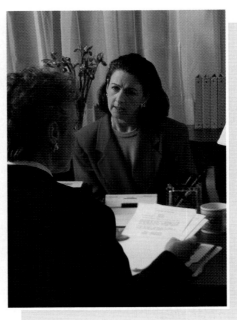 B

FIGURE 11.8

The medical area of the facility includes the examination rooms (A) and the physician's office or consultation room (B) for patient interviews and postexamination discussions.

modate the needs and comfort of patients. The arrangement of furniture is particularly important in small areas to give the illusion of more space. Attention also should be given to lighting for safety and reading comfort.

Colors. The colors selected for the walls, carpet, and furnishings should not only be functional but also cheerful and soothing. The use of artwork throughout the office is particularly pleasing. It can be a diversion for those who are waiting and also lessens the impersonal appearance of the medical environment. Artwork may be loaned, leased, or rented from a local artist, museum, or gallery. The assistant and physician also should see that current publications and magazines are available, not only in the reception area but also in the examination and treatment rooms. Another positive aspect is the use of music in the examination rooms. Music normally should not be piped into the reception area since it adds to the overall noise.

Traffic Patterns. The corridors through which patients travel to gain access to the various areas of an office should be evaluated to be certain that privacy and confidentiality are provided. Attention also should be directed at timing movement so that bottlenecks do not occur in any one area. This is most likely to occur at the reception window or in the control area, where several people may arrive at one time. Staggering patients at the reception and appointment desk will enhance privacy and confidentiality.

Maintenance. The major portion of the maintenance functions will be carried out by a janitorial service that has a written or verbal agreement with the employer or office manager. One employee should be assigned to monitor the

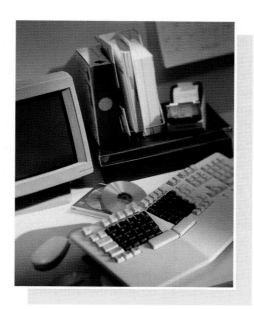

FIGURE 11.9

Administrative capital equipment denotes items needed to fulfill the administrative office duties. Copy machines and computers fall into this category.

efficiency of the service and communicate the needs of the office to the service personnel. You may wish to restrict some areas within the office from the janitorial service, such as those containing sterile equipment, confidential information, or personal work areas. Responsibility for maintaining the restricted areas then must be assigned to office staff, usually divided along administrative and clinical lines.

Capital Equipment

Capital equipment is the term applied to items that are considered major and involve the expenditure funds above a dollar value predetermined by the employer and the accountant. Although the amount that represents a capital expenditure varies, it often is placed at or near $500. Items are classified as capital when they are purchased. The accounting differences are handled by the office accountant.

Types of Capital Equipment

Items that are categorized as general capital equipment include the office furnishings, artwork, automobiles purchased by the practice, carpeting, and so forth. Remodeling of the premises also is considered a capital expenditure and often is referred to as leasehold improvement for an office rented in a medical building. Administrative capital equipment denotes items needed to fulfill the administrative office duties (Figure 11.9). Typewriters, word processors, copy machines, and computer terminals and printers all fall into this category. In the clinical area, the capital purchases will include the examination room furnishings, particularly the tables, which can be very expensive. Examination and treatment items include major equipment used by specialists such as ophthalmologists, neurologists, radiologists, and gynecologists. Other specialists, such as internists and otorhinolaryngologists, require little capital equipment and more expendable equipment, which will be discussed later. Regardless of the specialty, most offices also maintain equipment used to sterilize clinical supplies, prepare laboratory specimens, or perform some laboratory studies. Most also have a refrigerator to store perishable supplies.

Care and Maintenance of Capital Equipment

All equipment, capital or otherwise, should be handled carefully and used properly to preserve it in the best operating condition for the longest period possible. Before using any piece of equipment, thoroughly read the operating instructions and understand its functions. If in doubt, seek the help of another employee familiar with the equipment or an employee of the firm from which the equipment was purchased.

Equipment that is used extensively and has many moving parts or functions capable of breaking down can be covered by a maintenance contract. Typewriters, computers, and copy machines commonly fall into this category. A maintenance contract is a sort of insurance policy purchased to cover parts and labor charges incurred when a piece of equipment breaks or malfunctions. Maintenance contracts are renewed annually and should be reviewed to determine if the predicted cost of service calls exceeds the cost of the contract. This is more likely to be the case as the equipment ages.

Your responsibility for the office equipment includes using it properly, following maintenance instructions, and acquiring appropriate service when necessary. Because capital equipment is expensive, it is unlikely that you will have comparable backup items in the event of equipment failure. Therefore it is in your best interest to maintain the equipment properly and seek professional services at the first sign of a problem. This should help reduce the amount of time that you must be without the failed equipment.

Expendable Equipment and Supplies

Expendable equipment and supplies include items that you expect to use up within a short period and are relatively inexpensive, especially when considered at unit cost. Expendable administrative equipment and supplies include the following:

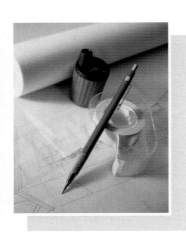

- Paper goods—stationery, typing paper, photocopy paper, insurance forms, chart folders, labels, medical record forms, laboratory and radiology request forms, appointment books
- Writing instruments—pens, pencils, color highlighters, correcting tape or fluid
- Typewriter and copy supplies—ribbons, cleaning fluids, copy ink or toners
- Accounting supplies—statements, ledgers, printouts, computer paper, accounting forms, adding machine tapes, receipt books or forms, and day sheets

In the clinical area, expendable items include the following:

- Linens—pillowcases, towels, drapes, laboratory coats, gowns that are used once and laundered
- Paper supplies—examining-table paper, disposable gowns, drapes, paper towels, wraps and bags for equipment sterilization
- Examination equipment—ear and nose speculum covers, disposable vaginal specula, disposable proctoscopes and sigmoidoscopes, lubricant, catheters, tongue blades, cotton-tipped applicators
- Treatment equipment—needles, syringes, cautery tips, suture material, dressings, elastic bandages, tape and cast materials

Ordering Systems

Because expendable supplies and equipment must be replaced relatively often, you will need to develop a system to keep an adequate supply on hand.

First, determine a reorder point for the various items. This is the point in time that takes into consideration the amount of supplies remaining and the amount of time needed to order replacement supplies and have them delivered. The object is never to reach the point at which all supplies are depleted before replacements arrive.

Second, develop a method of noting ordering needs. The responsibility may be delegated to one employee or divided according to administrative and clinical areas. A supply ordering notebook can be maintained and divided by type of supply or ordering source. As supplies are placed in the storage area, the boxes can be numbered. The box that indicates the reorder point can be marked in a manner recognized by all personnel. The person who removes the reorder-point item is responsible for noting this in the reorder book.

Third, the person or persons responsible for ordering supplies should be aware of the time required to place the order and the anticipated delivery time. Orders need to be placed far enough in advance of actual need. A copy of the order form should be retained to check against the order when it arrives or to check on the order if it does not arrive within the expected time.

Fourth, some basic considerations should be kept in mind when ordering supplies. A unit-cost saving usually can be realized by ordering in large quantities rather than by single item. For example, if one box of 100 syringes is ordered at a cost of $10, then each syringe costs 10 cents. The same supplier might reduce the cost per box to $8 if you purchase five boxes at one time, which will reduce your unit cost to 8 cents per syringe. Aside from cost, also consider available storage space and the expiration date of some items when you order in quantity. The storage problem could interfere with safety and efficiency, and ordering items that will be outdated before they can be used will be a waste of money rather than a savings.

Suppliers

You will need several suppliers to maintain an office, since administrative and clinical items usually are not available from a single source. Local suppliers provide the convenience of quick delivery and personalized service, whereas mail-order firms may provide a cost savings. The preference of the employer and the service capability demonstrated usually are the final deciding factors in selecting a supplier.

FIGURE 11.10

Special consideration must be given to the storage of drugs, particularly narcotics.

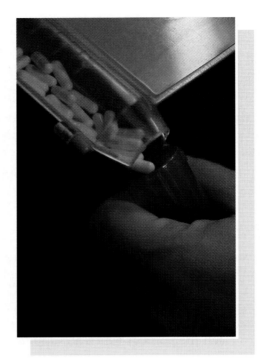

Receiving Supplies

A single location should be designated as the receiving area within the medical office. All deliveries should be deposited in this location and held until they can be checked for completeness. One person should be assigned the responsibility of receiving and signing for deliveries. The subsequent duties can be divided between administrative and clinical areas, with one person from each area being responsible for checking invoices or packing slips against the items delivered and distributing goods to the proper storage area.

Storage of Supplies

As supplies are placed in the storage area, supplies already on hand should be rotated to a position in which they will be used first. Items that have just arrived should be placed for subsequent use. Storage areas should be arranged so the most commonly used items are within the closest reach. Conversely, infrequently used items can be stored in less accessible sites. Special consideration must be given to the storage of drugs, particularly narcotics (Figure 11.10). The law requires that narcotics be locked up and that each item be accounted for as either currently in storage or dispensed.

Office Security

Some areas of the office are considered to be high security; these are areas where narcotics, medications, and syringes are stored. Another high-risk area is where the staff members place their personal belongings such as handbags, book bags, or backpacks.

It is important that all areas have secure locks. All windows should have locks, and all doors should have good double locks installed by a reliable locksmith. It is not easy to make an office completely burglar-proof; you may consider consulting with a professional security service.

It is important to have the areas around the building illuminated with sensor lights that have unbreakable shields. During the winter, as daylight fades much earlier, check to see that these lights are well maintained and work properly.

Alarms are helpful for security. However, if you are in a remote area, or if the alarm is easily accessible and can be disconnected by an expert, the practice should install an alarm system that will ring in the local police station or at an independent security office when disconnected.

Before leaving the office each evening, all windows and doors should be double checked, particularly in practices with many areas to check.

Fire exits should be clearly marked and the staff instructed on evacuation proceedings in case of fire. Smoke alarms are required in all new buildings, and should be installed in older offices. Fire extinguishers are required regardless of the age of the building.

The physician who maintains controlled substances (narcotics) on the premises must keep these drugs in a locked cabinet or safe. Any loss of controlled substances by theft must be reported to the regional office of the Drug Enforcement Agency (DEA) at the time the theft is discovered. The local police department and the state Bureau of Narcotics also should be notified.

OSHA Requirements

The Occupational Safety and Health Administration (OSHA) issued safety standards in 1984 to handle gas sterilization in the medical office. Since then more and more emphasis has been placed not just on safety in the office but also in the disposal of medically related materials. Most states have begun to adopt laws pertaining to the treatment and disposal of waste from all business offices, including medial offices. These laws will affect physicians who generate, store, move, or treat biohazardous waste. Medical waste includes blood products, cultures, specimens, and sharps (blades, glass, needles, and items with rigid corners or edges [Figure 11.11]). These items might be generated as a result of diagnosis, treatment, testing, or immunization. In some states physicians are required to register as either a small- or a large-quantity generator. Usually, accumulation of more than 200 pounds of waste per month would be considered a large-volume generator.

Waste could be treated on site but usually is treated at an approved medical waste treatment facility. Some firms specialize in this type of disposal, by incineration, discharge into the public sewage system if it meets specific requirements, or steam sterilizations. It is important that all biohazardous waste for disposal be properly identified using heavy-duty bags and sharps containers that are leakproof and sturdy. All waste containers in treatment rooms must be kept out of the reach of children. When waste is turned over to an outside firm, the firm must be a registered hauler or an approved person, and the waste must be properly identified.

FIGURE 11.11

Medical waste includes blood products, cultures, specimens, and sharps (blades, needles, and items with rigid corners or edges).

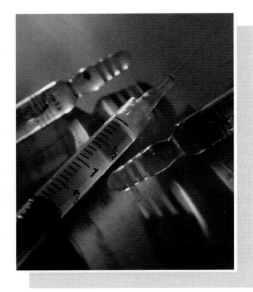

As of 1991 OSHA also issued guidelines that affect all health care workers. Private physicians must provide nurses and other health care workers with protective clothing, vaccinations, and protection against bloodborne diseases such as acquired immunodeficiency syndrome (AIDS) and hepatitis B. Protective clothing or equipment includes gowns, latex gloves, mouth guards, and other protective gear.

OSHA continues to update requirements each year, and the medical office must remain in compliance with the directives.

Conclusion

This chapter has introduced the medical assistant student to the organization of the administrative aspects of a medical practice or facility through a systems approach. In viewing the operation of a medical practice as a series of systems, you will be able to study each system independently while developing an understanding of how the systems affect one another. The orderly management of the office facilities and equipment provides an atmosphere of comfort for patients and efficiency for employees. Evaluating each unique situation, planing for the needs of the various areas within the facility, and maintaining the system in a consistent manner will enhance public image and provide a pleasant working environment. The development of systems makes for an orderly dispensation in all areas. Maintenance of all equipment and disposal of hazardous waste ensures that the office is always in compliance with current OSHA regulations.

Review QUESTIONS

1. Describe the role of the office manager.

2. What is systems management? Name and describe the systems involved in the medical practice.

3. Name and discuss the four steps of the process used to select new employees for a practice.

4. List and discuss the four possible levels of employment status.

5. Describe the purpose of the policy manual. Describe a procedures manual, and explain how it is used to train personnel.

6. Describe your responsibilities to patients regarding comfort, safety, and security, and to co-workers regarding equipment accessibility.

7. List and describe the four areas of internal office space.

8. Describe capital equipment, and give three examples of capital items.

9. Define expendable equipment and supplies, and give four examples each of expendable administrative and clinical equipment.

10. Describe the reorder point, and give an example.

11. Develop an efficient possible plan for reordering expendable supplies.

12. How should supplies be stored?

SUGGESTED READINGS

American Medical Association: *OSHA regulations: a prescription for compliance,* Chicago, AMA, 1992 (12-minute video).

American Medical Association: *Planning guide for physician's medical facilities,* Chicago, AMA, 1989.

Cody JP: Materials management: developing an inventory system, *The Professional Medical Assistant,* January/February: 11-14, 1991.

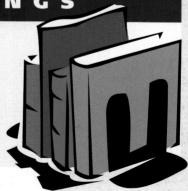

Medications

On completion of Chapter 12 the administrative medical assistant student should be able to:

1 Define the key terms listed in this chapter.

2 Explain the three types of medication names.

3 Define the five schedules of controlled substances.

4 Know how to read a prescription.

K E Y   T E R M S

Brand name	The trade name of a medication as copyrighted by the manufacturer.
Chemical name	The industrial name for the medication describing the main chemical contents of the medication.
Drug Enforcement Agency (DEA)	The federal agency responsible for the enforcement of laws regulating the distribution and sale of drugs.
DEA number	A federal monitoring tool issued by the DEA to physicians to regulate narcotic and hypnotic licenses.
Generic name	The established or official name by which the medication is known as an independent substance regardless of the manufacturer.
Pharmaceutical	Pertaining to pharmacies, drugs, and medications.
Pharmacist	A person trained in the art or practice of preparing and dispensing drugs; also known as a *druggist, apothecary,* and in some areas, as a *chemist.*
Physician's Desk Reference (PDR)	The reference book used by physicians and health care staff to review information regarding prescription medications; it contains information regarding components of the medication, uses of the medication, normal dosage, and adverse reactions. Sometimes a photograph of the actual medication is given.
Prescription	The description and directions for use of a particular medication for the patient, written by the physician to give directives to the pharmacist.

edication is an important element in medical practice. Many patients who have appointments with the physician will receive a prescription for medication. Other patients will telephone the practice and ask for prescriptions or ask to have their prescriptions refilled. Although medical assistants are not permitted to write prescriptions or to dispense medications, you will play an important role in helping the physician make certain that the medications are administered and safeguarded properly.

The Role of the Administrative Medical Assistant

Administrative medical assistants can be helpful to physicians by being knowledgeable about state and federal guidelines regarding medications, assisting patients in understanding medication instructions, and documenting medication information.

Knowledge of Medication Guidelines

The administrative medical assistant can schedule time periodically for the physician to meet with pharmaceutical representatives to learn about new medications on the market that would be useful to the physician in his or her practice. It is a good idea to schedule these meetings during the lunch hour or as the last appointment in the afternoon.

Patient Education

A policy of many medical practices is to require new patients to sign an informed consent regarding the use of medication and possible side effects. Food, beverages, and other medications taken in conjunction with the new medication could possible produce adverse side effects. If a patient taking medication calls the office with one or more complaints, such as blurred vision, constipation, dizziness, drowsiness, headache, hemorrhaging, nausea, rash, respiratory trouble, sleeplessness, vomiting, or weight loss, the medical assistant should immediately notify the physician. The medical assistant cannot legally tell the patient to stop taking the medication because this would constitute practicing medicine without a license.

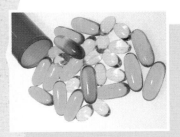

If a patient calls the office after taking an overdose of medication, the medical assistant should immediately call 9-1-1 so that the dispatcher can coordinate the personnel and services best suited to assist the patient in distress. If the patient is not in an area with 9-1-1 service, contact the nearest fire department.

Occasionally, physicians will request that the medical assistants instruct the patients about medication dosages and schedules. The assistant must be sure that the patient understands the directions and should request that the patient repeat them back to the assistant. With elderly patients it is helpful to have a large typed sheet for each medication in which the assistant can fill in certain

PERSPECTIVES ON MEDICAL ASSISTING

Drug Reactions

There is no drug that does not affect some patient adversely. Drugs are taken to produce good pharmacological effects, but allergic or toxic reactions are always possible. A comparison of a toxic vs. an allergic reaction follows:

- Toxic—may occur with any drug. The dosage usually is high. It may occur with the first dose or may be the result of a cumulative effect. The symptoms may be similar to the regular action of the drug, and there are no associated disorders.
- Allergic—occurs infrequently. The dosage usually is therapeutic, that is, a normal dose. It usually happens on reexposure to the drug, but some drugs cross-react with chemicals in other drugs of similar structure. The symptoms are not similar to the regular actions of the drug. Associated disorders are asthma and hay fever.

WHAT DO YOU THINK?

The patient was given a prescription for Cafergot suppositories to treat her migraine headaches. The prescription was for 12 suppositories to be inserted every 4 hours for headaches. Neither the physician nor the pharmacist cautioned the patient that no more than two suppositories should be used per headache and that no more than five per week should be used. The patient used the suppositories as directed but was unaware of the limitations so she overused them and experienced toxic effects as a result.

Who is at fault in this case? How can a situation like this be avoided? As an administrative medical assistant, what type of instructions can you give the patient?

blanks in large letters, while going over the information verbally. This will help prevent confusion when the patient is taking several medications. If a family member or friend has accompanied the patient to the office and assists with the patient's care, that person should be included when instructions are given.

When the physician provides the patient with samples of medications, the patient also should be given the insert from the pharmaceutical company. The physician can be held liable if the patient suffers an undisclosed side effect and does not have the insert.

Documenting Medication Information

The medical assistant should see that the information regarding the adverse medication reaction is well documented in the patient's chart and kept near the front of the medical record. If this information is not accessible to the physician, the patient's health could be jeopardized. For example, in some cases a patient was known to be allergic to a particular drug, such as penicillin, but the information was buried in the patient's chart. In one case the physician was not able to ask the patient, who was comatose, if he was allergic to penicillin, and a lethal dose was administered, resulting in the patient's death.

It is the medical assistant's responsibility to see that verbal prescriptions and refills are promptly documented in the patient's medical records. It always is helpful to have the name and telephone number of the patient's pharmacist listed on the front of the chart. It provides the medical assistant and physician with immediate access for telephoning a prescription or refill. To eliminate the possibility of errors when telephoning in a prescription, request that the pharmacist read back each prescription. Patients must be instructed to bring all medications to the office when being seen for the first time or before being admitted to a hospital.

The administrative medical assistant also is responsible for keeping well-documented records of narcotic prescriptions and for ensuring that the physician's narcotic license renewal through the Drug Enforcement Agency (DEA) is sent in a timely manner.

Names of Medications

The Food and Drug Administration (FDA) under the direction of the Department of Health and Human Services (DHHS) is responsible for monitoring and enforcing all drug legislation and for protecting the public and keeping them informed of the potential dangers of many medications. It also is the responsibility of the FDA to determine that medications are safe before allowing them to be marketed to the public. The FDA monitors strength, quality, and identification of medications before allowing them to be shipped throughout the country. This process results in the standardization of medications throughout the United States. The FDA also sees that information regarding new medications is gathered and published for public safety.

The administrative medical assistant must be extremely careful when documenting medications to use the exact name and spelling for the medication. Drug references, such as the *Physician's Desk Reference (PDR), Mosby's GenRx,* or *Facts and Comparisons,* are very helpful in determining the correct spelling. The assistant should be familiar with the format of several drug references and should know how to look up medications under the manufacturer's name, brand or generic name, product category, or product information, and how to use the references' product identification guide. The most commonly used sections of drug reference books are the brand or generic name and product information sections (Table 12.1). Sometimes a medication is listed in the PDR under three names, which are as follows:

1. Generic name—the established official name by which a medication is known as an isolated substance, regardless of the manufacturer. When a medication is licensed under its generic name, it also is given a brand name by the manufacturer (Figure 12.1). The generic name is assigned by the United States Adopted Names (USAN) Council. When typed or written, a generic medication name is not capitalized, unless the generic name is identical to the brand name.

TABLE 12-1

Examples of Drugs as Commonly Listed in Reference Books

Generic name	Brand*/trade name	Product information
Tetracycline	Tetracyn	Pfizer
Meprobamate	Equanil	Wyeth
	Meprotabs	Wallace
	Miltown	Wallace
Penicillin G	Bicillin	Wyeth
Penicillin G procaine	Crysticillin	Squibb

*A typical drug may be known by as many as three names.

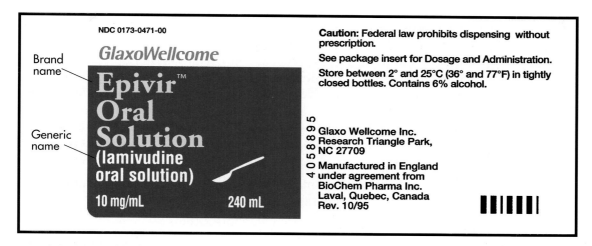

FIGURE 12.1

A drug's generic name is the official name by which it is known as an isolated substance regardless of its manufacturer; the brand name indicates ownership by the manufacturer and serves as a trademark. (From Gray D: *Calculate with confidence*, ed 2, St. Louis, 1998, Mosby.)

2. Chemical name—Indicates the chemical content of the medication.
3. Brand name—Indicates ownership by the manufacturer and serves as a trademark protected from competition. A superscript "R" to the right of the name indicates that the trademark has been registered with the U.S. Patent and Trademark Office. A "TM" to the right of the name indicates it is being used as a trademark but is not federally registered. The medications are named in various ways. Sometimes only the first letter is capitalized (for example, Restoril) or will have capital letters in the name (for example, pHisoHex). Some have hyphens in the name; others do not. Some medications, such as penicillin, may appear either capitalized or not.

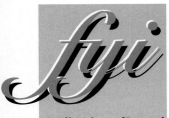

Medications (Drugs)

Most modern medications are composed of manufactured or synthetic drugs; however, about 40% of prescribed drugs still are natural substances or are semi-synthetic. Examples of natural medicinal sources are:

1. Alkaloids—alkaline substances from the poppy (for example, morphine) and from the tobacco plant (for example, nicotine)
2. Glycosides (also known as glucosides)—most common are digitalis from the digitalis (foxglove) plant, and strophanthin from the Strophanthus plant
3. Oxalates—oxalic acid comes from rhubarb leaves
4. Resins—come from milkweeds and laurels
5. Phytotoxin proteins—come from castor beans

It is very interesting to study medications and see how they are formed. Alternative medicine has brought about more information and use of natural or herbal medicine.

Legislation in most states allows patients to request that their prescriptions be filled with the generic equivalent of the medication. If the prescription does not specify a particular brand, the pharmacists can substitute generic for brand-name medications if they have the patient's and/or the physician's permission and if the substitution does not increase the pharmacist's dollar profit. For example, the generic medication oxytetracycline might be substituted for its brand name Terramycin. Generic medications are always less expensive; thus, it is likely that most patients will request generic medications on their prescriptions.

Medication References

For years very little published information was available on the uniformity or strength of medications. The United States Pharmacopeia (USP) was published in the late 1800s to provide medication standards for identification, to indicate the purity of medications, and to ensure uniformity of strength. Another reference is the National Formulary (NF), which contains formulas for medication mixtures as published by the American Pharmaceutical Association (APA). The medications included in this reference are selected based on therapeutic value.

Probably the most utilized reference in the physician's office is the PDR, published annually with supplements during the year by Medical Economics Company, Inc. in Montvale, New Jersey. This reference book provides essential prescription information on major pharmaceutical products. It lists only those medications the pharmaceutical companies pay to have listed, thus not all medications are shown. Still, only a few are missing. This reference book is divided into six sections:

1. Alphabetical index by manufacturer (white)—includes the manufacturer's name, address, and telephone number.
2. Alphabetical brand and generic name index (pink)—includes the name of the manufacturer and reference for a description of each product. This section can be used to check for the correct spelling of the medication name.
3. Product Category Index (blue)—useful as a reference if the assistant is not sure of the name of the medication but knows the category, that is, antibiotic, laxative.
4. Product Identification Guide (gray)—color reproductions of the products by manufacturer.
5. Product Information (white)—a large section of the book, well over 2750 medications and products alphabetized by manufacturer and then by product name within each manufacturer's list. This section contains detailed information on use, dosage, composition, actions, and side effects. The generic name of the medication is included in the description.
6. Diagnostic Product Information (green)—a list of injectable materials used in radiographic diagnostic procedures and brand names of products used for laboratory and skin diagnostic tests.

The PDR also is available for the personal computer equipped with a CD-ROM drive.

Other drug references are available that list medications by brand and generic names. Most of these are inexpensive, compact, and contain the same information as the PDR. Products also are available in electronic format, such as *Mosby's GenRx,* which can be accessed on CD-ROM, over the Internet, or through an office computer network or Intranet. A product like this is quick and easy to use and can be utilized by office staff for tasks such as researching drug interactions and costs of therapies.

Types of Medications

1970 Controlled Substances Act

As part of the Controlled Substances Act of 1970, physicians are required to register or reregister their narcotic license by June 30 each year with the DEA, an agency that is part of the U.S. Department of Justice. The DEA regulates the manufacturing and dispensing of dangerous medication or medication with the potential for abuse. If physicians have offices in more than one state, they are required to register with the DEA office for each region.

Should the physician be late in renewing his or her registration, there is a 3-month grace period after the registration expires during which the physician can continue to prescribe controlled substances. The physician must keep a record for 2 years of the drugs dispensed as listed in the five schedules under the Act. Medical assistants also should be aware of laws in their state that may affect this Act.

Controlled medications have a high potential for abuse; federal controls are designed to minimize their availability and diminish the opportunities for abuse. These medications, which include both narcotics and some nonnarcotics, range from those most easily abused and habit forming, classified as Schedule I, to those less dangerous to the user and not subject to as much abuse, classified as Schedule V (see the box about controlled medications).

The controlled substance packaging and labeling must show clearly the medication's assigned schedule. This is written to the right of the medication name.

The physician's DEA number must appear on all physician narcotic prescription blanks, purchase orders, and any other documents of transfer (most physicians have the DEA numbers preprinted on their prescription blanks). Schedule II substances must be ordered with the Federal Triplicate Order Form (DEA-222). To prevent unauthorized use of controlled substances, orders for Schedules III, IV, and V substances need the physician's DEA registration number written on the prescription. In some states, when ordering Schedule II substances from out-of-state companies, a copy of the purchase agreement (not the Federal Triplicate Order Form) must be sent within 24 hours of placing the order to the office of the state attorney general.

Reading the Prescription

The greatest difficulty in reading prescriptions often is the physician's handwriting; however, certain abbreviations and symbols are identifiable (Table 12.2). Prescription pads can be obtained that are carbon-backed or have NCR

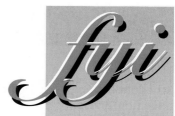

The History of Aspirin

Aspirin is the brand (trade) name for acetylsalicylic acid. It is a common analgesic and can be traced back to Hippocrates, who used the powder made from the bark of willows to treat pain and relieve fever. In 1829 the parent of the drug family, salicin, was isolated from the willow bark. In 1875 sodium salicylate was developed as a pain reliever, but it irritated the stomach so it was not very popular. In 1897 Felix Hoffman, a German chemist working for Bayer, decided to try to make a less acidic formula, and his work led to the synthesis of acetylsalicylic acid, or ASA. This became the popular pain killer among physicians worldwide.

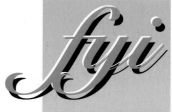

General Categories of Drugs

1. Antimicrobials—drugs that destroy or disable disease-causing microorganisms in the body
2. Pharmacodynamics—drugs that either stimulate or depress normal body functions so that the course of disease is changed
3. Chemotherapeutic—drugs used to treat cancer (uncontrolled growth of cells); these drugs have a selective effect

SCHEDULE OF CONTROLLED MEDICATIONS

Schedule I

Schedule I drugs, having the highest potential for addiction and abuse, have not been accepted for medical use in the United States. Their use is limited to research purposes only after the research facility has obtained government approval and agreement to research protocol to test drugs for medical indications. Examples are heroin, marijuana, lysergic acid diethylamide (LSD), and mescaline.

Schedule II

Schedule II drugs have a high potential for abuse and addiction but have an acceptable medical use for treatment in the United States. Examples are amobarbital, amphetamine, cocaine, codeine, meperidine, methadone, methamphetamine, morphine, opium, and secobarbital.

Schedule III

Schedule III drugs have a potential for abuse less than the drugs in Schedules I or II, and have a mod-erate or low addiction liability. They have an acceptable medical use for treatment in the United States. Examples are APC with codeine, butabarbital, methyprylon, nalorphine, and paregoric.

Schedule IV

Schedule IV drugs have a lower potential for abuse and limited addiction liability relative to drugs in Schedule III. They have an acceptable medical use for treatment in the United States. Examples are chloral hydrate, diazepam, meprobamate, paralde-hyde, and phenobarbital.

Schedule V

Schedule V drugs have a low potential for abuse and a limited addiction liability relative to drugs in Schedule IV. They have an acceptable medical use for treatment in the United States. Examples are drugs of primarily low-strength codeine (less than those compounds included in Schedule III) combined with other medicinal ingredients.

---

paper, thereby creating a copy of the prescription. However, most physicians and office staff find this system to be time consuming. Small pieces of paper tend to get misplaced, unless the chart is equipped with a special sheet with preadhesive backing on which to place the copy of the prescription. The physician is the only one who is approved to write the prescription and approve telephone requests for the prescription. If the handwriting is illegible, it is the responsibility of the pharmacist to telephone the physician for clarification. Many parts of the prescription may be misread. For example, 1.0 mg may be read as 10 mg, so instead write 1 mg; .3 mg may be read as 3 mg; so write 0.3 mg; U may be read as O, so write as Unit; every 3-4 hours may be read as 3/4 hr, so write as 3 to 4 hours.

In Texas and Iowa medical assistants may not call in prescriptions or refills; only physicians are allowed to call for controlled substances. The pharmacy is not allowed to accept the call from a nurse or assistant. Nonetheless, medical assistants should know prescription terms and abbreviations and understand the instructions regarding administration of medications because they will be used in telephone conversation (see Table 12.2). The abbreviations are a kind of medical shorthand that speeds taking telephone and other messages.

A prescription blank is preprinted with the physician's name, address, telephone number, state license number, and DEA number (Figure 12.2). There also is space for the patient's name, address, and the date issued by the physi-

TABLE 12-2

Common Prescription Abbreviations and Symbols

Abbreviation or symbol	Meaning	Abbreviation or symbol	Meaning
a	Before	NS	Normal saline
aa	Of each	noc(t)	Night
ac	Before meals	od	Daily or once a day
ad lib	As desired	OD	Right eye
amt	Amount	oint	Ointment
aq	Aqueous	OS	Left eye
bid	Twice a day	OU	Both eyes
c̄	With	oz	Ounce
cap(s)	Capsule(s)	ʒ	Ounce
cc	Cubic centimeter	p	After, past
dil	Dilute	per	By or with
Dx or Diag	Diagnosis	pc	After meals
D/C or d/c	Discontinue	po or per os	By mouth
D/W	Dextrose in water	prn	Whenever necessary
dr	Drain	pt	Pint (or patient)
ʒ	Dram	pulv	Powder
ʒ	One dram	q	Every
d	Day	qam	Every morning
Dr	Doctor	qd	Every day
fl or fld	Fluid	qh	Every hour
gal	Gallon	q2h or q2	Every 2 hours
g or gm	Gram	q3h or q3	Every 3 hours
gr	Grain	qhs	Every night
gt or gtt	Drop(s)	qid	Four times per day
H or hr	Hour	qod	Every other day
hs	Hour of sleep or bedtime	qs	Quantity sufficient
		Rx	Take thou
IM	Intramuscular	s̄	Without
IU	International units	sc or subq or SubQ	Subcutaneous
IV	Intravenous	Sig	Directions
kg	Kilogram	sol	Solution
L	Liter	ss	One half
liq	Liquid	subling	Sublingual (under tongue)
m or min	Minimum		
mgc	Microgram	stat	Immediate
mEq	Milliequivalent	tid	Three times a day
mEq/L	Milliequivalents per liter	tinc or tr	Tincture
		tab	Tablet
mg	Milligram	tsp	Teaspoon
ml or mL	Milliliter	Tbsp	Tablespoon
mm	Millimeter	ung or ungt	Ointment
npo (NPO)	Nothing by mouth	U	Units

THOMAS A. SCOTT, M.D.
General Practice

135 So. Elm St.
Sacramento, Ca. 94106
Telephone: (916) 344-5550

FOR _____ DATE _____

ADDRESS _____

R̷x

SAMPLE
DO NOT FILL

CAL. LIC. #G099914
DEA #AK08888888

REFILL_____TIMES   _____
#25-8294   *Thomas A. Scott, M.D.*

FIGURE 12.2

A prescription blank is preprinted with the physician's name, address, telephone number, state license number, and DEA number.

cian. In the remaining space the physician writes the four standard components of the prescription, which are as follows:

1. Superscription, which is the symbol Rx, signifying the Latin word for "take."
2. Inscription, which contains the name of the medication, quantity to be dispensed, and dose strength. The strength normally is given in mg (milligrams); the strength of creams, ointments, and topical liquids is given as a percentage. The strength of oral liquid medications is given as milligrams per milliliter.
3. Subscription, which gives directions to the pharmacist on the dosage, total quantity of the medication to be dispensed, and form of medication (for example, capsules, tablets).
4. Signature, which gives instructions to the patient. The pharmacist types the instructions on the label, so the patient will know how to take or apply the medication. (The instructions often are written using Latin abbreviations, which the pharmacist must translate.) Sometimes, written instructions are supplemented with verbal directions to the patient, for example, whether to take the medication around the clock or only during awake hours.

The physician's signature always is required in ink. If the prescription is not imprinted with the physician's narcotic number and the prescription is for a narcotic, the number must be written on the prescription. The bottom of the prescription blank has a space for the physician to indicate the number of refills

AT WORK TODAY

Parts of the Prescription

The various parts of a prescription blank are identified as follows:
1. Superscription—Rx, meaning "take"
2. Inscription—the drug name, quantity, and dose
3. Subscription—directions to the pharmacist on the dosage, total quantity of the drug to be dispensed, and the form of the medication
4. Signature—the instructions to the patient that the pharmacist is to print on the label

MEDICAL ASSISTING STEP-BY-STEP

Routes of Drug Administration

Drugs are administered through various routes to modify their effect on the body. Some drugs are suited for only one route of administration; others may be given using one of several possible routes. Drugs generally are administered one of two ways: locally or systemically. These are important categories to know so that you understand drugs more thoroughly.

Local
- Topical drugs
- Mucous membrane drugs
- Suppositories
- Nasal drugs
- Ophthalmic drugs
- Ear drugs

Systemic
- Oral drugs
- Sublingual drugs
- Parenteral drugs (injections)
  - Intradermal
  - Subcutaneous
  - Intramuscular
  - Intravenous

allowed. Some physicians sometimes will write on their prescriptions, "Do not substitute," "Dispense as written," or "Brand medically necessary," referring to the substitution of a generic medication for the specific brand-name medication.

Preventing Prescription Abuse

In some areas physicians often are approached by people exhibiting varying extremes of drug-seeking behavior. The administrative medical assistant should be able to recognize those patients who might be medication misusers or abusers. The stories these individuals present can be quite creative. For instance, they may say that they are from out of town, and accidently dropped their prescription down the toilet or that they lost their prescription on the way to the pharmacy. Someone unfamiliar to the medical assistant may state that he or she is a patient of the physician's colleague and needs to have a prescription for a controlled substance renewed. In such situations, the medical assistant should ask the patient for the name of his or her regular physician and attempt to verify the story. Be cautious when a patient avoids questions or hesitates in answering; such behavior may indicate a problem.

The physician's office is the prime target for medication abusers. The medical assistant can help protect the office and the physician by:

1. Storing unused prescription blanks under lock and key
2. Giving the physician one pad to carry with him or her and keeping one in a locked drawer
3. Not leaving prescription pads in examination rooms or treatment areas, and definitely not in the physician's automobile
4. Not using preprinted prescription blanks
5. Never having the physician sign prescription blanks in advance
6. Being sure the physician always writes the prescriptions in ink to prevent alteration
7. Checking to make sure the quantity of medications prescribed is written out as well as expressed numerically in a manner that cannot be changed, that is, 30 to 80 capsules.
8. Never allowing the prescription blanks to be used as scratch pads or notepads.
9. Using tamper-proof prescription pads that are tinted so erasures or whiteout ink is easily noticeable. All prescription copies should have the word "void" printed across them.

Should you discover a prescription pad missing, it might be a good idea to mark the remaining pads (perhaps clipping off the righthand lower corner) and notify local pharmacists to reject or double-check all prescriptions that appear as whole sheets. Many communities have set up a telephone network in which a pharmacist calls two pharmacists, those two then each call two other pharmacists, and so on, so that the entire community can be informed quickly when prescription blanks are stolen.

Disposal of Medications
Uncontrolled Substances

According to individual state laws governing disposal of uncontrolled substances, small quantities of syrups, tablets, or capsules may be flushed down the toilet, and the containers they came in may be put out in the normal trash bins. For injectables and topical preparations, it is preferable that they be incinerated. Companies are available in most areas that are licensed to incinerate drugs, or perhaps the medical assistant can ask the local hospital if it is possible to use its incinerator provided state laws permit that.

Controlled Substances

To dispose of controlled substances, one must obtain DEA Form 41, "Inventory of Drugs Surrendered," from the nearest DEA office. Complete the form and have the physician sign it to verify its accuracy. Call the nearest DEA office for any further instructions, since not all offices have facilities for storing and destroying controlled substances. To ship the medication, use registered mail.

After the drugs are destroyed, the DEA (or whoever is appointed by the DEA) should send the physician a receipt. File the receipt in a safe.

Conclusion

Administrative medical assistant students should understand the importance of medications, the need for protection of the prescription blanks, the need for clarity of handwriting on the prescription, and the difference between controlled and uncontrolled medications.

Review QUESTIONS

1. List the three types of medication names.
2. What are the five schedules of controlled substances?
3. How often must physicians renew their registration with the DEA?
4. What is the DEA?
5. Which is the best medication reference book?
6. What does qid. mean?
7. What is the best method of disposal for uncontrolled medications?
8. What is the best method of disposal for controlled medications?

SUGGESTED READINGS

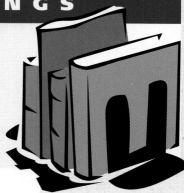

Facts and comparisons (a looseleaf subscription drug reference product providing monthly updates), Wolters Kluwer.

Mosby's GenRx (print and electronic editions published yearly, with quarterly updates available), St. Louis, Mosby.

Physician's desk reference (published each year), Montvale, NJ, Medical Economics.

Coding, Billing, and Claims Processing

OBJECTIVES

On completion of chapter 13 the administrative medical assistant student should be able to:

1. Define the key terms listed in this chapter.

2. Code procedures correctly.

3. Code diagnoses correctly.

4. Understand the assignment of benefits.

5. Define billing requirements for Medicare.

6. Complete a claim form.

7. Give the steps of working with rejected or lost claims.

KEY TERMS

Assignment of benefits The transfer of one's right to collect an amount payable under an insurance contract.

Benefit The amount payable by the insurance carrier toward the cost of various covered medical or dental services.

Claim A demand presented to an insurance carrier or intermediary to pay for services provided to the insured.

Copayment The portion of a service fee that the insured must pay.

CPT-4 *Physicians' Current Procedural Terminology, Fourth Edition;* a listing of procedure codes for all recognized physician services. This manual is updated every year and published by the American Medical Association (AMA).

Continued

K E Y   T E R M S

(Continued)

Deductible The insured's annual, initial, specific cost of health care as set by the terms of the health insurance policy required prior to insurance benefits being paid.

Fee for service The method of billing by a physician in private practice, whereby the physician charges for each professional service performed.

Indigent A person unable to secure the financial means to meet his or her basic needs.

Insured A person protected against financial loss by an insurance policy. In medicine, this may be the patient or the person (a separate individual) to whom the insurance policy belongs.

Provider Supplier, physician, or the one providing services to the insured or the insured's beneficiary (patient).

Reimbursement Payment to an individual for expenses previously paid.

ealth care professionals provide valuable, even life-saving, services to patients. The medical practice must generate revenue to continue providing those services. Correct coding, billing, and claims submission is crucial for the medical practice to be paid appropriately for services rendered. As the administrative medical assistant, you play a vital role in obtaining reimbursement for physician services. You must understand how to code claims correctly, how to assist patients with billing information, and how to submit claims for reimbursement (Figure 13.1). Your expertise in these areas will help the practice maintain a steady stream of revenue.

Procedural Coding

Physicians' Current Procedural Terminology, Fourth Edition (CPT-4)

Physicians' Current Procedural Terminology, Fourth Edition (CPT-4) is a listing of descriptive terms and corresponding five-digit identification codes for reporting medical and physician services and procedures. The purpose of the terminology is to provide a uniform language that will accurately describe medical, surgical, and diagnostic services, and provide an effective means for reliable nationwide communication among physicians, patients, and third parties. The CPT was first published in 1966 by the American Medical Association (AMA) and is updated annually. Each year the AMA deletes outdated codes, adds new codes, and occasionally changes the description applied to a code number (Figure 13.2). The new edition for the upcoming year is available in

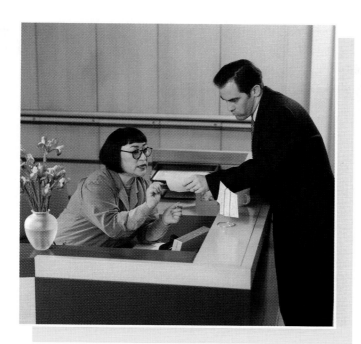

You must understand how to code claims correctly, how to assist patients with billing information, and how to submit claims for reimbursement.

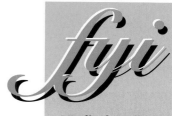

October of the current year. For example, the 1997 edition is available in October of 1996.

CPT descriptive terms and identification codes currently serve various important functions in medical nomenclature. This system of terminology is the most widely accepted nomenclature for reporting of physician procedures and services under government and private health insurance programs. CPT also is useful for administrative management purposes, such as claims processing, and for the development of guidelines for medical care review. The uniform language likewise is applicable to medical education and research by providing a useful basis for local, regional, and national utilization comparisons. With the introduction of almost 2000 new codes for evaluation and management services in the CPT 1992, important changes were made in the way that physicians report many of their services. These revisions were responsive to changes in the medical practice environment. All government and most third-party payers require the CPT-4 codes for claim purposes. The CPT is broken into six categories as presented in the box on p. 314.

Relative Value Studies (RVS)

Relative value studies (RVS), such as the California Relative Value Study (CRVS), are designed to describe medical/surgical services specifically for reimbursement purposes. The CRVS was first developed by the California Medical Association in 1956 to identify physician services and assign unit values to indicate a relative value scale within each individual section of the services described.

The CRVS was updated periodically to maintain continued use in a changing scientific environment and economy. In the mid-1970s the Federal Trade Commission (FTC) ruled that the use of the relative values was in viola-

Medical Coding

Coding has become a very important subject for the administrative medical assistant. There are two types of coding: procedure and diagnostic. The older type, diagnostic, was created in Europe in the seventeenth century and was used for reporting illness and causes of death. ICD (International Classification of Diseases) is a system developed by the World Health Organization of the United Nations to code the diagnosis (the problem). This system uses a three-digit number, which can be expanded up to five digits for specific diagnoses, injuries, and symptoms. Procedural coding uses five-digit numbers to represent medical procedures (the visit and what was done during that visit). This newer system was created in 1964 for the RVS (Relative Value Study), updated in 1975 for CPT (Current Procedural Terminology), and currently is updated annually by the AMA.

FIGURE 13.2

Responsibility falls on the administrative medical assistant to assist physicians in learning about new and updated codes.

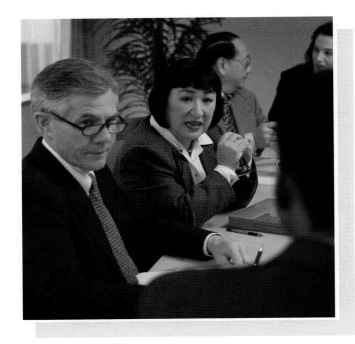

THE SIX CATEGORIES OF THE CPT

99201-99499: Evaluation and Management

These services include patient visits to the office, hospital, home, nursing home, emergency center, and skilled nursing facility; counseling/intervention; critical care; and observation.

00100-01999: Anesthesia

All anesthesia services are reported using a designated five-digit procedural code plus a physical status modifier. Certain carriers may request the use of other modifiers.

10040-69979: Surgical codes

These codes include the operation; local infiltration; metacarpal/digital block or topical anesthesia, when used; and normal, uncomplicated follow-up care. This concept is referred to as a *package* for surgical procedures. Some of the listed procedures commonly carried out are an integral part of a total service and as such do not warrant a separate identification. However, a procedure that is performed independently and is not immediately related to another service may be listed as a *"separate."*

Subheadings for surgical/diagnostic procedures are as follows:

- 10040-19499: Integumentary system
- 20000-29909: Musculoskeletal system
- 30000-37799: Cardiovascular system
- 38100-38999: Hemic and lymphatic systems
- 39000-39599: Mediastinum and diaphragm
- 40490-49999: Digestive system
- 50010-53899: Urinary system
- 54000-55980: Male genital system
- 56300-56300: Laparoscopy/peritoneoscopy/ hysteroscopy
- 56405-58999: Female genital system
- 59000-59899: Maternity care and delivery
- 60000-60699: Endocrine system
- 61000-64999: Nervous system
- 65091-68899: Eye and ocular adnexa
- 69000-69979: Auditory system

70010-79999: Radiology

These codes include diagnostic radiology services, ultrasound, nuclear medicine, radiation oncology, and therapeutic services.

80002-89399: Pathology and laboratory

These codes cover all pathology and laboratory services.

90700-99199

These codes cover a myriad of miscellaneous special services.

HCPCS CODES

A—used for medical and surgical supplies
B—used for enteral and parenteral therapy
D—used for dental procedures
E—used for durable medical equipment
J—used for injectable drugs

K—used for DMERCS use only
L—used for orthotic procedures
M—used for certain medical procedures
R—used for certain radiology services
V—used for ophthalmology and vision services

tion of price fixing regulations and therefore could no longer be used. The procedure description feature of the CRVS, however, has survived and was updated as recently as 1985. It is now known as the *California Standard Nomenclature.* Despite the FTC ruling, some state medical associations continued to publish their respective RVS. For example, the Florida Relative Value Study was published as late as 1986. The CRVS coding system still is used by some Workers' Compensation carriers, although the Workers' Compensation Board has been promising since 1992 that they eventually will utilize the CPT-4.

Health Care Financing Administration Common Procedural Coding System (HCPCS)

The *Health Care Financing Administration Common Procedural Coding System, National Level II,* commonly referred to as *HCPCS,* is a listing of codes and descriptive terminology used for reporting the provision of supplies, materials, injections, and certain services and procedures to Medicare and most Blue Cross carriers (see the box above). HCPCS 1996 is an annual publication based on the most recent revision of the HCPCS National Level II codes. The changes usually are made by October of each year, thus the new codes are effective on January 1 of each year. The use of HCPCS may vary from carrier to carrier. This variance causes some confusion regarding the use of the HCPCS; use according to "carrier discretion." There also is an HCPCS Local Level III; however, this has been largely ignored by the carriers. Notification for its use comes from bulletins published by the individual carrier.

The HCPCS is a five-digit code that begins with an alphabetical character (for example, A4550 is for surgical trays).

HCPCS comprises the following three distinct levels of procedural codes plus the series of modifiers:

Level 1. CPT-4, a listing of descriptive terms and identification codes for reporting medical services and procedures, is the basis for reporting most medical/surgical services performed by physicians.

Level 2. The HCFA developed additional alpha-numerical codes (A0000-V5999) to identify nonphysician (supplier), as well as additional physician services and procedures, not found in the CPT-4.

Level 3. Where there is no appropriate national code assignment (Level II codes) for a given service or procedure, the Medicare carrier may opt to assign an alpha-numerical code within the range W1000-Y9999. These codes allow the carrier the flexibility to code a particular service or item that may be unique to that service area or currently only seen in that local level. The HCFA evaluates Level 3 codes from all carriers periodically to determine if a national code should be assigned. It is therefore possible that services and procedures in the local code category will be moved to the national category and assigned a different number.

Modifiers

Modifiers permit a provider to indicate the circumstances under which a procedure as performed differs from the description by using a five-digit code.

Five advantages to using modifiers are as follows:

- They eliminate the need for a lengthy report
- They give a more accurate description of services
- They may increase or decrease the fee
- They may indicate a component of service or adjunctive service
- The physician's fee profile will not be affected as a result of fees being lowered

Modifiers are added as suffixes to the procedural code when additional information regarding the circumstances, setting, patient condition, and so on is required. Use modifiers when:

- The service or procedure being rendered has either a professional or a technical component, or both
- The service or procedure is performed by more than one physician and/or in more than one location
- The service or procedure has been increased/reduced
- The service or procedure was repeated
- Part of the service was performed in conjunction with another service
- Unusual events occurred

As with procedural coding, both national and local modifiers are utilized.

In addition to the two-digit modifiers identified in the CPT-4, other two-digit alpha-numerical and two-digit alpha modifiers are assigned nationally. These national modifiers are in ranges of A1-V9 and AA-VZ. Where there is no appropriate CPT-4 national modifier, carriers will assign a two-digit alpha-numerical or alpha modifier to identify certain billings. Local modifiers are in ranges W1-Z9 and WA-ZZ.

Diagnostic Coding

International Classification of Diseases, Ninth Revision, Clinical Modification (ICD9-CM)

The *International Classification of Diseases, Ninth Revision, Clinical Modification* (ICD9-CM) is published annually in cooperation with the HCFA. It originally was published by the World Health Organization (WHO), which developed the foundation for the ICD9-CM. The WHO Collaborating Center for Classification of Diseases in North America serves as a liaison between the international obligations for comparable classifications and the national health data needs of the United States.

The ICD9-CM is recommended for use in all clinical settings but is required for reporting diagnoses and diseases to all U.S. Public Health Service and HCFA programs. Continuous maintenance of the ICD9-CM is the responsibility of the federal government. The ICD9-CM is revised annually and usually is published as a three-volume set as follows:

Volume 1—*Diseases: Tabular List* (number followed by description)
Volume 2—*Diseases: Alphabetic Index* (description followed by assigned number)
Volume 3—*Procedures: Tabular List and Alphabetic Index*

Volumes 1 and 2 are the most commonly used in the medical office. Volume 1 also contains five appendices, which are as follows:

Appendix A—"Morphology of Neoplasms"
Appendix B—"Glossary of Mental Disorders"
Appendix C—"Classification of Drugs by American Hospital Formulary Service"
Appendix D—"Classification of Industrial Accident According to Agency"
Appendix E—"List of Three-Digit Categories"

Diagnostic and Statistical Manual, Third Edition (DSM-III)

The *Diagnostic and Statistical Manual, Third Edition,* is a diagnosis coding system used primarily by psychologists and psychiatrists. DSM-III was developed by the American Psychiatric Association's Task Force on Nomenclature and Statistics. The codes in DSM-III are somewhat compatible with the ICD9-CM; however, included is additional diagnostic information that is specific to the psychiatric specialty and also is used for data collection purposes.

AT WORK TODAY

Certified Coder

This is the world of specialization. If you find that you enjoy the challenge of coding (a type of detective work), then you may want to consider becoming a certified coder. The two organizations that provide coding certification are as follows:

Certified Procedural Coder (CPC)
American Academy of Procedural Coders
145 West Crystal Avenue
Salt Lake City, UT 84115

Certified Coding Specialist (CCS)
American Health Information Management Association (AHIMA)
119 North Michigan Avenue
Chicago, IL 60690

Billing Requirements

For the practice to be reimbursed properly, the front office staff must be aware of and understand insurance billing requirements. The administrative medical assistant plays a very important role by obtaining the correct patient information, reviewing the codes the physician has selected, assisting the physician in learning about new and updated codes, and seeing that the practice or the patient is reimbursed properly. Each carrier has special requirements; therefore, the administrative medical assistant must constantly review carrier bulletins and maintain a file for each carrier in order to file claims appropriately. This is especially time consuming if the physician or group belongs to numerous insurance panels, independent physician associations (IPAs), and preferred provider organizations (PPOs). These groups contract with numerous carriers, resulting in many carriers and claims requirements to keep track of.

The Role of the Administrative Medical Assistant

Obtaining Necessary Information

The first role the administrative medical assistant plays in helping both the physician and the patient be reimbursed for services is to obtain all pertinent information.

When the appointment is first made and if time allows, the medical assistant should ask the patient for all insurance information, including the following:

- If the patient has an identification card, it should be checked to see that the information is current, and then copied for the office record.
- When more than one insurance policy is involved, obtain the name, address, and group and policy number of each company.

MEDICAL ASSISTING STEP-BY-STEP

Quick Insurance Rules

1. Acquire all of the necessary insurance information. This will come from the patient information form in the medical record and from the patient's insurance card. Be sure to copy the card for your files.

2. Check to be certain that all information is correct and current.

3. When the patient has more than one insurance coverage, additional information will be needed.

4. Verify the insurance coverage when necessary for billing purposes.

5. Help patients fill out their own forms when necessary but do not advise them on coverage or plans.

- Make sure that the patient information sheet is filled out completely (Figure 13.3). If it has any open blanks, return the form to the patient and request that he or she complete all questions asked.
- Obtain the name of the subscriber, if it is someone other than the patient.
- Secure an assignment of benefits (Figure 13.4) for releasing information and securing payment if you are submitting the claim for the patient.

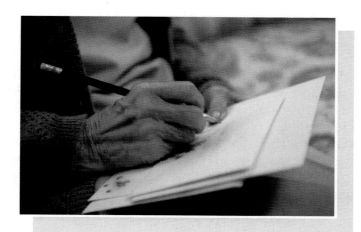

FIGURE 13.3

Make sure that the patient information sheet is filled out completely.

Assignment of Benefits and What It Means

When you accept the assignment of benefits from either Medicare or CHAMPUS, the check will come to you, and you are agreeing that you will accept as total payment what the government recognizes or allows. For example, the charge is $100, Medicare or CHAMPUS recognizes $80 and pays you $64. You then are expected to bill the patient the difference between the $64 and the $80, but you must write off the difference between the $80 and $100.

With other insurance companies, when you accept the assignment, it only means that the check comes to the physician office. You are expected to collect the difference between what is billed and paid from the responsible party.

Example:
I hereby assign all medical and/or surgical benefits, to include major medical benefits to which I am entitled, including private insurance, and any other health plans to:

(put in your physician's name)

This assignment will remain in effect until revoked by me in writing. A photocopy of this assignment is to be considered as valid as an original. I understand that I am financially responsible for all charges whether or not paid by said insurance. I hereby authorize said assignee to release all information necessary to secure the payment.

Signed _____ Date _____

FIGURE 13.4

Examples of the wording for an assignment of benefits. (Courtesy De A. Eggers & Associates, Sonoma, Calif.)

When verifying a patient's insurance, you must remember that many patients do not know or understand the type or extent of the coverage they have. Most patients expect the administrative medical assistant to be familiar with every insurance plan and type of coverage available. Trying to understand all polices and plans is impossible; however, you should set up a book detailing all of the information available for each plan in which the physician has enrolled. It is important that you verify the patient's coverage if you are unfamiliar with the plan or the patient requires unusual services.

Assisting with Billing Insurance

Some physicians who have been in practice a long time have had trouble adjusting to the rapid pace of changes in the health care field that has occurred since the early 1990s. Some physicians, particularly in rural areas, have been accustomed to charging patients based on their ability to pay, thus the fee may vary for a particular service. This has become a problem in that the HCFA has set forth a directive regarding waiver of deductibles and co-insurance amounts.

To help physicians and patients be reimbursed for services you first must obtain all important information. Do not attempt to be an intermediary between patients and their insurance carriers. Doing so is time consuming and prevents the patient from learning from the experience. You might keep the claims inquiry telephone numbers of the major insurance carriers on file to give to patients; this will show your willingness to be of help.

Most administrative medical assistants will assist patients with insurance billing by automatically providing the data necessary to file a claim, either in the monthly statement or on a superbill given at each visit. Many offices also complete the appropriate insurance forms for patients. This is an extra service provided for patients; most carriers, particularly the federal and state programs, require that the physician's office complete and submit the claim.

Some elderly patients have supplemental policies and rely on the medical assistant to submit various forms for them (Figure 13.5). This can become a problem, particularly if the forms are brought or sent in at different times or if the carrier requires their form instead of a standard HCFA-1500. If this is done, the chart or financial records must be retrieved several times for one patient. To discourage this practice, the office can provide the patient with several copies of the claim form (HCFA-1500) at one time, and each can be sent to a different company.

Another alternative is to charge for completing multiple insurance forms. The AMA states that charging for completing insurance forms is not unethical. It suggests, however, that if you wish to charge, it is in the best interest of public relations that the first form be completed at no charge and that a nominal fee be charged for subsequent forms billing for the same procedures.

Helping Patients With Their Insurance

When possible it is to your advantage to encourage patients to file their own insurance claims. However, because of constant changes in the health care field and the fact that patients switch carriers far more often than was previously the case, the number of patients filing their own claims has dwindled significantly. Regardless, some people maintain private insurance and prefer to file their own

STATIONARY ENGINEERS LOCAL 39 HEALTH AND WELFARE FUND

IMPORTANT: To assure payment of Benefits, this form should be FULLY COMPLETED and submitted to the Claim Settlement Office IMMEDIATELY following injury or commencement of treatment.

S.F. ADMINISTRATORS
501 SECOND STREET, ROOM 212
SAN FRANCISCO, CA 94107-1431
(415) 777-3707 • (800) 660-9989

STATEMENT OF MEDICAL CLAIM

Read instructions on back before completing form.

TYPE OR PRINT

CHECK IF YOUR ADDRESS HAS CHANGED SINCE YOUR LAST CLAIM ☐

PART I   PATIENT & PLAN MEMBER (EMPLOYEE) INFORMATION

1. Employee's Name (First, Middle, Last Name): JACK W

2. Address (Street) (City) (State) (Zip Code)

3. Name of Company Where You Work and Date of Hire: JOHNSON CONTROLS - BANK OF AMERICA 8-94

4. Employee's Social Security Number

5. Union Local No. 39

6. Employee's Date of Birth

7. Home Phone Number (Area Code Number)

8. Patient's Name: TARA

9. Patient's Date of Birth: 10-5-87

10. Patient's Sex   ☐ Male ☒ Female

11. Patient's Address (Street) (City) (State) (Zip Code)

12. Patient's Relationship To Employee: DAUGHTER

13. If patient not member, list patient occupation and Name of Employer

14. MUST BE ANSWERED IF PATIENT INJURED
A. Date of Injury
B. Where did the injury occur?
C. How did the injury occur?

15. Was Illness or Injury Work Related   Yes ☐   No ☒

16. Is Any Member of Your Family Covered by any Other Health Insurance, Group Plan, Medicare or Other Government Plan?   Yes ☐   No ☒
If Answer is Yes, complete questions 16a through 16g. If Answer is No, proceed to No. 17.

16a. Please provide name and address of OTHER Plan or Group:

16b. Group No. or Policy No.

16c. PLAN TYPE Active ☐ Retiree ☐

16d. Name of Employer or Organization Providing Other Coverage

16e. Name of Primary Person Covered Under Other Plan

16f. Identifying No. /SS No. of Primary Person Covered Under Other Plan

16g. Primary Person's Date of Birth

17. I AUTHORIZE ANY MEDICAL INFORMATION RELATING TO THIS CLAIM TO BE DISCLOSED TO AND ACQUIRED BY THE ADMINISTRATOR OF THIS PLAN AND SUCH AGENTS OF THE ADMINISTRATOR AS ARE NECESSARY TO PROCESS THIS CLAIM. SUCH INFORMATION MAY BE DISCLOSED BY A HEALTH CARE PROVIDER OR OTHER PLAN ADMINISTRATOR, AND WILL BE USED FOR THE PURPOSE OF PROCESSING THIS CLAIM. THIS AUTHORIZATION SHALL REMAIN VALID UNTIL THE CLAIM IS PAID, PROVIDED, SUCH INFORMATION SHALL BE RETAINED BY THE ADMINISTRATOR IF REQUIRED BY LAW.

Patient's Signature (Parent or Guardian's Signature, if Patient is a minor)
X
Upon request, the patient shall be furnished with a copy of this authorization.

18. EMPLOYEE'S SIGNATURE (I hereby certify that the foregoing statements including any accompanying statements are to the best of my knowledge and belief true and correct. CHECK: ☑ I DO ☐ I DO NOT ☐ authorize the administrator, in his sole discretion, to pay directly to the below named physician or any other supplier of services, any benefits otherwise payable to me, but not to exceed any of the charges by the physician or other supplier of services. I understand that I am financially responsible for any charges not covered by this authorization.)

X _____   DATE _____

PART II   PHYSICIAN OR SUPPLIER INFORMATION
TO BE COMPLETED BY PHYSICIAN OR SUPPLIER—OR YOU MAY ATTACH AN ITEMIZED BILL INCLUDING DIAGNOSIS

19. DATE OF:
☐ ILLNESS (FIRST SYMPTOM) OR
☐ INJURY (ACCIDENT) OR
☐ PREGNANCY (LMP)

20. DATE FIRST CONSULTED YOU FOR THIS CONDITION

21. HAS PATIENT EVER HAD SAME OR SIMILAR SYMPTOMS?   YES ☐   NO ☐

WORK RELATED?   YES ☐   NO ☐

22. DATE PATIENT ABLE TO RETURN TO WORK

23. DATES OF TOTAL DISABILITY   FROM   THROUGH

DATES OF PARTIAL DISABILITY   FROM   THROUGH

24. NAME OF REFERRING PHYSICIAN

25. FOR SERVICES RELATED TO HOSPITALIZATION GIVE HOSPITALIZATION DATES   ADMITTED   DISCHARGED

26. NAME & ADDRESS OF FACILITY WHERE SERVICES RENDERED (if other than home or office)

27. WAS LABORATORY WORK PERFORMED OUTSIDE YOUR OFFICE?   YES ☐   NO ☐   CHARGES:

28. DIAGNOSIS OR NATURE OF ILLNESS OR INJURY. RELATE DIAGNOSIS TO PROCEDURE IN COLUMN D BY REFERENCE TO NUMBERS 1, 2, 3, ETC. OR DX CODE
1.
2.
3.

FIGURE 13.5

Statement of Medical Claim form. (Used with permission from Stationary Engineers Local 39 Health and Welfare Fund, San Francisco, Calif.)

claims. Because patients may not submit claims in a timely manner, you will need to instruct them that they must pay at the time of service or on receipt of their statement rather than waiting for the insurance company to pay. You also will need to spend extra time educating patients about the process, but doing so will save time in the future.

The most appropriate claims that can be filed by the patients involve simple services, such as office or hospital visits for medical care. Claims that require supporting documentation should be filed by office personnel, because it is inappropriate to give patients copies of operative reports, pathology reports, and so on without the physician's approval.

Superbills are the simplest method of providing patients with the information they need to file claims. You may have the filing instructions printed on the back of the form to reinforce the verbal instructions given to patients. An alternative is to produce a statement with all the necessary information, including diagnosis. This can be accomplished with computer-generated statements.

Answering Patients' Questions

Patients may ask questions regarding their current health insurance or insurance they are considering. This is time consuming and beyond the scope of your responsibility, but be prepared to offer patients the courtesy of suggesting information resources to them. The most frequent inquiries will involve whether the patient's insurance will cover a service or procedure and how much of the cost the insurance company will pay. Because insurance cards contain minimal information, do not make any statement about the coverage. Instead, suggest that the patient contact his or her insurance company or benefits department at work, where there usually is an employee who handles health benefits.

Another common question about health insurance involves insurance options. The patient may ask either, "What is the best insurance I can get?" or "I have been offered two plans at work—which one would be better for me to take?" It is not appropriate for you to answer these questions, but you can suggest that the patient acquire the insurance that will best meet his or her needs. You might suggest that the patient contact an insurance broker, who can compare policies and help the patient assess the various options.

The final question patients often ask involves what they should look for when purchasing insurance coverage. You can suggest that they contact the major reputable insurance companies, whose representatives should be willing to answer questions and supply literature. Contacting an insurance broker, who will have access to information about policies issued by many companies, is an alternative to contacting insurance carriers independently. You can suggest that patients read a policy carefully, check the policy limits, and ask their agent questions before purchasing insurance.

Explaining Responsibility for the Unpaid Portion

Most insurance policies are written based on an 80/20 ratio. This means that the insurance company will pay 80% of the allowable charges and the patient can expect to be responsible for the remaining amount (this could be more than

OPERATING ENGINEERS PUBLIC EMPLOYEES 852635
P O BOX 23980 OAKLAND CA 94623-0980 (800) 844-8392 (510) 433-4422

	MEMBER NAME					SOCIAL SECURITY NO.			PATIENT NAME			CLAIM NO.	DATE ISSUED
								W BETTY		11172-----		55899	06/12/97

Benefit Category	No. or Z	Date(s) of Service	Fee or Rate	Less Discount	Other	Code	Plan Allows	Less Deduct	Member Copay	Other Insuran.	Basic Benefit	Major Med Benefit
OFFICE VISIT	1	02/04/97	150.00				150.00		30.00			120.00
X-RAY OR LAB	1	02/07/97	600.00				600.00		120.00			480.00
X-RAY OR LAB	1	02/07/97	100.00				100.00		20.00			80.00
X-RAY OR LAB	1	02/07/97	100.00				100.00		20.00			80.00
PROVIDER MINOTTI, J B MD			950.00				950.00		190.00			760.00

S075409413 CHECK NO. 7030762 ISSUED TO PROVIDER | MM Deductibles Remaining | TOTAL PAYMENT 760.00
PATIENT OBLIGATION   190.00

8450011

148   C-55 (R7-95)

PLEASE KEEP THIS VOUCHER FOR YOUR RECORDS

───── REMOVE DOCUMENT ALONG THIS PERFORATION ─────

IF AN ITEM HAS BEEN DENIED

If you are not satisfied or do not agree with the reasons for denial
and you wish to have your claim reconsidered, you may request
an appeal in writing stating clearly the reasons why your claim
should not be denied, within 60 days after the date of this notice.

FIGURE 13.6

Sample of EOB. (Used with permission from Operating Engineers Public
Employer, Oakland, Calif.)

20%) (Figure 13.6). In reality this is not always the end result, and you will need to explain why to the patient. The word "allowable" is the key to understanding the situation.

Most often the physician's fee and the fee allowable by the insurance company for procedure are not equal; the allowable fee usually will be less. The dollar and percentage differences caused by this situation mean that the patient may pay more than expected. You may need to use an example to explain the situation. Whatever method you use, you must convey to patients that they are responsible for the total amount billed, not the amount allowed by the insurance company. The one exception to this rule will be discussed under Medicare payment options.

HCFA Memorandum No. 85 (Figure 13.7) requires that the physician or supplier make a reasonable attempt (three billings) to collect the difference from the subscriber between what was paid by the insurance carrier and the original bill. The HCFA mandates that if a physician or supplier consistently writes off the difference between the amount paid and the billed amount, then the carrier (private or public), should reduce that provider's profile to the accepted payment amount. For example, the physician's fee for a particular service is always $1000, the carrier allows $800, and pays $640 (80%). If the physician regularly accepts the fee of $640 as payment in full and the carrier finds out, then the physician's fee for that service with that carrier will be reduced to $640, and the carrier will have to pay only 80% of the $640. If this happens frequently, the medical assistant should inform the physician that an excessive number of patients are not paying the full fee.

Assignment of Benefits

An assignment of benefits is an instruction to the insurance carrier about where to send the payment for services rendered.

Assignment By Patient to Physician

Method of Assignment

Most individual and group insurance plans will automatically reimburse the doctor if they do not receive specific instructions to do otherwise. To speed the reimbursement process and protect income by having the carrier pay the physician directly, many offices and facilities have the patients complete an assignment of benefits form, the assignment section of an insurance form, or a superbill designed with an assignment section. To incorporate all areas of the policy, the assignment should stipulate to include major medical benefits (see Figure 13.4). In many states this ensures that both the basic policy benefits and the major medical benefits will be paid to the physician.

Patient Instructions

The assignment of benefits by the patient to the physician does not absolve the patient of future financial responsibility. You will need to explain to patients that they will be billed and considered responsible for the difference between the amount charged by the physician and the amount paid by the insurance company.

PROGRAM MEMORANDUM

Reprinted HCFA-BO A/B
Transmittal No. A-85-4
                   B-85-3

Health Care Financing
Administration

Date: March 1985

SUBJECT: Routine Waiver of Deductible and Co-insurance Amounts

It has been recently brought to our attention that the volume and seriousness of the cases involving the routine waiver of deductibles and co-insurance by certain physicians and suppliers has grown dramatically. As a result, we believe there is a need at this time for carriers to aggressively seek out instances of routine waiver and to make specific reductions in charge screens for these providers. (In essence drop their reimbursement levels.)

As you know, current program instructions (section 5220 of the Medicare Carriers Manual) indicate that a billed amount that is not reasonably related to an expectation of payment should not be considered as the "actual charge" for processing a current claim or determining customary charge screens. Carriers have been expected to thoroughly review all situations that come to their attention when a physician or supplier routinely and consistently waives the collection of deductibles and co-insurance to determine whether their actual and customary charges should be reduced.

It appears, however, that carriers have not actively sought out specific instances of routine waiver, and that specific reductions in actual and customary charges once a routine waiver has been discovered have not been made on a consistent basis.

While we are developing a stronger range of sanctions against those who routinely waive deductible and co-insurance amounts, we believe carriers currently need to aggressively seek out instances of routine waiver and diligently enforce existing sanctions. Among other actions, carriers should review any advertising by suppliers designed to waive Medicare deductibles and co-insurance and alert such providers that they are in potential violation of the law, at risk of having their customary charges reduced and an overpayment assessed, and subject to criminal prosecution by the Department of Justice.

FIGURE 13.7

HCFA Memorandum No. 85.

Physician Accepts Assignment

Physician's Choice

In some instances, physicians may choose to accept assignment. This indicates that the physician will expect all payments from all carriers, other than those programs in which the physician is an enrolled (or contract) provider, to be paid directly to him or her. The physician, in this instance, is required to make a reasonable attempt to collect the balance of the amount originally billed from the subscriber or responsible party. In Box 13 of the standard claim form, the insurance biller should either have the subscriber sign or indicate "signature on file." An area on each insurance form near where the physician signs the document states "Accepts Assignment" and is followed by boxes in which to check yes or no. With Medicare claims it is mandatory that one of the boxes be checked. When the physician accepts assignment, the insurance company determines the allowed fee and pays the physician the percentage the carrier stipulates based on the insured's policy benefits. The physician then is expected to bill the patient the amount not paid by the carrier. Only in Massachusetts is the physician expected to accept the insurance carrier's payment as payment in full when the physician accepts assignment. The physician may accept the insurance carrier's payment as payment in full if it is evident that the patient is living on a fixed income or is experiencing financial hardship. If this is the case, the physician's office is required to have a "Waiver Due to Economic Hardship" signed. This also may occur if the patient is another physician or a member of his or her family. In this instance the balance is adjusted as a result of "Prior Agreement."

No-Option Situations

In certain instances physicians do not have a choice on assignment; by accepting the patient they agree to the fee paid by the insurance company or intermediary as payment in full. This occurs with Workers' Compensation cases, Medicaid or Medicare-Medicaid patients, and certain Blue Shield plans, if the physician is a participating provider.

Completing Claim Forms

Forms Completed By Office Staff

Necessary Equipment

If some or all of the insurance forms are completed by the administrative office personnel, minimal equipment is needed to complete the job. Supplies of forms from insurance companies with which you communicate regularly should be kept on hand. Because universal claim forms can be substituted for most insurance carriers' forms, you may wish to use this option. The universal form (HCFA-1500) reduces the amount of searching you must do to locate the various spaces in which information is to be entered. You also will need the patient's account information, the patient's medical record, a calculator or adding machine, and pens.

Administrative Medical Assistant's Responsibilities

You will be expected to complete as much of the claim form as possible from the medical record and the patient account information. The components of the HCFA-1500 Universal Claim Form are shown in Figure 13.8.

Block 1: Check the available program box at the top of the form. If more than one insurance program is involved (for example, Medicare and Medicaid), check more than one box.

Block 1a: Indicate insured's identification number.

Block 2: Patient's name. Copy the spelling of the patient's name exactly as it appears on the subscriber's insurance identification card. For Medicare benefi-

PICA

HEALTH INSURANCE CLAIM FORM

PICA

1. MEDICARE (Medicare#) MEDICAID (Medicaid #) CHAMPUS (Sponsor's SSN) CHAMPVA (VA File #) GROUP HEALTH PLAN (SSN or ID) FECA BLK LUNG (SSN) OTHER (ID)

1a. INSURED'S I.D. NUMBER (FOR PROGRAM IN ITEM 1)

2. PATIENT'S NAME (Last Name, First Name, Middle Initial)

3. PATIENT'S BIRTH DATE MM DD YY SEX M F

4. INSURED'S NAME (Last Name, First Name, Middle Initial)

5. PATIENT'S ADDRESS (No., Street)

6. PATIENT RELATIONSHIP TO INSURED Self Spouse Child Other

7. INSURED'S ADDRESS (No., Street)

CITY STATE

8. PATIENT STATUS Single Married Other

CITY STATE

ZIP CODE TELEPHONE (Include Area Code) ( )

Employed Full-Time Student Part-Time Student

ZIP CODE TELEPHONE (INCLUDE AREA CODE) ( )

9. OTHER INSURED'S NAME (Last Name, First Name, Middle Initial)

10. IS PATIENT'S CONDITION RELATED TO:

11. INSURED'S POLICY GROUP OR FECA NUMBER

a. OTHER INSURED'S POLICY OR GROUP NUMBER

a. EMPLOYMENT? (CURRENT OR PREVIOUS) YES NO

a. INSURED'S DATE OF BIRTH MM DD YY SEX M F

b. OTHER INSURED'S DATE OF BIRTH MM DD YY SEX M F

b. AUTO ACCIDENT? YES NO PLACE (State)

b. EMPLOYER'S NAME OR SCHOOL NAME

c. EMPLOYER'S NAME OR SCHOOL NAME

c. OTHER ACCIDENT? YES NO

c. INSURANCE PLAN NAME OR PROGRAM NAME

d. INSURANCE PLAN NAME OR PROGRAM NAME

10d. RESERVED FOR LOCAL USE

d. IS THERE ANOTHER HEALTH BENEFIT PLAN? YES NO *If yes,* return to and complete item 9 a-d.

READ BACK OF FORM BEFORE COMPLETING & SIGNING THIS FORM.

12. PATIENT'S OR AUTHORIZED PERSON'S SIGNATURE I authorize the release of any medical or other information necessary to process this claim. I also request payment of government benefits either to myself or to the party who accepts assignment below.

SIGNED DATE

13. INSURED'S OR AUTHORIZED PERSON'S SIGNATURE I authorize payment of medical benefits to the undersigned physician or supplier for services described below.

SIGNED

14. DATE OF CURRENT: MM DD YY ILLNESS (First symptom) OR INJURY (Accident) OR PREGNANCY (LMP)

15. IF PATIENT HAS HAD SAME OR SIMILAR ILLNESS, GIVE FIRST DATE MM DD YY

16. DATES PATIENT UNABLE TO WORK IN CURRENT OCCUPATION FROM MM DD YY TO MM DD YY

17. NAME OF REFERRING PHYSICIAN OR OTHER SOURCE

17a. I.D. NUMBER OF REFERRING PHYSICIAN

18. HOSPITALIZATION DATES RELATED TO CURRENT SERVICES FROM MM DD YY TO MM DD YY

19. RESERVED FOR LOCAL USE

20. OUTSIDE LAB? YES NO $ CHARGES

21. DIAGNOSIS OR NATURE OF ILLNESS OR INJURY. (RELATE ITEMS 1,2,3 OR 4 TO ITEM 24E BY LINE)

1. ___ . ___ 3. ___ . ___

2. ___ . ___ 4. ___ . ___

22. MEDICAID RESUBMISSION CODE ORIGINAL REF. NO.

23. PRIOR AUTHORIZATION NUMBER

24. A DATE(S) OF SERVICE From MM DD YY To MM DD YY	B Place of Service	C Type of Service	D PROCEDURES, SERVICES, OR SUPPLIES (Explain Unusual Circumstances) CPT/HCPCS MODIFIER	E DIAGNOSIS CODE	F $ CHARGES	G DAYS OR UNITS	H EPSDT Family Plan	I EMG	J COB	K RESERVED FOR LOCAL USE
1										
2										
3										
4										
5										
6										

25. FEDERAL TAX I.D. NUMBER SSN EIN

26. PATIENT'S ACCOUNT NO.

27. ACCEPT ASSIGNMENT? (For govt. claims, see back) YES NO

28. TOTAL CHARGE $

29. AMOUNT PAID $

30. BALANCE DUE $

31. SIGNATURE OF PHYSICIAN OR SUPPLIER INCLUDING DEGREES OR CREDENTIALS (I certify that the statements on the reverse apply to this bill and are made a part thereof.)

SIGNED DATE

32. NAME AND ADDRESS OF FACILITY WHERE SERVICES WERE RENDERED (If other than home or office)

33. PHYSICIAN'S, SUPPLIER'S BILLING NAME, ADDRESS, ZIP CODE & PHONE #

PIN# GRP#

(APPROVED BY AMA COUNCIL ON MEDICAL SERVICE 8/88) WHCFA-1500-CS-N90

PLEASE PRINT OR TYPE

FORM HCFA-1500 (12-90) FORM OWCP-1500 FORM RRB-1500

FIGURE 13.8

HCFA-1500. (Used with permission from the American Medical Association Council on Medical Service.)

MEDICAL ASSISTING STEP-BY-STEP

Insurance Forms

1. Have a specific place to work and a definite time to do it.

2. Use the HCFA-1500 form as much as possible.

3. Keep a binder with specific information for filling out the forms for various types of insurance.

4. Have the medical record and insurance card handy.

5. Check for necessary signatures, for example, release of information and assignment of benefits (if applicable).

6. Fill out forms accurately and neatly.

7. Proofread forms and make the corrections necessary.

8. Submit claims either by paper or electronically.

---

ciaries, request the red, white, and blue Medicare card. For Medicaid information, enter the last name first, then the first name followed by the middle initial.

Block 3: Patient's date of birth. Indicate month, day, and year, if available. Check the correct box indicating the patient's sex.

Block 4: Insured's name. If the patient is covered by employment-related health insurance, show the full name of the employed person. This name also should appear in Block 9.

Block 5: Patient's address. Give the patient's current mailing address (include apartment number and Zip code). Furnish the patient's telephone number, if available. If the patient resides in a convalescent facility or nursing home, indicate the name of the facility in addition to the address.

Block 6: Patient relationship to the insured. If the patient had health insurance based on his or her own or spouse's current employment, check the appropriate box.

Block 7: Insured's address. Provide the street, street number, city, state, and Zip code.

Block 8: Patient status. Check the appropriate box.

Block 9: Other insured's coverage. Indicate the patient's Medicaid identification number for cross-over claims or policy number for other coverage if Medicare is the primary payer. The federal intermediaries now are automatically submitting the claim and Medicare allowed amount and paid amount to a significant number of secondary carriers.

If Medicare is the secondary payer because of employment-related insurance, show the patient's name and health insurance claim number. If this insurance is based on the spouse's employment, also show his or her name and health insurance claim numbers.

If Medicare is a secondary payer because of employment-related insurance (ESRD or working aged), enter the name and health insurance claim number of the policy holder and the name and address of the employer plan.

If Medicare is the secondary payer because of automobile no-fault liability insurance, show the name and address of the automobile no-fault liability insurer.

Should any of the carriers just mentioned pay the *same* or *more* than Medicare would normally allow, then do not expect further payment from Medicare. Write off the remaining balance.

Block 10: Check the appropriate box.

Block 11: Provide the primary insured's policy or group number.

Block 12: Print "Patient signature on file" in this box (make sure you have this information). Obtain the signature of the beneficiary or an authorized representative. If a lifetime signature has been obtained (see Figure 13.4), indicate the patient's payment authorization on file.

Block 13: Print "Insured's signature on file" in this box (make sure you have the signature on a patient information sheet).

Block 14: Indicate the date of first symptom, injury, or date of pregnancy.

Block 15: You usually will leave this block blank.

Block 16: If work related, fill in this block.

Block 17: Indicate the referring physician, if appropriate. The name and complete address of the referring physician is required by Medicare for consultation.

Block 17a: Indicate the referring physician's UPIN (universal personal identification number) as assigned by the Medicare carrier, as a directive given from the HCFA.

Block 18: Indicate dates of hospitalization, if appropriate.

Block 19: Leave blank.

Block 20: Indicate if services you are billing for were processed by an outside laboratory; list fees charged by the laboratory.

Block 21: Indicate the diagnosis for the services rendered, or diagnoses, if appropriate. Describe the nature of the illness or injury treated. ICD9-CM diagnosis coding is required in all states for relating this information; however, narrative should be utilized.

Block 22: Indicate the Medicaid resubmission code, if appropriate.

Block 23: Indicate the prior authorization number as required by any number of carriers.

Block 24: This section is for the charges and services rendered. Make sure that all blocks, (that is, A, B, C, D, E, F, G, H, I, J, and K) are filled out. Use a separate line for each service and particularly for each month. Do not include two months together on the same form, particularly December of one year and January of the next year. In Box 24a indicate the dates of service to and from. The place of service is important and listed in Box 24b as follows:

- 11 signifies inpatient hospitalization
- 22 signifies outpatient hospital services (including ambulatory surgical centers [ASC]; hospital-affiliated clinics and dialysis centers, emergency services, and certified outpatient rehabilitation facilities [CORF])
- 33 signifies office services

In Box 24c indicate the type of service as follows:

- 11 signifies office, 22 signifies hospital, and so forth

Utilize the appropriate CPT, HCPCS, or RVS code number, with modifier if required, in Box 24d. In Box 24e indicate the appropriate ICD9-CM diagnosis code for each service rendered. Indicate the fee for the service in Box 24f, and show days for units of service in Box 24g. Use Block 24h only for EPSDT, primarily for Medicaid programs. Blocks 24i and 24j currently are left blank. Block 24k normally is used to indicate the provider's UPIN number.

Block 25: Place the physician or group tax ID number in this area, and check the appropriate box for the Social Security number (SSN) or EIN (employer identification number [from the IRS]).

Block 26: If you have a patient account number, place it in this area and it will print on the Explanation of Benefits (EOB) the amount paid by most carriers.

Block 27: This box must be checked for government programs; most other carriers do not pay attention to this box. You must always check the "yes" box if your physician is a participating provider and for Medicaid programs. If your physician is a nonparticipating provider, you may check the "no" box and the payment will be sent directly to the patient.

Block 28: Indicate the total of all charges for this page only.

Block 29: You do not need to fill in this blank unless you are billing a secondary coverage; at that point you will show what the primary carrier has paid, and attach a copy of the primary coverage EOB.

Block 30: You need not fill in this block unless it is to show the balance due after payment by the primary carrier.

Block 31: Signature of the physician. This may be a signature stamp for carriers other than Medicaid.

You may have your signature on file with the Medicaid carrier to sign claims for the physician. Someone must sign the Medicaid claims; they cannot have a signature stamp.

Block 32: Indicate the name and address of the facility where the services are rendered. The facility name, city, and provider identification number must be listed if the services were rendered in a place other than an office or home. Facilities included are independent laboratories; ASCs; dialysis centers, CORFs; skilled nursing facilities (SNF), nursing homes, and hospitals.

Block 33: Indicate the physician's or supplier's billing name, address, Zip code, and phone number. You must also include the physician's provider number.

If there are items that do not apply to the particular case being reported you may leave them blank. It is not necessary to indicate N/A (not applicable). If there are some questions you cannot answer from the resources available, put a check using red ink next to the item as a quick locator when you review the forms with the physician.

Once you have completed as much of each form as possible, clip the forms to the appropriate patient's chart and present them to the physician for review and signature. When the physician is finished with them, the forms can be separated from the chart and the copies placed in the appropriate section of the patient's medical record. The originals then are prepared for submission to the insurance carrier. Once each form is ready, it should be mailed to the appropriate insurance intermediary.

Submission of Hardcopy Claims

With the advent of really good computerized billing programs, much of the guesswork is taken out of submitting hardcopy, or paper, claims. With the appropriate computer billing system, the majority of your claims should be submitted electronically. However, physicians frequently develop new procedures or provide a service that requires a report to be submitted with the claim. Operative reports still are necessary for the majority of major surgeries and unusual services (for example, heart, kidney, liver, or lung transplants, or fetal care). When submitting a claim that has an attachment, you should indicate on the claim that there is an attachment and what it is. When a claim arrives at the carrier's processing unit, the first thing that happens after the envelope is opened is that all attachments are removed and everything (that is, the claim and attachments) is microfilmed. This is where data frequently are lost, and the report does not get reattached before being sent to processing. Thus the claims processor returns the claim to you for the information that you already supplied. To prevent this, highlight that there is an attachment to your claim. When submitting paper claims, do not fold them; it is best if you send them in a 9 x 12 envelope to prevent having to fold them. Claims that are folded are sent to processing much later than unfolded claims. This is because folded claims must be unfolded and smoothed out before being microfilmed. Therefore the microfilmer will stack folded claims until pressure from the piled-up claims removes the folds.

Remaining Current on Claims Processing

The methods used to process insurance claims are changing rapidly because of computers, and the information required to complete claims also will change as cost-containment mechanisms are introduced. You will need to keep abreast of these changes. Several resources are available to help in this endeavor. Six common sources of information are as follows:

- Bulletins from insurance carriers. Some major carriers, especially Blue Cross, Blue Shield, and Medicare/Medicaid intermediaries, send routine updates on claims processing. These updates should be read immediately and retained for future use. For easy reference use a large, three-ring binder to store the bulletins. Use a separate binder for each carrier that sends you bulletins.
- Articles in *The Professional Medical Assistant*, the official journal of the American Association of Medical Assistants
- Articles in *Medical Economics*, a magazine for physicians and staff
- *Part B News*, which is produced by United Communications for both physicians and staff
- Professional relations representatives from Medicare and Medicaid
- Courses that provide updated information. Be very careful in selecting the courses or seminars to attend since some provide no information useful to

WHAT DO YOU THINK?

As an administrative medical assistant, you process all of the insurance forms—paper and electronic—for Dr. Renky's office. Besides his office patients, the doctor regularly sees his convalescent patients, whom you bill after he has visited them. This month the doctor was ill and did not make his rounds at the convalescent hospital. The office manager told you to bill for visits anyway, using the amount that was charged last month as a guide. Most of these patients receive Medicare with Medicaid supplement.

Should you bill using last month's fees? Is this illegal? Could your doctor get in trouble if you did this?

the profession. You should find out from the company sponsoring the seminar whether the person giving the seminar had any hands-on experience in the medical front office.

Local medical societies offer useful information in their publications and may hold periodic "brown-bag" lunches to inform office personnel of recent administrative changes, including insurance billing.

One of the best sources for continuing education and information is to join a local chapter of the Medical Group Manager's Association (MGMA). You do not have to be a group manager to join; you may be the only person in the office, a receptionist, or any other staff member. This group has grown rapidly and is gaining a very strong presence in the medical field. It also has been influential with regard to the passage of new state and federal legislation.

You will want to take advantage of all available resources to keep current on methods to speed up claims processing.

Electronic Submission

When selecting a medical billing program, you must ask whether the programming is cleared for American National Standards Institute (ANSI) transmission. All good medical billing systems or programs will have in place the ANSI criteria for submission of electronic claims to Medicare, Medicaid, and through the eight clearinghouses. The clearinghouse then transmits the claims to approximately 93 carriers. Some HMOs, IPAs, and PPOs also have developed the programming to accept electronic submission.

The medical practice that is computerized may transmit claims via modem or by submitting a disk or tape to the carrier or intermediary (Figure 13.9).

The obvious advantage of electronic billing is the overall savings in time, cost of claim forms, envelopes, and postage. An added advantage is that you become aware quickly of problems because the system rejects the transmission of claims that are incorrect or do not have all of the information required for proper payment. You will know immediately if the carrier has received the transmission, how many claims were transmitted, the patient name, and the dollar amount, allowing you time to correct certain claims and have them ready for the next transmission.

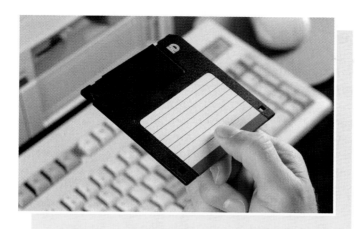

FIGURE 13.9

The medical practice that is computerized may transmit claims via modem or by submitting a disk or tape to the carrier or intermediary.

AT WORK TODAY

Electronic Claims (EMC)

Advantages	Disadvantages	Route of Submission
Claims can be filed immediately	Claims have to meet certain criteria	The medical office ↓
Payment time is reduced	Cannot submit claims that are complicated or have attachments	The clearinghouse ↓
Processing expense is reduced	Requires computer equipment/ personnel trained to operate it	Different insurance companies ↓
		Paid ↓
		Denied ↓
		Paperwork generated ↓
		Electronic remittance advice/ explanation of benefits

Turnaround time for reimbursement also is faster with electronic submission of claims. When claims are submitted electronically, they are read by the carrier's computer, and thus are paid much faster, typically in 14 to 17 days instead of 30 to 45 days for hardcopy claims. Many carriers also are developing automatic transfer of reimbursement directly to the physician's bank. The carrier then sends to the physician office a copy of which claims were paid and for how much, for tracking by the office. In many geographical areas this part of the system still has some major obstacles; sometimes all of the transmitted claims do not show as paid on the printout. A very strict accounting must be kept of claims transmitted and paid per carrier.

The HCFA has pushed hard for the development of electronic claims, requiring that all physician offices be tied into a billing service or have an in-house computer system by 1997.

Again, not all claims are suitable for electronic submission. Any claim that is complicated or out of the ordinary must be submitted on hard copy.

Rejected Claims

If claims are improperly processed, insurance companies will return them for resubmission. Your office should avoid this, if possible. Claims that can be processed on receipt by the carrier will improve the accounts receivable figures in the office, because they will be paid faster. This is particularly true of major fees for complicated diagnostic and treatment services. Avoiding returned claims also reduces the workload of the administrative personnel. If a claim is returned, you will have to determine the reason for the return, retrieve the appropriate records, and resubmit the corrected form to the insurance carrier.

Common Reasons for Rejected Claims

Four common reasons that claims are rejected by the insurance carrier are as follows:

- Erroneous or missing data
- Missing attachments
- Incorrect carrier
- Illegibility

Erroneous or Missing Data

Before you transmit or submit a claim to the insurance carrier for processing, spend an extra moment to double-check that all data are present and correct. Trouble spots often involve:

- Missing or incorrect insurance identification numbers
- Incomplete or missing diagnosis
- Missing physician's signature
- Missing or incorrectly multiplied fees for services
- Dates of treatment that do not correspond with the support documents

The limited time you spend confirming these items will save time in the end by avoiding rejected claims.

Missing Attachments

Claims for certain services require the submission of documents to support or describe the claims made by the physician. Although insurance carriers may not include a statement of this requirement with the claim forms, you should assume that the documents are necessary. Always submit support documents necessary to support unusual services of By Report (BR) procedures; these may include unusually complex consultations, treadmill reports, extensive operative reports, and pathology reports for cases involving malignancies (since the fees will be much higher than in cases of benign pathology).

Incorrect Carrier

Claims submitted to the incorrect insurance carrier will delay payments because of the time spent trying to determine the patient's eligibility before the claims are returned. Most errors of this type can be avoided by frequently checking with patients about the status of their insurance coverage. Most insured individuals have their policies reviewed and updated once a year through their employment, and the employer may even change insurance companies at a review. However, because patients may not remember to tell you of any changes, you must take the responsibility for asking.

Illegibility

Insurance forms and superbills that are handwritten require special attention with regard to legibility. If completing these forms by hand, you should print, using a pen that will imprint through all copies. If the physician writes in the diagnosis and there is any doubt that it can be clearly understood, you may reprint it, enclosed in parentheses and immediately following the physician's notation.

Lost Claims

Methods of Monitoring Claims Processed

To avoid overlooking or losing claims forms that must be processed, set up separate file folders for each type of insurance you handle. The method you choose will depend on the volume of forms you process. Doctor's First Reports for Workers' Compensation forms should always be kept with the patient's record, and be processed immediately after the first visit because of the legal requirements.

For all other claims, select the appropriate form as the patient arrives for a visit or when you are notified that the physician has seen a patient at another facility. Office patients should sign the authorization to release information and authorization to pay at the time of the visit. The form should then be dated and placed in the folder(s) in chronological order. Then process the forms, in the order in which they were initiated, at preplanned times during each filing period.

Insurance Log

You may develop a log for insurance forms to be processed. It can consist of a single sheet in a spiral notebook, with separate columns for the patient's name, type of insurance, date entered in log, and date completed. An alternative way to develop a log is to maintain separate sheets in a ring binder, with one sheet set aside for each type of insurance. Each sheet can be divided into columns for the patient's name, date entered, and date the form is completed and sent. If an insurance log is used, you may choose one of these methods or design a log that fits the needs of your office or facility. If you are using a well-configured computerized billing system (either a service or an in-house system) the computer system will keep this for you automatically.

Claims Processed Daily

Computer systems allow you to process claims each and every day, which means that claims are transmitted every evening. Thus the income is much

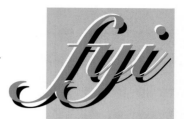

Errors/Problems Caused

Errors that can cause your claim to be rejected include:

- **Diagnosis that does not match the treatment**
- **Charges that are not itemized properly**
- **Patient's portion is not completed**
- **Dates that are incorrect**
- **Claim was sent to the wrong company**
- **Numbers that are incorrect or missing**
- **Referring physician's UPIN is missing**

Problems caused by the errors include:

- **Work must be repeated**
- **Lower reimbursement amount**
- **Denied claim**
- **Delayed payment**
- **Patient complaints**

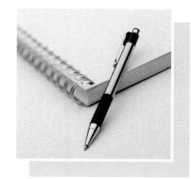

more stable because it is generated regularly, rather than irregularly, which would be the case if you only ran transmissions once a month or weekly. It is to your advantage to see that claims are processed daily (for large clinics) or at least weekly. Collecting payment for services is primary to your position as a medical assistant responsible for insurance. You must monitor the transmission to see that all claims were transmitted, correcting and retransmitting those that were not received. You also must monitor to ensure that all claims either transmitted or submitted on paper were paid appropriately. You will probably have to wait at least 30 days after submission or transmission to call the carrier and check where the processing of the claim stands. Should the carrier's representative indicate that the claim was not received, request the fax number for the carrier, the representative's name, and submit a copy of the claim through the fax. Also call the carrier and confirm that the person did indeed receive the faxed claim. This is a fast and easy way to monitor all claims. Most claims are lost in mailing, which is all the more reason to send claims electronically. If you are told that there is no record of the claim and you have a copy of the transmittal log but no payment, fax the information again immediately to prevent nonpayment for services rendered.

Conclusion

The subject of coding, billing, and claims processing is extensive and evolutionary. Coding correctly is an absolute skill that must not be overlooked. Understanding the types of insurance available to patients helps you in providing the correct information to the patient. You must continually monitor office policies and procedures regarding billing, as well as the reimbursement of claims by each carrier. You must control all aspects of coding, billing, and claims processing to ensure that the practice is reimbursed properly and fully for the services rendered.

Review QUESTIONS

1. Describe in your own words how you would explain to patients their responsibilities regarding their health insurance.

2. How would you explain to a patient the difference between assignment of benefits by the patient and acceptance of assignment by the physician?

3. Describe Medicare's role as a secondary carrier.

4. Describe in logical sequence an effective method of processing insurance claims for patients.

5. What will patients need to file their own claims?

6. What are the advantages of electronic claims transmission?

7. Which coding systems do Medicare and Medicaid use?

8. Should the diagnosis support the procedure?

9. How should you submit a claim that requires a report?

10. How do you know if the claim sent electronically was actually received by the carrier?

SUGGESTED READING

American Medical Association: *The business side of medical practice,* Chicago, 1989, The Association.

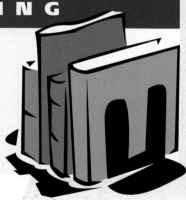

Health and Accident Insurance

OUTLINE

OUTLINE

OBJECTIVES

On completion of Chapter 14 the administrative medical assistant student should be able to:

1 Define the key terms listed in this chapter.

2 Discuss the purpose of health insurance and the patient's responsibility when using health care coverage.

3 List the five methods of access to health insurance and the types of plans available.

4 List and describe the three government-mandated sources of insurance and the four sources of private plans.

5 Discuss utilization review and the role of the medical assistant in the process.

6 List the type of insurance a physician needs for his or her practice.

7 List and discuss reimbursement levels.

8 Discuss the types of health plans available.

KEY TERMS

Benefit   The amount payable by the carrier toward the cost of covered benefits, liability losses, malpractice, or medical benefits.

Broker   An individual licensed by the state to sell insurance; brokers represent multiple insurance companies rather than a single firm.

Capitation rate   A fee determined by a prepaid health plan and applied to each person insured; the fee is expected to cover the expenses of providing necessary health care for 1 year.

Carrier   A term applied to companies that provide insurance to protect individuals from financial loss.

Claim   A demand presented to an insurance company to pay for services provided for an insured person.

Clause   An element of a contract that states a single feature or restriction of the document.

Copayment   The portion of a service fee that the insured must pay.

Deductible   An amount the insured person must pay before policy benefits begin.

Experience rate   The number of claims submitted for payment of services compared with the total number of individuals covered by an insurance policy.

Fiscal year   A 12-month period that begins on the same predetermined date each year and is selected for financial purposes.

Indigent   A person unable to secure the financial means to meet his or her basic needs.

Insured   The person protected against financial loss by an insurance policy.

Mandate   A law or order from a legislative government body.

Peer   An individual or group that is similar to another individual or group; professionally, an individual with the same educational preparation and credentials as another.

Policy   A document or contract that describes the insurance coverage for an individual or a property.

Private sector   The business and industry owned and operated by a private citizen.

Public sector   The area of operation that is controlled by a government agency and funded by public money.

Subscriber   The individual named as the primary person covered by an insurance policy.

Variance   Deviation from the expected.

*I*nsurance is an integral part of everyone's life, so you can expect to encounter various types of insurance in the course of your professional responsibilities. Your employer will see patients with a variety of health insurance coverage, and the medical practice will receive a significant portion of its income from insurance payments. Although you may not know the details of every available plan, your office will be more efficient if you understand the purpose, potential, and methods of processing transactions covered by insurance policies.

Insurance Basics

Insurance is protection against financial loss caused by possible but unplanned events that can affect an individual or business. Depending on the protection you want or anticipate needing, insurance can be acquired from two sources: private companies or, in special situations, government agencies.

Premiums are the fees paid to a carrier to be protected by an insurance policy. Premiums are determined after consideration of several factors by the insurance company. These factors include the likelihood that the insured will need financial reimbursement, the likelihood that an event will occur, and the

PERSPECTIVES ON MEDICAL ASSISTING

Insurance

Insurance was first used for accidents in the mid-1800s. Early medical insurance was set up to cover income loss rather than to cover expenses. By the 1930s, medical insurance generally was used for hospital expenses and surgical/obstetrical procedures performed by physicians in hospitals. Blue Cross originated in Texas in 1929 when a group of schoolteachers made arrangements for prepaid hospital insurance with Baylor Hospital. Government insurance started with CHAMPUS in 1956, followed by Medicaid in 1965 and Medicare in 1966.

Insurance has changed so greatly that offices struggle to keep current. Until the 1980s, most people had indemnity plans that paid some or all of the expenses for covered services for illnesses or accidents for the policyholder and covered dependents. Benefits were decided on a fee-for-service basis, which meant that they were based on what the physician charged for the services. In the 1980s, more employers offered group insurance, which people began to use more frequently, causing health care costs to rise dramatically. Consequently, managed care was developed to ensure that patients received cost-effective health care. Managed care, with HMOs, IPAs, PPOs, and PHOs, now has become the norm in health care.

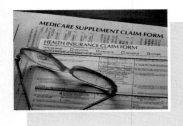

company's past experience with claims. Premiums are determined for a fixed period, usually 1 year in advance, and may be paid all at once or divided into partial payments to be made throughout the coverage period. The policy is evaluated at the end of the period to determine if the premium should be adjusted. Excessive claims against an insurance policy may result in an increase in an individual premium. If the insured is part of a group (several people who need the same type of insurance), the cost of protection can be shared, since members of the group will make varying demands on the policy.

Insurance Benefits

It is rare that a patient seeking care in your medical office or facility will not have some form of health care coverage. Patients may be part of a group plan where they work, may be protected at work by another policy in case they are injured or become ill because of their job, may have a personal health insurance policy, or may be protected by a government program.

You also will encounter various insurance policies that are acquired to protect the office or facility against financial loss. It is important for you to understand the types of insurance policies your office purchases so that you will know to which company to submit a claim in the event of a loss. The possible insurance policies protecting a business are classified as property insurance, legal liability insurance, criminal loss insurance, and package policies.

Patient Health Insurance

The purpose of patient health insurance is to defray or reduce the amount of personal money that an individual must pay for health care services. Health insurance is a form of protection that is becoming increasingly necessary because of the constantly rising cost of health care. Health insurance has evolved to keep pace with the increasing cost of complex health services and the personnel who provide them.

Some people will require extensive health care services, while others will need few or none. Because it is impossible to predict future needs, health insurance is purchased in the event that services are necessary. The insurance carrier estimates the total claims that will be made during the period covered by an insurance policy, and the cost then is shared, in the form of a premium, by all the people insured by the company.

Patient Responsibility

Each individual or group insurance policy is unique. A policy may be written to cover only some services or a broad range of possible health needs. Ideally, patients will have read their insurance plan literature and understand which services are covered by the insurance company. Unfortunately, this is not always the case, and many patients do not understand their coverage. Because each plan is different, you must avoid making statements such as, "I'm sure your insurance will pay for this," when you cannot be certain that it will. You also must avoid the time-consuming task of reviewing a patient's insurance literature to determine coverage. You might misinterpret it and assure a patient that

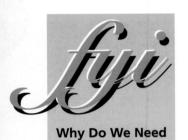

Why Do We Need Medical Insurance?

We need insurance to cover medical office visits.

We need insurance to pay for surgical/obstetrical procedures.

We need insurance to pay for hospital care.

We need insurance for emergency room visits.

We need insurance for prolonged illness and long-term care.

We need insurance for laboratory tests/x-rays.

We need insurance for convalescent care.

We need insurance for on-the-job injury or illness.

We need insurance for durable medical equipment/vision care/orthotic appliances.

We need insurance for home health care.

We need insurance for special tests/procedures.

We need insurance for mental health care.

Medical insurance is very important.

a service is covered when it is not. Patients will undoubtedly feel differently toward you when they discover that they must pay for services they thought the insurance company would cover. Instead, you should tell patients that since each contract is different it would be better if they called their insurance carrier to find out what will be covered.

Insurance Information Cards

Patients with health insurance coverage are issued identification cards, which usually state the following:

- The carrier's name
- The patient's name
- The patient's group number and personal subscriber identification number
- Where to submit claims
- A brief description of covered services
- Telephone number for prior authorization

Patients who have an independent plan rather than one through a group of their choice still are assigned a subscriber identification number. This number indicates to the carrier that they are an independent subscriber.

You should request to see the identification card of all insured patients at the time of the first visit and make a photocopy of the card for your records. The photocopy will provide verification in case a number is transposed on the record of an insurance claim form. The patient's insurance should be verified periodically, especially when you recheck the patient's address, telephone number, and employment information. If the patient's place of employment changes, you can expect the insurance coverage to change and the patient may not remember to show you the new card.

Insurance Verification

If you are working in a practice that provides services that frequently come under the major medical portion of the policy (that is, hospital services, surgery, obstetrics, psychiatry, and so on), it is important that the insurance be verified. Identify yourself and the physician, indicate the patient's name, subscriber name, and all identifying numbers. Although some insurance cards contain the number to call on the back, many do not, and you may have to call the employer to obtain the telephone number of the carrier.

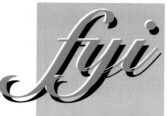

Insurance Tips

1. Patients always are ultimately responsible for paying their accounts in full.
2. When a patient is treated, some type of payment must be made—either from the patient or facility.
3. Always keep a copy of the patient's current insurance card, and verify coverage when necessary.
4. When filing claims, keep a copy and insurance log to track claims more easily.
5. The claim process can be complicated so use proper documentation, claims preparation, submission methods, and timely follow-up.

Coordination of Benefits

When a patient has more than one insurance carrier, coordination of benefits assures that the patient does not receive funds over and above the cost of the services provided. Do not assume that the patients will understand the details of working with the insurance companies and their payment methods. If both spouses work, both may have coverage. Also, many people carry a second or third policy for coverage. This means that benefits will have to be coordinated between the carriers. Except for children in those states that have the "birthday rule," the primary carrier will be the policy held by the person receiving the services. The secondary carrier would then be the spouse's policy. Medicare is the primary carrier in most instances, with other coverage being called *secondary* or *supplemental*. However, if a person is older than age 65, is eligible for Medicare but is still working, and the company has more than 20 employees, then the employer must provide the same coverage for that person as is provided to the other employees. Thus the employer's policy becomes the primary carrier and Medicare becomes the secondary.

Types of Insurance
Access to Health Insurance
As an Individual
Anyone with money to pay the insurance premium can contract with a carrier for any insurance plan available. Premiums for individual plans generally cost more than other policies but allow each individual to select the plan he or she wants.

As Part of a Group
Patients can gain access to group insurance plans in various ways. The most common group is formed by people who work together or belong to the same labor union. Other group plans are available through education or social organizations formed to meet a common goal.

Components of Health Insurance Policies

There are many possible components of a health insurance policy, and the insurance subscriber may select one or more of these components when developing a health coverage policy.

Basic Benefits
A basic health plan will provide varying coverage for patients using the nonsurgical services of a physician for office, hospital, home, and emergency room visits. Also a basic plan usually covers laboratory and radiological diagnostic studies. Most basic plans do not cover routine physical examinations, eye examinations, family planning services, or medically necessary equipment such as artificial limbs. They may have a maximum annual benefit allowed, stated in dollar amounts, such as "X-ray examinations covered to a maximum benefit of $400 annually." Plans that state maximum benefits allowed (regardless of possible complications) are referred to as *indemnity plans*.

Major Medical Benefits
Major medical plans often are acquired to supplement basic benefits or are offered as a combined plan. These plans provide coverage to a much higher dollar amount. Major medical coverage begins where the basic plan leaves off, paying for expenses incurred because of a very serious or prolonged illness. These plans frequently cover many of the items disallowed by the basic coverage. The major medical plan frequently covers hospitalization, surgery, radiation, or oncology treatment.

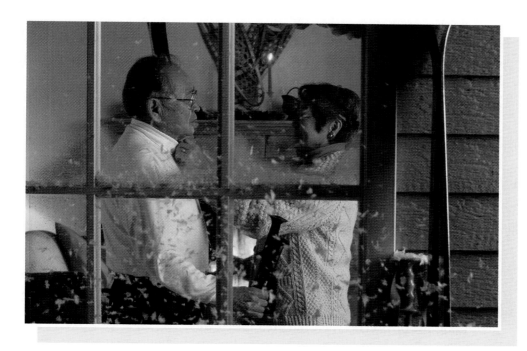

FIGURE 14.1

Many elderly persons carry what is known as catastrophic benefits to cover long-term illnesses.

Catastrophic Benefits

Many elderly persons carry what is known as *catastrophic benefits* to cover long-term illnesses (Figure 14.1). These policies usually have a $5000 or $10,000 deductible. They will cover long-term recovery from a transplant, a long-term kidney ailment where transplant may not be viable (thus the patient must have dialysis), and services and long-term care that would not be covered under the usual basic or major medical coverage. This type of policy also would cover long-term services for a person who has experienced a severely debilitating vehicular accident and needs long-term ventilation, respiratory, physical, or occupational therapy.

This coverage takes over when the major medical plan is maximized to its dollar limit, usually $1 million. This coverage also will assist in meeting expenses for inpatient services in an acute-care facility. The policy can kick in, for instance, when a patient must be isolated in a private room because of an infection. There are many variations to these plans. If the patient does not completely understand his or her coverage, suggest that they talk with their insurance representative or broker and have that person outline the plan and its coverage in full.

Supplemental Plans

Many insurance companies offer plans designed to pick up the payment of the 20% not paid by conventional insurance plans. These companion plans are available to the patient or subscriber as a supplement to Medicare. However, many of these plans incorporate many exclusions or limitations that usually are not apparent to the patient or subscriber. Thus the subscriber must be very cautious to check out all the plan's exclusions. Frequently the patient will expect you to know and understand the exclusions or limitations of their plan.

Special Automobile Insurance

Many automobile insurance policies include a clause to cover injuries incurred as a result of vehicular accident. This clause usually is referred to as *bodily injury coverage*. People may pay for this type of insurance to provide coverage for passengers in their car, regardless of who causes the accident, or for the occupants of any other vehicles if the insured is responsible for the accident.

Insurance for the Medical Office

Physicians also must carry several types of insurance for their office. The basic reason for insurance in a medical practice is the same as for any insurance: to protect against financial loss. Your responsibilities for the various insurances required probably will be limited to storing and retrieving policies and reminding the physician when the premium is due.

Policies should be stored in a safe, fireproof environment. The most common location is in a safety deposit box in a local bank. If policies are kept on the office premises, they should be stored in a fireproof cabinet, preferably locked for additional security. To make policy retrieval easy, you should keep a master list of all office insurance policies in an accessible place in your work area. The list should include the following information:

- Type of policy
- Insurance company
- Policy number
- Annual renewal date

Because policies are only in effect if insurance premiums are paid, you will need to establish a means to ensure that payment dates are not missed. The eas-

AT WORK TODAY

The Physician's Office Insurance

The physician has several types of insurance to be concerned about in this day and age. He or she must carry property insurance to protect against loss of office furnishings, equipment, and business/medical records, as well as for loss incurred because of embezzlement.

He or she also must carry personal liability insurance to cover injuries on the premises such as from a fall on an ice-covered sidewalk or a trip on carpeting. By law, the physician must carry Workers' Compensation insurance for his or her employees and may also carry income loss, disability, and life insurance for himself or herself.

Malpractice, or professional liability, insurance is important because lawsuits against physicians have reached astronomical proportions. Physicians in some types of practices and in some areas pay as much as $50,000 or more per year just for this coverage. "Practicing medicine" takes a large part of the physician's budget.

iest method is to use a master calendar or tickler file. Insurance companies typically send renewal notices in advance of the due date, but to prevent problems should the notice be lost, either before or after reaching your office, you should have a back-up reminder system. The date noted in the reminder file should be 2 to 4 weeks before the renewal date. If you have not received a renewal notice by 2 weeks before the renewal date, contact the insurance company or the office insurance broker.

Although you will not be responsible for the investigation or acquisition of insurance policies for the office, it is to your professional and personal advantage to understand the basics of protective insurance. Insurance policies are classified as follows:

- Property
- Criminal loss
- Disability
- Liability
- Life
- Overhead
- Bonding

Medical offices usually have one or more of these policies to protect the physician from financial loss.

Property Insurance

There are many policies that can be purchased to protect against property loss; only the more common will be described here.

Damage to Owned Building and Contents Coverage. This type of policy provides basic coverage for loss from fire and may be extended to include loss from vandalism or malicious mischief (Figure 14.2). The latter often is necessary, because medical offices are common targets for burglars in search of cash and drugs.

Consequential Loss Coverage. This coverage can be very important to a medical practice, because the loss of property or contents may result in loss of

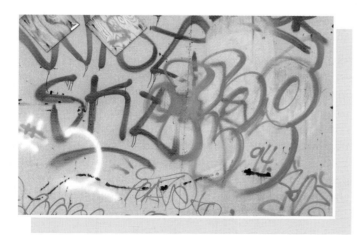

FIGURE 14.2

Property insurance can provide basic coverage for loss from fire and may be extended to include loss from vandalism or malicious mischief.

the ability to conduct business during the course of rebuilding property or replacing furnishings or equipment.

Broad-Form Coverage. This type of policy may be a way to cover a practice for all of the items just discussed and all potential risks, but you should be aware that most policies still contain some exclusions such as floods, earthquakes, and tornadoes. Careful reading of insurance policies is always wise but is particularly important with this type of coverage.

Special Area Needs Coverage. This coverage will depend on the area in which the practice is located. Insurance may be obtained for specific possible needs, such as protection against loss because of hurricane, earthquake, or flood. In areas where there is a high risk of these events, the insurance premium can be expected to be particularly high.

One thing to keep in mind when acquiring property insurance is that the policy can be written at actual cash value or for replacement value. Replacement value is more appropriate, because inflation will make the cost of replacing any item higher than it was at the time of purchase.

Criminal Loss Insurance

Criminal loss in a medical practice usually is related to the loss of funds or property from theft by employees. Protection against this type of loss is classified as fidelity bonds, which can be purchased in three forms. Individual fidelity bonds protect the employer against losses from any dishonest act by an employee. Each employee must complete an application for this type of bond. The employees then will be named individually with the insurance bonding company. Scheduled fidelity bonds may be purchased to cover individual employees or specific positions for a stated dollar amount. A blanket fidelity bond covers all employees automatically, regardless of position, for a dollar limit established by the employer. The blanket bond has the additional advantage of payment for the loss even if the responsible employee cannot be identified.

Disability Insurance

There are several types of disability insurance, which usually is designed to provide protection should the physician become disabled and be unable to perform his or her duties and function as a physician. Normally the physician must be disabled for a specified period before insurance benefits begin. This time frame normally is 90 days and requires that the treating physician submit a report that will assist the carrier in determining future reimbursement for disability.

Liability Insurance

Comprehensive General Liability. There are numerous types of liability insurance. First is comprehensive general liability, a broad form of coverage designed to protect the policy holder from financial losses resulting from injury caused by a condition or defect on the premises or by operation hazards. It also provides protection for building owners against claims as a result of conditions created by renters. This policy is similar to the public liability commonly held by homeowners and renters, except that the dollar amounts for a business generally are higher because of the number of people who visit the office.

Professional Liability. Professional liability was discussed at length in Chapter 4. The professional liability insurance carried by physicians to cover their acts and omissions and those of their employees is basically related to claims for bodily injury and issues related to patient care.

Workers' Compensation. States have mandated that insurance coverage be provided for employees in the event that they are injured or become ill in the course of their work. In many states the physician-employer also can be covered under the same policy as the employees, because the physician is subject to the same exposure. Although some states do not require coverage from employers with fewer than 10 employees, most medical practices carry Workers' Compensation regardless of the number of employees because of the possible exposures in the medical environment.

Excess Liability and Umbrella Policies. Excess liability and umbrella forms of legal liability coverage are available for unexpected claims or events. Excess liability extends the dollar coverage provided by basic liability policies to assist with exceptionally large claims. An umbrella policy may be purchased to serve as "catch-all" coverage to protect the policyholder against all of the possible hazards not covered by or excluded from basis liability policies.

Life Insurance

Almost everyone has some type of life insurance policy. The physician-employer normally has a significant amount of life insurance. Some of this insurance may be designated to pay off loans against the practice (perhaps the physician's student loans). Occasionally, physician-employers will provide life insurance for their employees, along with their health insurance.

Overhead Insurance

Overhead insurance can incorporate both disability and coverage to see that the practice's costs are covered while the physician is disabled. In this day and age, it is particularly important that the physician obtain and maintain overhead insurance. Such insurance allows the practice to hire a locum tenums physician to continue the practice while the physician is disabled and provides the income necessary to support the day-to-day costs of running a practice.

Bonding Insurance

This type of insurance guarantees that a background check has been made on each employee, particularly those who handle funds in the practice. Should an employee ever embezzle from the physician office, the practice can be reimbursed for the funds found to missing.

Carrier Reimbursement Types

Indemnity Schedules

Indemnity schedules are set by each individual carrier based on reimbursement rates. The carrier agrees to pay the subscriber a set amount of money for a particular service or procedure. The insured person is given a fee schedule when the policy is purchased.

Indemnity plans do not pay for the total amount charged for the services rendered. Many times there is a difference in the amount paid by the carrier and the amount of the physician's fee. For example, the carrier may agree to pay up to $1000 for a specific procedure, with no consideration for the time or complications of the surgery. If the physician charges $1200, the difference of $200 is then billed to the patient as his or her responsibility.

This type of plan takes the major expense out of medical bills and helps to keep the premiums lower. The amount of the premium often determines the amount at which the procedures are paid. Indemnity benefits usually are paid to the person insured unless the person has signed the assignment of benefits that includes major medical services.

Service Benefit Plans

With service benefit plans, the carrier agrees to pay for certain surgical and/or medical services without additional expense to the person insured. There is no set fee schedule.

In a service benefit plan, a surgery with complications may determine a higher fee than a relatively straightforward surgical procedure. Occasionally the premiums for this type of coverage may be higher; however, the payments usually are higher. The assignment of benefits to the physician is honored, and the payment is sent directly to the physician. However, other than in Massachusetts, the physician is required to bill the difference between what was paid and what was billed. In Massachusetts the physician must accept the payment from the carrier as payment in full.

Workers' Compensation Schedules

Each state has a Workers' Compensation panel that sets the reimbursement fees for a Workers' Compensation claim (Figure 14.3). Workers' Compensation is a difficult group to bill, because in many areas they are still using the old 1974 Relative Value Study (RVS) on which to base reimbursement. That means that many of the services provided must be indicated with an unlisted procedural code, which means a report must accompany the claim. This is considered a delay tactic by the carriers. The Workers' Compensation fee schedules are far below the standards of reimbursement, even at times below Medicare. Updated coding and reimbursement systems have been promised; however, the Workers' Compensation agencies have yet to come forth with the changes.

Usual, Customary, and Reasonable Fees

You often will hear physicians refer to their profile when discussing patient-care insurance payments. A profile is a numerical image of a physician's patterns of charging for various services as monitored by insurance companies that are billed for reimbursement. The individual profiles physicians refer to represent usual fees. Comparative profiles are developed from all fees submitted by any physician in the geographical area for each service code. These profiles set the standards for usual, customary, and reasonable (UCR) standards and determine the maximum charges the insurance carrier will allow. This profile then becomes a determining factor for reimbursement rates for multiple types of policies.

Usual Fees

Usual fees for each physician are calculated by computer and represent the fees routinely charged by a physician for each service. The profile is calculated for a

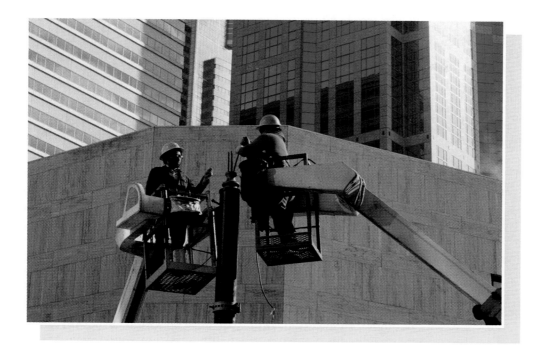

FIGURE 14.3

Each state has a Workers' Compensation panel that sets the reimbursement fees for a Workers' Compensation claim.

specific period, usually 1 year. This becomes the base year that determines the fees paid. Physicians may feel that the system is unfair to claimants, because the base year may be several years earlier than the one in which the services are billed.

Fees may change over time because the costs of maintaining an office will increase, requiring more income. If you want to determine a physician's usual fee, you select a specific period, at least 1 year, and check the fees for a specific procedure at various times throughout the year. The fee that occurs most often is the usual fee. For example, if your survey reveals charges for a specific procedure to include $10, $12, $12, $14, and $16, the usual fee would be $12.

Customary Fees

Fees are considered customary if they fall within the upper and lower profile limits for physicians of the same specialty or practice type who practice within a geographical area determined by the insurance company. If the upper limit profile is $18 for a specific service code and the lower limit is $14, the physician who submits a bill for $16 will have the fee recognized as customary.

Reasonable Fees

Fees are commonly declared reasonable if they meet criteria for usual and customary fees. In some cases, multiple problems can exist that make the services more complex and warrant a higher fee. Physicians submitting a higher-than-average fee should attach a statement and documents to support the extra fee. The claim will be reviewed by a panel of the physician's peers, and the appropriate fee will be determined.

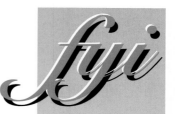

Usual, Customary, and Reasonable

Usual, customary, and reasonable is a process that has been used for indemnity plans starting with Blue Shield/Blue Cross. It is important that the physician's "profile" is correct or the payments may be calculated incorrectly by the insurance carrier. The physician's profile is studied to see what has been his or her usual charge for a procedure over the past year. This represents the *usual* in the fee schedule. The *customary* fee is what most physicians charge in the same type of practice and in the same community. *Reasonable* means the first two criteria for usual and customary fees are acceptable and the physician will need to attach documentation of a problem that results in an additional fee.

Types of Health Plans

Blue Cross

History

The concept of Blue Cross originated during the Great Depression of the 1930s when hospitals were left with empty beds and unpaid bills. The American Hospital Association has played a major role in the development of Blue Cross, and today there are more than 200 for-profit and nonprofit Blue Cross plans throughout the United States that provide financial assistance for health care services.

Possible Plans

Depending on the geographical area, Blue Cross plans may be available for coverage of hospital, medical, or surgical services or for any combination of the three. In some instances Blue Cross has teamed with Blue Shield to provide a combination plan, wherein Blue Cross pays for hospitalization and Blue Shield pays for the physician portion; this is evident in the Federal Employee Plan of Blue Cross/Blue Shield. In addition, Blue Cross has developed a "Companion Care" plan that provides supplementary benefits to patients who have Medicare. Several companion options are available, including those that pay for the 20% of hospitalization that is not paid by Medicare. Most supplementary plans do not pick up the deductible.

Eligibility

It is possible to acquire Blue Cross insurance as an individual or as part of a group. Individual plans cover one person and, if appropriate, his or her family (Figure 14.4). Group plans are available through employers or associations for employees or members and their families. The primary insured person is the subscriber, and eligible family members are dependents. If the insurance is an employment benefit, the employer may pay all or a major part of the subscriber's premium; if dependents are covered, the employee pays for the additional coverage, often through payroll deductions.

FIGURE 14.4

Individual plans cover one person and, if appropriate, his or her family.

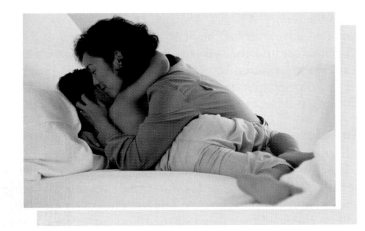

Benefit Payments

When a physician's services are billed to Blue Cross and the patient signs the assignment of benefits or authorization, the payment of the carrier's portion will be sent directly to the physician. The patient is responsible for the remainder of the fee. If the patient assignment is not signed, the benefits check will be sent to the patient, often with both the physician and the patient listed as the payee. Theoretically this check would require both signatures to be cashed, but if this is not enforced, the physician may have difficulty securing payment.

Blue Shield

History

Like Blue Cross, the first Blue Shield organizations were born of the Depression and the need of physicians to protect their incomes. Blue Shield plans are nonprofit and are local or statewide corporations. There are approximately 100 Blue Shield plans covering almost 20% of the population in the United States. Because the original intent was to pay for physician services, Blue Shield plans were known as *physician's service organizations*. Blue Shield has since diversified, like Blue Cross, and dropped the word "physician" from its title. Blue Shield is no longer considered physician sponsored.

Possible Plans

Blue Shield offers the same options available through Blue Cross, including a Medicare companion plan to supplement both Parts A and B of the Medicare program.

Eligibility

Blue Shield also is available under individual and group contracts that are paid for in the same manner as Blue Cross. As is usually the case, a group plan premium is less costly for the subscriber.

Benefit Payment

Blue Shield develops fee profiles of physicians just as other insurance companies do. These profiles influence the determination of UCR fees. Physicians may elect to be members of the local Blue Shield organization. As members they agree to accept the UCR fee as payment in full for services on some specific plans; other plans may allow the physician to bill the patient for the stated allowed amount on the Explanation of Benefits (EOB). Patients of Blue Shield physician-members are responsible, however, for the annual deductible and for uncovered services. Nonmember physician services also will be covered, but the patient can be billed for the difference between the UCR payment and the physician's actual fees in addition to the deductible and uncovered services. Payment is automatically sent to physician-members and will not be sent to nonmember physicians. Payment then is sent to the patient.

CHAMPUS

CHAMPUS is the abbreviation for Civilian Health and Medical Program of the Uniformed Services. This is a congressionally funded, comprehensive health benefits program designed to provide families of uniformed services personnel and service retirees a supplement to medical care in military and public health service facilities. Beneficiaries may receive a fairly wide range of civilian health care services, with a significant share of the cost or amount paid for by the federal government. Usually these patients seek care from military medical facilities near their homes. However, there are times when they can seek care through a private physician's office or hospital. When beneficiaries live within a 40-mile radius of a military facility where they could receive the same level of service or the same service, they must provide the physician's office with a Form DD1251, "Non-availability Statement" from either the commanding officer of the military facility or the CHAMPUS advisers.

Eligibility

Public Law 569, enacted in 1956 and subsequently expanded in 1996 by the Military Medical Benefits Amendment Act, allows treatment in nonmilitary facilities for select individuals. CHAMPUS benefits are available for the following:

- Dependents of military personnel
- Military retirees
- Dependents of military retirees
- Dependents of deceased military personnel or deceased retirees

Benefit Payments

CHAMPUS allows eligible beneficiaries to receive many types of inpatient and outpatient services through private-sector providers. These services are paid for in part by the federal government. The payment schedules are similar to those of private insurance in that they have a deductible and copayments that are the patient's responsibility. After the deductible is paid, which currently is $50 per patient with a combined total per family of $100, dependents of military personnel are responsible for a copayment of 20%; all others eligible for benefits pay a 25% copayment.

CHAMPVA

CHAMPVA was established in 1973 for the spouses and dependents of individuals considered by the Veterans Administration (VA) to be permanently disabled or who are deceased as a result of service-related duties. Once eligibility is established and cards are issued, potential patients may seek care from private-sector providers.

Claims for CHAMPUS and CHAMPVA services must be filed either on the CHAMPUS 500 form or on the HCFA-1500 Standard Claim Form (see Figure 13.8). The top half, items 1 through 18, is to be completed and signed by the patient or his or her legal guardian; the bottom half, items 19 through 32, is to be completed by the medical assistant; and item 33 is to be signed only by the physician. A signature stamp or the medical assistant's signature as the physician's representative may not be substituted for the personal signature of the physician.

The benefits and payment schedules for CHAMPVA patients are the same as for CHAMPUS patients. As with other government programs, the rules are relatively rigid and may change periodically. The office manual on eligibility,

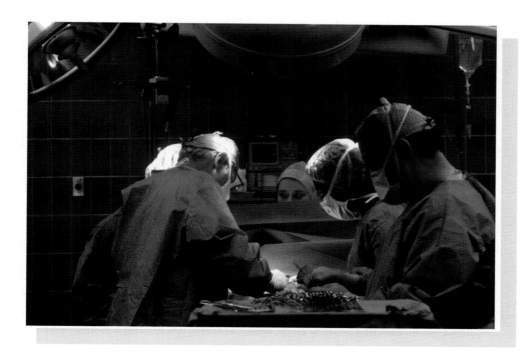

FIGURE 14.5

Rapid advances in medical technology and the accompanying sharp escalation of medical care costs have motivated the public to find a way to protect itself through insurance coverage.

services, and billing is available through your regional CHAMPUS office or by writing to O'CHAMPUS, Fitzsimmons Army Base, Aurora, Colorado.

Commercial Carriers

Development

Approximately 750 private insurance companies currently provide health policies. After World War II independent insurance carriers entered the health care field because of public need and improvements within the insurance industry. Rapid advances in medical technology and the accompanying sharp escalation of medical care costs motivated the public to find a way to protect itself against rising expenses (Figure 14.5). The relative prosperity of the economy at the same time allowed the insurance industry to introduce broad forms of insurance coverage, including major medical, that previously were unavailable.

Commercial companies may offer service plans, which pay on the UCR schedule, or indemnity plans, which pay a fixed amount for various injuries or treatments. The greater the amount of the indemnity or benefits, the higher the premium.

Plans Available

An individual health insurance plan is purchased directly by the individual receiving the benefits. The policy is issued to the individual and/or eligible dependents. As determined under COBRA legislation enacted in 1987, an individual covered by a group health plan through his or her employer may convert to an individual policy when he or she terminates employment. Usually an individual plan will have higher premiums and fewer benefits compared with the same group plan.

Group Health Plans

A group health plan is purchased for individuals by an employer or administrator of an association. This plan is written for any group of participants and their eligible dependents under a single policy issued to the employer or group. Individual certificates of membership in the group plan are issued to the individuals and dependents, with equal coverage to each person in the plan.

Commercial Health Insurance Carriers

Commercial health insurance carriers are for-profit companies that provide group and/or individual plans. These plans are paid for through premiums. Coverage and benefits of an insurance plan underwritten by a commercial carrier will vary widely from plan to plan and carrier to carrier. The type and amount of payment also will vary greatly. The plans are governed by the state insurance commissioner since they include both life insurance and medical insurance.

Eligibility

Carriers have many methods and guidelines to determine eligibility; each contract or policy may have different requirements.

Reimbursement

Payment of benefits through policies held with independent carriers generally is made directly to the insured and not to the provider unless the patient authorizes an assignment of benefits. The patient is responsible for the physician's entire bill regardless of what the insurance policy pays.

Employer-Sponsored Plans

Employers may choose to establish their own in-house benefit plan that is underwritten by one of the major insurance companies. Usually this allows employers to develop a specific plan that they feel will meet the needs of their employees. Normally only very large companies can afford to develop their own plans, yet companies that use such a plan may realize cost savings. For example, companies can give incentives to those employees and their families who have a relatively low incidence of illness. It has been found that many of the larger companies that provide this type of coverage and administer their own claims have, in fact, saved a significant amount compared with what they might have paid for a PPO, HMO, or commercial insurance.

Foundations for Medical Care

A foundation to provide medical care is a management system for community health services that normally is backed by Blue Cross or in some areas by carriers, such as Sutter Health, that have developed foundation status. A foundation can take the form of an organization created either by a hospital group of physicians or perhaps through a medical society. This type of coverage concerns itself with the quality and cost of care (almost every service must have a prior authorization). Under the foundation concept, the foundation contracts with a major insurance carrier to sell and negotiate the policy. The carrier collects all premiums, assumes all of the risk, and reimburses the foundation through a claims office.

The foundation sets policy standards; receives, reviews, and processes the claims; sets reimbursement based on their own internal profile for each specialty; elects physician-members yearly; and continues to study local medical economic problems. Member physicians agree to accept the foundation reimbursement as payment in full, other than the copayment (anywhere from $5 to $20) the patient is required to make. The local medical society normally controls the foundation legally and selects the foundation trustees.

The patient then selects the physician of his or her choice; the patient or the patient's organization (for example, labor union or employer) pays the premium directly to the insurance carrier.

Health Maintenance Organizations (HMOs)

Development

By the early 1970s the federal government recognized that health care costs were rising dramatically and that there was growing public pressure to do something about the situation. In addition, the federal government saw that although health insurance programs generally paid for services required for illness or injury, few would cover preventive service. In evaluating possible solutions, the federal government identified prepaid group practice as one mechanism that had a proven record for controlling costs. Doctor Paul Ellwood, a presidential adviser, coined the phrase "health maintenance organization" (HMO) to describe this mechanism, and federal support was proposed to create a national network of HMOs.

In 1973 the federal HMO Act (Public Law 93-222) was signed into law. It authorized federal funds for 5 years to establish and develop new HMOs. According to this law, an HMO provides or arranges for a comprehensive range of inpatient and outpatient health care services based on a fixed, prepaid fee. If the HMO is administered properly and its services provided appropriately, the plan will function within the budget. If not monitored properly, the plan will go over budget and have to provide care throughout the premium period without reimbursement, since the reimbursement rate was calculated in advance. This puts the emphasis on keeping patients well and treating them early, in the hopes of preventing the need for major medical care.

Methods

By 1978 laws had been amended twice to promote the survival of the HMO concept. Additional grants were made available to qualifying groups wishing to continue or develop efficient HMOs. Under this concept, physician services may be delivered through staff or group models.

Staff Model. Physicians involved in the staff model type of HMO work in a group-practice clinic that is owned by the HMO and that employs its own physicians on a salaried basis.

Group Model. Physicians who work in a group practice clinic enter into an agreement to provide services to the HMO subscribers. Based on a medical service agreement, the physicians' group accepts as fee for service a predetermined capitation rate. This means that each month the group receives a flat fee for each subscriber to the HMO. Some members will not see the physicians at any time during the month, while others will require many services. If the capitation rate has been calculated properly and the physicians carefully select the methods of care, the physicians should be able to provide all needed services and still earn an income. Involved physicians may continue to treat nonmembers of the HMO on the usual fee-for-service basis.

Medical Assistants and HMOs

As an administrative medical assistant you may choose to work in an HMO. If you work in a group or IPA type practice, you will use both fee-for-service and HMO billing techniques. Each HMO functions according to a unique set of rules as long as it meets the federal criteria as an organization. If you are working in a practice associated with an HMO, familiarize yourself with the details of billing for services. Some group and IPA models require that a deductible, typically $1 to $20, be paid by the patient for each visit.

Independent Physicians Association (IPA)

The Independent Physicians Association (IPA) model is a legal entity organized and operated by physicians to promote the preservation of the private-practice concept. Through this mechanism, physicians join together to enter into contractual arrangements with other parties, such as HMOs and other prepaid health plans, to provide medical services from private offices and in hospitals to a specific population of subscribers. Membership in an IPA does not limit a physician's practice to the treatment of patients covered under an IPA or HMO contract. As the individual IPA physicians provide services to the HMO subscribers, they submit their claims to the IPA for reimbursement on a predetermined fee-for-service basis. The fund available to pay for care also is based on a capitation rate. If care has been provided prudently, the funds will be adequate to pay all claims submitted throughout the prepaid time period; if not, physicians must continue to provide care without reimbursement. This is termed an *at-risk* form of insurance, because the physician is at risk of not being paid; the patient is not at risk, because care must be provided without prejudice.

Medicaid

Indigent Aid

Medicaid is available to assist persons who qualify to acquire necessary medical care. It is available to eligible persons who have no access to care or to those who have Medicare but are unable to pay the difference between the allowed Medicare fees and the amount paid by Medicare (Figure 14.6).

Combined Effort

Medicaid is a cooperative arrangement between each state and the federal government and was initiated by the Social Security Act amendments of 1966. It receives its authority from Title XIX of Public Law 89-97. The federal government provides a major portion of the funds for the program, with the

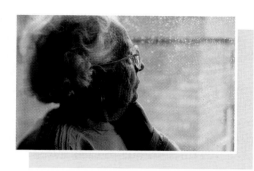

remainder of the funds provided by each state. In addition, each state accepts responsibility for administering the program.

State Responsibilities

Each state makes independent determinations on details of the Medicaid program regarding an applicant's eligibility, available services, and maximum payments that will be made to providers for services rendered. Each state issues to eligible patients an official identification card. Although each state administers a Medicaid program, the state may use different terminology to name the program, thus leading to confusion for the medical assistant when out-of-state patients refer to the Medicaid programs by the name used in their state. Medicaid may be referred to as Medical Assistance, Public Assistance, DPW, Welfare, Medicaid, Title XIX, MediCal (California), SAMI (Nevada), and ACCESS (Arizona).

Physician Options and Responsibilities

Physicians may choose whether to accept Medicaid patients. An office policy should be established and the guidelines for accepting Medicaid patients made known to all employees. Physicians may accept patients with the Medicare/Medicaid combination, or they may choose to accept Medicaid patients only on referral from another provider, only from the hospital emergency department when they are on rotation, or only for consultation.

Often the physician will have to restrict the percentage of Medicaid patients in the practice, since patients with Medicaid frequently require a much greater level of service and the low reimbursement for services can be almost prohibitive (as low as 30% of the physician's usual fee). Physicians must then write off the unpaid portion. In other words, physicians who accept Medicaid patients must accept the state's schedule as payment in full and may not bill the patient for the remaining portion. Many states have imposed stringent guidelines on the actual billing requirements, prior authorization requirements, and/or time frames fro claims submission. Consequently, the additional paper work and staff time required makes the reimbursement amount virtually negligible.

If it is office policy not to accept Medicaid patients, you will be responsible for screening new patients and informing them of office policy. You may be able to suggest physicians who accept Medicaid or refer individuals needing care to the county medical society, where a list of physicians who accept Medicaid patients is kept.

If Medicaid patients are accepted, you will need to check identification cards before the first visits each month. At this time, you should photocopy the card for your records. Some states now have machines to dial into the Medicaid program and obtain eligibility status, whether or not the patient has a share of cost (including whether it has been met), and authorization for services for which some states have a requirement. You also will need to keep abreast of program changes and covered services, which usually are communicated in printed bulletins mailed periodically to all providers. Also be careful to bill according to the very specific program rules unique to each state.

Medicare

Medicare was established in 1966 through an amendment to the Social Security Act. It is available to elderly or disabled persons and is designed to assist patients with a major portion of their medical bills. Citizens become eligible for Medicare beginning with their sixty-fifth birthday and should register with a local Social Security office at least 3 months before that date. Medicare also is available to individuals of any age who have been declared permanently disabled and have been receiving financial disability assistance for 2 years. Determination of eligibility ultimately is made by program evaluators. Hospital services are provided under Part A of the Medicare program and are paid from a fund contributed to by the self-employed or by working individuals and their employers. These contributions are made in the form of a tax levied under the Federal Insurance Contributions Act (FICA). Anyone eligible for Medicare may receive Part A benefits. Railroad employees, federal employees, and state employees are not part of the Social Security system and receive their old-age hospital and physician benefits from other sources. Railroad retirement funds administer their Medicare separately from Social Security Medicare; federal and state employees have an independent benefits program.

Physician medical services are provided under Part B of Medicare, a voluntary program that requires the payment of a monthly premium. The monthly premium is nominal compared with other insurance and usually is withheld from monthly Social Security checks. In the past few years, the premium and deductible have been rising rapidly; additionally, few supplemental plans will pay this portion.

Employers with more than 20 employees must offer those of their employees older than age 65 the same insurance coverage as the younger employees. This then makes that insurance carrier the primary coverage and Medicare the secondary coverage. If the primary carrier pays more for the service than Medicare would allow in the first place, then there will be no further payment from Medicare. Should the patient retire or terminate employment, the process reverses and Medicare again becomes the primary carrier. It is best to request that the patient provide the physician's office with a letter stating the date of retirement or the date termination will be effective.

Social Security Income (SSI) patients qualify for Medicare benefits even though they are not over age 65. In such cases it has been determined through physician documentation that the patient has had either a physical or mental illness for 2 or more years. In many instances patients will not have worked enough to have contributed sufficient funds into the Medicare program to qualify for benefits. Such patients will be qualified to utilize benefits through their parents.

Immigrants or aliens also may qualify for Medicare benefits if they are over age 65 and have resided in the United States for more than 5 years. If the patient has not resided in the United States for 5 years, then request that the patient secure a form from the Social Security office stipulating the date the patient will be eligible for Medicare benefits.

Physician Options and Responsibilities

Physicians may opt whether to participate in the Medicare program. If the physician chooses to participate, then the physician's office must file all claims to Medicare and must accept assignment of benefits for all claims. If the physician chooses not to participate, then he or she may opt to accept assignment on some claims but perhaps not on others. In any case the practice must file the claim with Medicare. If a physician chooses not to participate and provides elective surgical services that are more than $500, the physician's office must apprise the patient of the fee for the surgery, the amount Medicare is expected to pay, and what the expected amount due from the patient will be. This must be in writing and acknowledged with the patient's signature. Medicare may request proof of such acknowledgement (Figure 14.7).

Whether or not the physician chooses to participate, there may be some services that are either not a benefit of the Medicare program or may not be considered "medically necessary" by Medicare. In either case the physician's office is required to notify the patient that Medicare may consider the service not a benefit of the program or not medical necessary; See Figure 14.8 for an example of the form that must be sighed by the patient. Should the physician's office not apprise the patient of this information, the Medicare program may consider the lack of such notification to be an attempt to defraud the government.

Other situations considered by Medicare to be fraudulent include the following:

- False representation with intent to gain
- Billing for services not rendered
- Duplicate billing
- Upgrading/using procedure codes higher than services actually rendered
- Receiving "kickbacks" from laboratories or imaging facilities

The Medicare program has various methods for compiling the above data. They are as follows:

- Computer comparison of billings for that practice
- Beneficiary complaints
- Physician-employee complaints
- Anonymous telephone calls

Any of the fraudulent practices just discussed may result in the following for the physician:

1. Sanctions
   1 year to lifetime removal from the Medicare or Medicaid program
   Notice published in local newspapers for 3 weeks after sanctions
   Notice published in the national bulletins

How to Calculate the Medicare Estimated Payment for Elective Surgery and the Medicare Beneficiary Obligation

1. Your actual charge for the service.   _____
   (If less than $500 no notification to the patient is necessary.)

2. The Medicare-approved charge.   _____
   This is the lowest of your actual charge, your customary charge, or the area prevailing charge. (If you have accepted assignment on a claim for the same service, the Medicare-approved charge was provided to you. If you do not know this information, contact your carrier.)

3. Enter the difference between your charge and the Medicare-approved amount (line 1 minus line 2).

4. Enter the 20% co-insurance on the Medicare allowable charge.   _____

5. The beneficiary's out-of-pocket expense.   _____

You must provide the beneficiary the information on lines 1, 2, and 5 (assume that the Part B deductible has been met).

Draft Notice to the Patient

Date:

Because I do not plan to accept assignment for your case, federal law requires me to provide you information on the amount that I intend to charge you for your surgery, the amount that Medicare will pay you, and the amount (including the Medicare-required co-insurance) that you will be responsible for. (You may have other insurance that will cover all or part of this difference.)

Type of Surgery _____

Estimate of my fee: _____ (from line 1)

What Medicare should pay: _____ (from line 2)

The out-of-pocket costs for which
   you will be responsible:_____ (from line 5)
   (including Medicare required co-insurance)

You should obtain your patient's signature on this form and retain it for your records.

FIGURE 14.7

Outline of the procedure for calculating the Medicare estimated payment for elective surgery and the Medicare beneficiary obligation as required by the HCFA. (Courtesy De A. Eggers & Associates, Sonoma, Calif.)

Not Medically Necessary Form

Medicare will only pay for services that it determines to be "reasonable and necessary" under section 1862(a)(1) of the Medicare law. If Medicare determines that a particular service, although it would otherwise be covered, is "not reasonable or necessary" under the Medicare program standards, Medicare will deny payment for that service. I believe that, in your case, Medicare is likely to deny payment for:

Date: Reason: Service:

_____   _____   _____

Fee: Signature:

_____   _____

I have been notified by my provider that he or she believes that in my case Medicare is likely to deny payment for the items or services identified above, for the reason # stated. If Medicare denies payment I agree to be personally and fully responsible for payment.

_____

Patient Signature

1. Medicare does not usually pay for this many visits or treatments.
2. Medicare usually does not pay for this service.
3. Medicare usually pays for only one nursing home visit per month.
4. Medicare usually does not pay for this injection.
5. Medicare usually does not pay for this many injections.
6. Medicare does not pay for this because it is a treatment that has yet to be proved effective.
7. Medicare does not pay for this office visit unless it was needed because of an emergency.
8. Medicare usually does not pay for services by more than one physician during the same period.
9. Medicare does not pay for this many services within this period of time.
10. Medicare usually does not pay for more than one visit per day.
11. Medicare usually does not pay for such extensive procedures.
12. Medicare usually does not pay for like services by more than one physician of the same specialty.
13. Medicare usually does not pay for this equipment.
14. Medicare usually does not pay for this lab test.

FIGURE 14.8

Not Medically Necessary form. (Courtesy De A. Eggers & Associates, Sonoma, Calif.)

2. Civil monetary penalty law:
   Assessment of up to $2000 per line item on the claim
3. Civil suit
4. Criminal suit (imprisonment)

Preferred Provider Organization (PPO)

The Preferred Provider Organization (PPO) concept is a legal entity that has been organized by various promoters (for example, hospitals, physicians, and insurance carriers). Through this mechanism, physicians and hospitals join together to enter into contractual arrangements with other parties, such as employers, unions, and associations, to provide medical services in private offices and in hospitals to that specific population of enrollees or subscribers. Membership in a PPO does not limit a physician's practice to the treatment of patients covered under the PPO contract. As the PPO physicians and hospitals provide services to their subscribers, they submit their claims to the specific entity for reimbursement on a predetermined fee-for-service basis. The funds available to pay for care also are based on a predetermined rate. If care has been provided prudently, the funds will be adequate to pay for all claims submitted throughout the paid time period. If not, the physicians and hospitals must continue to provide care without reimbursement. This is another type of at-risk form of medical coverage, since the physician and hospital are at risk of not being paid.

The physician should evaluate each contract (be it a modified HMO, IPA, or PPO) very carefully before agreeing to participate. The assistant must be aware that with many of these contracts a greater burden of paperwork is placed on the insurance assistant because of the many variations of requirements for second opinions, prior authorizations (Figure 14.9), and predeterminations prior to treatment.

Workers' Compensation

Availability

Every state possesses its own Workers' Compensation law, and the basic purposes of each law are the same: that employees who are injured or become ill as a result of their employment will have adequate means of support if they are unable to work and that they will be free from the cost of any medical services.

Employers must provide for these benefits and usually do so through a Workers' Compensation policy paid solely by the employer. Because the guidelines in each state vary, be aware of those unique to your area. For example, some states do not require that employers have coverage if they have fewer than 10 employees.

Administered by the State

The laws of each state indicate who is eligible for Workers' Compensation benefits but usually leave the determination to the physician treating the patient. If an employer, insurance company, or the state is in doubt about a patient's claim, they may request a determination from the Workers' Compensation Board or Industrial Relations Board.

REFERRAL REQUEST

Authorization

REFERRAL # ___149515___

MIPA
Marin Individual Practice Association

125 E. Sir Francis Drake Blvd., Suite 400
Larkspur, CA 94939
Phone: (415) 464-8181
Fax: (415) 925-6560

☐ **URGENT**

☐ Aetna Select Choice
☐ California Care
  ☐ Blue Cross Plus
  ☐ HMO / USA
☐ Cigna
☐ FHP / TakeCare
☐ FHP / TakeCare Senior Program
☐ Other _____

☐ HPR
☐ Health Net
☐ Health Net Seniority Plus
☐ Lifeguard
☐ OMNI
☐ PruCare
☐ PruCare Plus

QUICK REFERRAL TO MARIN IPA PHYSICIAN ONLY (COMPLETE SECTION 1-4)

1 PATIENT'S NAME (LAST)   (FIRST)   (M. INITIAL)   I.D. NO.:   DATE OF BIRTH   M   D   Y

ADDRESS

2 REFERRING PCP: TELEPHONE NO.

3 SPECIALIST'S / FACILITY NAME   TELEPHONE NO.

ADDRESS   CITY

4 Dx: ICD 9   DATE LAST SEEN BY PCP: REASON FOR REFERRAL / TREATMENT TO DATE:

NUMBER OF VISITS REQUESTED ☐ SINGLE / CONSULT ONLY   ☐ 2

SIGNATURE - REFERRING PHYSICIAN / PCP   DATE REQUESTED

SINGLE VISIT EXPIRES 45 DAYS AFTER ISSUE DATE. MULTIPLE VISITS EXPIRE 90 DAYS AFTER ISSUE DATE.

THIS REFERRAL ONLY VALID FOR MARIN IPA MEMBER PHYSICIANS.
PRIOR AUTHORIZATION IS REQUIRED FOR ALL NON MARIN IPA PHYSICIANS OR CONTRACT PHYSICIANS.

5 **PRE-AUTHORIZATION REQUEST**
MANDATORY PRIOR TO ALL SERVICES LISTED BELOW

☐ OUT OF PLAN / NON MARIN IPA OR CONTRACT PROVIDERS
(Requires Chart Notes)

☐ PHYSICAL / OCCUPATIONAL / SPEECH THERAPY

☐ PSYCHOTHERAPY / PSYCHIATRY / MENTAL HEALTH

☐ COST OF SERVICE EXCEEDS $450.00

☐ MRI / CT (HNSP/Lifeguard)

☐ BENEFIT REVIEW / PATIENT REQUEST

☐ EXTENDED SERVICE (exceeds 3 mos., e.g.; Chemo/Rad Treatment)

☐ INFERTILITY STUDIES / TREATMENT (requires infertility worksheet)

☐ RETRO REFERRAL DOS: _____
(include supporting documentation)

☐ WORKERS COMPENSATION / THIRD PARTY LIABILITY (e.g. MVA)
Date of Injury _____

☐ MGH - OUTPATIENT SERVICES (including Lab & X-ray)

☐ OTHER _____

6 **SPECIALIST SECTION:**
REFERRAL TO NON-MARIN IPA OR CONTRACT PROVIDER VALID ONLY IF PRE-AUTHORIZED (SECTION 5) SPECIALIST REPORT, DIAGNOSIS & TREATMENT MUST BE INCLUDED. ALL ANCILLARY SERVICES MUST BE PRE-AUTHORIZED (SECTION 5).

REASON FOR EXTENSION / TREATMENT PLAN:

MARIN IPA USE ONLY: ☐ APPROVED   ☐ DENIED

SIGNATURE - MEDICAL DIRECTOR   DATE

NUMBER OF VISITS REQUESTED BY SPECIALIST: _____

NON MARIN IPA PHYSICIAN EXTENSION VALID ONLY IF PRE-AUTHORIZED BY MEDICAL DIRECTOR.

A COPY OF THIS REFERRAL MUST ACCOMPANY ALL BILLINGS.
This authorization certifies medical necessity only. This guarantees payment only if the member proves to be eligible at the time services were rendered.

FORM #U1001 (REV 11/96)

FIGURE 14.9

Example of a referral request form. (Courtesy Marin IPA, Larkspur, Calif.)

The Workers' Compensation Board also established a fee schedule that sets the maximum amount payable for each health care service. The maximum amount allowed usually is less than the physician's standard fees. However, physicians who accept a Workers' Compensation case, sometimes referred to as an *industrial* case, agree to accept the predetermined fees. In essence, they are accepting assignment.

Insurance Coverage

Some employers who have a relatively low risk of an employee suffering an injury or illness prefer to pay necessary expenses directly in the event that they occur. These employers are referred to as *self-insured*. In this situation the bills for services are sent directly to the employer. Most often, however, the employer acquires a specific insurance policy to cover such events. The annual premium is relatively low and calculated according to the combined salaries of covered employees and the previous experience rate.

Claims made

Claims may be made for any illness or injury that is the result of a job or the work environment, regardless of cause and including employee carelessness. Before Workers' Compensation laws were passed in the 1930s the prevailing attitude was that employees should protect themselves. However, the laws presume employer responsibility and guide employers in educating and providing a safe environment for employees.

Benefits to Patients

Patients with work-related injuries or illness have a right to expect payment of all necessary medical services, including hospitalization, rehabilitation, and occupational therapy. Patients also will receive their regular salary during the period that they are unable to work. In cases of permanent disability, a hearing is held and a settlement determined. This settlement represents the total compensation for the illness or injury. In the event of a work-related death, the Workers' Compensation Board will determine the total benefits to be paid to the survivors.

Filing Claims

Two types of forms are necessary to file Workers' Compensation claims. The first time a physician sees a patient in a Workers' Compensation case, the physician must complete a Doctor's First Report of Occupational Injury or Illness form (Figure 14.10). You will probably be responsible for acquiring the information for items 1 through 11 on this form. The information may be typed or written in by hand.

Be as precise as possible when acquiring this information. The employee may be uncertain of the Workers' Compensation insurance carrier or confuse it with his or her private health insurance carrier. If there is any doubt, call the employer's personnel department. Also pay particular attention to item 11, the patient's statement of the cause of the injury or illness. It should be written in the first person in the patient's own words and in quotes for the greatest validity. For example, the entry might read: "I was entering the cafeteria when I slipped on a wet spot. I twisted my left ankle outwardly before I fell to the ground." The entry should not read, "Twisted left ankle laterally after contact with wet spot on cafeteria floor."

DOCTOR'S FIRST REPORT OF
OCCUPATIONAL INJURY OR ILLNESS
STATE OF CALIFORNIA

Immediately after first examination, mail original to insurer or self-insured employer. Failure to file a doctor's report is a misdemeanor (Labor Code 6413.5). In addition, in the case of diagnosed or suspected pesticide poisioning, you are required to: Send one copy of this report directly to the Division of Labor Statistics and Research, P.O. Box 603, San Francisco, Ca. 94101; send one copy to your local health officer; notify your local health officer by telephone within 24 hours.

A. INSURER

1. EMPLOYER NAME	DO NOT WRITE IN THIS SPACE

2. Address: No. & Street   City   Zip

3. Nature of business (e.g., food manufacturer, building construction, retailer of women's clothes)

4. PATIENT NAME (First name, middle initial, last name)	5. Sex ☐ Male ☐ Female	6. Date of birth

7. Address: No. & Street City Zip	8. Telephone number ( )

9. Occupation (Specific Job Title)	10. Social Security No.

11. Injured At: No. & Street City	County

12. Date & hour of injury or onset of illness	13. Date & hour of first exam or treatment	14. Date last Worked	15. Have you (or your office) previously treated patient? ☐ Yes ☐ No

16. HISTORY (History of injury or onset of illness. If occupational illness, specify exposures, chemicals &/or compounds)

17. MEDICAL FINDINGS (Use reverse side if more space is required & for remarks, if any.)
  A. Subjective complaints

  B. Objective findings

    X-Ray & Laboratory findings (State if none.)

  C. Diagnosis (If occupational illness, identify etiologic agent.)

18. Are your findings and diagnosis consistent with history of injury or onset of illness If "No", please explain.	☐ Yes ☐ No

19. Is there any other current condition that will impede or delay patient's recovery? If "Yes", please explain.	☐ Yes ☐ No

20. TREATMENT ☐ Office ☐ Hospital out-patient ☐ Hospital in-patient	Treatment Rendered	Further treatment required? ☐ Yes ☐ No Physical Therapy? ☐ Yes ☐ No

If in-patient, give Hospital name & location	Date admitted	Estimated stay

21. WORK STATUS Is patient able to perform usual work? ☐ Yes ☐ No	If no, give date when you estimate patient will be able to return to:	Usual work?	Modified work?

DOCTOR (Name & degree) (Type or print)   No. & Street   City   Zip

Doctor's Signature	IRS Number	Telephone number ( )	Report Date

FORM 5021 (Rev. 2)
(May 1980)

PLEASE SUBMIT YOUR REPORT WITHIN FIVE DAYS OF YOUR EXAMINATION
DELAY IN SUBMITTING THIS REPORT MAY CAUSE A DELAY IN BENEFITS TO YOUR PATIENT

CARRIER'S COPY

FIGURE 14.10

Doctor's First Report of Occupational Injury or Illness form for use in Workers' Compensation cases.

The form then should be clipped or stapled to the front cover of the chart to alert the physician of the need to complete the form. The physician's notes for items 12 through 20 usually are handwritten.

Each state establishes the time limits within which Workers' Compensation cases must be reported. Employers must notify the insurance company, often within 48 hours, on a special form that details the circumstances and conditions at the time the claim originated. Physicians must also file timely reports, usually within 5 days of the patient's first visit. After the physician completes the initial report, type an original and four copies of the claim. These will be distributed as follows:

- The original and one copy to the insurance carrier
- One copy to the employer
- One copy to the state compensation board
- One copy retained for the physician's files

If only one visit is required, prepare a statement immediately and submit it with the Doctor's First Report. If several visits are involved, which will be indicted on your initial report, send your routine office statement for subsequent visits. If the visits are beyond the original estimate or complications develop, submit a Doctor's Monthly (or final) Report and a bill. In any case all bills must be sent directly to the employer, if self-insured, or to the insurance carrier. Patients must never be billed for any services for care in a work-related case.

Controlling Utilization
Monitoring Quality of Care

The rapidly growing variety of available health care services and the number of providers have caused concern among many groups regarding the quality of health care being given. These groups include patient advocates, providers (peers), and the federal government. They are seeking methods of monitoring the care patients receive and the need for ancillary services based on the premise that each individual has the right to the best care possible.

Cost Containment

Hand in hand with the need for quality control is the growing concern over the costs of medical care. The availability of insurance and facilities has sometimes resulted in the overuse or improper use of health care services. In 1972 the federal government took the initiative to control the costs of medical care, since a large portion of those costs was paid for through government programs. The Social Security Act was amended to allow the formation of professional standards review organizations (PSROs) to monitor both the quality and cost of health care services provided with government funds. Other payers have since become equally interested in controlling the cost of health care.

PERSPECTIVES ON MEDICAL ASSISTING

What Are the Differences?

1. Blue Cross/Blue Shield—Oldest indemnity plans. They are mainly non-profit community service organizations, although some have converted to for-profit status. There are different types of plans, including HMOs, in some localities. They assist federal and state governments in the administration of Medicare and Medicaid.

2. CHAMPUS—Civilian Health and Medical Program of the Uniformed Services. It uses the Defense Enrollment Eligibility Reporting System (DEERS), which is a worldwide database of the people covered. CHAMPUS is divided into three parts: TriCare Standard, which is no cost and provides basic care; TriCare Prime, which is the HMO with an annual fee; and TriCare Extra, which is a PPO (a provider network from which patients can choose physicians and pay a reduced fee).

3. Medicaid—A plan sponsored by federal, state, and local governments. Eligibility varies from state to state, but it generally is designed for low-income families, persons who are blind or have disabilities, and members of families with dependent children. Coverage originally was through offices or clinics but now HMO coverage has been added in some areas.

4. Medicare—Originally created under an amendment of the Social Security Act, people 65 years of age or older are eligible if they have paid into the system. Part A is for hospitalization and is provided automatically; Part B is for physician and other services for which coverage the patient pays a monthly charge or a yearly deductible. Medicare also covers people who are blind or have disabilities regardless of age. A person may be covered under a parent's Social Security number.

5. Workers' Compensation—Coverage required by law for the worker for on-the-job injury or illness. It is paid by the employer, and rehabilitation of the patient is the goal.

6. Commercial carriers—These are private companies that enroll patients for premiums. Many plans are available. Examples of carriers are Aetna and Travelers.

7. HMOs—Health maintenance organizations. These are prepaid medical services and are either a closed panel HMO, which has its own facilities complete with physicians and services, or an open panel HMO, which contracts with physicians on a fixed-fee basis. Patients may choose their physician from a list, and they usually are charged a copayment for routine office visits and medications purchased from the pharmacy.

Involvement in Utilization Review

Government Insurance Programs

Through the PSROs the government has established certain mechanisms to control costs under the common term *utilization review (UR)*. The purpose of UR is to ensure and document that care is necessary and is provided at the appropriate level. The UR activities with which you will come into contact involve prior authorization for elective hospitalization and concurrent review during hospitalization.

WHAT DO YOU THINK?

Medical costs have been steadily rising for the past 20 to 25 years. Advances in treatments and technology are costly. The money to pay for them must come from somewhere or someone—usually the patient. Different methods to cut or control costs are being used. The Peer Review Organization (PRO) uses a group of physicians to monitor hospital admissions, treatment expenses, and even check the medical records of hospitals for compliance in cost effectiveness.

Diagnostic-related groups (DRGs) is a method that classifies patients according to their primary diagnosis rather than the length of stay. It was developed to monitor quality of care and utilization of services in the hospital. Fixed payments to the hospital are based on DRGs for Medicare payment.

What suggestions could you make to improve this situation? Is managed care the solution for all patients? Is our quality of care as good or better than it was 5 years ago? How should technology be limited to cut our expenses, or should it be limited at all?

Prior Authorization

When a patient is to be admitted to a hospital for elective (nonemergency) medical or surgical care, permission must be obtained in advance. A review coordinator or physician associated with the PSRO will, based on the information provided, determine the necessity of hospitalization. If the services can be safely provided in an outpatient setting, the request for hospitalization will be denied. Outpatient services cost much less than inpatient care and therefore are encouraged (Figure 14.11).

Concurrent Review

Concurrent review is a method of monitoring patients who have been admitted to the hospital for care. Their charts are reviewed on admission and every few days thereafter to determine if they need to stay in an acute-care hospital or if their care can be continued at a nursing facility or at home.

HMOs/Primary Care

UR is built into the HMO concept from the perspective of centralized control. Many HMOs conduct patient care through a concentration of primary care. Each patient selects or is assigned a primary care physician who manages the patient's needs and refers patients to specialists or for hospitalization as needed. This helps monitor activity, and since other services may not be paid without primary physician referral, avoids unnecessary services or self-referral by the patient to specialists.

Emphasis of Care

Care through HMOs stresses health maintenance and preventive care. It is based on the principle that patients should seek care before problems begin or before they require major care. Through early intervention, care can be provided at a reduced cost and on an outpatient basis rather than at costly, inpatient hospital rates.

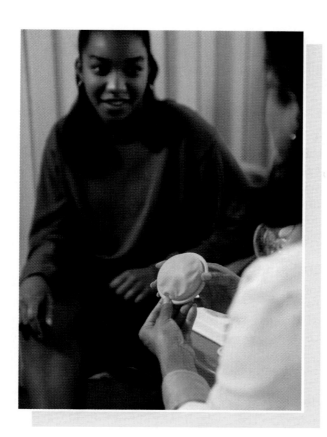

FIGURE 14.11

Outpatient services cost much less than inpatient care and therefore are encouraged.

Other Insurance Companies/Employer's Request

Because employers pay a majority portion of the health premiums for their employees, they are now requesting stricter guidelines by the carriers. Insurance premiums are steadily rising because of increased utilization of service. In other words, patients request and use more sophisticated services than may be considered necessary for appropriate, effective care. In an effort to curb health care costs, employers are encouraging insurance carriers to assist in cost containment. Many times this results in carriers requesting that certain types of services be reviewed by a utilization review organization prior to authorization being given to proceed with the planned treatment. Some insurance carriers are trying to educate patients regarding proper utilization by putting an emphasis on primary care physicians to direct patient care, including all referrals to specialists, and monitoring hospitalization to minimize the length of stay.

Second Opinion for Elective Surgery

Some insurance companies are requiring a second opinion when elective surgery is recommended. In these cases the patient must be seen by another surgeon, who is selected by the insurance company. If the second surgeon concurs with the original recommendation, then the surgery may be performed by the original surgeon. If the surgeons disagree, then the insurance company may choose not to pay for the procedure or may request a third opinion. The insurance company will pay the entire fee for the second opinion. The second-opinion physician is strictly an independent consultant and may not accept the patient for treatment, even if the patient prefers him or her.

The Medical Assistant's Role in Utilization Review

Your role in UR is to know the restrictions. The government and private insurance restrictions for cost containment will vary from one area to another. Learn the rules and regulations that apply in your area, and be alert to the changes that take place. Government agencies and insurance companies usually will mail announcements to each physician's office regarding program changes. Arrange a system with your employer to ensure that these announcements are shared with all employees.

Necessary Permissions

If advance permission is needed for certain referrals or hospitalizations, you will be responsible for filing the proper forms and notifying the appropriate agencies or facilities. Being aware of the necessary advance steps and following established procedure will make the process simple and reduce the stress on you and on patients. These rules need not interfere with other responsibilities if you have planned an efficient procedure.

Hospital Reviewers

On occasion you may receive a telephone call from the hospital UR coordinator. He or she will need to speak with the physician for information regarding a hospitalized patient. The coordinator works with the physician to see that the patient does not stay in the hospital any longer than is medically necessary. If the patient needs convalescent care, the hospital discharge planner will locate the appropriate facility and notify the physician of the planned transfer. These services provided by hospital personnel relieve you of duties that in the past often were performed by medical assistants working with the patient's family members.

Filing Claim Forms

In some instances claim forms for Medicaid may be supplied by the intermediary; however, it is easier and faster to order claim forms through local supply houses, PMIC, or Med-Index. The majority of all carriers now have authorized the HCFA-1500 1990 version. The HCFA has required that carriers try to standardize the claim forms and code numbers. Some private companies insist that their own form be used; some providers believe that this is a delay tactic to hold up paying the claim. It is best to enlist the patient's or subscriber's assistance in calling the carrier. When you are forced to file claims to independent insurance carriers using their forms, you will find that the variation in the forms will require more of your time. Most are not adaptable to the computer.

Conclusion

The subject of insurance is extensive and evolutionary. The types of insurance coverage and cost-containment requirements will influence the methods you use to remain knowledgeable about the subject so that effective and efficient insurance processing procedures can be maintained. Continued monitoring of office policy and procedures will ensure the least disruption of reimbursement for services and the efficient control of policies required to protect the medical practice.

Review QUESTIONS

1. Describe in your own words how you would explain to patients their responsibilities regarding their health insurance.

2. Explain three of the several types of health coverage available.

3. How would you explain to a patient the difference between assignment of benefits by the patient and acceptance of assignment by the physician?

4. What is the difference between Medicare and Medicaid?

5. What is the difference between CHAMPUS and CHAMPVA?

6. Who is eligible for Workers' Compensation?

7. Describe Medicare's role as a secondary payer.

8. Describe how the need for adequate documentation affects utilization review.

9. Describe in logical sequence an efficient method for processing insurance claims for patients.

10. What will patients need to file their own insurance claims?

11. What types of insurance policies are needed to protect the medical practice?

12. What are your responsibilities with regard to office policies?

SUGGESTED READINGS

American Medical Association: *Current procedural terminology,* ed 4, Chicago, 1996, The Association.
International classification of diseases, ninth revision, clinical modification (ICD9-CM), Pittsburgh, 1996.
Medicare Part B. Produced monthly by United Communications, Bethesda, Md.

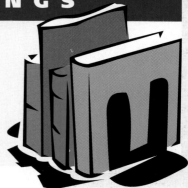

Managed Care

On completion of Chapter 15 the administrative medical assistant student should be able to:

1. Define the key terms listed in this chapter.

2. Describe the types of managed care plans.

3. List basic skills for evaluating managed care plans.

4. List areas of service and education the plans should provide to the physician provider.

5. Describe expected changes in the managed care programs.

6. Describe the amount of administrative support needed for the physician office.

K E Y   T E R M S

Balance billing   A process in which the physician office is required to bill the patient for the difference between the original physician charge and the amount the physician has received from the third-party payer (the insurance plan).

Capitation   A method of payment for health care services in which the physician accepts a prearranged fixed payment per patient per month in exchange for health care services to be provided.

CMP   Competive medical plans.

Copay   The amount of payment that the insured or member pays directly to the physician office at the time of services rendered.

Eligibility   Patient status with the carrier to receive health care services as covered benefits.

EPO   Exclusive provider organization.

HMO   Health maintenance organization.

IPA   Independent Physicians Association.

Medically necessary   Covered services that are required to maintain the health status of a member or eligible person in compliance with area standards of medical practice.

PHO   Physician hospital organization.

POS   Point of service.

PPA   Preferred provider arrangements.

PPO   Preferred provider organization.

Continued

KEY TERMS

(Continued)

Primary care physician   A physician (normally a family practitioner, pediatrician, internist, general practitioner, and sometimes an obstetrician/gynecologist) who typically provides primary care services for all body systems.

Prior authorization   A method of controlling utilization by the carrier to evaluate the need and provide approval for health care services before the service is rendered.

Utilization review   Medical review of information regarding the patient, usually conducted by trained or professional personnel to assess the appropriateness, quality of, and need for services provided to the patient.

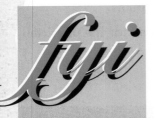

What's the Difference? Traditional vs. Managed Care

Traditional care is what most people have received over the years and find difficult to change from. Patients had a physician whom they would see as needed with minimal expense and insurance paying its part. Insurance premiums were paid by the employer in most cases. The method of payment was known as *fee-for-service*.

Managed care is a general term covering several types of organizations (for example, HMOs and PPOs). This type of health care developed in response to spiraling medical costs that resulted because of patient demand for attention, technological advances, longer life expectancies, and higher malpractice expenses resulting from an increase in the number of lawsuits. It developed as a way to give adequate medical care and yet control the cost of that care. Care is controlled by using a primary care physician (PCP), who is responsible for the patient and any referrals, tests, or prescriptions needed.

Vast changes have occurred within the health care delivery system over the past 25 years, including a shift to a managed care system of delivery in recent years. Administrative medical assistants need to be aware of the changes within the scope of medical services provided in their place of employment. The administrative medical assistant also must be knowledgeable regarding local plans in order to provide the physician with information about the plans and to help the physician judge whether membership in the plan is appropriate for his or her practice.

Background of Managed Care

In 1972, when a prominent multispecialty medical group first contemplated pursuing the health maintenance organization (HMO) business, the managed care market share in its community stood at zero. At that time the group included one part-time true primary care physician, as well as six or seven internists and pediatricians whose practices involved both primary and subspecialty care. All of the other members of its almost 70-physician staff were subspecialists. Twenty years later, when the local managed care market share had increased to 40 percent, more than half of the group's patients were participants. The staff had grown from about 70 physicians to more than 200; however, the shift was significantly to primary care physicians. This was just the beginning of significant changes in health care delivery.

Because the cost to provide medical care was rising rapidly, a federal law was enacted in 1973 to bring about extended changes in health care delivery. Congress enacted Public Law 93-222, the Health Maintenance Organization Act of 1973, which sought to shorten hospital stays. That goal has been achieved. The changes brought about by these legislative acts have been tracked very carefully. Although most changes have taken place within the hospital setting, one can expect outpatient services or ambulatory care to be challenged in the late 1990s (Figure 15.1). In this regard the administrative medical assistant

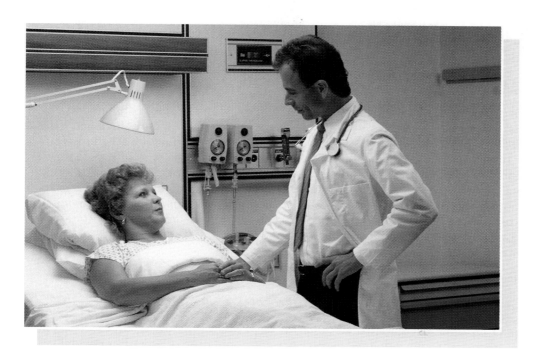

FIGURE 15.1

The HMO Act reduced the length of hospital stays.

will have to be aware of the changes within the scope of medical services provided at their place of employment. The medical administrative assistant also must be knowledgeable regarding local plans in order to provide the physician with information about them and allow the physician to judge competently whether membership with the plan is appropriate for their practice.

In all reality it is society's demand for better value and greater access that is determining the shape of the health care industry in general and the managed care component in particular. There are no simple solutions to these social and economic issues, nor is managed care the only approach that has merit.

Understanding the Types of Plans

Before assisting the physician or practice in evaluating plans, the administrative medical assistant must understand the many types of plans available.

Capitation

Under the capitation system, a fixed amount of payment per eligible beneficiary in a specific geographical region is determined. The amount paid is a prospective per eligible beneficiary amount regardless of weather the beneficiary uses the services. Capitation works best with large enrollee populations. The plan may set a capitation rate and then recruit physicians or providers to serve the specified area. Providers also may be selected first and then the capi-

AT WORK TODAY

Managed Care—the New System

Although "managed care" began in the early 1970s, it did not become an official player in the health care game until the mid-1980s. The concept advanced significantly in the 1990s, and millions of people now receive health care in this way.

The idea of managed care came about when it became increasingly important that patients obtain needed services in a more cost-effective setting to control skyrocketing health care costs. New organizations have formed under managed care that offer services through joint venture agreements or through a single source. The new managed care organizations work toward quality patient care but also must be involved in some type of cost containment such as a second opinion before surgery or preauthorization for nonemergency procedures. In this setting, you will hear some new terminology—gatekeepers, participating provider, and capitation to name a few.

tation rate is negotiated secondarily. Capitation provides a consistent revenue stream, through a defined captive patient population. Capitation normally will require less paperwork than the fee-for-service process. Capitation usually has a copayment that must be collected at the time service is provided.

Competitive Medical Plans (CMPs)

Competitive medical plans (CMPs) are a type of managed care organization that was created by the 1982 TEFRA legislation to facilitate the enrollment of Medicare beneficiaries into managed care plans. Most CMPs are organized and have a financial base much like the HMOs but are not bound by as many of the regulatory requirements of the HMOs. While in the early stages of organization, these plans maintained a much slower growth pattern. As the federal government has continued to pursue more successful means of controlling the cost and quality of health care services provided to elderly people, it is very evident that the managed care industry has and will become more aggressive in the enrollment of Medicare beneficiaries. Many times elderly patients have attended what was to be an informational meeting regarding the plan, and have found themselves enrolled in it. You will need to check the patients' eligibility with Medicare every time they are seen in your office. You will soon recognize some of the names of the plans, for example, Secure Horizons, Senior Security Plan, and MediPrime.

Exclusive Provider Organizations (EPOs)

Exclusive provider organizations (EPOs) are very similar to PPOs in their organizational style and purpose. However, EPOs are allowed to limit their beneficiaries to participating providers for their health care services. In this case the beneficiaries covered by an EPO are required to receive all of the covered services from providers that participate in the EPO (similar to many Blue Cross and Blue Shield plans). The EPO usually will not cover or pay for services received from providers who are not members of the EPO. Most EPOs utilize a PCP or "gatekeeper" approach to authorize any nonprimary health care services. These plans will require that an administrative medical assistant and the physician educate patients as to the services available to them.

Health Maintenance Organizations (HMOs)

Health maintenance organizations (HMOs) are responsible for both financing and providing a previously agreed upon set of comprehensive health maintenance and treatment services to a specifically defined and voluntarily enrolled population for a prepaid, fixed sum. The HMO serves as both the insurer and provider (or arranger) of health care services. As opposed to traditional indemnity health insurance, which simply reimburses the covered individual or provider of service, the close relationship between insuring and providing health care services requires HMOs and their providers to carefully monitor and manage both the quantity and quality of care.

Independent Physicians Associations (IPAs)

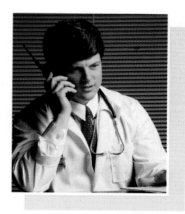

An independent physicians association (IPA) is a health maintenance type organization in which the HMO contracts with a physician association or organization, which in turn contracts with individual physicians. The IPA physicians practice in their own offices and continue to see other fee-for-service patients. The HMO usually reimburses the IPA on a capitated basis; however, the IPA normally will reimburse the physicians on a fee-for-service basis. This type of coverage combines prepayment with the traditional means of delivering health care services. Most of these plans require a copayment and a deductible from the patient.

Physician Hospital Organizations (PHOs)

In a physician hospital organization (PHOs) a hospital and a physician organization form a joint venture structure to create a health care delivery system that can contract with other types of plans, insurance companies, or directly with employers. However, PHOs remain primarily delivery systems, rather than insurance programs.

Point of Service Plans (POSs)

Point of service plans (POSs) are one of the fastest growing managed care plans today. The POS plan combines some of the features of an HMO with the provider selection flexibility of a PPO. Although there are many plan variations, in most cases members select a primary care physician who manages the patient's care. However, this type of plan allows members to seek care from outside the POS network and have less coverage. Most HMOs are introducing POS products as a means of attracting a greater market share than they can with the traditional "locked-in" (to HMO providers) type of care.

WHAT DO YOU THINK?

Match the Abbreviations with Their Information

1. CMP _c_
2. EPO _d_
3. HMO _a_
4. IPA _b_
5. POS _f_
6. PPO _e_

a. An organization that is both an insurer and provider of health care

b. An HMO that contracts with a physician group, which in turn contracts with individual physicians

c. Managed care organization created to assist in the enrollment of Medicare beneficiaries. Secure Horizons is an example of this type of organization.

d. Similar to a PPO but limit their beneficiaries to participating providers for health care

e. Organizations represent arrangements between groups of physicians, hospitals, and other providers and a health insurance carrier, third-party payer, or a self-insured employer to provide medical services for a specified patient group

f. Members select a primary care physician to manage their care. Members may seek care outside the network but less coverage

Preferred Provider Arrangements (PPAs)

Preferred provider arrangements (PPAs) involve contractual arrangements very similar to PPOs, except that the contracts are arranged without the establishment of a separate organization to act as the contracting agent. With PPAs an insurance carrier contracts directly with individual physicians and other providers. This type of arrangement or structure has not become as popular as the HMOs and PPOs.

Preferred Provider Organizations (PPOs)

Preferred provider organizations (PPOs) represent arrangements between groups of physicians, hospitals, and other providers, and either a health insurance carrier, a third-party payer, or a self-insured employer. These preferred providers, as those selected providers are known, enter into a contract with the PPO, which can be an insurance company, a Blue Cross/Blue Shield plan, a third-party administrator, a large employer, an HMO, or an organization of physicians that has been created specifically for this purpose. Under the contract the providers agree to abide by certain rules, regulations, and procedures, such as utilization review, preauthorizations or precertifications, and certain reimbursement agreements, in exchange for an anticipated increased volume of patients. These groups normally provide beneficiaries with financial incentives, such as lower copayments and deductibles, and request that they seek care through the preferred providers. In most instances these beneficiaries may seek care from either a preferred provider or a provider of their choice, if they are willing to pay the extra cost.

Evaluating the Managed Care Plans

Before the physician or group signs a provider contract, the knowledgeable administrative medical assistant can provide the physician(s) with information to make an intelligent decision regarding whether the plan is appropriate or will be an asset to the practice. To do this, both the physicians and the administrative medical assistant should have in place a checklist of information, such as the list that follows, required from and about the plan.

1. Who owns the plan? (Do physicians provide a strong representation on the board?)

2. Is the plan operating at a profit? (You may ask for a financial statement.)

3. How long has this plan been in operation?

4. What is the current number of enrollees or potential patient base?

5. Are there withholds (an amount held by the plan for future administrative cost over-runs)? If so, what is the average amount, and has the plan ever returned them?

6. Request a list of the participating physicians and hospitals.

7. Are other physicians of your specialty providers for the plan?

8. Are the physicians that cover for your physicians members of the plan?

9. Request a list of employers who offer the plan. Many times it is to the physician's advantage to know which employers of the community are offering the plan.

10. What is the duration of the contract? (It usually is 1 year.)

11. Must you pay a fee to join? Is that a one-time or yearly fee?

12. Must each physician pay a fee or is there a flat fee for the whole group?

13. If a group practice, is every member required to join?

14. What is the reimbursement structure to the physician office? Is it a discounted fee-for-service, based on usual, customary, and reasonable (UCR)? Resource-Based Relative Value Study (RBRVS)? Capitation? If the plan sets its own UCR rate, then you should request a copy of the rate, as it may be well below the community standards, and drastically lower than your current fee.

15. Request and review the reimbursement schedule for at least 25 of the most frequent services by CPT code that are rendered in your practice.

16. Request a list of services that require prior authorization.

17. Is there a capitation component to the plan?

18. Is there a copayment or deductible? What are the billing requirements if the beneficiary does not pay at the time of service? Physicians should be allowed to bill patients for copayments, noncovered services, and those services not deemed medically necessary, where the patient agrees in advance to make such payment.

19. Is there a requirement that if he beneficiary or patient does not pay the copayment at time of service, the plan is not required to pay for the services rendered? Plans frequently mail questionnaires to beneficiaries asking

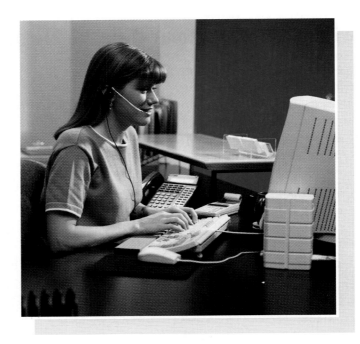

FIGURE 15.2

In evaluating a managed
care plan, ask whether the
plan accepts electronically
submitted claims.

whether they were treated with courtesy and in a timely manner, whether
they liked the physician and staff, and whether they paid their copayment
at time of service. Plans then use the information to inform of nonpayment for services rendered, citing a clause in the contract that stipulates
that the copayment must be collected at the time services were provided.

20. Request a copy of the explanation of benefits (EOB). If the EOB includes
    nothing more than the patient's name, date of service, and amount paid,
    then tracking adjustments and receivables becomes almost impossible.
    The EOB should show this information, as well as the amount billed,
    amount allowed, any withholds, deductibles, or copayments.

21. What is the turnaround time for reimbursement of claims? An average
    turnaround time of 45 or more days indicates a poorly run plan. Federal
    law requires that third-party payers (other than HMOs or prepaid plans)
    must pay providers for "clean," or undisputed, claims within 30 days of
    receipt. Anything over 45 days must bear interest of 10 percent per year. Is
    there a clause in the contract in which the physician waives this statutory
    right by contractual agreement?

22. Does the plan accept electronically submitted claims, and are their criteria
    based on the standard ANSI requirements (Figure 15.2).

23. Does the plan provide a training program for the physician's office staff?
    The better plans provide team training with a very complete manual.

Physicians will have many additional questions regarding covered services,
noncovered services, emergencies, medical necessity, out-of-area care, group
coverage, and utilization review. The contracts have become very complicated,
and the physician may choose to have a contracting firm review all of the contracts that are provided. However, if the questions just listed are answered to

the physician's satisfaction, the administrative medical assistant will have saved valuable time for the physician(s) and the contracting entity. Many of the IPAs and PPOs now provide this service to preassess all contracts from carriers, self-insured employers, and employer groups.

Managed Care Contracts

Because managed care now accounts for a significant number of patients (approximately 70% in certain areas) in the physician practice, the contractual terms of managed care plans become increasingly important to the physician practice. These contracts affect payment, office organization, procedures, and clinical decision making. Contractual terms of plans that are particularly significant to a medical practice can affect the degree of success of the physicians involved. Solo practitioners may choose to only participate through their local IPA or PPO, rather than individually. However, each contract from any of the sources just mentioned will have some basic components and requirements.

The administrative medical assistant should highlight each area for the physician to review before sending the contract to the attorney or consultant. If all questions have been satisfactorily answered, there will be additional questions regarding financial, clinical, legal, and operational issues; responsibilities of the physician; relationship with the contracting agency, physician's rights in dispute resolution; provisions for termination by either party; and others.

Basic Components of the Contract

Contract Terms

The contract is valid for a set period (usually 1 year). Check whether the contract renews automatically unless one party gives notice of a desire to terminate or does it terminate with renegotiation required? Contracts usually stipulate that the plan may transfer the contract and the physician may not, or that neither party may transfer the contract without the consent of the other. It is better when the contract specifically states that neither party may transfer or assign the contract without the written consent of the other. Words to watch for are: "Plan may assign."

Physician Responsibilities

The contract should indicate the basic responsibilities of the physician, including covered services, accessibility, and primary care gatekeeping. The contract should clearly indicate whether primary care or specialist services are involved. If primary care is specified, does the contract require the physician to meet availability requirements such as specific office hour and telephone availability and emergency services? The contract may require the physician to accept all patients assigned. As a gatekeeper the physician must preauthorize or deny either specialty or elective care. The contract may indicate that the physician must manage, monitor, and coordinate all care of assigned patients, including other physicians and ancillary care.

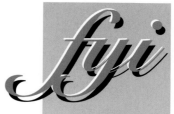

Contracts

In traditional patient care the "contract" often in force was verbal or just assumed by the actions of the patient and physician. Care often was basic and so were the expectations of the patient. Modern medical practice is not only more sophisticated but much more at risk from the threat of lawsuits.

The term *contract* means a written or spoken agreement between two or more parties that is intended to be enforced. It also can be called a deal, understanding, arrangement, or pact.

Managed care is set up with contracts, and the physician will need to understand what is required and what type of contract he or she is entering into. If the physician does not understand the contract, he or she should consult with his or her attorney for interpretation.

General Clauses

General clauses should be included regarding coverage, duration of contract and termination, liability and indemnification, and boilerplate provisions including notice, severability, and assignment. The contract should show which type of entity is involved (for example, HMO, PPO). All parties should be clearly identified so that there is no confusion over the respective roles and responsibilities of additional parties whose involvement is implied (for example, as in an IPA model in which the contract may be with an IPA that then contracts with an HMO). It is important that all parties are stipulated in the contract.

The contract should indicate which services are covered as basic benefits and which are clearly excluded or might be considered not medically necessary.

The contract should have some specific language as to whether it requires the physician to hold the managed care organization harmless and indemnify the organization for claims or liabilities made against it for the failures of the physician, such as malpractice or other types of negligence. Or the contract may specify that the contracting managed care organization agrees to indemnify and hold the physician harmless for its own failures, including negligent utilization standards and negligent selection of other providers. Boilerplate contracts must be reviewed very carefully, and it is best to leave it to an expert, although the basics may well be covered. The contract should indicate that it will provide the physician with notice of changes in procedures in advance of their effective date by the managed care organization.

All contracts should specify the initial qualifications required of the physician, for example, licensure, Drug Enforcement Agency (DEA) registration, board certification(s), hospital staff privileges, malpractice insurance at specific levels, geographical location of the office, professional references, work history, malpractice claims experience, sanction experience, and occasionally, a photograph.

Utilization Management Issues

If the contract does not specify the required standard of care, the law requires the physician to provide reasonable care in accordance with what other similarly situated physicians would provide.

The contract should specify quality assurance requirements and performance standards or protocols. Further, it should specify utilization management issues, and describe what techniques are used (for example, prior authorization, concurrent review, case management, or gatekeeping). The contract should indicate the requirements regarding clinical practice guidelines, protocols, pathways, parameters, or other statements that affect approved utilization.

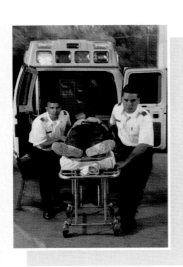

Financial Matters

The contract should specify financial matters. For instance, what is the compensation method (UCR, fee schedule, capitation rate)? How is the physician placed "at risk" if at all (withhold, risk/incentive pool, or capitation alone)? How are emergency services paid? Is there a stop loss or reinsurance against high-cost patients? May the physician collect for copayments, coinsurance, or deductibles from the patients? Is there a specified time within which the physician office must submit claims? Does the contract specify the managed care organization to pay claims within a specified timeframe? What happens to payments owed to the physician if the contract terminates?

Operational Requirements

The contract should specify operational requirements such as audits of the physician practice regarding quality performance, member grievances, provider grievances, economic performance, or utilization behavior. The contract should specify the recordkeeping requirements with regard to medical records, consents, referral forms, and completion of claim forms for other carriers for coordination of benefits.

The contract should specify the allowance by the managed care organization for the physician to affiliate with other HMOs, PPOs, or groups.

Before the physician signs the contract, the administrative medical assistant at the direction of the physician should arrange to have the contract reviewed by an expert (for example, attorney, certified public accountant) to see that all is within the specified guidelines of a good and fair contract for both parties.

Working with Capitation

In the past most physicians and staff viewed managed care as a necessary evil. Today, attitudes are changing. Some offices, particularly in largely rural areas (for example, Montana or Wyoming) may never participate in managed care, either because the physicians may retire before it is imperative to do so, or because the physicians believe they can carve out a market of their own. However, the likelihood of most physicians practicing in managed care will be very significant, and for a number of them managed care will constitute a major portion of their practice. To date, capitation has been applied almost exclusively to primary care physicians, multispecialty group practices, fully integrated health care systems, and certain services such as mental health, prescription drugs, and laboratory services. Because capitation requires relating a specific panel of patients to a specific physician, subspecialists (with a few exceptions) are still most commonly paid based on some variation of the fee-for-service method. However, in California, Arizona, Florida, and Virginia, managed care programs are experimenting with capitation in a significant number of subspecialties, for example, gastroenterology, orthopedics, ophthalmology, and mental health. Capitation is a method of payment under which providers are reimbursed at a fixed amount per member per month, in other words, per capita. As such, it represents a significant shift in the basic economics of medical practice in which the focus changes from how much the physician will be paid, as is the case in fee-for-service care, to how much it will cost the physician to provide the services specified in the capitation agreement. Physicians generally have responded very negatively to capitation, because early capitation programs caused undue risk and economic hardship to the practice.

The physician office risk under capitation can, and should be evaluated, managed, and limited both to the physician and the capitation program. The medical assistant will have to work with the appointment system to schedule patients appropriately. The physician and clinical staff will have to be very careful in the use of time, given that it is an extremely limited and valuable commodity. It also is important to be careful of capitation contracts that place the physician at risk for services provided outside the office, unless those services are included as part of the overall capitation program incentive system, which spreads part of this risk among other participating physicians. Where capitation is used to reimburse a multispecialty group practice or integrated heath service, the scope of services for which the group is at risk increases substantially.

It also is essential to understand exactly what services are included in a capitation rate, regardless of whether the capitation applies only to services provided by the individual physician or is more broadly based. Additional risk is not necessarily undesirable, however, depending on how the risk is structured and whether the physician and staff have a reasonable opportunity to manage that risk. Do not accept risks the practice cannot afford.

It needs to be understood that Capitation rates can be structured in ways that will make capitation extremely attractive to the practice. Many capitation arrangements allow a more favorable economic outcome than payment on a fee-for-service basis.

Learn how to evaluate a capitation rate, and if possible, equate it to fee-for-service revenue. For example, if the practice has 2000 capitation patients and if the capitation reimbursement is $8 per patient per month, the result would be a gross of $192,000 per year. Although this does not take into consideration patient mix, it at least provides some basis against which a capitation rate can be measured. Before the physician signs the contract request, the capitation rates based on age and sex for each member should be provided by the managed care organization.

Read the contract and highlight what specific services are included in the capitation rate, the anticipated frequency in terms of units of service per member per month, and the estimated unit cost for each of those services. These are basic calculations that the managed care organization should already have developed, and which it should be willing to share so that the practice can evaluate the adequacy of the capitation rate. It is impossible to evaluate the adequacy of a capitation rate until both the services to be included and the population to be served have been precisely identified. Be very careful when evaluating contracts that indicate low-frequency patient contract with high-cost services. This type of contract can end up costing the practice money rather than generating additional income.

Talk with other practices that have experience with the managed care organization you are evaluating. They should be able to provide you with information regarding physician support, reimbursement timeframes, and other operational issues.

It is becoming increasingly common for managed care organizations to add a factor for case management for primary care physicians in addition to the basic services included in the capitation rate. This is a set rate per enrolled patient per month. As the value of the patient case manager's cognitive skills increases, it is likely that this line item with the capitation rate, or the unit cost projections contained in the capitation rate, or both, will increase, thus covering the salary increases for the case manager.

The broader the scope of services available in the practice, the broader the capitation, because more services (for example, laboratory, x-ray, and mammograms, as well as primary care) can be managed by the practice (Figure 15.3). Age and sex variations in capitation rates also must be taken into consideration because of the predictably higher use rates of certain members of the panel base.

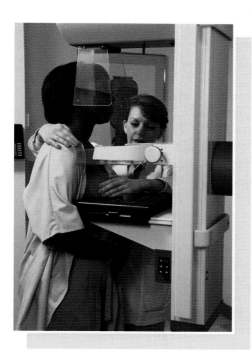

FIGURE 15.3

The broader the scope of services in the practice, such as laboratory work, x-ray, and mammography, the broader the capitation.

Always request information about how members are enrolled. Normally you will receive a list of plan members who have enrolled with the practice as soon as your physician is a provider for the plan. The frequency with which this list is updated will depend on the plan and is something you will want to have your physician or the attorney clarify during negotiations. For large-volume practices, many capitation plans are beginning to provide on-line terminal access to the capitation database. Of course, the more often you receive the information or can access the database, the less administrative time will be spent checking the member status of new patients who are not yet on the list (retroactive list) and billing patients who are no longer members but who remain on the list. The procedure for contacting the plan to verify enrollment and the terms of the contract regarding retroactive terminations are areas that should be included in the contract negotiation. Enrollment should be verified at the time the appointment is scheduled. The procedure for verification will be similar to what the practice already requires for insurance verification; however, an emphasis should be placed on copayments and coordination of benefits.

The future is likely to see the development of more capitation-like reimbursement systems as the managed care industry becomes more sophisticated in developing equitable capitation rates and in providing capitated physicians with the management tools through which they can succeed in this kind of reimbursement program. The practice should make every effort to know and understand the programs with which they are involved.

Improving Practice Productivity

The administrative medical assistant will need to learn every aspect of assisting the physician in controlling the costs of patient care while providing quality service to the patient. The use of paraprofessionals and medical assistants will provide additional staff and services to the patients without cutting the quality of care. The use of physician assistants to take medical histories, perform basic physical examinations, make and record the assessment, and present it to the physician also will contain costs. Physician assistants may also help with routine screening and tests including, but not limited to, drawing blood; performing catheterization and routine urinalysis; giving pelvic examinations (including Pap smears); giving injections and immunizations; debridement and care of superficial wounds; strapping, casting, and splinting of sprains; and incision and drainage of superficial skin infections. They may recognize and evaluate situations that call for the immediate attention of the primary care physician, or as necessary, institute emergency treatment procedures essential for the life of the patient. Physician assistants and clinical medical assistants may help instruct and counsel patients regarding physical health, diets, social habits, family planning, growth and development, and the aging process. These assistants may also help physicians arrange hospital admissions, provide continuing care services, review treatment and therapy plans, evaluate patients, and perform procedures and tasks as specified by the physician.

Costs may be trimmed by expanding clinic hours to include weekends, thereby reducing emergency room care, which is always more expensive in time and effort.

The practice should work to avoid duplication of ancillary services when tests are performed in the clinic or on an outpatient basis and then repeated in the hospital on an inpatient basis.

The staff and physician(s) should review the scheduling practices for higher productivity. They also should remember to offer and schedule appointments for patients who need to be reminded for monthly, bi-yearly, and yearly examinations. The computer system that provides a flexible recall standard is extremely useful in this case. Other practices find it particularly helpful when patients fill out the recall notices in their own handwriting; these then are kept on file until the appropriate mailing time arrives.

Many short appointments will require more examination rooms, thus they should be worked in with the long and medium-level appointments. It is helpful if a consultation room is located close to the examination rooms, because that helps free the examination rooms for the next patient. The staff should take data and supplies to the physician (although supplies should be stocked each evening); this keeps the physician in the examination area treating patients, providing a more economical system. Work with the system to keep patients flowing in and out of the examination rooms, x-ray, and laboratory without undue delay.

The Administrative Medical Assistant's Role in Managed Care

Managed care is expected to become a significant aspect of medical practice, and the well trained, interested, and knowledgeable administrative medical assistant will play an enormous role in carrying out all the responsibilities this will entail. The practice may require a managed care staff with clearly differentiated responsibilities or perhaps one individual will carry out all responsibilities. This will depend entirely on the size of the practice, the patient volume, and the sophistication of the contracts or market the practice serves.

Accepting the risk of providing care for a particular group of patients through managed care puts the practice in the position of running a mini-insurance company in addition to practicing medicine. The capitation payment the practice accepts every month is analogous to the premium a health insurance plan would receive. In return for the payment, the physician ensures that the patient will receive the services covered under the insurance contract as required by the enrollee. Of course, there are some internal administrative requirements for accepting capitation that are similar to those you would find in a health plan or insurance carrier rather than the physician's office. These requirements may include reconciliation of payments, claims processing, and financial reporting.

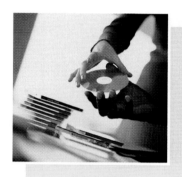

Administrative medical assistants most likely will require a computer system equipped with a managed care or capitation software program. They will need to be able to track the number of times a patient is seen per year and in what setting (for example, hospital, outpatient, skilled nursing). They will need to track the number of times the patient did not make a copayment, or pay for deductibles for services that are either noncovered or considered medically unnecessary, so that they might bill the patient for these items.

Capitation payments usually come at the same time monthly as the enrollment list. An administrative medical assistant should be assigned to reconcile the capitation with the number of enrollees. The number of patients for whom the practice provides services, but who are not yet on the enrollee list, should be tracked so that retroactive payment may be requested (additional capitation payments for that member may or may not be included in the next check). The practice should receive capitation from the time the member enrolled with the plan or selected your physician as their primary care provider. If the plan's procedures for primary care physician assignment are weak, be sure to include a requirement in the contract for payment to your group for a share of the "unassigned" patients. These patients are a source of profitability for both the plan and the practice, and the plan may keep payments for these patients unless so stipulated in the contract.

Depending on the services covered under the capitation, you may be required to pay claims submitted by other providers. This requires having staff trained to perform this function. If you will be receiving many claims, this function also will require claims processing information system capabilities. The staff assigned to this area will need to have a complete understanding of the services and terms of coverage to pay claims properly. They also will need to be able to communicate with the billing offices of other providers who are submitting the claims, as well as with patients to explain claim denials when necessary. Groups or IPAs may also elect to pay an administrative fee to have the plan or a third party pay claims for them. Many plans will do this without an additional fee to avoid patient complaints. These arrangements require administration through careful reviews of the financial reports provided by the third-party administrator.

As the administrative medical assistant, you may be required to track your group's financial performance under contracts. This information will significantly affect your physician's financial status, and it is vital that the information is correct. This information may well affect future contracting with the group of managed care organizations with whom the practice currently is involved, or may determine which contracts to eliminate. Finance reporting should be presented not only on a cash basis but also should include an estimate of the incurred-but-not-reported claim liability of the group. It is important that the practice have sufficient retrospective payment under fee-for-service; capitation is prepayment for a future benefit. Accrual rather than cash accounting must be used when capitation is material to the practice. Financial reports need to show use of services by specialty or in as much detail as possible. These reports will be used for future negotiations and may also be used to evaluate the income distribution to the practice members. The administrative medical assistant may be required to monitor financial performance for certain services in order to recommend operational change, and assist with data to renegotiate subcapitation agreements. Normally, instruction on this type of reporting will be given by the medical practice's bookkeeper and with the assistance of a certified public accountant (CPA).

Administrative medical assistants, as well as the physician, often are responsible for patient education. Success in managed care requires an enormous amount of education on the part of all involved: the physicians, the administrative medical assistants, the patients, and the managed care organization. The potential of resistance exists from some consumers and physicians to managed care organizations that limit flexibility (restricting patients to seeing only physicians in their geographical location). It is easier when the physician or group elects to start with a loosely structured program. However, one must be aware that managed care organizations are becoming more tightly structured as they attempt to have a greater impact on the cost and quality of care. The administrative medical assistant may well be placed in the role of explaining to patients the limits of their care. The assistant needs to work with the patient to explain that most times less care does not mean a loss of quality of care. The assistant must explain that although visits may seem to be limited, the fact is that because of additional auxiliary staff (for example, physician assistants, certified medical assistants), the care provided is even greater than when the physician did everything. The team is ready to see that all is in place and that the team's primary concern is the patient's welfare (Figure 15.4).

The Future of Managed Care

The future of managed care is really a local business that depends on local physicians and what occurs during the physician-patient interface. The physician's relationship with the rest of the delivery system also is a local variable. Such relationships must be developed based on laws and regulations that may be enacted at a national level. The federal government is attempting to stipulate guidelines for nationwide healthcare; these guidelines will determine much of the access to medical care and how it is provided.

It is anticipated that there will be significant geographical variations in the provision and acceptance of managed care. Although in many instances managed care offers very special opportunities, this does not apply in rural areas. It

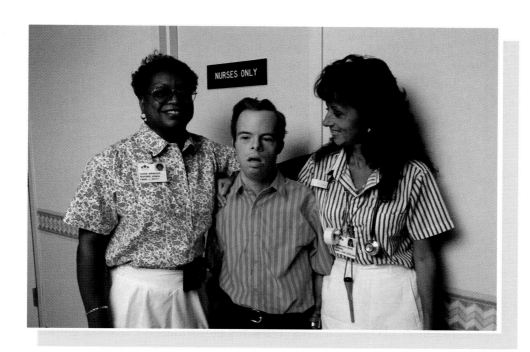

FIGURE 15.4

The expanding health care team can provide greater care then the physician working alone; the team's primary concern is the patient's welfare.

is expected that managed care in nonmetropolitan and rural areas will continue to lag behind the growth anticipated for the more urban areas. However, a number of very successful rural HMOs currently operate in the United States, which suggests that we can anticipate a steady increase in managed care activity during the next decade. Allowances must be anticipated, of course, for such variables as local economics and geographical barriers. However, understanding the growth strategies of existing managed care organizations makes it clear why greater affiliation with rural areas is inevitable.

As metropolitan markets become saturated, managed care organizations will target what they typically call "secondary markets" as their area for potential growth. These secondary markets are located beyond the immediate metropolitan market where the managed care organization began. Once the secondary market has been penetrated, managed care organizations will expand to a third-tier market, which sometimes will include rural areas. Therefore, given the current level of saturation within a given market, the likelihood of a managed care organization expanding into the adjacent market can be determined.

Current trends indicate that the bulk of the entire health care system will be converted to some type of managed care on a national basis. The following trends will depend on variables within the physician's location and the current health system reform proposals favored by government health policy makers, which indicate that the majority of the entire health care system would be converted to managed care:

- In view of the volatility of the health care industry, many experts predict that 70% to 80% or perhaps more of Americans may be receiving their health care service through some type of managed care by the end of the century, even if major reforms are not in place.

- Unrestricted indemnity insurance is being phased out and will probably represent no more than 5% to 10% of the marketplace in the next 5 years.

- The focus on managed care will shift even more closely to controlling the cost of care, particularly in ambulatory or outpatient areas.

- The patient will have restricted choice of providers, unless willing to pay out of pocket for the level of care.

- Physicians and other providers will have less independence in making decisions regarding patient care.

- Larger corporations will move away from defined benefit plans to defined contribution plans.

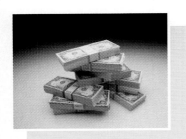

This last trend warrants some explanation.

Under a defined benefit plan, an employer pays the full amount of the employee's health benefits. Under a defined contribution plan, the employer contributes a fixed amount but offers a selection of health plans to the employees, some of which cost more than others, but also may offer more benefits to the employees. The employee then is free to select the more costly coverage but must pay the difference between the defined contribution and the cost of the coverage. Thus, if an employee were to choose a more costly health benefits plan, he or she then would pay more out of pocket than if a less costly option had been selected. The intent, of course, is to encourage employees to become more aware of the best value for the dollar among their options and, as a result, evaluate their options from the perspective of a prudent buyer.

It is expected that the distinctions between HMOs, PPOs, and other managed care plans will blur, and that this blurring will continue to accelerate in the coming years. PPOs already are beginning to look more like HMOs in terms of the degree of influence they have over the delivery of care, and as markets mature, there likely will be movement away from such plans and toward more tightly controlled plans. It already is evident that Medicare and Medicaid beneficiaries will be required to receive their care through some form of managed care.

It is anticipated that the United States will experience a shortage of primary care physicians as the market share for managed care increases. The resulting demand for physicians probably will encourage the shift of a larger percentage of the health care dollar toward acquiring certain cognitive skills that are essential to effective patient management. However, this good news for primary care physicians cannot be delivered without a qualifier. Most managed care organizations have developed or are developing databases that will permit them to objectively evaluate provider performance. Those physicians who do not develop the skills required to practice effective, high-quality primary care can expect the demand to pass them by.

Prospects for subspecialists in many areas will be diminished; as a result it is realistic to anticipate a significant surplus of subspecialists as the demand for their services is eroded by the managed care organizations. Subspecialists must learn how to measure and prove the value of their services.

Carriers or third-party payers, as well as the public and employers, will demand greater value from the health care dollar. Physicians and health care providers should not lose sight of the fact that employers and individual purchasers of health care coverage are willing to evaluate the cost of the care based on someone else's calculations. Many consumers are now viewing the costs in terms of the total costs per person per year. This much more comprehensive focus in turn demands a much more comprehensive approach to managing the cost of all of the care an individual may receive during the year. However, it is safe to assume that, whatever approaches are eventually developed, whatever they are called, they will inevitably be built on what has been learned and is still being learned as the managed care industry continues to develop.

As mentioned previously, as the shift in focus from inpatient to ambulatory or outpatient services intensifies, pressure will build to control costs in that segment of the health care services industry. This challenge will not easily be met, because there are many more and varied sites at which ambulatory services may be provided and a far greater number of individual services involved. It is likely that an entirely new level of management technology will be required to successfully achieve this particular goal, much of it involving physician, clinical, and automated clinical databases, and automated clinical decision-making support systems.

The shift in underwriting risk from insurers to providers is expected to continue. Before managed care, providers were reimbursed on a fee-for-service basis. Employers and insurers assumed all of the risk for the care their employees and beneficiaries would need. Managed care plans tend to shift this underwriting risk to providers, particularly if capitation is the method of reimbursement used by the payers. Capitation may become the most prevalent form of physician/provider payment during this decade. As the risk is shifted, certain tools will be required, most importantly, the reporting mechanisms to provide essential information and databases that will allow comparisons of actual performance by individual physicians to established standards. Other important tools will include provider incentive systems and utilization and quality management systems. Managed care organizations that are committed to long-term success must also be committed to making their physician providers successful by equipping them with these tools. The physicians and their practices will have to do their part by learning the value of services and using the tools provided effectively.

To the physician/practice concerned with affiliating with organizations that promise the greatest likelihood of success, an HMO's size is not necessarily the best indicator. Some of the largest managed care organizations to date have produced some of the largest failures. Conversely, some smaller local and regional companies are operating effectively and will probably enjoy considerable success in the future. Each managed care organization must be evaluated on its own merit.

As the blending of delivery system models occurs (for example, IPAs, PPOs, HMOs), the managed care organizations may attempt to compete with one another for additional patient loads by developing more effective cost and quality management systems. This may allow an increased opportunity for the physician/practice to participate individually with the managed care organization rather than through a closed-panel structure.

PERSPECTIVES ON MEDICAL ASSISTING

Managed Care—The Future

The future is happening now and accompanying it are changes, no matter how we might feel about that. Managed care is regulated by law so there is more government control. Several states already have as much as 70% of their population in some type of managed care plan.

If you are a skilled and responsible administrative medical assistant, different job opportunities will be available to you. You must be able to learn quickly but be able to adapt to the various plans and endless changes that are occurring in the medical arena. Education will become even more important to you as more will be expected of you in the new managed care world.

It is not expected that indemnity insurance plans will ever attain the same level of efficiency as the tightly structured managed care organizations, nor is it likely that the presence of managed care organizations is the only reason for declining hospital utilization. The shift in utilization will continue to occur as physicians learn new practice styles.

The continued pressure on health care costs will occur as a result of normal economic cycles. This means that the physician/practice will have to continue to monitor their cost effectiveness, as well as the effectiveness of the managed care organizations with whom they are affiliated. It is expected that the majority of well-run managed care organizations will most likely take the appropriate steps to support both the patient and the provider in delivering high quality, cost-effective care and will be in a position to survive the natural gain/loss cycles.

Conclusion

Managed care will bring constant changes to the practice of medicine. Both the administrative medical assistant staff and the physicians will need to be prepared for that. The growth of the managed care plans and the delivery of service will be monitored from many levels. The administrative medical assistant will be required to obtain as much knowledge as possible about each plan in which the physician participates, in order to achieve quality of care to the patient and maximum reimbursement to the physician.

Review QUESTIONS

1. What are the different types of managed care plans?

2. How can you assist your physician in reviewing the managed care plans?

3. Are you allowed to request a financial statement from the managed care plan?

4. Explain how managed care plans are becoming important to the physician/practice?

5. List at least six basic components of a managed care contract.

6. Explain in your own words the meaning of capitation.

7. How do you evaluate the capitation rate?

8. Give three examples of how to improve practice productivity.

9. How important will the administrative medical assistant's role be in managed care?

SUGGESTED READINGS

American Medical Association: Doctors Resource Service, *Medicine in transition* (videotapes, audio tapes, and books), Chicago, 1993, The Association.
Denning Jeffrey: *Coping with managed care.* Seminar published by Practice Performance Seminars, Long Beach, Calif, 1993.

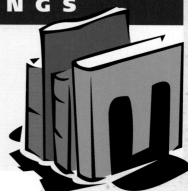

Credit, Billing, and Collection

(Continued)

■ **Collection Maintenance**
Current Accounts Receivable
Charge Slips or Superbills
Payment at the Time of Visit
Credit Cards
Billing Patients for Services

■ **Collection Techniques**
Legal Considerations
Collection Goal
Personal Interview
Telephone
Written Notices

■ **Using a Collection Agency**
When to Use Collection Agencies
Responsibility for Agency Actions
Fees Associated with Agencies
Patient Care after Collection Action

■ **Special Collection Problems**
Disputed Charges
Claims Against Estates
Bankruptcy
Options to Sue
Loss of Accounts Receivable Records

OBJECTIVES

On completion of Chapter 16 the administrative medical assistant student should be able to:

❶ Define the key terms listed in this chapter.

❷ Describe the importance of accounts receivable and the administrative medical assistant's responsibilities to the office and patients with regard to the billing system.

❸ List the basic information needed from the patient and the information provided by the office to form the foundation of an effective billing system.

❹ List and describe the three basic in-office methods and the two methods from outside the office of providing bills to patients.

Continued

OBJECTIVES

(Continued)

5 Compare the three options for computerized services.

6 Discuss the special considerations necessary for preparing a patient's statement, selecting a billing cycle, billing minors, or billing third-party payers.

7 Describe the reasons for establishing a credit and collection policy, the methods of informing patients of the policies, and the medical assistant's role in effective collection of accounts.

8 Discuss the three major components of an account collection system and the elements of each.

9 State the five special collection problems and the methods of managing each situation.

KEY TERMS

Accounts receivable   A figure that represents the total dollars due to the physician who has provided services or goods.

Asset   Anything of value that belongs to a person or business and can be evaluated in dollar amounts.

Charges   The fees for professional services rendered. In most offices charges are referred to as *fees.*

Charge slip   A transaction slip completed by the physician at the time a patient receives medical services.

Computer memory bank   The section of a computer that accepts the information you enter (type) into it and stores the data until you need it.

Credit   An extension of time allowed a customer or client to pay after a service has been provided.

Data   An organized collection of facts that can be analyzed and used to produce reports and documents.

Debtor   A person who owes money to an individual or a business.

Emissary   A person who acts as the representative or agent for another individual, particularly when diplomacy is needed.

Fee schedule   A listing of procedure codes and the fees assigned to each code.

Intermediary   Situated or coming between; for example, Blue Shield is the intermediary between HCFA and the provider of service.

Professional courtesy   A discount for services provided to another health care provider and/or his or her family.

Superbill   A billing slip that is given to the patient to submit to an insurance carrier.

Third party   Someone other than the provider or the recipient of a service.

*P*atient credit, billing, and collection provide the foundation for all financial functions and indeed for the survival of a medical practice. Payment for medical services is the source of income for the physician, the practice, and ultimately you. Administrative medical assistants are responsible for maintaining accurate billing procedures and fee structures and collecting outstanding accounts receivable. Administrative medical assistants also are responsible for educating patients about specific charges on their statements and about the office policy on fee establishment, account collection, and credit. The ability of the health care team to continue to provide medical services depends on the income generated by these services.

Administrative Medical Assistant's Responsibilities

To Office

The primary responsibilities of the medical assistant in relation to the billing system are to maintain accurate billing procedures and fee structures, and to collect outstanding accounts receivable. The ability of the health care team to continue to provide medical services depends on the income generated by those services. The process is a complete cycle that must be monitored constantly for potential breaks.

To Patients

The medical assistant primarily responsible for billing also is responsible for educating the patient. This often involves explaining specific items noted on individual statements, since patients may be confused by the terminology or concerned about the fee. The educational process should actually begin before medical services are provided, at which time the medical assistant can explain to each new patient the office policy on fee establishment, account collection, and credit. Specific techniques of patient education are discussed later in the chapter.

Setting Fees

Setting fees in a physician's office or for a group requires understanding of the RBRVS (Resource-Based Relative Value Study, as determined by Harvard Research for the Department of Health and Human Services) in addition to knowledge of the "limiting charges" set by the HCFA (Health Care Financing Agency, which functions under the Department of Health and Human Services) for Medicare reimbursement by geographical location. On average, one takes the limiting charge per CPT procedural code, multiplies that charge by two, and divides by the unit value assigned by the RBRVS (Figure 16.1). This

CPT[1]/ HCPCs[2]	MOD	Status	Description	Physician work RVUs[3]	Practice expense RVUs	Mal-practice RVUs	Total	Global[2]	Update
23395	....	A	Muscle transfer, shoulder/arm..................	16.00	11.13	1.84	28.97	090	S
23397	....	A	Muscle transfers.........	15.23	13.97	2.34	31.54	090	S
23400	....	A	Fixation of shoulder blade.....................	12.96	9.84	1.68	24.48	090	S
23405	....	A	Incision of tendon & muscle...................	7.97	7.49	0.99	16.45	090	S
23406	....	A	Incise tendon(s) & muscle(s)	10.33	9.41	1.58	21.32	090	S
23410	....	A	Repair of tendon(s)........	11.90	10.94	1.75	24.59	090	S
23412	....	A	Repair of tendon(s)........	12.69	13.37	2.16	28.22	090	S
23415	....	A	Release of shoulder ligament.................	9.51	5.18	0.83	15.52	090	S
23420	....	A	Repair of shoulder.........	12.60	14.68	2.34	29.62	090	S
23430	....	A	Repair biceps tendon......	9.56	7.34	1.19	18.09	090	S
23440	....	A	Removal/transplant tendon...............	10.08	7.17	1.17	18.42	090	S
23450	....	A	Repair shoulder capsule.....	12.85	12.75	2.04	27.64	090	S
23455	....	A	Repair shoulder capsule.....	13.82	15.56	2.50	31.88	090	S
23460	....	A	Repair shoulder capsule.....	14.66	14.07	2.24	30.97	090	S
23462	....	A	Repair shoulder capsule.....	14.62	15.13	2.48	32.23	090	S
23465	....	A	Repair shoulder capsule.....	15.14	14.15	2.27	31.56	090	S
23466	....	A	Repair shoulder capsule.....	13.65	16.53	2.67	32.85	090	S
23470	....	A	Reconstruct shoulder joint....	16.12	16.76	2.65	35.53	090	S
23472	....	A	Reconstruct shoulder joint....	16.09	20.60	4.89	41.58	090	S
23480	....	A	Revision of collarbone.......	10.56	6.59	1.02	18.17	090	S
23485	....	A	Revision of collarbone.......	12.68	11.35	1.87	25.90	090	S
23490	....	A	Reinforce clavicle..........	11.31	9.98	0.80	22.09	090	S
23491	....	A	Reinforce shoulder bones.....	13.63	12.70	2.11	28.44	090	S
23500	....	A	Treat clavicle fracture......	1.95	1.65	0.21	3.81	090	S
23505	....	A	Treat clavicle fracture......	3.54	2.57	0.38	6.49	090	S
23515	....	A	Repair clavicle fracture.....	7.01	6.93	1.12	15.06	090	S
23520	....	A	Treat clavicle dislocation....	2.03	1.38	0.19	3.60	090	S
23525	....	A	Treat clavicle dislocation....	3.40	1.98	0.27	5.65	090	S
23530	....	A	Repair clavicle dislocation...	7.02	6.58	0.91	14.51	090	S
23532	....	A	Repair clavicle dislocation...	7.59	7.23	1.19	16.01	090	S
23540	....	A	Treat clavicle dislocation....	2.10	1.55	0.19	3.84	090	S
23545	....	A	Treat clavicle dislocation....	3.07	1.98	0.29	5.34	090	S
23550	....	A	Repair clavicle dislocation...	6.65	8.51	1.46	16.62	090	S
23552	....	A	Repair clavicle dislocation...	7.83	7.29	1.17	16.29	090	S
23570	....	A	Treat shoulderblade fracture..	2.10	1.70	0.25	4.05	090	S
23575	....	A	Treat shoulderblade fracture..	3.88	2.75	0.43	7.06	090	S
23585	....	A	Repair scapula fracture.....	8.41	7.70	1.29	17.40	090	S
23600	....	A	Treat humerus fracture......	2.75	2.90	0.43	6.08	090	S
23605	....	A	Treat humerus fracture......	4.56	4.76	0.76	10.08	090	S
23615	....	A	Repair humerus fracture.....	8.38	10.72	1.78	20.88	090	S
23616	....	A	Repair humerus fracture.....	19.88	22.32	3.54	45.74	090	S
23620	....	A	Treat humerus fracture......	2.25	2.88	0.46	5.59	090	S
23625	....	A	Treat humerus fracture......	3.64	3.82	0.60	8.06	090	S
23630	....	A	Repair humerus fracture.....	6.89	8.82	1.40	17.11	090	S
23650	....	A	Treat shoulder dislocation....	3.24	2.10	0.24	5.58	090	S
23655	....	A	Treat shoulder dislocation....	4.26	2.93	0.44	7.63	090	S
23660	....	A	Repair shoulder dislocation...	7.09	9.07	1.40	17.56	090	S
23665	....	A	Treat dislocation/fracture....	4.16	3.35	0.51	8.02	090	S
23670	....	A	Repair dislocation/fracture...	7.44	9.52	1.85	18.81	090	S
23675	....	A	Treat dislocation/fracture....	5.60	3.93	0.61	10.14	090	S
23680	....	A	Repair dislocation/fracture...	9.44	12.09	2.13	23.66	090	S
23700	....	A	Fixation of shoulder........	2.47	2.09	0.34	4.90	010	S
23800	....	A	Fusion of shoulder joint.....	13.32	16.35	2.63	32.30	090	S
23802	....	A	Fusion of shoulder joint.....	15.62	14.07	2.24	31.93	090	S
23900	....	A	Amputation of arm & girdle...	18.40	12.57	2.40	33.37	090	S
23920	....	A	Amputation at shoulder joint..	13.60	13.85	2.54	29.99	090	S
23921	....	A	Amputation follow-up surgery..	5.03	4.27	0.74	10.04	090	S
23929	....	C	Shoulder surgery procedure ...	0.00	0.00	0.00	0.00	YYY	S
23930	....	A	Drainage of arm lesion.......	2.78	1.61	0.24	4.63	010	S
23931	....	A	Drainage of arm bursa	1.63	0.75	0.11	2.49	010	S
23935	....	A	Drain arm/elbow bone lesion...	5.56	4.69	0.78	11.03	090	S
24000	....	A	Exploratory elbow surgery.....	5.32	6.81	1.44	13.57	090	S
24006	....	A	Release elbow joint.........	8.70	7.14	1.17	17.01	090	S
24065	....	A	Biopsy arm/elbow soft tissue...	2.03	0.79	0.10	2.92	010	S
24066	....	A	Biopsy arm/elbow soft tissue...	4.95	2.71	0.41	8.07	090	S
24075	....	A	Remove arm/elbow lesion......	3.79	1.98	0.35	6.12	090	S
24076	....	A	Remove arm/elbow lesion......	6.01	3.68	0.67	10.36	090	S

[1]All CPT codes and descriptors copyright 1996 American Medical Association.
[2]Copyright 1994 American Dental Association. All rights reserved.
[3]+Indicates RVUs are not used for Medicare payment.

FIGURE 16.1

Example of relative value units used to set fees in a physician's office. (From the Federal Register, Vol. 61, No. 227, Rules and Regulations, 1996, U.S. Government Printing Office.)

is called the *practice conversion factor*. For example, for Code 99214, Expanded Problem office visit, the unit value is 1.78, the limiting charge is $59.70, and the practice fee is $120. Dividing by the unit value of 1.78 equals a conversion rate of $67.42. Thus all of the fees for the practice would be set at $67 times the unit value for each procedural code. The information is provided by either the RBRVS (which can be ordered through Medi-Code, PMIC, or other sources of medical books) or the Federal Register (which can be ordered through the Government Printing Office in Philadelphia). The RBRVS and the Federal Register provide the procedural code, a brief description, unit value, and days of follow-up if a CPT code is a surgical procedure. The Medicare limiting charge schedule usually is sent to the physician's office in November of each year and provides the conversion factor by locality, according to Medicare. The Medicare limiting charge provides the procedural code, participating provider fee, nonparticipating provider fee, and charge limit. Participating and nonparticipating providers are explained in Chapter 13.

Physician Fee Profile

You often will hear physicians refer to their profile when discussing patient care insurance payments. A profile is a numerical image of a physician's patterns for charging for various services as monitored by insurance companies that are billed for reimbursement. The individual profiles physicians refer to represent usual fees. Comparative profiles are developed from all fees submitted by any physician in the geographical area for each service code. These profiles set the standards for usual, customary, and reasonable (UCR) fees and determine the maximum charges an insurance carrier will allow.

Usual Fees

Usual fees for each physician are calculated by computer and represent the fees routinely charged by a physician for each service. The profile is calculated by a computer for a specific period, usually 1 year. This becomes the base year that determines the fees paid. Physicians may feel that the system is unfair to claimants, because the base year may be several years earlier than the one in which the services are billed.

Fees may change over time because the costs of maintaining an office will increase, requiring more income. To determine a physician's usual fee, select a specific time period (at least 1 year), and check the fees for a specific procedure at the various times throughout the year. The fee that occurs most often is the usual fee. For example, if your survey reveals charges for a specific procedure to include $10, $12, $12, $14, and $16, the usual fee would be $12.

Customary Fees

Fees are considered customary if they fall within the upper and lower profile limits for physicians of the same specialty or practice type who practice within a geographical area determined by the insurance company. If the upper limit profile is $18 for a specific service code and the lower limit is $14, the physician who submits a bill for $16 will have the fee recognized as customary.

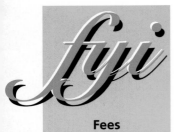

Reasonable Fees

Fees commonly are declared reasonable if they meet the criteria for usual and customary fees. In some cases, there can be multiple problems that make the services more complex and warrant a higher fee. Physicians submitting a higher-than-average fee to the insurance carriers should attach a statement and documents to support the extra fee. A panel of physicians peers will review the claim, and the appropriate fee will be determined.

Resource-Based Relative Value Study (RBRVS)

In 1988 Congress allotted some $2.5 million to Harvard University to establish a relative value for each procedure performed. This is very similar to the Relative Value Study (RVS) that was established in 1964 by the California Medical Association (CMA) and the Florida Medical Association (FMA). At one time the Federal Trade Commission (FTC) considered the RVS as price fixing and ruled it illegal. However, the Medicare and Medicaid programs under directives from the HCFA continued to reimburse under a unit value system since the state and federal programs are exempt from FTC rules. The FTC reversed its ruling and most all carriers use a blend of RBRVS units and usual and customary fees. Only the government continues to use a straight unit value reimbursement.

Discussing Fees with Patients

Discussing fees is not always the easiest part of working with patients, but it is necessary. The medical assistant should think of fees as the income that pays his or her salary. If the fees are not paid, then the assistant's salary will not be paid. When an assistant views asking for payment of fees as his or her salary, then discussing fees becomes much easier.

The majority of patients who come to the office seeking medical care are more concerned about their health problems than with payment for services. The assistant must listen to the patient's medical problem but should be prepared to discuss the expense, if the patient requests information about the fee. After the patient explains the medical problem, the assistant should tactfully inquire as to whether the patient has health insurance coverage; this initial office visit begins the credit process and establishes a credit relationship. The majority of patients have some type of medical insurance coverage that will offset some of the office and hospital expense. Sometimes patients will indicate that they do not wish for their insurance carrier to know about certain services and would like to pay cash (for example, for HIV tests). In these instances they should pay for the test before it is performed. Many patients who do not have any type of insurance coverage wait until the problem has become severe enough that they go to a hospital emergency room.

A patient should never be judged by his or her outward appearance. Even if the patient is poorly dressed and conveys the impression that he or she cannot afford to pay, the medical assistant may not ask embarrassing questions. The rule is that the assistant must never assume anything about a patient's financial status. Tact is called for in all instances, whether the person has the ability to pay or not.

Fees for medical service should be stated clearly and matter of factly. When a fee is misquoted, the patient usually will become angry. The assistant should never apologize or act guilty about the fees. If the patient has a financial problem, the patient should be interviewed by the office manager in a separate room to avoid the embarrassment of discussing the issue in front of other people. The physician usually expects the assistant to handle all financial discussions, other than when surgery is recommended or for the delivery of a baby.

On occasion a patient becomes emotionally upset over the discussion of fees. It is wise for the assistant to ask, "Would you like to know more about the expense of your treatment?" This allows the patient to feel more comfortable about discussing the fees. There will be times when nothing you say will be accepted by the patient. You then must refer to the policy manual, office manager, or the physician.

The administrative medical assistant must be alert to certain signs that indicate that the patient may not choose to pay for services or treatment. These signs are:

- No employment record
- No home or work telephone number
- A motel address
- No referral
- No insurance

It is best to ask the patient who cannot supply the above information to pay at time of service. Refer to the office policy manual.

PERSPECTIVES ON MEDICAL ASSISTING

Talk About Money

The money (patient fees) will need to be collected in a timely manner for the physician to be able to continue his or her practice. Discussing money (fees) with people is not an easy task but one that probably will fall on the administrative medical assistant's shoulders.

The primary concern of both the physician and the patient is that there be good quality medical care. In a sense the physician's fee will be secondary but the patient has thought or is thinking about it. It is best that fees be discussed openly and a full explanation provided. Answer any questions that the patient has, because when the patient has a good understanding of the fees and knows what to expect he or she is more likely to pay the fees without complaint.

Just remember that it is a good practice to discuss the fees (charges) in advance with new patients. If necessary, discuss the fees in private with new patients on their first visit so that any questions can be answered at the beginning of the new "contract."

Credit and Collection Policies and Procedures

Reasons for a Policy

The subject of credit, the accumulation of debt, and the collection of accounts is a delicate situation that must be handled tactfully and legally by the medical assistant. An established policy will guide the medical assistant in this important function.

The most important reasons for a policy are that it does the following:

- Establishes guidelines for informing the patient of payment procedures
- Standardizes the information given by all employees to all patients
- Reduces the overall costs to all patients by avoiding the expense of repeated billing and possibly collection agency fees

Some physicians choose to convey their policy to patients in writing by providing them with an information pamphlet. Other physicians may be timid about discussing financial issues in the pamphlet. Physicians should be reminded of the importance of finances to the office, and the subject should be discussed frankly in staff meetings with the physicians present. Because the pamphlet will discuss a number of policies, a discussion of finances will not appear out of place.

Another method of introducing the patient to office credit policies is to discuss policies privately with the patient at the time of the first visit. It is interesting to note that the medical assistant, rather than the physician, often is viewed as the financial manager. This perception can be used to the benefit of the office, since the patient perceives the discussion is taking place with a person of authority.

It may be effective to reinforce the office policy by giving the patient a copy of the policy pamphlet after the discussion (Figure 16.2). The patient can read it at his or her leisure and keep it for future reference. The pamphlet also eliminates a patient claim of lack of knowledge of the policy. See the box on p. 406 for an example of credit and collection policies and procedures.

Billing Systems

Data Necessary for Effective Billing

To establish a billing system you will need two specific blocks of information. One of these is provided by the patient, and one is generated by the physician and the medical assistant.

Patient Information

Gathering information from the patient is the first step in establishing an account and integrating the patient into the billing system. This information includes the following:

- Patient's name, spelled correctly
- Name of the person responsible for payment, if other than the patient

---

OUR FINANCIAL POLICY

CASH PATIENTS

FULL PAYMENT AT THE TIME OF SERVICE.
We accept cash and checks.

HMO/PPO

COPAYMENT AND DEDUCTIBLE AT THE TIME OF SERVICE.

PRIVATE INSURANCE

First visit is to be paid in cash at time of service. However, when we are provided with insurance information we will submit the visit to your insurance company for you.

On subsequent visits we will bill your insurance, although you must pay at least 20% of total charges at the time of service. If your insurance company has not paid the **FULL BALANCE** within 45 days, you have 15 days to pay the balance.

Insurance is a contract between you and your insurance company. We are **NOT** a party to this contract, in most cases. (We will inform you if we are a party to your insurance contract, and will handle your claims according to our agreement with the insurance company, if one exists.) We file insurance claims as a courtesy to our patients. We will not become involved in disputes between you and your insurance company regarding deductibles, copayments, etc. other than to supply factual information as necessary. You are responsible for the timely payment of your account.

MEDICARE/WORKERS' COMPENSATION

If you are covered by Medicare, Workers' Compensation, or any other government-sponsored program, please discuss payment situation with our office staff.

Thank you for understanding our financial policy. Please let us know if you have any questions or concerns.

Responsible Party_____ Date _____

FIGURE 16.2

Example of an office financial policy used to educate patients about expectations regarding payment for services. (Courtesy De A. Eggers & Associates, Sonoma, Calif.)

- Complete billing address (home)
- Complete medical insurance information
- Data for collection purposes

The first four items are self-explanatory. The fifth, collection data, involves information that might be helpful in evaluating the patient's ability to pay or

MEDICAL ASSISTING STEP-BY-STEP

Credit Collection

De A. Eggers & Associates
Credit and Collection Policies and Procedures
Purpose: It is the intent of this practice to require payment at the time services are rendered for patients who have no insurance coverage. All staff will inform patients of the policy. Appropriate staff will collect full fees from patients who have no insurance, copays from patients with HMO/PPO coverage, and deductibles due as indicated by carriers. We will always be courteous and kind foremost to our patients in enforcing this policy.

I. Prevention

New patients:

1. At the time the appointment is made for the new patient, state the basic estimated copay, etc., that is to be paid on the date of service (we cannot know about additional tests to be ordered). This includes all copays or deductibles; payments can be made in cash, by money order, or check.

2. If patients have more than one insurance company, inform them that it is our policy to bill all carriers. The patient will then always be responsible for any unpaid balance.

3. New patients should be asked to call their carriers (Medicare and Medicaid patients excluded) to verify their benefits coverage. This is particularly important for the PPO/HMO caseload.

4. New patients should be asked to bring in their insurance coverage cards, in order that we might copy them front and back for our records. We should stress that we need to know the address where the insurance claims are to be submitted, and we need to know the phone number of their insurance company benefits office.

5. Any new patient requesting "terms" should be referred to the manager immediately.

6. New patients with a Workers' Compensation injury should be advised that they must bring in the name, address, phone number, and policy identification of their employer's compensation insurance carrier with them. Failure to provide this information at the time of the visit means that the patient will be responsible for payment of the visit in full at the time of service. Any patient question or concern with this policy should be referred to the manager.

7. New Medicaid patients should be informed that they must bring in their current card indicating eligibility or pay for the visit until the card is provided.

8. For new patients who are students or possibly children whose parents are responsible for payment but who will not be with the student or child at the time of the first visit, parents are to be informed that payment for service is due at the time of the visit. The student or child must bring payment at the time of the visit.

9. When the new patient arrives, provide a copy of the office financial policy. Ask the patient to read it, sign it, and return it to you. (This signed copy is to go into the patient's record.) When the patient returns the signed copy to the front desk, he or she should be specifically asked if they have any questions concerning the office payment policy.

10. Any new patient requesting "terms" at the time of the first visit is to be referred to the manager.

11. Any Medicaid patient presenting without a current Medicaid card is to be referred to the manager. Most states now have the on-site verification machine that transmits directly into the Medicaid program to verify eligibility.

Credit Collection (cont'd)

II. Established Patients

1. When established patients call in for visits, inform them that the physician or clinic is establishing a stricter payment policy. Inform them as you do the new patients. Inform them that we expect that they will not be inconvenienced by this change in policy. We want them to know that from now on payment for deductibles, copays, or insurance denials is expected at the time of service. All private-pay patients (patients with no insurance) will now be responsible for paying for their service at the time the service is provided or at the time the next statement is sent out. Explain to patients that they may wish to contact their insurance company to verify the family deductible or copay due.

2. Physicians will preferably not engage in any discussion with patients regarding this policy, expect to reinforce the collections policy and that patients discuss concerns for terms with the manager.

3. Established patients should be asked to bring in their insurance benefit cards so that we can duplicate them, front and back, and update our records. This should be done annually at the very least.

4. Established patients should be provided a demographical printout and asked to update it annually.

III. When All Patients Leave

1. Total the Superbill with the adding machine and collect the amount due. Do not offer a choice; do not negotiate except as indicated below. Refer anyone who gives you a problem to the manager immediately.

2. Established patients with an outstanding balance are to be informed of this when they call to set up their appointments. They are to be informed that payment in full is now due and that a minimum payment of $50 is expected. Anyone not capable of complying must settle terms with the manager or billing office. (The outstanding balance is not reflected in the insurance pending. This is the amount due to the practice.)

3. Any account in which terms have been established will have a note placed in the person's account in the comments section. All staff are to note this information.

IV. Exceptions

1. Physician courtesy or insurance-only patients (that is, family of other physicians or other persons as designated by the doctor).

2. Patients who are seen first in the hospital. These patients should have their benefits verified by the office, before their first office visit, so that if there are copays or deductibles, these can be discussed with the patient at the time of the first visit.

V. Billing and Collection Procedures by Billing Office

1. First month—any unpaid balance is billed in regular format. May have the following stamped on the statement if requested by the client: "Balance due from responsible party" or "Please pay balance."

2. Second month—a handwritten note preferably, or a sticker or stamp requesting payment in full now. See stamp that may be placed on statement if requested by the client.

3. Third month—a handwritten note on statement that balance is due in 10 to 15 days, stating specific date (not a Saturday or Sunday). Flag the account in the system for tickler follow-up. All flagged accounts will be called for payment due now. See stamp that may be placed on the statement if requested by the client.

4. Fourth month—if no payment or agreement for payment is achieved through phone calls, then the billing office will work in the following manner, depending on the nature and amount of the account and working the highest amount balance due first:
   Certified letter—return receipt requested
   Collection agency—after approved by the physician

Continued

MEDICAL ASSISTING STEP-BY-STEP

Credit Collection (cont'd)

VI. Mail Returns

❶ The billing office will first try to find from records or any other source available another address and send the statement out again.

❷ If this is determined to definitely be a "skip," the billing office will request authorization to send the account immediately to collection.

VII. Contracts

The billing office will have patients sign contracts on all large accounts to be paid off. Will monitor payments, accounts with agreements, and no payments according to the plan: first month skipped will be called; second month skipped will be advised in writing of 10-day due or turned over to a collection agency. If no payment or contact with the office is achieved by the third month the account will be turned over to a collection agency after approval by the physician.

VIII. Billing and Collection Procedures, Other Than Above

❶ Medicare, Medicaid and Medi/Medi billing will be done each week.

❷ Workers' Compensation billing will be done each week.

❸ Surgery billing will be done on receipt of charges but held until an operative report is received to support the claim.

❹ Other insurance forms will be processed on a weekly basis.

in locating a patient "lost to the practice," that is, difficult to find to collect overdue payment. Collection data includes employment status, name and location of employer, and unique identifying numbers such as Social Security or driver's license numbers. This method of obtaining billing information is discussed in Chapter 9.

Office-Generated Information

Once an account has been established and medical services begun, the remaining data needed to produce a bill is generated by the physician and introduced into the billing system by the medical assistant. This information, known as *transaction data,* includes the following:

- The date of the visit or procedure
- The five-digit insurance billing code that identifies each specific medical service
- The fee for the service
- The diagnosis, stated or by diagnosis code number

Without both kinds of information—that provided by the patient and that generated by the provider—a statement of services cannot be sent.

AT WORK TODAY

External vs. Internal Billing

External billing, or *out-sourced billing,* refers to the use of a billing service to prepare and mail patient bills. Although this is an expense, there are advantages: it eliminates a time-consuming job for the staff, the bills will be sent on time because it is the billing service's business, and it saves the physician money by not having to maintain expensive billing equipment, especially for programs that require constant updating as a result of government directives.

Internal billing refers to the normal types of billing that take place in the office setting. The size of the practice will determine the best method to use. Billing will range from the superbill, a statement that is given to the patient as he or she leaves the office, to ledger card copies for statements to computerized statements. In some offices, credit card billing is accepted for services rendered.

In-Office Billing Procedures

Typed Statements

In the past, statements for medical care services were individually typed by the medical assistant each month (some offices still use this system). The process was and is extremely time consuming and eliminates the possibility for the medical assistant to assume more challenging responsibilities. This system is all but outmoded today except in practices that involve a limited number of patients such as some psychiatric practices and some very rural practices. Practices of this type either do not require much income or charge a substantial fee for each service.

Another consideration in the use of this billing system is the changes that have occurred in the education of the administrative medical assistant. Today's medical assistants are prepared to assume a wide variety of duties, and their time and talents would be wasted on this type of billing system. However, the physician will determine the type of system used for the practice.

Ledger Cards

Ledger cards are forms printed on firm paper that are designed to record the financial activity of an individual patient. The card provides spaces for the patient's name and address and then a series of columns in which to record the date and type of transaction and the current balance due. Transactions may be typed or handwritten onto the ledger card as they occur so that the balance in the last column is always current.

Ledger cards used alone are processed monthly by the medical assistant, who must photocopy each ledger card with a balance, fold the copies, insert them along with a return envelope into a window envelope, affix the postage, and mail them. It is possible to lease equipment that will fold, stuff, seal, and apply postage automatically, but it is relatively expensive. It might be wiser to apply the money to a billing service that also will assist you with cumulative accounting information and status reports to help monitor the efficiency of the billing system. This type of billing is almost as outmoded as the typed statement.

Pegboard Systems

Pegboard systems are unique in that they allow you to retain control of your billing system within the office while adding insurance and accounting features. Because it can perform several functions at once, the pegboard also is referred to as the *Write-It-Once system.*

The term *pegboard* is derived from the appearance of the equipment used to hold the various forms. The board is made of lightweight metal and is appropriately sized for the average desk. The pegs extend down the left-hand edge to hold the corresponding perforations on the accounting sheets.

Pegboard systems still are used, but because of federal electronic requirements, they are fast becoming outdated.

The cost to establish a pegboard system can vary from approximately $200 to $750, depending on the features you select and the printing of fees. The basic system includes the following:

- Patient charge slip and receipt
- Ledger cards
- Journal page
- Folding pegboard

You may choose to include a feature called the *superbill* (Figure 16.3, *A* to *C*). This multicopy slip is a patient charge slip, a receipt, and a form that the patient can use to bill his or her insurance carrier. You may select from standard superbills or design one to meet your needs. The initial imprinting adds to the cost of establishing the system and is proportional to the complexity of superbill design.

The superbill saves you time that would be spent billing patients' insurance carriers. The overall cost of the system can be quickly recovered in time that might otherwise have been spent collecting past-due accounts. However, the pegboard system is still more time consuming than the computerized system.

Alternative Billing Systems

Microfilm Billing

Microfilm billing is almost, but not completely, outdated. Microfilm billing is a service that may be used in conjunction with the ledger card or pegboard type systems. A representative of a microfilm company comes to your office at least once a month and uses a portable microfilm camera to photograph each of your ledger cards that has an active balance. The filming process generally takes no more than 20 minutes. The film then is forwarded to the company plant for processing. Most of these companies have gone a step further and now enter the information into a computer system, transmit the claims electronically, and produce a statement for the patient. This system has allowed some offices to remain on their ledger system, yet have available to them the electronic submission as required by the federal government.

Computerized Billing

As a practice grows, either because of caring for greater numbers of patients or perhaps adding more physicians to the group, the billing system will need to be updated. Manual systems, such as typed statements or ledger cards, may be too

| DATE | | DESCRIPTION | TOTAL FEE | PAYMENT | ADJ. | BALANCE | PREVIOUS BALANCE | NAME |
| FAMILY MEMBER | | | | CREDITS | | | | |

EXPLANATION OF CHARGES

1. OFFICE VISITS CPT FEE
( ) New Patient, Compreh. 92004(-AP)
( ) Estab. Compreh. 92014(-AP)
( ) New Patient, Intermediate 92002(-AP)
( ) Visual Supplies 92358
( ) Refraction 92015
( ) _____
( ) _____
( ) _____
( ) _____

2. CONSULTATIONS
( ) Consult. Comp 90620
( ) Consult. Ext. (New) 90610
( ) Consult. Inter. (New) 90605
( ) Follow-Up Intermediate 90642
( ) Follow-Up, Limited 90641
( ) _____
( ) _____

3. OFFICE VISIT-NEW PAT., MEDICARE CPT FEE
( ) New Lmt. 99201
( ) New Int. 99202
( ) New Ext. 99203
( ) New Comp. 99204
( ) New Comp. 99205

4. OFFICE VISIT-ESTABLISHED MEDICARE
( ) Lmt. 99211
( ) Lmt. 99212
( ) Int. 99213
( ) Ext. 99214
( ) Comp. 99215

5. CONSULTATIONS-NEW MEDICARE
( ) Lmt. 99241
( ) Int. 99242
( ) Ext. 99243
( ) Comp. 99244

6. SPECIAL STUDIES
( ) Gonioscopy 92020
( ) Tonometry 92100

6. SPECIAL STUDIES CONT. CPT FEE
( ) Fluor. Angio Reading 92235
( ) Ophthalmoscopy, Mono 92225
( ) Ophthalmoscopy Bilat. 92225-50
( ) A/Scan Ultrasonography 76519-TC
( ) A/Scan Calculation 76519-26

7. OFFICE SURGERY
( ) Diag. Scraping of Cornea 65430
( ) Subconjunctival Injection 68200
( ) Subtenons Injection 67515
( ) Chalazion Injection 68200
( ) Prob./Dil Canaliculus 68840
( ) Dilation, Lacrimal Punctum 68800
( ) Epilation, Simple 67820
( ) Excision Chalazion, Single 67800
( ) Removal Corneal Foreign Body/Slit Lamp 65222
( ) Removal Conjunctival FB 65210
( ) Perm. Punctal Plugs A4263
( ) Temp. Punctal Closure w/Implants 68830
( ) Surgical Tray 99070

DIAGNOSTIC CODES

☐ 373.13	ABSCESS EYELID	☐ 371.57	CORNEAL DYST/DEG.	☐ 364.05	HYPOPYON	☐ 372.51	PINGUECULUM
☐ 995.2	ALLERGIC REACTION - MEDICATION	☐ 371.50	CORNEAL DYSTROPHY	☐ 377.41	ISCHEMIC OPTIC NEUROPATHY	☐ 362.33	PLAQUENIL SCREENING
☐ 362.34	AMAUROSIS FUGAX	☐ 371.2	CORNEAL EDEMA	☐ 714.30	JUVENILE RHEUMATOID ARTHRITIS	☐ 367.4	PRESBYOPIA
☐ 368.0	AMBLYOPIA	☐ 371.42	CORNEAL EROSION	☐ 370.9	KERATITIS - ANY	☐ V43.1	PSEUDOPHAKIA
☐ 367.32	ANISEIKONIA	☐ 370.60	CORNEAL NEOVASCULARIZATION	☐ 370.40	KERATOCONJUNCTIVITIS	☐ 348.2	PSEUDOTUMOR CEREBRI
☐ 367.31	ANISOMETROPIA	☐ 371.00	CORNEAL OPACITY	☐ 371.6	KERATOCONUS	☐ 372.4	PTERYGIUM
☐ 379.41	ANISOCORIA	☐ 370.0	CORNEAL ULCER	☐ 870.0	LACERATION - EYELID	☐ 374.3	PTOSIS
☐ 379.31	APHAKIA	☐ 375.3	DACRYOCYSTITIS	☐ 362.63	LATTICE RETINAL DEGENERATION	☐ 375.52	PUNCT. STENOSIS
☐ 367.2	ASTIGMATISM	☐ 133.8	DEMODEX	☐ 369.4	LEGAL BLINDNESS	☐ 961.4	R/O PLAQUENIL TOXICITY
☐ 714.0	ARTHRITIS, RHEUMATOID	☐ 692.9	DERMATITIS	☐ V80.2	LOVASTATIN SCREENING FOR CATARACT	☐ 361.9	RETINAL DETACHMENT
☐ 362.32	B.R.A.O.	☐ 222.2	DERMOID CYST - BENIGN NEOPLASM	☐ 017.0	LUPUS	☐ 362.60	RETINAL DEGENERATION
☐ 362.36	B.R.V.O.	☐ 250.0	DIABETES MELLITUS	☐ 362.5	MACULAR DEGENERATION	☐ 362.81	RETINAL HEMORRHAGE
☐ 351.0	BELLS PALSY	☐ 362.01	DIABETIC RETINOPATHY	☐ 362.57	MACULAR DRUSEN-DEGENERATION	☐ 362.54	RETINAL HOLE
☐ 373.0	BLEPHARITIS	☐ 362.02	DIABETIC RETINOPATHY - PROLIF.	☐ 362.77	MACULAR DRUSEN-HEREDITARY	☐ 361.01	RETINAL TEAR
☐ 374.30	BLEPHAROPTOSIS	☐ 388.2	DIPLOPIA	☐ 371.55	MACULAR DYSTROPHY	☐ 362.18	RETINAL VASCULITIS
☐ 333.81	BLEPHAROSPASM	☐ 375.15	DRY EYE	☐ 362.83	MACULAR EDEMA	☐ 362.74	RETINITIS PIGMENTOSA
☐ 362.31	C.R.A.O.	☐ 374.1	ECTROPION	☐ 362.51	MACULAR HOLE	☐ 362.11	RETINO. HYPERTENSIVE
☐ 362.35	C.R.V.O.	☐ 360.0	ENDOPHTHALMITIS	☐ 371.02	MACULAR SCAR	☐ 362.1	RETINOPATHY - OTHER
☐ 375.53	CAN. STENOSIS	☐ 374.0	ENTROPION	☐ 373.12	MEIBOMITIS	☐ 364.42	RUBEOSIS IRIDIS
☐ 366.9	CATARACT	☐ 375.2	EPIPHORA	☐ 346.8	MIGRAINE - OPHTHALMOPLEGIC	☐ 368.12	SCINTILLAT. SCOTOMA
☐ 362.41	CENTRAL SEROUS RETINOPATHY	☐ 378.41	ESOPHORIA	☐ 346.2	MIGRAINE SYNDROME	☐ 379.0	SCLERITIS/EPISCIERITIS
☐ 373.2	CHALAZION	☐ 378.0	ESOTROPIA	☐ 367.1	MYOPIA	☐ 710.2	SICCA SYNDROME
☐ 363.13	CHORIORETINITIS	☐ 378.42	EXOPHORIA	☐ 375.56	NASOLAC. DUCT OBSTRUCTION	☐ 378.54	SIXTH NERVE PALSY
☐ 363.30	CHORIORETINAL SCARS	☐ 378.10	EXOTROPIA	☐ 224.9	NEOPLASM - BENIGN	☐ 378.9	STRABISMUS
☐ 363.8	CHOROIDAL NEVUS	☐ 216.1	EYELID - BENIGN LESION	☐ 379.50	NYSTAGMUS	☐ 372.72	SUBCONJUNCTIVAL HEMORRHAGE
☐ 372.30	CONJUNCTIVITIS-ALLERGIC	☐ 368.4	FIELD DEFECT	☐ 365.05	OCULAR CONTUSION	☐ 378.52	THIRD NERVE PALSY
☐ 372.03	CONJUNCTIVITIS - BACTERIAL	☐ 930.1	FOREIGN BODY - CONJUNCTIVAL	☐ 695.3	OCULAR ROSACEA	☐ 376.21	THYROID EXOPH.
☐ 372.13	CONJUNCTIVITIS - VERNAL	☐ 930.0	FOREIGN BODY - CORNEAL	☐ 743.42	OPACITY - INTERFERING WITH VISION	☐ 374.05	TRICHIASIS
☐ 224.3	CONJUNCTIVAL - BENIGN NEOPLASM	☐ 378.53	FOURTH NERVE PALSY	☐ 377.1	OPTIC ATROPHY	☐ 364.3	UVEITIS - ANTERIOR
☐ 940.4	CONJUNCTIVAL - BURN	☐ 365.9	GLAUCOMA	☐ 377.21	OPTIC NERVE DRUSEN	☐ 365.00	UVEITIS - ACUTE
☐ 372.75	CONJUNCTIVAL - CYST	☐ 355.11	GLAUCOMA - OPEN ANGLE	☐ 377.30	OPTIC NEURITIS	☐ 364.10	UVEITIS - CHRONIC
☐ 372.9	CONJUNCTIVAL - LESION/MASS	☐ 365.0	GLAUCOMA SUSPECT.	☐ 362.84	OPTIC NEUROPATHY - ISCHEMIC	☐ 363.20	UVEITIS - POSTERIOR
☐ 077.9	CONJUNCTIVITIS - VIRAL	☐ 054.43	H. SIMPLEX KERATITIS	☐ 802.8	ORBITAL FRACTURE	☐ 360.11	UVEITIS DUE TO SURGERY
☐ 918.1	CORNEAL ABRASION	☐ 053.9	H. ZOSTER	☐ 379.91	PAIN AROUND EYE	☐ 368.8	VISION BLURRED
☐ 921.3	CORNEAL CONTUSION	☐ 373.1	HORDEOLUM	☐ 377.00	PAPILLEDEMA	☐ 369.9	VISION LOSS
☐ 371.40	CORNEAL DEGENERATION	☐ 367.0	HYPEROPIA	☐ 368.15	PHOTOPSIA	☐ 379.29	VITREOUS DETACHMENT
☐ 371.10	CORNEAL DEPOSITS	☐ 364.41	HYPHEMA	☐ 360.41	PHTHISIS	☐ 379.24	VITREOUS FLOATERS
						☐ 379.23	VITREOUS HEMORRHAGE

OTHER DIAGNOSES/SYMPTOMS _____

Doctor's Signature _____

RETURN: _____ Days _____ Weeks _____ Months _____ Year

6526

Continued

FIGURE 16.3

A to C, Examples of superbills.

ACCOUNT NO.	AUTHORIZATION NO.	DATE
130,344		

PATIENT NAME — LAST / FIRST

MEDICARE/SOCIAL SECURITY NO.

CONDITION — Illness 1 □ / Injury 2 □ / Pregnancy 3 □

SEX — M □ / F □

BIRTH DATE

PATIENT ADDRESS — STREET / CITY AND STATE / ZIP CODE

TELEPHONE — AREA / NUMBER

GUARANTOR OR SUBSCRIBER — LAST / FIRST

POLICY NO. / GROUP NO. / COVG. CODE

RELATION — Self 1 □ / Spouse 2 □ / Child 3 □

INSURANCE CO. NAME / INSURANCE CO. ADDRESS

HOSPITAL / RECALL DATE / PATIENT REFERRED — DOCTOR / CITY

DIAGNOSIS / CONT. CASE

B

PLACE OF TREATMENT: 1-I.P. Hosp. 2-O.P. Hosp. 3-Office 4-Home 6-Laboratory 7-ECF 8-Nursing Home

DESCRIPTION	Code		Unit Mod	AMOUNT	PT	DESCRIPTION	Code		Unit Mod	AMOUNT	PT
Complex Consultation	01/29	99245				CVP Line	24/51	36491			1
Comprehensive Consultation	03/28	99244				Arterial Line	25/52	36620			1
Intermediate Consultation	0/30	99243				Paracentesis (abd)	26/53	49080			1
Initial Office Visit	04/31	99205			3	Pulmonary Artery Cath.	27/54	93505			1
Initial Office Visit Intermediate	05/32	99204			3	Critical Care Inter.	89	99292			1
Initial Office Visit Limited	06/33	99203			3	Art Line Placement	90	36625			1
Office Visit Intermediate	07/34	99214			3	CV Line Placement	91	36491			1
Office Visit Limited	08/35	99213			3	Pul Line Placement	92	36010			1
Office Visit Extended	09/36	99215			3	Swan Ganz	93	93503			1
Office Visit Re-Examination	10/37	99214			3	Vas Cath		36489			1
Volume Flow Study	11/38	94001			3						
Volume Flow Post Brondl	12/39	94004			3						
Hospital Admit Comprehensive	13/40	99223			1						
Hospital Admit Intermediate	14/41	99222			1						
Hospital Extended	15/42	99233			1						
Hospital Intermediate	16/43	99232			1						
F/U Consultation	17/44	99262			1						
Critical Care		99261			1						
Spirometry	18/45	94010			1						
Endotrachael Intub.	19/46	31500			1						
Laryngoscopy	20/47	31535			1						
Bronchoscopy w. Biopsy	21/48	31625			1						
Thoracentesis	22/49	32000			1						
Needle Biopsy/Pleara	23/50	32420			1						

PAYMENT: □ CASH □ M/C □ VISA

ASSIGNMENT OF BENEFITS: I hereby assign all medical and/or surgical benefits, to include major medical benefits to which I am entitled, including Medicare, private insurance and any other health plans to:

This assignment will remain in effect until revoked by me in writing. A photocopy of this assignment is to be considered as valid as an original. I understand that I am financially responsible for all charges whether or not paid by said insurance. I hereby authorize said assignee to release information necessary to secure the payment.

SIGNED: _____ DATE: _____

FIGURE 16.3, cont'd

Examples of superbills.

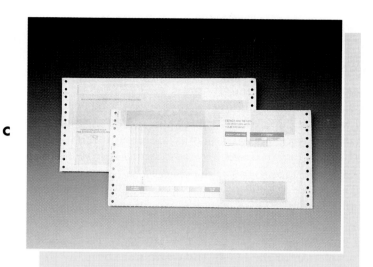

FIGURE 16.3, cont'd

Examples of superbills.

C

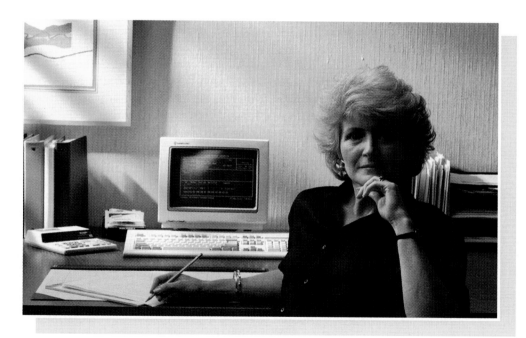

FIGURE 16.4

Because all claims to Medicare and Medicaid programs must be transmitted electronically, it is important to choose a system with this capability.

time consuming to be profitable. Computer systems (Figure 16.4) or services are recognized as an efficient alternative. There are four basic computerized billing services that readily adapt to a medical practice:

- Batch systems
- Full-service systems
- On-line systems
- In-house mini or microprocessors

When a practice uses a computer system, each patient usually is assigned an account number. This number then becomes another element in the transaction data and must be used to process any transaction for that patient.

Batch Systems. The *batch* method of computerized billing involves compiling all new patient information and each day's transactions (charges, payments, plus adjustments, and minus adjustments). The batch may be made up of one copy from the superbill or charge slip of each patient seen during that day. The charge slips are checked against the appointment book or list to see that one has been turned in for each patient seen. These will be clipped together with adding machine tape for all of the charges for the day. An additional group of forms will be used to record all payments and adjustments for the day. Again, these should be clipped together with adding machine tape, totaling all payments and adjustments. When the batch arrives at the computer billing company, a data entry operator will enter the data into the physician-client's data bank. On completion of the batch, the computer company then will generate claim forms, statements, and electronic transmission of claims. The computer company will return to the office the reports as requested by the physician or office manager, usually accounts receivable listing, an alphabetical listing, and a collection listing.

Full-Service System. The *full-service system* of computerized billing involves the same data collection compilation as the batch. Usually with this type of service the service bureau will process all charges, payments, and adjustments and will produce all statements, insurance forms, electronic submission of claims, reports, and recall notices. The practice will be provided with the reports as agreed on with the physician-client. The service bureau will monitor all patient accounts with the patient and/or third-party payer. With this type of system the service bureau follows the account through collection. Sometimes as a result of the physician's type of practice, the service bureau will receive, record, bank, and report all payments to the physician-client. Usually the payments will be received and recorded by the physician's office, with the service bureau receiving a percentage of the collected income for this service. A variation of this might be that the service bureau charges the physician-client by the number of transactions recorded per month.

On-Line Computer System (In-House CRT [Terminal] With Direct Transmission). *On-line computer systems* do not eliminate the need for writing out the transaction data. There must always be a source document, that is, a charge slip or payment record. The office is equipped with a computer terminal. A cathode ray tube (CRT) screen/monitor usually rests above the terminal when not in use. There typically are three pieces of equipment: CRT, keyboard, and modem. Together they look like a typewriter with a small television screen. This is linked to a computer that may be in a building many miles away. There are two methods of connecting the CRT to the computer. One method may be to dial a specific number at the computer center. You will wait to hear a high-pitched tone and then will be linked directly into the main computer. The other method is called *hard wire,* which means that the CRT and the computer are directly connected using a modem, and may be used as needed. No matter which method is utilized, you will need a password to communicate with the computer processing unit. Each physician-client will be provided with a password or a series of passwords. After typing the password, you will be allowed to communicate with the computer. Anything keyed (typed) into the computer usually appears on the screen immediately. This is how each patient transaction is recorded. You also may request to see data previously stored in the computer, and it will appear on screen.

Mini-Microprocessor. The basic equipment of the mini or microprocessor includes the CRT, computer, memory bank, printer, and modem. The printer allows the office to print as needed on paper the data entered into the system. This is considered an in-house system and does not require that there be outside connection by telephone to another computer. However, with the advent of federal requirements that all claims to the Medicare and Medicaid programs be transmitted electronically by 1997, it is important to choose a system that has this capability. To transmit electronically one must have the ANSI programs as specified by the HCFA. Claims are transmitted through the modem into the government intermediary. "Clearinghouses," such as GTE and NEIC, allow transmission of claims for another 93 insurance carriers. Unless the claim is for services that are out of the ordinary (for example, liver, heart, or kidney transplants, which require a report), the claims should be sent through the clearinghouse. Using a clearinghouse saves processing time and expense, plus it saves postage and reduces the amount of time from the usual 30 to 45 days to 17 to 20 days for the carrier to pay the claim.

Billing Considerations

Regardless of the type of billing service used, many considerations need to be taken into account. If you are the medical assistant receptionist, you often will be responsible for obtaining all information needed to complete accurate billing.

Statement Preparation

It is important to the office records and particularly to the patient that the data on the statement be completely accurate. Any error in the information will be upsetting to the patient and will require that office records be corrected. Accuracy must be ensured for all elements of the transaction data but particularly for the procedural code and fee. It also is important that itemization of services provided be precise and easily understood. If the statement is clear, the number of telephone calls to the office requesting explanations will be lessened.

Billing Cycle

Planning and Preparation

Generally, the term *billing cycle* refers to the time lapse between statements. To initiate the cycle you should select the date on which you wish the statement to arrive at the patient's home. Financial consultants frequently suggest that statements arrive 3 to 5 days before the end of the month to take advantage of first-of-the-month paydays. Next, determine the cut-off date. The cut-off date represents the last day of patient transactions that will appear on the statement. Each billing system requires a different number of days to prepare the statements for mailing. If you will be typing 25 statements, a 1-day task, your cut-

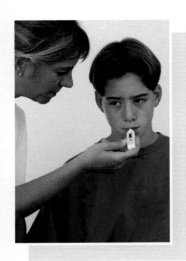

off date will be the day before the statement should arrive. Microfilm and batch computer services usually require 5 days; therefore, the cut-off date will be 5 working days before the delivery date. Depending on the cycle you have chosen and the demands of your billing service, you can plan the advance time needed to prepare or submit the data needed for statements.

Cycles Based on Practice Needs

The once-a-month billing cycle is the one most commonly used in medical practices. Physicians and medical assistants find this system the least disruptive and the most responsive to advance planning.

Intermittent-cycle billing refers to the technique of billing predetermined segments of the account receivable at various times throughout the month. This system usually is used by companies with credit card customers because of the extremely large volume of statements they handle. The account segments usually are decided alphabetically. An office might decide on four billings each month, so that cycle 1 statements would be sent in the first week to patients whose names begin with the letters A through F, cycle 2 statements would be sent in the second week to patients whose names begin with the letters G through L, and so forth.

The major advantage of intermittent-cycle billing is that the income from payments occurs relatively evenly throughout the month. Once-a-month cycles tend to generate the greatest amount of income during the first week after statements are received, and income dwindles down to nothing the week before statements are to be sent. The disadvantage to intermittent-cycle billing is that the medical assistant responsible for the billing system feels constant pressure about meeting deadlines and handling patient financial issues.

Billing Minors or Third-Party Payers

Minors

Billing for services provided to minors requires special attention to certain legal details. You will be expected to make determinations on financial responsibility and appropriate preparation of statements

Determination of Responsible Party. Because a minor cannot legally be held responsible for any financial statement, you must determine at the time of the first visit the person legally responsible for the child. You must remember that this is not always the child's parents; even children with living parents can be in the legal guardianship of another adult. You might pay particular attention to the child who is brought in for care by someone other than the parent. If you are billing an insurance company for the minor, note that many states have implemented the coordination of benefits "birthday rule." Except for cases of dependent children of divorces or separated parents, the rule stipulates that the health plan of the person whose birthday falls earlier in the year (month/day/not year) will pay first and the plan of the other person covering the dependent will be the second payer.

If the persons with the two plans covering the same dependent have the same birthday, then the plan of the person who has had the coverage longer is the primary payer. If either of the two plans has not adopted the birthday rule (that is, if one of the plans is in another state), the rules of the plan without the birthday rule will determine which plan is primary and which is secondary.

Address Statement to Responsible Party. The account and the statement should not be addressed to the minor, even with an "in care of" notation (c/o) naming the responsible party. The appropriate method is to fully address the statement to the responsible party with an "Re:" notation naming the minor.

Separated or Divorced Parents. A legal determination of custody and legal responsibility will have been made in the case of a child of divorced or legally separated parents. The parent with legal custody is responsible for the child's debts. In the event of joint custody, the parents are jointly responsible.

Emancipated Minors. Emancipated minors are individuals who are 16 years of age or older but not yet 18, live outside of their parents' residence, are independent financially, and are legally responsible for the debts they incur.

Third-Party Payers

In some instances an individual or organization will request that a patient be given a special examination or evaluation. The one who requests the service accepts financial responsibility and is termed the *payer.* Because the payer is not the patient or the physician, this person is considered a third party in the arrangement, thus the term *third-party payer.* Some of the organizations or individuals in this classification are discussed in the sections that follow.

Examinations Requested by Insurance Companies. Insurance companies frequently request the services of an independent physician, one unknown to the patient, for an objective evaluation of the patient's health status or a determination of the degree of disability. Individuals who apply for life insurance or who are to be insured as a benefit of their jobs often are given physical examinations that are paid for by the insurance company.

Workers' Compensation. Workers' Compensation cases involve individuals who are injured or acquire an illness in the course of their job. Financial settlements often are determined on the basis of the physician's opinion. Some physicians even limit their practices to Workers' Compensation cases, and their fees are paid by the Workers' Compensation insurance company.

Examinations Requested by Social Services. Some claims for federal disability benefits are made by individuals with complex problems. In an effort to determine the degree of disability, social services agencies may pay a physician for an independent evaluation. This is particularly likely to occur if the claimant disagrees with a previous determination by the agency.

Examinations Ordered by the Court. Numerous cases have occurred, particularly in custody battles, in which one parent is trying to prove that placing the child with the other parent is detrimental to the child's welfare. Thus a judge may order either a physical or psychological evaluation of the child and/or parents. Usually the judge will stipulate who is responsible for payment of the evaluation (Figure 16.5). You then will coordinate billing with the attorney or attorneys for the designated responsible party.

Aging Accounts Receivable
Definition of Aging

Aging is a term applied to the technique of classifying each account with a balance due by the length of time the amount has been owed to the office. Because

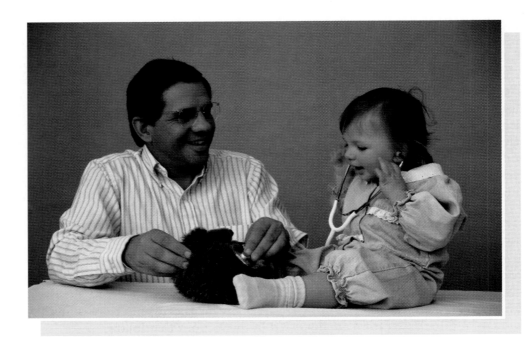

FIGURE 16.5

When the courts order an evaluation of a child, the judge usually will stipulate who is responsible for payment.

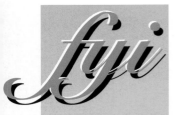

Example of Aging Code

Although colored tabs can be used on the ledger cards to denote 30, 60, 90, or 120 days, you also can use a marking system. An example follows:

S—Superbill given to patient

1—Ledger card copy mailed at 30 days

2—Ledger card copy mailed at 60 days

3—Ledger card copy with letter stating, "We have not received payment" at 90 days

4—Ledger card copy with letter stating, "Your account is overdue" at 120 days

5—Letter stating, "Your account is being turned over to collection" at 5 months

statements usually are sent once a month, the aging segments are stated in terms of 30, 60, 90, and over 90 days, averaging all months out to 30 days each.

The amount on a patient's statement that represents new services provided during the present month are classified as current or "this-month" charges. The day statements are sent to patients for current charges is day 1 or the day aging begins. If the charges have not been paid by the time the next statement is sent, the account is considered 30 days old because the patient has had 30 days in which to pay the fees. Each time statements are sent and the fees have not been paid, the amount ages 30 more days. You might think of it as you do your birthday; you become age 1 by starting to count from the day you were born. A financial account reaches a new category by counting 30 days from the day the statement was first sent.

Reasons for Aging Accounts

Evaluating the Collection System

Separating accounts into aging categories allows you to see at a glance the effectiveness of your collection system. Once each account has been classified and the appropriate dollar amount has been entered in the correct category, you will be able to calculate the total amount due in each aging bracket. You also may determine the percentage each age category represents.

Statistics, in the form of dollar totals and percentages, help you and the physician decide if your collection techniques are working. The largest percentages should be in the current month's charges, next largest in the 30-day

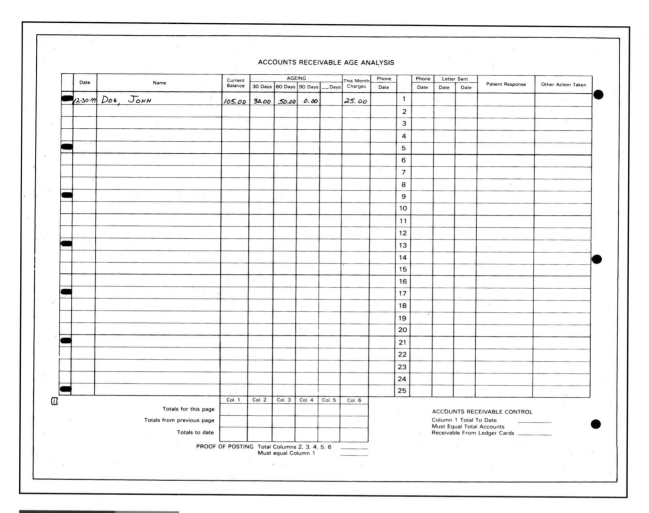

ACCOUNTS RECEIVABLE AGE ANALYSIS

	Date	Name	Current Balance	AGEING				This Month Charges	Phone Date		Phone Date	Letter Sent Date	Date	Patient Response	Other Action Taken	
				30 Days	60 Days	90 Days	__Days									
	12-30-99	Doe, John	105.00	30.00	50.00	0.00		25.00	1							
									2							
									3							
									4							
									5							
									6							
									7							
									8							
									9							
									10							
									11							
									12							
									13							
									14							
									15							
									16							
									17							
									18							
									19							
									20							
									21							
									22							
									23							
									24							
									25							

	Col. 1	Col. 2	Col. 3	Col. 4	Col. 5	Col. 6
Totals for this page						
Totals from previous page						
Totals to date						

PROOF OF POSTING Total Columns 2, 3, 4, 5, 6 _____
Must equal Column 1

ACCOUNTS RECEIVABLE CONTROL
Column 1 Total To Date _____
Must Equal Total Accounts
Receivable From Ledger Cards _____

FIGURE 16.6

Accounts receivable age analysis. (Courtesy Bibbero Systems Inc., Petaluma, Calif.)

category, and so forth; the smallest percentage should be in the "over 90 days" group. Collection experts agree that you can consider it a problem if 10% or more of the accounts receivable are 90 days or older. The office accountant can help you and the physician determine appropriate percentages for each category and make changes in the collection system to improve the situation.

Alerting Personnel

Aging techniques will alert you to the specific accounts that require your attention. Using a form such as the one shown in Figure 16.6 is one method you can use to make this determination easily and note the specific action taken to collect the account.

FIGURE 16.7

Patient account card showing the account aged by hand. (Courtesy Meg Master Systems, St. Louis, Mo.)

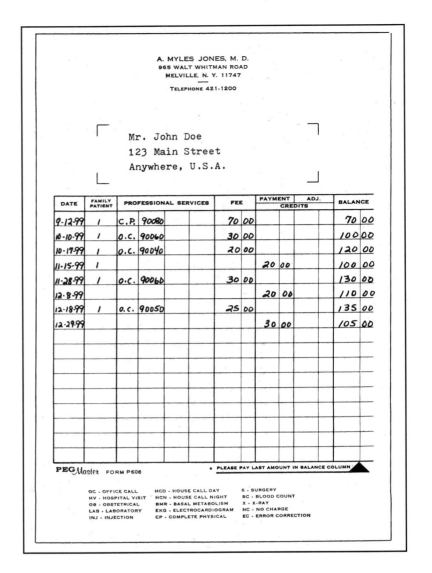

Aging by Hand

If you use an in-office billing system, such as typed statements or ledger cards, you will need to age the accounts by hand. This can be accomplished by using a sheet such as the patient account card shown in Figure 16.7.

As you can see, it is possible for one account to have amounts due in several age categories if charges for services provided in previous months remain unpaid. Figure 16.7 demonstrates how the dollar amounts shown in Figure 16.6 were determined. Any partial payment made is subtracted from the oldest portion of the account. When the $20 was paid on 11/15/99, it was applied toward the $70 debt incurred on 9/12/99, only partially reducing the oldest segment of the account.

To complete the process, you will need to determine the total dollars represented in each column and calculate the percentages they represent. The dollar totals are determined by simply adding together the amounts in each column. The percentages are determined by separately dividing the total of each column by the accounts receivable total.

The formula is as follows:

$$\frac{\text{Age category total}}{\text{All accounts receivable total}} = \text{Category percentage}$$

Example:

$$\frac{\$500}{\$5000} = 10\%$$

In other words, if your accounts receivable total is $5000 and your 90-day-old accounts total is $500, 10% of the total accounts receivable has been overdue from patients for 90 days.

Computer Systems

If you use a computer-assisted billing service, the computer will produce an aging report for you on demand or request. This report is separated from the report of all accounts and may list only those accounts with balances 30 days old or older. If an account has only current amounts due, it usually will be listed as current. The configuration of this report can have many variations depending on the computer system.

Account Age and Collectibility

Experience has shown that the longer an account exists without any payment being made on it, the less likely it is that the account will ever be collected. Some experts believe that if an account reaches 90 days without any payment there is only a 50% chance that any of the money will ever be collected. This will vary depending on the general state of the economy and sometimes the location of the practice. For example, in a town that depends on one industry, a plant strike that suddenly puts everyone out of work will influence the payment of bills. If the decision is between rent and food or the physician's bill, the latter will be ignored. A practice in this environment may want to set a stricter policy on cash at the time of service to prepare for such potential problems. Although such an event represents the extreme, it serves as a reminder of the need for constant attention to the accounts receivable situation.

In addition, everyone is aware that each day a dollar is worth less than it was the day before. Therefore each day that elapses until a bill is paid means that, in the end, less than the amount charged will actually be collected.

In general, accounts should be considered for beginning collection attention at approximately 45 days of aging, before the third statement.

Collection Maintenance
Current Accounts Receivable

The most effective techniques for managing accounts with unpaid balances are to give close attention to each account as each fee is entered and also to make the patient aware of how much owed.

Charge Slips or Superbills

Using a charge slip or a superbill is one method of making patients immediately aware of the fees incurred during a visit. The administrative assistant gives the patient the slip at the end of each visit to hold as a receipt or to submit to their insurance company for reimbursement. Because the slip includes the charges of the day in addition to any outstanding amounts, patients are reminded of the total amount due to the office. Personally receiving the slip from the administrative medical assistant subtly reminds patients that the staff is equally aware of the balance due.

Payment at the Time of Visit

Many offices or facilities request payment at the time services are rendered. This is possible in some types of practices, such as internal medicine, pediatrics, psychiatry, or family practice, in which the fee is predictable. It may not be possible when major fees for services are involved, such as in surgery or orthopedics, and the patient usually cannot be expected to be financially prepared.

If office policy directs you to collect at the time of service, you will need to be diplomatic but direct with the patient. Because the policy will have been described to the patient in an information pamphlet or discussed in advance of the first visit, it will not be a surprise, but it may need reinforcing. It is particularly important if the patient is to be seen only once or is an out-of-town visitor. Some offices post a sign, clearly visible to waiting patients, that states, "Payment is expected at the time service is rendered." Another technique is to remind the patient of the fee when he or she stops at your desk with the superbill that the physician has signed after checking off the appropriate services. After you have calculated the fee from a prepared list corresponding to the service codes, you may return the slip to the patient and simply state, "The charge for today, Ms. Smith, is $20." This message is clear yet professional.

Credit Cards

Credit cards have become a common method of acquiring and paying for goods and services. Some cards, such as Visa, Mastercard, and Discovery, are known as bank cards and can be used for many things. Responding to patient requests and the wish to improve collections, some physicians accept bank cards as a method of payment for services. When the charge slip is sent to the card company, the physician is paid the amount due minus a fee (1% to 3% of the total due) for the card company's services. The card company must then collect the amount due from the person who charged the services. All credit card companies charge the patient interest or finance charges on the amount due.

Billing Patients for Services

In practices in which patients are allowed to accumulate the charges for services and are billed at the end of the cycle, you will need to inform them of the policy associated with this method. Patients must understand that this is an added service and that the account should be paid in full each month.

Although physicians usually are willing to recognize special situations and accept partial payments each month until the account is paid off, usually

10/3/99

Dear Patient:

Effective Jan. 1, 2000, this office will add an interest of $\frac{1}{2}$ of 1% to the balance of all accounts receivable. Although we do not like taking this step, we must do so to cover the costs of maintaining the accounts receivable.

Sincerely,

The business office of
James A. Burdick, M.D.

FIGURE 16.8

Sample letter informing patients that a finance charge will be added to any unpaid balance.

without a finance charge, the practice should not be encouraged. If a finance charge is to be added to the unpaid balance, the patient must be notified in advance, in writing, based on the "Truth In Lending" laws (Figure 16.8).

Some patients feel that it is acceptable to wait for payment from insurance companies and expect you to keep track of their claims. You must explain that help with filing patients' insurance claims is an added service, and that you cannot act as an intermediary between patients and their insurance companies. Doing so could become very time consuming, and some insurance companies feel that your inquiry is a breach of client confidentiality. You may print a simple statement explaining this on the back of the patient's receipt or super-bill.

Collection Techniques
Legal Considerations

When you attempt to collect overdue accounts, you must observe certain legal limitations on your collection methods. These limitations exist to protect the patient. If you must contact debtors at their place of employment because their mail is being returned or their telephone number has been changed without a forwarding number, you must observe extreme caution. If the debtor's calls are screened, you must not reveal to anyone other than the debtor the reason for the call. Merely state your name and ask for the person with whom you need to speak.

If you contact debtors at work, you must respect the fact that they may not have adequate privacy to speak with you (Figure 16.9). When this is obvious to you because of the answers given or you detect an effort to conceal the conversation (such as whispering), you should retreat, and tell the patient you understand but that you must discuss the problem soon. Leave your name and telephone number and firmly but politely state that it is important the call be returned. Persisting in continuing the call when it may jeopardize the patient's privacy or job can result in legal action against the caller for harassment.

FIGURE 16.9

If you call debtors at work, you must respect the fact that they may not have adequate privacy to speak with you.

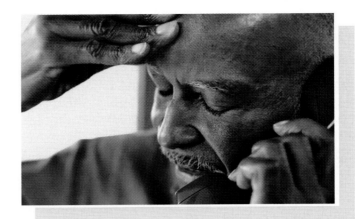

MEDICAL ASSISTING STEP-BY-STEP

Rules for Debt Collection

Although the Fair Debt Collection Practices Act generally does not apply to those not part of the collection industry, it still is a good idea to use the law as your guide.

1. Do not call the debtor before 8 AM or after 9 PM.

2. Do not use improper language.

3. Do not make the debt public knowledge.

4. Do not make threats you do not plan to pursue.

5. Do not call the debtor at work unless necessary.

WHAT DO YOU THINK?

Emily Frank was employed as an administrative medical assistant in a small-town medical office for Doctor James Dogood. The office also was staffed with a nurse practitioner and a clinical medical assistant. It was a busy office, and Emily kept busy with appointments, telephones, and referrals. It was the end of the month, and she had just completed her computerized billing. The computer had printed a list of overdue accounts to contact for collection. She decided to make her collection calls during the lunch break, since the schedule did not give her enough time to do it in the afternoon. The first call was to Jim Boone at his workplace, since it was the only number she had that was correct (his home number had been disconnected). She asked the receptionist if she could speak to Mr. Boone and was told that Jim could not take personal calls. Emily got angry and said that it was imperative that she talk to him immediately. The receptionist asked her the reason for her call, and in her anger Emily said, "A bill." The receptionist put Jim on the phone, who was angry for being contacted at work and told her so. Emily then told him that she was turning him over for collection if he did not pay his bill today, and she hung up on him.

1. What went wrong with this conversation?

2. Did Emily violate the Fair Debt Collection Practices Act?

3. What suggestions would you make to improve this call?

If you must contact the reference sources of patients to locate them, the same considerations apply. Revealing to the reference the reason for calling also is considered a breach of confidentiality.

Collection Goal

The primary goal of account collection policies is to keep the percentage of accounts receivable 60 days and older as low as possible. It also is important to develop collection procedures that will meet this goal in the most tactful and discreet manner and with as little staff time as is possible to perform the task efficiently. Each office uses different specific techniques. You will need to experiment to determine which techniques will work best in your situation. Sometimes a combination of techniques is necessary. It may be impossible for the patient to pay in full, in which case you must be flexible and willing to arrange a payment schedule. Collecting an account in a series of payments is preferable to not collecting it at all. Any collection contact and subsequent information or arrangements should be noted in writing, and the patient should be made aware of the notation. This reinforces your seriousness in following through.

Personal Interview

You may choose to speak to the patient in person as a first attempt to collect an account. This may be possible on a follow-up visit to the office. As always, the discussion should be tactful and diplomatic but factual. You must be certain to conduct the interview in absolute privacy and allow the patient the opportunity to explain any extenuating circumstances. Mutually acceptable payment schedules should be noted in the accounting record, and the patient should be aware of the notation.

The personal interview is time consuming if you have many accounts to deal with. It is dependent on the patient's arrival in the office and contingent on the opportunity for private time with the patient when it is convenient for you. Place a reminder note on the chart so that the opportunity is not forgotten and inadvertently missed.

Telephone

Most collection specialists believe the use of the telephone is the most effective technique in managing the collections system. Because you can approach most patients as you encounter them on your list of telephone calls to make, you remove the element of chance while retaining the advantage of personal contact. Patients often respond more quickly to personal contact than to written notices. The legal considerations of telephone contact have previously been discussed and must be observed.

Written Notices

Personal Notes

Sending a special note to each patient with a delinquent account is costly, particularly in terms of employee time. However, handwritten notes on the statements have proven to be very effective. If an individual letter is written, it

FIGURE 16.10

Example of a collection
notice. (Courtesy De A.
Eggers & Associates,
Sonoma, Calif.)

James J. Jones, M.D.
1234 Any Street, Suite 204
Anytown, KS 87152

(316) 555-1212

M _____ March 1, 1999

_____

We have been as lenient as we can about your delinquent
account; however, we have had no response from you
regarding your balance of _____.
Payment is expected at once. We will consider this your
final notice. If we have not received full and final payment
by _____ the account will be assigned to an outside
agency and record of same placed on your credit file with
national agencies.

should be tactful and direct, requesting that the amount due be paid or that the
patient contact the office to make arrangements. Sign the letter, "Administrative Assistant to Dr. Jones" or your appropriate title below the typed signature.
The tone of personal collections letters should be checked with the physician,
since ultimately the letters represent him or her.

Preprinted Form Letters

Most medical office suppliers can provide you with a five-part series of collection notices that increase in forcefulness of message (Figure 16.10). The most
gentle is used for the first attempt to collect; the last is used when all attempts
have been exhausted and the account is about to be referred to professional bill
collectors. The appropriate notice is sent with the statement from the office or
separately (10 days after the statement) as a reminder.

Messages on Statements

Microfilm and computer billing services can print collection messages directly
on the monthly statements. The possible messages are similar to, but briefer
than, the preprinted cards. The intensity of the message is chosen by a predetermined code that advises the service of the message you want.

Using a Collection Agency

When to Use Collection Agencies

When all in-office collection techniques fail, a decision must be made whether
to refer the account to a collection agency. If a patient indicates a willingness to
pay but there was a temporary hardship, the physician commonly holds the
account pending payment. However, if the debtor has not made any attempt
to contact the office and explain the situation or work out a payment plan, the
account may be turned over to a collection agency.

Responsibility for Agency Actions

Physicians usually wish to be involved in the decision regarding which accounts to turn over for collection and which collection agency to use, because they can be held legally responsible for the techniques used by the agency. Collection agencies or bureaus must observe the same legal restrictions discussed earlier. Therefore it is vital that physicians choose a conscientious and reputable collection agency. Some local medical societies develop their own collection bureaus to assist physicians, because this gives the physicians greater control over collection techniques. Other medical societies will evaluate the local collection bureaus and recommend or endorse one that is determined to be appropriate for handling the particularly delicate accounts associated with medical practices.

Fees Associated with Agencies

All collection agencies charge a fee for collecting delinquent accounts. Until recently it was not uncommon for an agency to retain 50% of the amount collected as its fee. However, agencies found that their high fees prevented many physicians from turning over accounts or caused them to wait until it was really too late to collect anything. To encourage account referrals within a reasonable period, collection agencies have developed various sliding scales or flat rates. A sliding scale means that the larger the dollar value of the account, the lower the percentage retained by the agency. Flat rates are based on the number of accounts referred rather than the dollar amount collected. Collection agencies also may provide what are called *precollection letters* for free. This means that you assign the account for precollection. If the account pays, then all funds are returned to the office with no charge; if the account is not paid within a specified period, then the account is turned directly to straight collection. This has become a very useful tool for the medical office, particularly for accounts with small balances. The precollection letter from the agency is just enough of a nudge to get the patient to pay.

Patient Care after Collection Action

An office policy must be established concerning the future association between patients and physicians after serious collection problems. Most physicians choose between two options: (1) terminating the patient-physician relationship or (2) requiring cash payment at the time the services are rendered.

Special Collection Problems

Disputed Charges

Administrative Medical Assistant's Responsibility

A disputed charge can exist when the patient does not agree with the amount billed or is billed for services not rendered. The latter may occur when you inadvertently post a visit for one patient to the account of another patient. The patient being charged usually will call the error to your attention. You must verify the error and post the visit to the proper account. Regardless of the billing service you use, you should immediately type and send a statement to the patient who should have received the bill. Otherwise an additional 30 days will elapse before the correct patient is billed.

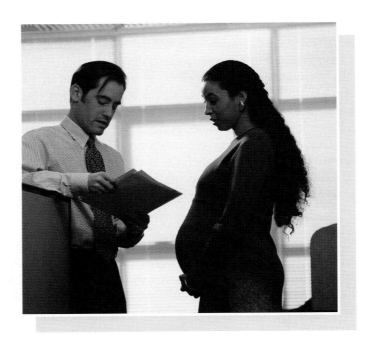

FIGURE 16.11

When it comes to special collection problems, it usually is better for the practice if you act as the patient's emissary with the physician.

Seeking the Physician-Manager's Advice

When the disputed charge is lowered from the amount billed for a service that was performed, the patient usually still believes that the fee is too high. You may attempt to discuss it with the patient and explain that the fee is usual for the area and approximately the amount charged by similar physicians. If you believe that the patient still is uncertain, you can offer to discuss it with the physician for the patient or suggest that the patient speak directly with the physician. It usually is better for the practice if you act as the patient's emissary with the physician (Figure 16.11). Physicians often feel uncomfortable discussing fees and will offer to lower a charge rather than discuss it. If you can privately discuss the issue with the physician, you can evaluate it objectively and without pressure. Each case must be examined separately, and if the patient's request is valid or brought on by inability to pay, you may determine an appropriate adjustment, as directed by the physician.

Medical Society Intervention

If a serious dispute exists, the patient or physician may request an objective determination from the local medical society. Most medical societies have a professional relations committee that will examine all of the pertinent facts, including the physician's records, and make a decision about the charges. The physician must abide if the decision is to reduce the charge.

Claims Against Estates

If an account has an outstanding balance at the time of the patient's death, you must file a claim against the estate to be paid. The form to be filed is called a *creditor's claim* and is merely an itemization of the charges, the total amount due, and the physician's signature. The physician's signature must be notarized, witnessed, and verified by a notary public before the claim is submitted for payment.

Filing a Creditor's Claim

Once a creditor's claim has been completed in triplicate, all the copies must be submitted for payment. A photocopy should be retained in your files. If you know the deceased patient's attorney or estate executor, the claim may be submitted to that person. Otherwise, the claim should be filed with the probate clerk of the county in which the patient lived. This should be done within the time specified by the county.

You will suspend your regular billing of the patient's account but must monitor the amount due from the estate. The executor or county clerk will notify you if funds are available to pay all or part of the claims. If you have not been notified within 60 days, you should inquire and follow up on the claim.

Bankruptcy

Bankruptcy is filed under federal laws when a business or individual has debts that exceed assets. The local division of the federal court will notify you in a legal document when a patient files bankruptcy under either Chapter 11 or Chapter 13 of the bankruptcy laws. Both attempt to reorganize and settle the filer's debts, but Chapter 13 protects a wage earner by preventing claimants from putting a lien on the wages. Putting a lien on the wages would defeat the purpose of reorganization, which is to evaluate all of the debtor's assets and, if possible, prepare a schedule to pay off the existing debts. Wages are considered part of the assets.

When you are notified of bankruptcy proceedings, you are advised of the amount the debtor claims to owe the physician. If you agree with the amount, you simply await the court's decision. If not, you must appear at the hearing or submit a notarized document itemizing the charges and balance due. In either case, you must immediately suspend direct billing of the patient and await the court decision. A physician's bill represents an unsecured debt (that is, one not backed by a specific asset) and it often is dismissed. If it is paid, payment may be at a nominal monthly rate, and it may take years to settle the account. Because you must accept the court's decision, you cannot collect by any other means, and you do not have to bear the cost of billing services, you should view these payments as better than the alternative of writing off the whole account.

Options to Sue

Small Claims Court

If all billing and collections methods have been conducted properly, the patient exhibits no intention to pay the debt, and you cannot determine any extenuating circumstances for nonpayment, the physician may consider filing a suit in small claims court to recover the money. Small claims courts are for claims of a limited amount, currently less than $5000. The limit changes periodically to remain in proportion to the cost of living. It usually is sufficient to cover a physician's claim.

The advantage of a small claims suit is the elimination of legal fees. The physician and the debtor state their own cases to a judge, who makes a decision and notifies each party of the binding court order within a short time. The physician often wins these suits.

Attorney-Directed Suit

Physicians rarely resort to a civil lawsuit handled by an attorney to collect any outstanding debt. This type of suit is very costly, often costing more than the

When it comes to a civil lawsuit, in every case the physician must consider the value of the amount to be collected in relation to the cost of collecting it.

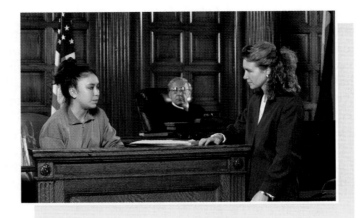

debt that is owed, and not worth the time necessary to complete the process. On occasion, physicians will have their attorneys write a letter to try to collect a debt. This may be effective, since it implies that further legal action is possible, and a letter will definitely cost less than a lawsuit. In every case, however, the physician must consider the value of the amount to be collected in relation to the cost of collecting it (Figure 16.12). If there is little to gain, the account might best be written off the accounts receivable records as a bad debt, that is, uncollectible.

Loss of Accounts Receivable Records

The details of accounts receivable are vital to the financial survival of a medical office or agency. If you utilize microfilm, an outside computer billing service, or an in-house computer system that has back-up tapes kept off premises or out of the office, and the records are lost, you can reconstruct the accounts, aging, and total due. If other billing methods are used and no copies of the records exist outside of the office, the loss of the accounts receivable data could be devastating. Because loss by fire or flood is possible, although unlikely, insurance premiums are paid on the average accounts receivable. You will need to report the accounts receivable amount monthly during the first year of the insurance policy so that the company can determine an appropriate premium rate.

The insurance carrier may require the logical precaution of storage in a closed, insulated metal cabinet and proof that security was observed if a claim is made. You will need to develop the habit of always returning the records to the storage area each evening before closing time.

Conclusion

Every aspect of billing and collection—from acquiring data necessary to produce a bill through explaining policy, charges, and managing special problems—requires your attention, tact, and understanding of available services. Special attention should be paid to the ever-changing laws that are designed to protect the rights of consumers and providers of services.

Review QUESTIONS

1. What are accounts receivable? What must you do to manage these accounts?

2. List and describe the minimum information necessary to establish a patient's account; list the information you or the physician must supply.

3. What billing service can you use in your office to produce bills to patients? How does each one work?

4. What should you keep in mind when preparing statements and when selecting a billing cycle?

5. What is different about billing minors and third-party payers? Where should the bills be sent for each?

6. How does a credit and collection policy help you in your work? How can you inform patients of these policies?

7. List and describe the four methods of collecting current accounts receivable. What could you say to encourage a patient to pay at the time of the visit?

8. What is accounts receivable aging, and how is it done by hand? Determine the age of the account entries as of 10-15-99 if the following visits were posted: 7-12-99, $40; 7-18-99, $25; 8-22-99, $25; 9-8-99, $20; and 10-12-99, $25; and charges were $40 on 8-15-99 and $20 on 9-8-99.

9. When should you become concerned with the age of an account?

10. What legal considerations should you keep in mind when attempting to collect an overdue account? State and describe the five methods.

11. What are your responsibilities when a charge is disputed, when the debtor dies, and when the debtor files bankruptcy?

SUGGESTED READINGS

PMIC: *Reimbursement manual for the medical office,* 1995, Salt Lake City, Majors.
PMIC: *Physician fees,* 1995, Salt Lake City, Matthew.
MedIndex: *Reimbursement strategies,* 1995, Salt Lake City, Matthew.
McGraw-Hill: *Managing reimbursement in the 90's;* 1989, McGraw-Hill.

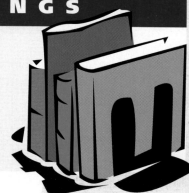

Basic Computer Use in the Medical Practice

On completion of Chapter 17 the administrative medical assistant student should be able to:

1 Define the key terms listed in this chapter.

2 List and describe key components of a computer and its system unit.

3 Describe the purpose and functions of a computer network.

4 Describe three basic types of application software used most often by medical offices.

5 Describe the hierarchical method for storing information and software within a computer.

K E Y   T E R M S

Applications	Individual programs, such as word processing or a spreadsheet, run on a computer.
Batch system	System in which patient information, registration, charges, payments, and adjustments are forwarded to a centralized service bureau that then provides the data entry and reports as requested.
CD-ROM drive	Component that enables computer to gain access to and use information available on a compact disk.
Central processing unit (CPU)	The "brain" of a computer; controls and coordinates the functions of all other components and processes information
Database program	Software designed to store and categorize large amounts of similar information.
Disk operating system (DOS)	Software language that allows the computer to perform basic functions.
Hard disk drive	Feature that holds the computer's internal memory and can store a vast amount of information within the computer on a permanent basis, including both application and data storage.
Keyboard	Letter and number pad similar to that of a typewriter and calculator combined that enables the user to input data and interact with the computer by typing in information or hitting special function keys.
Laptop computer	Portable personal computer.
Mainframe computer	Automated machine system capable of manipulating, maintaining, and storing large amounts of information. Largest of all computers; normally used in large facilities.
Microcomputer	Desktop computer, originally designed as a personal computer (PC).
Minicomputer	Computer with larger storage capacity than the microcomputer but much less bulky than the mainframe computer.

Continued

K E Y   T E R M S

(Continued)

Modem	Device that converts data for transmission to the data processing equipment, usually from a telephone; the term comes by merging the terms *modulator* and *demodulator.*
Monitor	Component similar to a television screen that allows the user to see what is occurring within the system at any given time.
Mouse	Device used to enter information into a computer by clicking on information or commands displayed on the monitor screen as well as selecting and moving data on screen; usually used in conjunction with the keyboard.
Network	Two or more computers connected either with special wiring or with telephone lines.
On-line service	System in which a practice inputs and transmits data from its computer via modem to the service bureau's computer system, which then handles printing and other requested services.
Random access memory (RAM)	Device that holds information temporarily for the applications being run; the individual applications are loaded into the RAM from the long-term storage device.
Removable media disk drive	Device that enables large amounts of information to be moved to and from the computer's hard drive from "floppy" (removable) disks or tape.
Scanner	Automated machine that "reads" and enters information from a document into the computer to prevent the need for typing large amounts of data; also can be used to copy images into the computer.
Spreadsheet	Financial software program.
System software	Information used by the CPU to control the basic functions of the computer.
System unit	Heart of the computer, consisting of all the basic parts of the machine itself, including the central processing unit, random access memory, hard drive, removable media disk drive, and connectors.
Word processing	Software program that allows the user to type and format documents.

*D*enise is an administrative medical assistant in a small, private pediatric office. One Tuesday morning, she has barely begun her usual routine when her employer, Dr. Jane Amata, asks her to write a letter to Ms. Hart about her daughter, Jill. The letter looks something like this:

Dear Ms. Hart:

After reviewing your daughter Jill's files, we are pleased to tell you that her routine care seems current, and we hope that Jill continues to exhibit such good health! In order to ensure that Jill remains healthy, we want to remind you that, as Dr. Amata said at your daughter's last checkup, Jill will need her third hepatitis vaccine sometime between now and November 22 to keep her immunization record up to date. Please call us any time it is convenient for you, and we will help you set up Jill's appointment at your convenience.

Sincerely,

Dr. Jane Amata
and the Hillside staff

Thanks to the clinic's computer, Denise is able to type this letter much faster than she could have using the clinic's old electric typewriter. First, of course, it is easier to correct her typos and other errors with the simple tap of a few keys. This not only makes Denise a faster typist than she was on the conventional typewriter, but also it makes every letter Denise types into an unblemished, perfect copy-no more slow, tedious, or messy corrections. Second, copies are as perfect as the original and can be made without the use of carbons. Third, copies can be stored in a much smaller space electronically (within the computer) or on a floppy disk than if she had to store them as a printed sheet of paper (the "hard" copy). And because a perfect copy is always available, once made, this letter can be used again and again; Denise has only to change the name and address of the patient, the dates, and any other details, rather than writing each letter from scratch. Each version of the original can be saved in a separate file. But, best of all, when Denise is finished, the program that helped her write her letter can be "stored" or put away within her computer, enabling her to use the computer for other things, such as patient scheduling programs, spreadsheets, billing programs, and database programs.

Types of Computers

Most physicians' offices today use computers. They are not only unavoidable, they are essential. If you are unfamiliar with computers—or even if you've always considered yourself a "computer-phobe"—once you've had the experience of doing the same job both with and without a computer, you'll no doubt change your mind. A computer makes all the difference in accomplishing any

FIGURE 17.1

Most physicians' offices today use computers for multiple tasks. A computer makes all the difference in accomplishing any task with greater speed and accuracy.

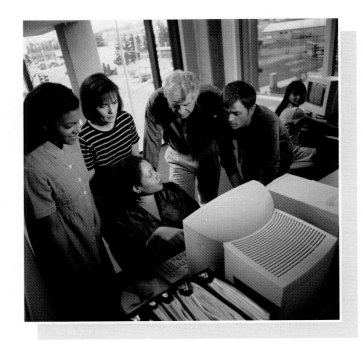

task with both maximum speed and accuracy (Figure 17.1). Billing becomes simpler and correspondence and storage become nearly instantaneous compared with the alternative. Just a few of the reasons for electing to computerize the office include the following:

- Office efficiency is increased
- Overall cost is lower than with manual processing of information
- Better management control and more current information will be available
- The physician may expand the practice more conveniently
- Collections may be improved
- Records are more secure

Contrary to what the uninitiated might assume, the type of computer system used will depend on the type of applications software needed. Choosing the software first provides the information necessary to select the type of computer, speed, and memory needed.

Mainframe Computers

Within the medical and allied health fields, mainframe computers—the largest of all computers—are normally used in large facilities such as hospitals, centralized clinics operating with several outlying clinics, research institutes, and universities. These very large computers are capable of manipulating, maintaining, and storing large amounts of information. Normally, this type of computer is placed in temperature- and humidity-controlled environments.

AT WORK TODAY

Computer Literacy

The computers that existed 45 years ago were enormous and expensive. They were used for science and military purposes, so most people did not expect to use them or even touch them.

The world has sped on at such a rate that almost every aspect of our lives is touched somehow by the computer. Think about it!

One day last week:

- You made travel arrangements
- You bought gasoline for your car
- You received a traffic ticket

- You went to the clinic for a tetanus injection
- You received your paycheck
- You went grocery shopping

This does not take into account the work world, which uses the computer in different ways every day to make everything more efficient. Computers have become an everyday working tool just like reading and writing, so we need to be able to operate a computer to keep up with the "Information Age" in which we live.

Laptop, Notebook, and Palmtop Computers

If mainframes are the largest computers, laptop, notebook, and palmtop computers are surely among the smallest. These computers act as portable personal computers (PC). Because they are lightweight and easy to carry (all three can fit into a briefcase—in some cases, at the same time), these computers are meant for traveling either long distances or to local meetings or seminars, and make it possible for the physician to take copies of certain kinds of files home or on trips. Laptops, in particular, are popular both because their keyboards, though considerably smaller, still feel similar to that of a PC keyboard and because they have as much power and as many options as the microcomputer. Some users have talked about the adjustments that must be made for the much smaller keys on the notebooks and palmtops.

Microcomputers

The microcomputer is a desktop computer. Although it originally was designed as a PC, today its widely expanded uses and user-friendly applications have made it very popular and accessible for a multitude of business applications, including the medical office. A great advantage is the PC's accessibility to networks and popular business-application software packages.

Minicomputers

Minicomputers frequently are found in health care facilities, since they normally have larger storage capacities than the popular, smaller microcomputers. They also have the advantage of multilocation terminals, although networking is quickly beginning to close the gap between the capabilities of mini- and microcomputers.

The vast majority of medical offices use either minicomputers or microcomputers (PCs). The two most popular types of microcomputers are

FIGURE 17.2

A computer is not a single entity but is actually made up of numerous components, each with a specific function.

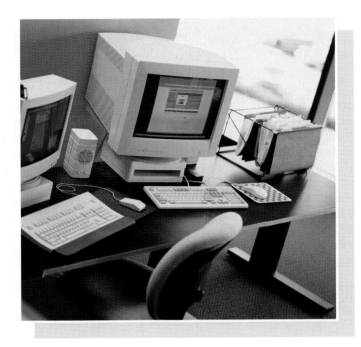

IBM-compatible computers and Macintosh computers. The application software for each type of computer is similar. In addition, your PC may or may not be networked to other computers.

In this chapter, we will examine a computer system most typical of the kind you may encounter in any medical office practice. This information may vary slightly, depending on the type of computer and software chosen, but the basic concepts are the same.

Basic Components of the Computer

New users may think a computer is a single entity, but it is actually made up of numerous components, each with a specific function (Figure 17.2). These components usually include the following: system unit, keyboard and mouse, monitor, printer, and removable storage devices. System software is needed to control the basic functions of the computer, and application software consists of the various programs used. Finally, many basic computer systems often are supplemented by such optional features as a scanner and modem.

System Unit

The system unit sometimes is referred to as the heart of the computer. This unit consists of all the basic parts of the machine itself—many of which you as a user will never see. The system unit can be broken down into the central processing unit, random access memory, hard drive, and removable media disk drive. Many system units also provide a CD-ROM drive.

ffyi

Basic Computer Organization

Input
- Keyboards
- Floppy disk
- Tape
- CD-ROM

Central Processing Unit
- Information stored here to make computer operate—usually connected with hard drive for storage

Output
- Monitor
- Printer
- Modem

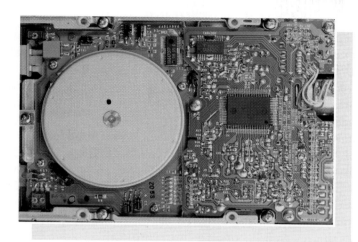

FIGURE 17.3

Hard drives can permanently store both application and data information within the computer.

Central Processing Unit (CPU)

The central processing unit (CPU) is really the "brain" of the computer. It controls all of the other components and processes information; it coordinates the functions of all parts. It is here that computations and words are processed. The *disk operating system (DOS)* refers to a software language that allows the computer to perform basic functions. DOS is dependent on specific microprocessors, and it is important to know which type of processor a system is using.

Random Access Memory (RAM)

This feature holds information temporarily for the *applications,* that is, the individual programs you want to run, such as word processing or a spreadsheet. Applications and databases are loaded into the RAM when needed from the storage device. The CPU gathers the information and codes it needs from the RAM. For instance, in the case scenario given at the beginning of this chapter, Denise needed to type a letter so she "loaded" or "opened" her computer's word processing program. Her computer stored this information within the RAM for quicker use. In this way, the RAM speeds things up. Once a program is loaded, all the tools needed to run that program are at hand-just as some of a physician's examination room equipment is set out for easy access, while unneeded instruments and supplies are stored in drawers and cabinets.

Many times a medical practice will grow, necessitating additional RAM for the system; RAM can be purchased and loaded easily.

Hard Drive

The hard disk drive, or hard drive, holds the computer's internal memory and can store a vast amount of information within the computer permanently; this includes both (1) *application* and (2) *data storage* (Figure 17.3). For instance, when Denise has finished writing her letter to Jill's mother, the word processing program (the application) is "put away" or stored on the hard drive, usually in an "applications folder" with other application software she uses. The contents of her letter also are stored, if Denise saves the letter, in a folder she has designated within data storage. Folders in data storage are set up by the user (in this case, Denise or the office manager) in much the same way as a regular filing system is set up. Only the user knows what names should be assigned to each folder and how those folders should be subdivided into other folders, to best fit the office's organizational needs. Then, each time a user saves a letter or spreadsheet or computerized bill, it becomes a file. The first time Denise saves that letter, the computer will help her assign it to a specific folder, creating that folder for her if she needs one. After that, this letter is automatically stored in the appropriate folder until the next time Denise needs it.

For instance, suppose that Denise has a correspondence file just for Jill Hart herself. Denise could create a folder called, "Hart, Jill"; this folder would in turn probably be stored in a larger folder titled, "Patient Correspondence"; or perhaps Denise's office keeps a general "Correspondence" folder, with a subdivision titled, "Patients." All of these folders are stored, stacked according to the hierarchy Denise has assigned them, within the hard drive. When Denise saves this letter, it becomes a "file" within Jill's folder. Denise may want to name the file "hepatitis notice" (or, in some PC systems, a shorter name, followed by the characters ".doc"). Or, as an alternative, she may choose to name each letter file according to the date it was written or sent. Naturally, a hard copy of this letter can also be printed out and stored in Jill's regular patient files.

But suppose further that Dr. Amata has a separate computer folder titled, "Immunizations," in which she is keeping track of immunizations given within her practice and charting the most effective means of engaging parents to be involved in keeping their children's immunizations up to date. How will Denise decide whether the file "hepatitis notice" should be filed under "Hart, Jill" or "Immunizations"? The answer is simple. Hard drives enable the user to store the same letter in more than one place every time the user gives it a new file name and places it in another folder.

Removable Media Disk Drive

It does not take long for a hard drive to get "full," as its storage space is filled up with new files, especially in a busy office that uses its computer for various applications and functions. That is why so much important information will need to be stored on "floppy," or removable, disks (or on tape). This is the function of the removable media disk drive. Denise can move immense amounts of information onto floppy disks to be carefully labeled and stored outside the computer's hard drive. In addition, if the office has more than one computer but these computers are not connected, Denise can move information from one computer to another by "copying" it onto a disk and then copying it a second time from the disk to the second computer's hard drive.

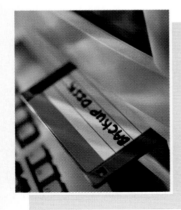

However, floppy disks do more than serve as excess storage sites or move files between computers. In any office, but especially in a medical practice, it is essential to maintain duplicate information storage outside the hard drive, in case the computer itself breaks down and its files are lost or damaged. The removable media disk drive does the work of copying files onto floppy disks while retaining the information, if desired, on the hard drive as well. As a safety precaution, information from the computer should be periodically stored on a larger *backup tape* to ensure that a complete, updated backup of the entire system exists for safekeeping. All backup information that is absolutely critical should be done each evening and removed to a safe deposit box away from the office site.

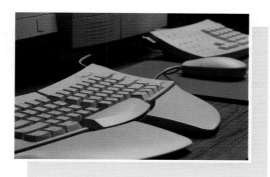

FIGURE 17.4

Computer keyboards have been altered to be more ergonomic. That is, they have been modified to provide minimal damage to the computer user.

CD-ROM Drive (Optional)

Until fairly recently, whenever a computer user purchased new application software, it came on a set of floppy disks. From these, the information was installed on the computer's hard drive for permanent storage and use. Now, however, even larger amounts of information can be stored on CD-ROM disks. As with the floppy disks, CD-ROM disks also are used to move information onto a computer. These disks have one important difference from the older "floppies": without special equipment the user cannot "write" or "copy" information *onto* these disks. This is easy to realize when comparing these CD disks with music CDs. So far, the music industry has not provided CDs that can be recorded over, while the older cassette tapes do have this capacity.

Keyboard and Mouse

The keyboard and mouse need little explanation. A computer *keyboard* is used both to communicate data into the system and to interact with the computer itself and its software by typing in information. Computer keyboards are set up much the same as that seen on typewriters, but with the addition of a 10-key number pad (which parallels that of an adding machine or calculator), as well as a series of function keys that streamline the commands made directly to the computer or a specific application program. Some of these function keys may be programmable in that they can be set by the user to perform specific functions.

Over the years, as the medical field has encountered more and more cases of carpal tunnel syndrome among typists and computer users, computer keyboards have been altered to be more ergonomic. That is, they have been modified to provide minimal damage to the computer user. Figure 17.4 is an example of one of today's new ergonomic keyboards. Obviously, this is a modification not yet achieved with typewriters and adding machines!

Some computers also make use of a *mouse,* a device used to enter information by clicking on information or commands displayed on the monitor, as well as selecting (highlighting) information seen there. A mouse makes it even easier to drag, move, copy, cut, and paste large sections of material, often in conjunction with the keyboard's use. This function has streamlined a number of medical office functions tremendously.

Monitor

Computer *monitors* communicate to the user exactly what is going on within the computer, allowing the user to see the immediate consequences of each interaction with the keyboard and mouse. Some computer screens provide full color, which can be handy when creating finance charts. Others can be swiveled to create either a horizontal or vertical display. This can be very helpful when working with spreadsheets or designing an office brochure—or even for providing more comfort to the user. Sometimes a vertical monitor is more ergonomic for the user than a horizontal one.

Printer

While not absolutely essential to the function and use of a computer, *printers,* like most monitors, are purchased separately. Unlike monitors, however, they are not essential for interacting with a PC system. At the same time, nearly every office that uses a PC system also uses a printer. And if you are producing spreadsheets or correspondence, eventually you are going to want a printer along the way, either to mail out correspondence or to print out financial information for meeting or tax purposes.

Printers come in a wide array of types and costs, ranging from the very simple dot matrix machines to state-of-the-art laser printers capable of producing camera-ready page quality. For the most part, routine reports can be produced on dot matrix printers, but high-speed, letter-quality printers are recommended, when affordable, for outside correspondence and more formal reports. This is because laser printers can print up to 600 or more lines per minute. They not only are faster and quieter than dot matrix printers but also they produce much higher-quality type. However, they are more expensive than dot matrix printers. Nonetheless, they are almost always the printer of choice for service bureaus or larger facilities.

Removable Storage Devices

Removable storage devices (floppy disks and CD-ROM disks) are essential for storage outside a computer. Removable media hold information just like a hard drive does, but the floppy disk can easily be physically removed and taken to another location or computer. Again, the importance of a daily backup, with a full system backup each week, cannot be overemphasized. If the backup procedure with disks and tapes seems cumbersome or time-consuming, consider the fact that even though these steps take time, the task of rekeying in all lost information in case of malfunction or damage far outweighs the time it takes to make a backup. Remember, too, that CD-ROM disks also serve a storage function, but without special equipment, information cannot be saved, copied, or written to these disks (Figure 17.5).

System Software

Finally, let's return for a moment to what we have said is the "brain" of the computer—the central processing unit. Just as our brains control almost all of our other components and functions, they also need information or knowledge with which to be able to function at higher levels. Similarly, the CPU needs information to act on—this information is the *system software.* The system software controls the basic functions of the computer, in conjunction with the CPU. The average user does not need to know much about this system software.

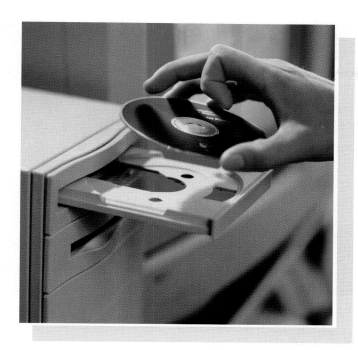

FIGURE 17.5

Large amounts of information can be stored on CD-ROM disks, but without special equipment, the user cannot "write" or "copy" information onto these disks.

Additional Hardware

Now that we are familiar with the basic components of a PC system, there are several other items frequently used in businesses and in some medical practices as well.

Scanner

Besides using a keyboard, another way users sometimes enter information into a computer is by using a *scanner*, although this is less common in the average office setting. A scanner is most useful to a medical practice if a large document or numerous documents are acquired by the office and would have to be typed in by hand because no disk is available that contains this same information. In such an instance, a scanner can be used to "read" and enter the information from paper.

Modem

The birth of the so-called information highway has brought the function of the *modem* to the fore. Adapted by merging the terms *modulator* and *demodulator*, the word *modem* refers to a device that can convert data for transmission to the data processing equipment, usually from a telephone. The modem connects a computer through telephone lines to other computers. A modem also can connect your computer to information services, such as America Online and Compuserve, or, through an Internet service provider, it enables you to access and communicate on the Internet and the World Wide Web.

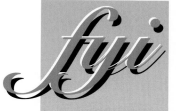

Computer Hardware vs. Software vs. Storage

Hardware comprises the "hard" pieces of your computer. It consists of your central processing unit, that is, your hard drive and the peripherals, which are the monitor, printer, modem, CD-ROM drive, tape drive, scanner, and so on.

Software refers to your computer's operating systems, such as Windows or DOS, and the applications, which are the different programs (for example, Word Perfect, Word, Excel, and Medisoft) that you operate on the computer.

Storage refers to saving information and is accomplished using the hard drive, magnetic tapes, and "floppy" disks.

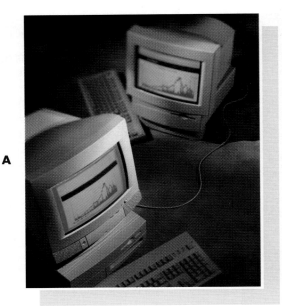
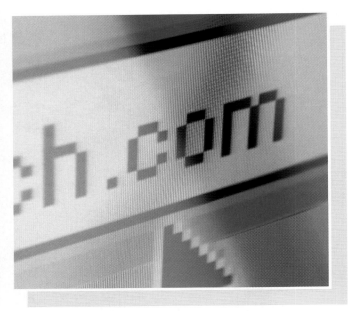

A

B

FIGURE 17.6

Networking can be done via modem from one computer to another (A) or over the Internet (B).

Computer Networks

Often two or more computers may be connected to form a *network*. These computers may be in close proximity to each other and connected with special wiring, or they may be physically distant and connected over telephone lines (Figure 17.6). In either case, being part of a network allows two or more computers to share the same information, resources, and printers, and increase productivity. Networking computers requires special hardware and software. It also requires special knowledge to install and maintain a network, and this usually is provided by a networking consultant. Still, it is worth this initial effort and investment because computer networks are now almost a must in a large medical practice.

Computer Service Systems

An in-house or office computer system is made up of equipment—hardware, software, documentation, and data—that together perform an important task. These components can be purchased or leased. If a medical practice purchases its own equipment, it will purchase software as well, products on floppy disk or CD that are designed to make a task easier. Sometimes, however, rather than the equipment itself, computer *services* are purchased from a service bureau; this enables the practice to avoid the expense and extra work of setting up and operating its own computer system. These out-of-office services generally fall into four types: batch systems, on-line time sharing, on-line service, or full service.

Batch System

Using a batch system, patient information, registration, charges, payments, and adjustments are forwarded to the service bureau daily or weekly. The service bureau provides the data entry and reports as requested.

On-Line Time Sharing

With this type of service, the practice may have one or more monitors connected directly to the service bureau's computers. The service bureau may lease out time or provide service to any number of customers; thus, the computer is not always available when needed. Usually the service bureau prints reports to be submitted to the office. However, some bureaus may provide printers for the practice.

On-Line Service

Using an on-line service, the practice inputs and transmits data from its computer via modem to the service bureau's computer system. The service bureau then handles the printing of all reports, statements, and anything else provided for in the contract. Again, with this type of service, the practice may or may not be provided with a printer.

Full Service

With a full-service contract, the service bureau receives data either daily or weekly and then provides most of the computer service to the practice. The service bureau provides all of the data entry, sends out all statements, produces all electronic data interchange (EDI) transmissions, produces forms and reports as required by the agreement, and processes all payments and adjustments. With full service, the service bureau then continues to monitor payments from patients, insurance carriers, and other third parties. The service bureau also will provide a certain number of collection procedures before sending the account to a collection agency.

Application Software

As we have seen, computers in a medical office are intended to make certain tasks much easier, more accurate, and more secure. However, the computer alone will not be able to satisfy all these tasks; that's why an almost unlimited variety of software is available to provide the inner workings that equip your computer for these specialized functions. In the scenario at the opening of this chapter, we saw Denise make use of a word processing program, a type of *software* used for writing and formatting documents. This word processing program is just one type of application software popular in most offices, including medical offices that own their own computer equipment.

How are software programs chosen? Asking the following questions should help the buyer cover the most important considerations once the software is in place.

- How compatible will this product be with our other programs?
- Do we need additional software or hardware to integrate more than one system?
- How available are, and what are the fees for, updates and enhancements?
- Do we need a license, and are there fees for this license?
- Is user training available, and if so, how much does it cost?
- How useful are the user manuals?
- Is there a customer service number? When is it available?

There are three main types of computer applications: word processing, spreadsheet, and database programs. Among the most likely applications are billing/accounts receivable, appointment scheduling, payroll, accounts payable, general ledger, word processing, medical records, EDI, patient reporting systems, and on-line systems. The particular applications you use will probably already have been selected, purchased, and installed on the computer for you.

Word Processing

Word processing programs allow the user to type and format documents. The most common examples would be the letter Denise wrote to Jill Hart's mother, or a report required by your physician's larger affiliations, or a research abstract your employer wishes to present at a medical convention. The most popular word processing programs on PCs are *Microsoft Word* and *WordPerfect*, though many others are available as well.

Spreadsheets

Spreadsheet programs are most often used for financial applications. Basic bookkeeping may be done using a spreadsheet program, although there are many new application programs that make basic financial tasks easier. *Lotus 1-2-3* and *Excel* are the most well-known spreadsheet programs.

Database Programs

Database programs are designed to store and categorize large amounts of similar information; they are at the heart of most computer applications used in a medical office. Customized applications in this category of application software are used for scheduling, patient records, billing systems, and others (Figure 17.7).

Billing Systems

Many offices now use computerized billing software. Although somewhat expensive, the time these systems save in both job performance and accuracy, and the storage space and security they provide, can certainly make it well worth the initial cost. Numerous products are on the market, depending on the type and brand of hardware you have.

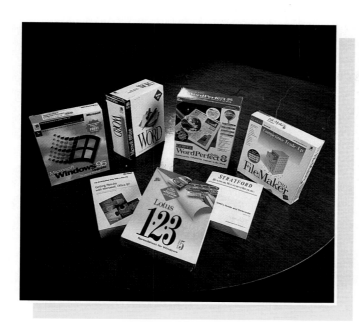

FIGURE 17.7

Three main types of computer application products are available: word processing, spreadsheets, and database programs.

Even more impressive is the fact that some of these products are made just for the health care market and are tailored to their needs. Some even specialize in meeting the needs of very specific kinds of health care services, such as dental, laboratory, or medical accounts receivable. For the purposes of this text, we have focused on one specific product, *Stratford Healthcare Management System.*

An Example—*Stratford Healthcare Management and EDI Software*

Although there are numerous billing software programs on the market, an advantage to incorporating information about *Stratford Healthcare Management System (SHS)* in this text is its flexibility for this text's purposes (Figure 17.8). *Stratford* can be adapted for a variety of health care settings beyond the physician's office and includes features that can be tailored to the needs of professional billing services, dentists, laboratories, anesthesiologists, and durable medical equipment suppliers (DMEs). It also can be applied in special facilities such as hospitals, dialysis units, and surgicenters.

Features. Included in the *Stratford* and similar products you may expect to find patient statements, day sheets, end-of-month reports, and collection reports. Many also have network capabilities that enable the program to have multiple users on various computers within a single facility.

In addition, more specialized products like *Stratford* may include electronic data interchange capabilities for most states, enabling easier compliance with specific government agency requirements. For instance, *Stratford* provides electronic data interchange for Medicare for all states and for Medicaid in most states. Another specialized feature is its use of specific diagnosis and procedural codes, and standard insurance forms including: HCFA-1500, HCFA-1450, PM160, and Doctor's First Report.

In addition to the statements, day sheets, and reports you might expect to find in any billing system, some of the more specialized products, including *Stratford,* include collection letter forms, patient recalls, and production reports

FIGURE 17.8

Patient billing is far more complex than it used to be, but software packages such as the *Stratford Healthcare Management System* billing system make it simpler and more accurate.

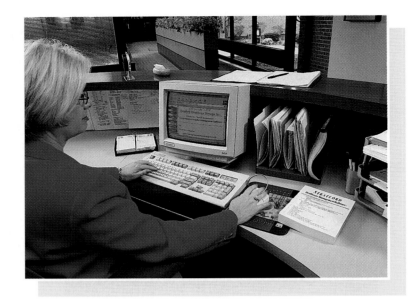

(by both provider and procedure). Finally, *Stratford* also enables the user to do specialized activities such as creating and printing insurance forms and creating an automatic transaction library; an automatic transaction library sets up special codes that let you eliminate all repetitive typing. Other features include: automatically pricing differently for different financial classes, creating a wide variety of statements, generating and monitoring a wide variety of business financial reports, customizing reports, generating recalls and service charges, batch processing and appointment scheduling, creating and monitoring statistics in various categories, and three methods for entering facility transactions.

Use. Naturally, the purpose of these software systems is to make billing easier. For that reason, once you have become familiar with computer use in general you should find that a well-written software package should be easy to follow. Pop-up screens like the kind encountered in the *Stratford* make it easy to get around.

Think of a software product as a hierarchy similar to that we have already described for computers. Earlier in this chapter we described a computer and its software as a sort of filing system. Every service application on your computer is stored in the hard drive, sorted into various folders. To get into a particular file, you must first open up the appropriate folder in which this particular file is stored. Similarly, billing software packages also begin with a main "menu" or "directory," which appears on the screen when the application is opened or loaded. From there, the user can select more specific parts of the program, depending on the task required.

If you have an opportunity to work with the software cited in this text, you will get a chance to move around within the *Stratford* program itself and become more familiar with its hierarchy. Again, the intent is to make things easier for the user.

For instance, suppose we return to Denise, the administrative medical assistant discussed earlier in this chapter; let us further suppose that her office uses the *Stratford* program. Any time Denise wants to work on billing, she simply selects or opens the *Stratford* program on her computer. A main directory appears with a list, or menu, of activity from which to choose. The screen will look something like this:

Accounts Receivable (Main) Directory

1 Finished with Patient's Receivables for Now
2 Change the Report/Default Date
3 Patient Information (Enter, Change, Inquire)
4 Statement Programs
5 Insurance Claim Form Programs
6 Report Programs
7 Statistics and Other Information
8 File and System Management

Suppose Denise must send a statement to Mr. Jensen. She will open or select option 4, Statement Programs. Once inside the Statement Programs menu, she will find more selections, depending on the types of statements her facility needs (Medicare, family account, etc.). If she is unsure what kind of coverage, if any, Mr. Jensen has, she may want to select option 3 first—Patient Information—to inquire. Appendix B and the student study guide will provide more in-depth opportunities to interact with the *Stratford* software.

Security for Data

The advent of computer technology in medical practice offices has made the security of data even more crucial. But when computers have made access to information so easy, how do we protect patient data? The first step in records security, of course, is to verify the authenticity of all confidential medical and personal information as it is entered into the database. The second step is to implement security levels or passwords that permit only authorized individuals into the system; these include all personnel and hospital carriers—anyone who must receive EDI or access to the database. Once an individual is granted a security level, he or she cannot necessarily use anything in the computer system. Each specific security level permits access only to areas appropriate to that user's needs. Procedures for adding or changing information on the database should indicate individuals authorized to make specific changes and time periods in which these changes will take place. Further, each should have a specifically designated password to the area of the database in which they will be working. Passwords should be changed regularly, and the passwords for all terminated or former employees should be eliminated from the system. If a practice uses a service bureau, all source documents, reports, and data should be returned to the practice when their contractual agreement is terminated.

Security guidelines or policies and procedures will become extremely important as more and more physician offices, clinics, and facilities place medical record information in the database, as the HCFA and government agencies will eventually require.

Making both patients and physicians aware of this security system will make your job easier by providing them with this necessary assurance of privacy.

WHAT DO YOU THINK?

Joan is an administrative medical assistant for the Gladstone Clinic. It is a very busy office, and the staff uses computers with practice management software so that most of their work is completed without paper. Joan's main station is patient checkout so she prepares their superbills and handles the insurance transmission. Her friend, Annie, comes to the clinic to see Dr. Green and spends time talking to her while she works with patient records on her computer. Annie also went to lunch with her one day and came back in while Joan logged on with her password.

What is wrong with this situation? Name the two security problems. How would you correct the situation? Why can security be a problem when using a computer?

FOCUS ON THE WORKPLACE

The "Paperless" Office

The goal of the future is to have a "paperless" office. This is something to keep in mind as time marches forward. In the world of computers, time seems to run!

John Jacobs calls to make an appointment. You use your computer to see what time slots are available and make an appointment for him for 2:30 PM on Tuesday. Mr. Jacobs arrives for his appointment, and you check him in on your computer. He is shown to an examining room. Before the physician enters the examining room, he obtains the results of laboratory tests that Mr. Jacobs had performed on Monday. After discussing the results with Mr. Jacobs, the physician uses the computer to obtain information on a new drug. He then uses his computerized patient charting system to input the current problem, test results, and medications prescribed. After being given instructions, Mr. Jacobs returns to the front office where you, the administrative medical assistant, print out the drug information for him and run the billing program to prepare and print out a superbill. Using the computer, you set a new appointment for him and print out a reminder of it to give him. After Mr. Jones leaves, you run his insurance information and transmit it through EDI to the insurance company. You also check your E-mail for messages from the office of a cardiologist while you wait for a report.

And so it goes in the nearly paperless medical office.

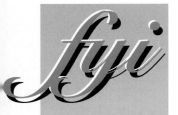

Computer Terms

Backup: To make copies of files

CD-ROM: Compact Disk–Read-Only-Memory. An optical disk capable of storing up to 1 gigabyte of data

Disk copy: To copy the files from one disk to another

Floppy disk: Small, magnetic, portable disks used to store data

GUI: Graphic User Interface. The use of icons to activate program operations (for example, Windows programs)

Mouse: Device used to control cursor on screen

RAM: Acronym for random access memory. Part of the inner computer memory

ROM: Acronym for Read Only Memory. The part of the computer memory that cannot be changed (instructions for starting the computer)

Conclusion

Computers make all processes done by an administrative medical assistant not only faster but also more accurate; this in turn makes many of these functions easier to perform. Most important, today's patients are better cared for as a result of a simple office PC. Referrals are done immediately, certain records are available much faster, and correspondence regarding patient needs is accomplished days sooner than would be possible without a computer. Finally, patient billing, which is far more complex than it used to be, is kept simpler and more accurate than ever before, thanks to spreadsheets and billing systems. Be sure to take advantage of all opportunities to learn new computer skills. These skills will not only keep you performing at peak efficiency (and with the greatest possible ease) but also will increase your marketability in this growing field. More exercises using the *Stratford* program can be found in Appendix B and in the student study guide.

Review QUESTIONS

1. What are some of the advantages of using computers in the medical or health care office?

2. What is the difference between a minicomputer and a microcomputer?

3. How do a system unit, a hard drive, and a central processing unit differ in function?

4. Describe how information is stored in a computer. What kind of hierarchy is assigned? What role does RAM play?

5. Explain the purpose and function of a computer network.

6. What are the four most common types of out-of-office computer services a medical practice might use?

7. Assume that you have been asked to purchase software for your office's computer system. What kinds of factors would influence your choices?

8. Name three types of software typically used in a health care office.

9. Denise is using the *Stratford Healthcare Management System* billing system. She is asked to print out an insurance claim form for Ms. Eliot; however, she does not remember what kind of coverage Ms. Eliot has. Finally, before she leaves today, her employer has asked her to print out statistics that break down the practice's clientele by insurance providers. Which items in the *Stratford* main directory will Denise use, and in what order?

SUGGESTED READING

Stratford healthcare management software: user's guide and reference. Stratford Healthcare Systems, Inc., Burlingame, Calif.

Banking

(Continued)

■ **Bank Reconciliation**
   Purpose
   Parts of a Statement
   Reconciling the Statement

■ **Other Banking Services**

OBJECTIVES

On completion of Chapter 18 the administrative medical assistant student should be able to:

1 Define the key terms listed in this chapter.

2 Discuss the basic functions of banking and the administrative medical assistant's responsibility for interaction with the bank.

3 Describe the uses and parts of a check.

4 List and describe the seven types of checks.

5 Describe efficient policies for accepting checks, including types and uses of endorsements, and policies for accepting cash payments.

6 Discuss techniques for preparing bank deposits accurately and depositing funds.

7 Discuss the three major reasons that checks are returned from a bank and the procedures for processing returned checks.

8 State the reason for reconciling a bank statement and an efficient related policy.

9 Reconcile a bank statement.

KEY TERMS

ABA number American Bankers Association number. The number printed in the upper-right corner of a check to identify the location of the bank at which the check is to be redeemed.

Accounts receivable The funds due to the practice for services rendered.

Continued

K E Y   T E R M S

(Continued)

Check   A written order to a bank to pay the bearer or presenter with the amount stated.

Magnetic ink character recognition   A series of numbers and characters printed in unalterable ink at the bottom of a check, including the checking account number of the payer and the amount of the check; these numbers are subsequently "read" by a machine for speedy processing.

Payee   The person named as the individual to whom the stated amount of a check is payable.

Payer   The person who signs the check to release the funds to the payee.

Reconcile   To make consistent or compatible; in banking, to make the necessary adjustments on a bank statement or check register to make the figures consistent.

anking and bookkeeping are interrelated and are critical to the medical practice. Your role in maintaining control of bank functions cannot be overemphasized. Attention to the smallest details will simplify all subsequent functions of reconciliation of funds and eventually the bookkeeping activities (Figure 18.1). The status of the banking and bookkeeping aspects of the medical office affects all of the basic functions needed to provide patient care. The availability of personnel, facilities, and equipment depends on financial security.

Banking Services
Banking Functions

The basic banking functions you will encounter involve the following activities:

- Depositing funds
- Withdrawing funds
- Reconciling statements
- Using auxiliary services

The funds deposited to checking and savings accounts are generated principally from the collection of accounts receivable. Funds are withdrawn by check or transferred from savings to checking for distribution and are used to pay business-related accounts payable. The distribution of funds must be conducted in a systematic manner, because the records are needed by the practice accountant and are subject to examination by government tax agencies. Statements of the checking account are sent from the bank every month and must

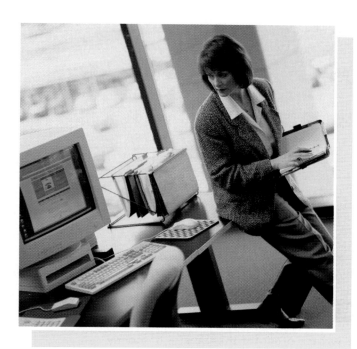

FIGURE 18.1

Attention to the smallest details will simplify all bookkeeping activities.

AT WORK TODAY

The New Banking World

The so-called information age has changed banking through advanced computerization. The *Electronic Funds Transfer (EFT)* system allows physicians to transfer money automatically from a savings account to a regular checking account whenever it is needed.

Another system, called *pay by phone,* allows the administrative medical assistant to call the bank to make the office payments. The bank writes the checks and mails the payment. A small fee may be charged for this service.

In still another system, autonomic bill paying, the bank pays itself from the office/physician's account. These funds are for mortgage payments, loans, insurance, and so on.

be reconciled immediately to verify the funds available to the practice. In addition to the basic services, banks offer other services such as safe deposit boxes, loans, and retirement plans that may be needed by a medical practice.

Checking

Checks have become the foundation for most banking services and virtually all business transactions. A check is a written order for the transfer of money (Figure 18.2). Checks are provided for a charge by the bank where funds are held in a checking account. Checks also may be purchased through office supply systems or computerized accounting programs such as Quicken or QuickBooks. Regardless of where the checks are purchased, all will include certain basic components, often preprinted on each check, and represent infor-

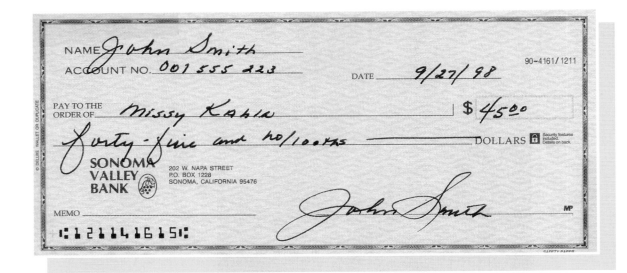

FIGURE 18.2

A check is a written order for the transfer of money.

mation that will not change. Checks must include the following information or space in which to enter the information:

- Preprinted name and address of payer
- Preprinted sequential number of the check
- American Bankers Association (ABA) number
- Space to enter the date the check is written
- "Pay to the order of" line and space to enter the payee name
- Space to enter the amount of the check in number form
- Space to enter the amount of the check in writing
- Preprinted name and address of the bank
- Magnetic ink character recognition (MICR) figures for bank processing of the check
- Line for payer's signature

All of the blank spaces must be filled in before a bank will process a check for payment.

Checking Account Types

Bank Checks

You are, of course most familiar with the standard form of bank check, which is supplied in pads and used by the public to complete transactions. Checks can be provided in other forms, however, and you should be familiar with them.

Why Write Checks?

1. Checks are a safe method of paying out money.
2. You can maintain a good record of the money.
3. You will have good tax records.
4. Money is protected while in the bank.
5. You receive monthly summaries of your account.
6. A "stop payment" option is available if you need the service.

Cashier's Checks

Cashier's checks are written by a bank on a bank form that represents guaranteed payment. The funds for payment of the check are debited from the payer's account at the time the check is written. A service charge is usually added.

Certified Checks

Certified checks are similar to cashier's checks in that the funds are guaranteed, but certified checks are written on the payer's own check form and verified by the bank with an official stamp. The stamp indicates that the bank certifies the availability of the funds.

Limited Checks

Limited checks are written on forms that are preprinted with a figure representing a maximum dollar amount for which the check can be written or a time limit during which the check is valid. This type of check often is used for payrolls or insurance payments.

Money Orders

Money orders represent guaranteed payment, because they are purchased for the cash value of the order plus a service charge. Domestic money orders can be purchased from post offices, banks, and authorized agents in retail stores. International money orders can be acquired in U.S. dollars to be cashed in foreign countries.

Traveler's Checks

Traveler's checks are preprinted with stated dollar amounts and represent assurance of payment to the payee, since the checks are prepaid. The face of each check contains space for the signature of the payer to appear twice. One space on each check is signed at the time of purchase in the presence of the seller; the other space is signed at the time the check is cashed. This precaution is to protect the payer in the event that the checks are stolen, because the payee can easily compare the signatures.

Voucher Checks

Voucher checks (Figure 18.3) provide three separate sections for complete information about the transaction represented in the check. The upper portion of the face of the check is the standard form, and the lower portion of the face provides room for details of the transaction, such as payroll deductions, reason for the check, or the bookkeeping account to which the check is to be credited. Once the check is completed, the face portion is detached and forwarded to the appropriate payee, the carbon is discarded, and a second sheet remains with the payee as a duplicate copy of the transaction. Supporting documents, such as receipts or invoices, can be attached to the copy for a complete, permanent record.

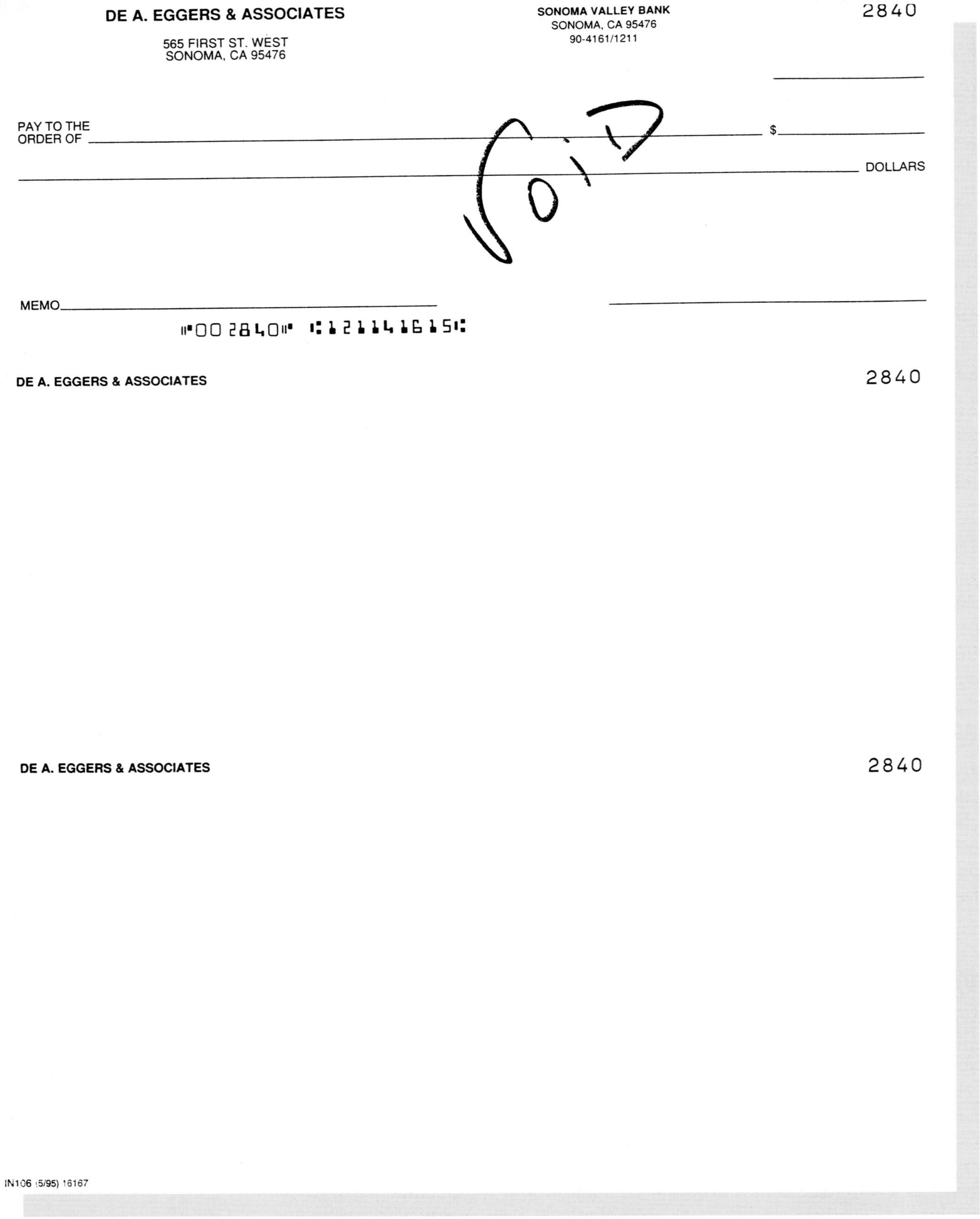

DE A. EGGERS & ASSOCIATES

565 FIRST ST. WEST
SONOMA, CA 95476

SONOMA VALLEY BANK
SONOMA, CA 95476
90-4161/1211

2840

PAY TO THE
ORDER OF _____ $ _____

_____ DOLLARS

Void

MEMO_____

⑈00 2840⑈ ⑆1211416 15⑈

DE A. EGGERS & ASSOCIATES

2840

DE A. EGGERS & ASSOCIATES

2840

IN106 (5/95) 16167

FIGURE 18.3

Voucher checks provide three sections for complete information about the transaction. (Courtesy Sonoma Valley Bank and De A. Eggers & Associates, Sonoma, Calif.)

Accepting Checks for Accounts Receivable

An office policy should be established to guide you with decisions about accepting checks for payment of accounts receivable. You will find that the majority of outstanding bills are paid by personal checks to be drawn on the bank accounts of patients. This is a common and accepted business practice.

You may wish to avoid accepting some checks in cases where the payer is unknown to you. These are known as *third-party checks,* because the payee is the third person in the process. A third-party check is one that is written by an unknown party to the payee, in this case your patient, who wishes to release the check to you for payment of an outstanding balance. Because you do not have contact or experience with the payer, you increase the risk that funds are not available to pay the face value of the check.

Government or payroll checks are another form of third-party checks. You may be inclined to accept these checks, because the payer appears reliable. You will find, however, that the amount of the check frequently is larger than the amount owed. This will require you to either refund the overpayment in cash or issue an office check for the difference, requiring additional work for you and increasing the risk of financial loss.

Occasionally, patients will send checks for payment that result in an overpayment on the account. This may occur if the check was written for an incorrect amount or an insurance carrier made a payment after the patient's statement was sent. You can handle this situation by either returning the incorrect check to the patient and requesting that a new check be written for the correct amount or depositing the check in the office account and writing a refund check to the patient for the amount of the overpayment. The second option is considered the soundest business practice, since it ensures payment of the account.

Finally, checks with the notation "in full" or "paid in full" written on the face indicate that the patient understands that their account will have a zero balance once the check is recorded. You will need to be certain that this is correct before depositing the check. By depositing a check with this notation, you are acknowledging that it is correct; if it is not correct you may have difficulty

WHAT DO YOU THINK?

Doctor Georgia Harris has two medical assistants: Tammy is the administrative assistant and Cass is the clinical assistant. They share some duties and cover for each other for breaks during the day. One day Cass was at the front desk covering for Tammy when a woman whom she did not recognize came in and said she was there to pay Sam Long's medical bill. Cass accepted a check in payment and gave the lady a receipt with the amount Sam owed on it. When Tammy returned, Cass told her about the woman, saying she did not recognize the name on the check. There was no imprinted telephone number to call and check on the woman.

What did Cass do wrong? What other information should she have gotten? What can she do if the check is returned?

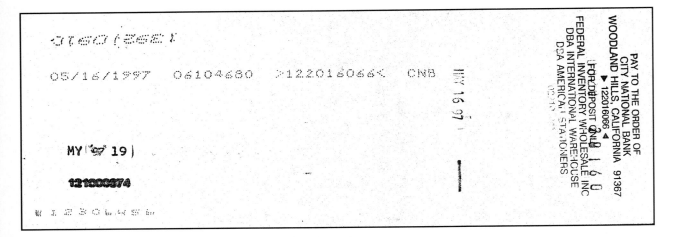

FIGURE 18.4

An endorsed check.

collecting the balance due. You may, however, cross out the notation, initial the area you crossed out, call the patient or person who paid the account, and then deposit the check.

Endorsement of Checks

A check must be endorsed (Figure 18.4) to transfer the funds from one person to another. This is accomplished by signing or rubber-stamping the back of the check in ink, at the left end, and perpendicular to the bottom of the check. Endorsements are regulated in all states by the Uniform Negotiable Instrument Act. Checks may be transferred to several individuals, as noted in the discussion of third-party checks. If a check is made payable to the physician but there is an error in the spelling of the name, have the physician sign his or her name as written on the face of the check, followed by the endorsement stamp.

Problem Checks

Occasionally, checks deposited for processing will be returned to the depositor by the bank. When a check is returned, it will be accompanied by a returned item notice (Figure 18.5). This may occur for various reasons, many of which you can identify before depositing and thereby avoid the extra bookkeeping required when an item is rejected.

Before submitting a check to the bank, you should examine all entries on the face for completeness and accuracy. Common errors include the following:

- Date missing
- Payee's name missing

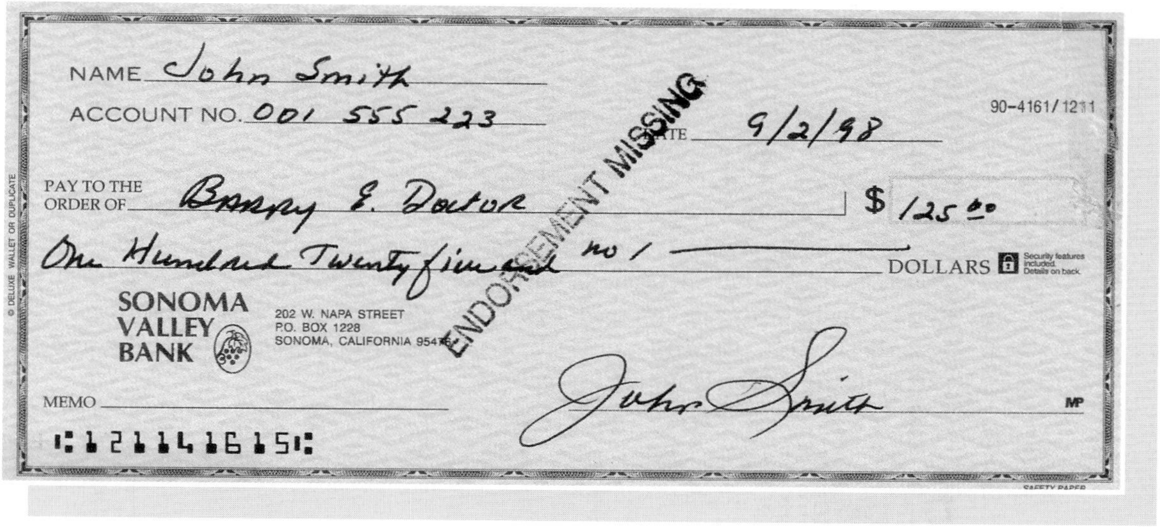

FIGURE 18.5

A returned check bearing a returned item notice.

- Signature missing
- Discrepancy between amount in numerals and amount written out

If the date or payee's name is missing, you may fill them in; if the signature is missing or the amounts do not match, the check must be returned to the payer. The bank also will reject a check that is not endorsed. Double-check the back of each check to be certain that the item has been stamped or signed before you deposit it.

The final reason the bank may return a check is difficulty with the payer. This is something you cannot predict or prevent. Returned checks in this group will be stamped with an explanation, usually one of the following:

- Refer to maker
- Nonsufficient funds (NSF)
- Other

"Refer to maker" indicates that you should contact the payer for an explanation. This notation may be because of a stop-payment order or a problem with the transfer of funds. "NSF" indicates that the payer's account does not contain sufficient funds to pay the amount stated on the check. "Other" rarely is noted, but when it is, there may be problems such as illegibility or a signature that does not match the one on file with the bank.

Checks that are incomplete or include errors can be handled in several ways. You can return the check to the payer with an explanation and request a new check, advise the payer that you will hold the incorrect check until a replacement arrives, or advise the payer to bring a correct check on the next visit if it is within the next few days.

When a check is returned with a "Refer to maker" or "NSF" notation, telephone the payer immediately. The payer may explain that an error was made and request that the check be resubmitted for payment. To accomplish this, cross out the notification stamp, write the word "resubmit" on the face and back of the check, and prepare a new deposit slip. You might want to call the payer's bank to verify that the funds are available before resubmitting the check.

If you have any doubts about the credibility of the check or if the patient is relatively new to the practice and you do not have a credit history, you may wish to pursue more aggressive collection measures. You may request that the patient send payment in the form of a cashier's check or money order or make payment by cash in person. In any case, hold the returned check until you receive the alternate payment. If payment is not received after attempts to work directly with the patient, notify the patient that you will transfer the account to a collection agency and do so.

Deposits

Patients occasionally will pay cash for services. When accepting cash, you need to be very careful that both you and the patient agree on the amount involved in the transaction. You should always count the payment in the presence of the payer. The higher total amount should be spoken aloud as each bill is counted, and the total amount restated to the patient for acknowledgment. You then should write a receipt for the patient, preferably using a receipt book that produces a copy that can be retained by the office as a permanent record. The original receipt is given to the patient.

General Policies

Policies and procedures will vary from office to office, but some considerations need to be incorporated into any business routine. When working with incoming funds, you should do the following:

- Keep daily receipts (cash and checks) in a single, safe location
- Prepare and make deposits daily
- Compare the deposit slip total with the day sheet
- Keep duplicates of deposit slips in the office
- Keep bank receipts of deposits
- Record the deposit total in the checkbook or master calendar

While cash and checks are in the office, they should be stored in a location that is not accessible to anyone other than employees. For additional security deposits should be made daily, especially if cash is involved. Most branch banks have locations that are convenient enough to include this activity in the daily routine. To ensure accuracy, you should compare the daily credits to accounts receivable with the total on the deposit slip. If they do not match, you will need to retrace the individual items to determine if they match.

Discrepancies often occur because of transposed numbers or an item omitted from one of the records. Duplicate deposit slips are automatically produced if the pegboard system is used. If you use the deposit slips provided by the bank, you may photocopy the slip before submitting it to the bank and retain the copies in chronological order. An alternative is to keep a stenographer's notebook and use

DEPOSIT TICKET

NAME _John Smith_

ACCOUNT NO. _001 555 223_

DATE _10/11/98_

DEPOSITS MAY NOT BE AVAILABLE FOR IMMEDIATE WITHDRAWAL

SIGN HERE FOR CASH RECEIVED (IF REQUIRED) ✱

SONOMA VALLEY BANK

202 W. NAPA STREET
P.O. BOX 1228
SONOMA, CALIFORNIA 95476

CHECKS AND OTHER ITEMS ARE RECEIVED FOR DEPOSIT SUBJECT TO THE PROVISIONS OF THE UNIFORM COMMERCIAL CODE OR ANY APPLICABLE COLLECTION AGREEMENT

© DELUXE   HD 101

☑ CASH ▶

90–4161/1211

_11.35_ ▶

_11.24_ ▶

_11.24_ ▶
(OR TOTAL FROM OTHER SIDE)

SUB TOTAL ▶

✱ LESS CASH RECEIVED ▶

$

_10.—_
_50.—_
_25.—_
_15.—_
_100.—_

_100.—_

⑈⑈12⑈⑈⑈4⑈⑈6⑈⑈5⑈⑈   ⑈0

FIGURE 18.6

A deposit slip.

carbon paper to imprint a copy of the deposit slip as you complete it onto consecutive pages of the book. After the deposit has been made, you can attach the bank deposit receipt to the corresponding page in the notebook to be retained as proof to check against deposits recorded on the monthly statement. And finally, you must know the daily balance in the account. This can be accomplished by adding each deposit to the current balance on the check stubs, or if you use voucher checks, by keeping a master calendar on which you enter all deposits and checks written daily. The deposit slip is the method of indicating to the bank the total dollar value in cash and checks to be credited to the physician's account (Figure 18.6). All entries on the deposit slip must be clearly printed in ink to ensure that they can be recorded correctly at the bank. The top section of the slip is devoted to the cash portion or the deposit. The total amount in currency (bills) is entered separately from the total amount in coins. The next section is for checks. Each check is recorded separately on numbered lines. The left-hand section of the check section provides space to record the ABA number of each check. If room is available, you may wish to note the last name of the payer above the ABA number to assist in locating errors. Directly opposite the ABA number is a section to enter the amount of the check in dollars and cents. Space is provided at the bottom of the slip for the total amount of the deposit. Double-check the total on an adding machine or calculator; the amount should equal the total receipts from your day sheet. If you have a computer, you can enter the payment amounts and then make a printout that indicates the amount of the deposit.

If the totals of the deposit slip and day sheet or computer printout do not agree, search for the error, which can occur in either document. First, recheck your addition. If the totals remain the same, check each item on the deposit slip to be sure you did not transpose any numbers. Next, subtract the lesser number from the greater to determine the amount of the error and search for missing item in that amount. The error can be one of omission (that is, an item is not recorded on the day sheet, or the computer printout or deposit slip) or one of commission (that is, an entry is recorded twice).

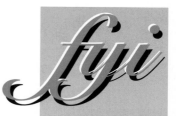

The Automated Teller Machine (ATM)

One innovation of the past 10 years is the automatic teller machine (ATM). These machines basically are computer terminals that allow customers to withdraw, deposit, or transfer money. They continue to become more sophisticated and offer more features. ATMs generally are located on the outside wall of a bank, although they now may be found in airports, train stations, shopping malls, and supermarkets. ATMs usually are open 24 hours a day, 7 days a week. Access is possible with a debit card and a personal identification number (PIN). It is important to exercise caution when using ATMs. Because these machines are not as protected as they would be if they were located inside the bank, robbery is a concern. When making a transaction, observe who is nearby, guard your PIN, and do not show any money!

Methods of Deposit

Deposits can be accomplished in three ways: in person, by mail, or at commercial night depositories. Automatic teller machines (ATMs) are not always adaptable to business (commercial) practices. Because ATM machines only dispense cash, most banks are not inclined to issue ATM cards for business accounts. Businesses therefore must carry out transactions by check to have a permanent record. Making deposits in person is the most direct method, and the teller immediately provides a receipt to verify the transaction. If you deposit by mail, cash payments cannot be included because of the risk of loss or theft. Mail deposits also delay credit to the account for at least 24 hours while the item is in transit. Some practices prefer this method, however, because it can be completed at the end of the business day and include all transactions. An alternative to mailing that fulfills this objective is the use of the night depository. Clients with business accounts can obtain a key to the night depository and a set of bags with security locks. Deposits can be prepared at the end of the day and brought to the bank after hours. Bags dropped in the night depository rest in a locked safe until bank employees retrieve them the next day. Your deposit is recorded and a receipt placed in the bag, which you may claim during bank business hours.

Savings Deposits

Funds not needed for current accounts payable should be transferred to a savings account, because the funds in savings will earn interest. It also is a sound business practice to retain sufficient funds to maintain the practice for at least 2 months, in the event that income ceases for any reason or the funds are needed for tax purposes.

Transfer of funds from a commercial checking account to a commercial savings account should be done by check. It ensures the safety of the funds and provides a record of the transaction to be posted in the ledger accounts. The savings account deposit slip (Figure 18.7) is completed in the same manner as a checking account deposit slip. The check ABA number is entered in the right-hand column and the check amount is in the space provided. You may wish to maintain a copy of the deposit slip for office records in the same manner as you do the checking account deposit slips.

The permanent record for a savings account is a passbook. You will take this book with you to the bank when conducting a transfer involving a savings account, and the bank teller will make a notation of the transaction. The passbook provides an up-to-date statement of deposits, interest earned, withdrawals, and account balance.

Checkbook Control

Controlling the checkbook is an absolute must. This allows adequate funds to remain in the checkbook to ensure that payroll, taxes, and bills are paid on time. Often the supplier will offer a discount if the account is paid either immediately or within a certain time frame.

Cash disbursement is a common bookkeeping term for the distribution of funds to suppliers and creditors. The use of the word *cash* can be confusing,

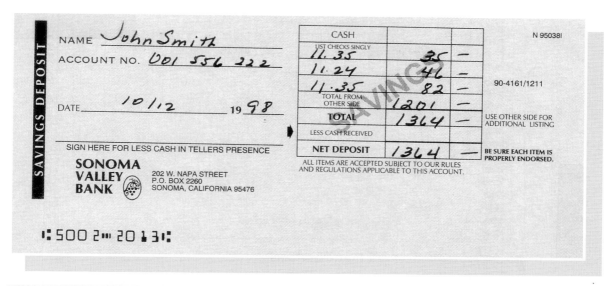

FIGURE 18.7

A savings account deposit slip.

because if it is taken literally, you would infer that cash is used to pay outstanding bills. In a business, you should consider the word *cash* to be synonymous with *check*. Only checks should be used for the disbursement of funds, because they provide proof of payment, produce a permanent record for documentation for tax purposes, and reduce the likelihood of embezzlement.

Check Writing Techniques

Although the basic components of checks are the same, the technique you use in preparing checks for signature will vary slightly with the type of check used. Your office may use a write-it-once system, a computerized system, prenumbered checks with stubs, or prenumbered voucher checks that produce a carbon copy.

Write-It-Once System

Check writing systems have been developed that produce a check and disbursement register through a carbon strip on the back of the check. This produces a record of the payee, date, check number, and net amount of the check (Figure 18.8). The remaining columns of the register are used to charge the expense to the appropriate account. Each check register contains space to record 25 checks.

Checks with Stubs

When using checks with stubs, fill out the stub portion first. This portion includes the following information:

- Date the check is written
- Payee's name

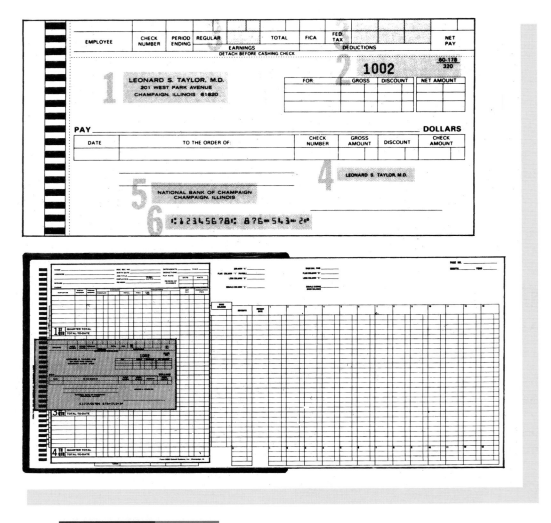

FIGURE 18.8

Write-it-once check cashing system. (Courtesy Colwell Systems.)

- Beginning account balance
- Amount of check
- New balance (previous balance minus amount of current check)

Completing the stub first ensures that the information available is an accurate reflection of the account balance. You should double-check the mathematical results for accuracy and write the new balance in the appropriate spot on the next stub in preparation for writing subsequent checks.

Voucher Checks without Stubs

Although voucher checks produce a carbon copy for a permanent record, you will need to develop a method of monitoring the daily bank balance. On a cal-

AT WORK TODAY

Advice for Checkwriters

1. Always keep the balance in your checkbook current.
2. Complete the stub before you fill out a check.
3. Make sure the date is correct.
4. Always use black or blue ink (black is preferable).
5. The amount of the check should always be written close to the dollar sign—draw a line through any blank space on the check.
6. Fill in the check amounts in words and numbers.
7. Make no major changes on the checks.
8. Have the physician sign unless you or someone else is authorized to sign.

endar with a 1- or 2-inch box for each date, enter the beginning balance each day, add the total of the daily deposit, subtract the total of all checks written each day, and arrive at the daily ending balance.

Computerized Check Writing Systems

Computerized check writing systems make life so much easier, because not only are the checks ready to print with all the pertinent information, but also they are already categorized to the appropriate designation for disbursement. In addition, there is a voucher section that can be attached to the invoice paid for further follow-up.

Method of Completing Checks

If you do not have a computerized system, checks must be written with materials that cannot be altered. They should be handwritten in ink or typewritten. Another option is to write out all information except the net amount of the check, which may be imprinted by a machine that perforates the paper. Any of these methods is acceptable. Write-it-once systems require the check to be handwritten. Checks with stubs may be typewritten if the check is detached from the stub, but you must be careful to complete the stub information. Voucher checks may be handwritten, using a pen that will imprint the copy, or typewritten to ensure legibility.

In most cases the checks will be prepared by you and presented to the physician-employer for signature. Complete the date, payee's name, check amount in numerals and handwriting, and memorandum portion with invoice numbers, if applicable. Any supporting documents and the envelope in which the check will be mailed should be attached before presenting the check for signature. The signee, usually the physician-employer, should verify the amount of the check with the document, usually an invoice or statement.

Errors on Checks

Occasionally an error is made when preparing a check. If the error is major, such as writing the name of the payee on the line provided for the handwritten dollar amount, the check becomes invalid. You will need to strike a line across the entire face of the check and, using ink, write the word "VOID" in large letters on it. The check is retained as proof of its invalid status. If the error is minor, such as writing the number 74 when you intended 84, you may change the 7 to 8; the authorized signee must initial the change.

Support Documents

Support documents are important to provide proof of payments made for valid business expenses and are subject to auditing by the Internal Revenue Service. These documents include invoices, statements for supplies and services, and vouchers for salaries and expenses. You will need to develop a method of retaining the supporting documents indefinitely and in an orderly manner. For stub or write-it-once systems, you can note the check number and date paid on each document and store the documents for each month in an envelope or manila file. For computerized systems, you need only to attach the voucher to the invoice and again store documents for each month in an envelope or manila file. You may also set up an accounts payable file and file invoices with the voucher attached by vendor. Should you elect to use the manila file system, you can file the corresponding monthly bank statement with the documents in each file. This only works well if the bank statement ends on the last day of the month. If you choose to attach the voucher directly to the invoice, the checks may also be arranged in batches by month and stored with the appropriate bank statement.

Account Hold

On rare occasions you will be notified by the bank that a hold has been placed on the checking account. This usually relates to a deposited item for which the bank needs assurance of redeemability. The check may be for an unusually large amount or from a bank in another geographical location. A hold means that the bank will not credit your office's account until the check has been processed and paid by the payer's bank. Your office's bank will indicate the specific period of time that the hold will be in effect, and until that time has elapsed you must treat that dollar amount as unavailable funds. You may not write checks that would involve those funds until the hold has been lifted.

Bank Reconciliation
Purpose

Banks provide monthly statements of checking accounts to determine if any errors have been made in office or bank accounting notations and confirm the financial status of the account. The statement includes the debits and credits noted by the bank and may be accompanied by the checks that have been processed and paid to creditors by the bank. Some accounts have the option of having the bank microfilm the checks, store the information, and provide the office only with the bank statement. The listing of checks by number or the physical presence of the paid checks allows you to ascertain those checks that have not been paid and may not have reached their intended destination.

Statements usually arrive on or about the same date each month. Office policy should include that bank statements be reconciled as soon as possible after arrival and may indicate a specific date by which this should be accomplished. It also should be office policy that the statement be reconciled by a person other than the one who makes deposits or prepares the checks for signature. This is a standard business practice designed to prevent embezzlement.

Parts of a Statement

Bank statements may vary in appearance, but they all contain certain basic information (Figure 18.9). The face of the statement includes the following information:

- Closing date
- Caption
- List of checks processed
- List of deposits

The caption is a synopsis of the account activity that has taken place during the month up to the closing date and includes the beginning balance, total value of checks processed, total amount of deposits made, service charges, and ending balance. The checks processed by the bank may be listed by check number, by the date they were paid, or by both, but the listing always includes the dollar value of the check. Finally, deposits are noted by the date the bank recorded the deposit and the dollar amount credited.

The back of bank statements is printed with the regulations governing the responsibilities of both parties, the instructions for reconciling the statement, and a worksheet for accomplishing the reconciliation.

Reconciling the Statement

The task of reconciling a bank statement can be relatively simple if it is approached in an orderly manner. Working with the face of the statement, first compare the beginning balance of the current statement with the ending balance of the previous statement. They should always agree. Next, compare the deposits noted by the bank with your records or receipts, placing a check mark next to each correctly recorded deposit. Deposits submitted toward the end of the month may not be posted by the closing date of the statement. The deposits not credited but recorded in your office records for the calendar month involved should be noted in the appropriate space on the back of the statement.

Next, compare the face value of the checks enclosed (or use your checkbook entries) with the corresponding value of the checks noted on the statement, again placing a check mark next to the correctly listed ones. The returned checks should then be put in numerical order. You will be able to determine which checks are outstanding by the numbers missing from the sequence. You also may check against the checkbook to see if a check was in fact voided. Each outstanding check is listed by number on the back of the statement; the dollar value of each is traced through the check stubs or copies, and the amount is

SONOMA VALLEY BANK

202 WEST NAPA STREET
SONOMA CALIFORNIA 95476

6-18-97
PAGE 1
1411667

```
********    LOAN RATES ARE DOWN!! TALK TO SONOMA VALLEY BANK'S     ******
********    LOAN OFFICERS ABOUT CONSTRUCTION AND EQUITY LOANS NOW! ******
********     COMMERCIAL LOAN PROGRAMS AS LOW AS 8.50%-FIXED!!      ******
********          CALL 707-935-3200 FOR MORE INFORMATION!          ******

            VINTAGE 50 CHECKING              ENCLOSURE COUNT      6
            PREVIOUS BALANCE      5-18-97        919.34
            +DEPOSITS/CREDITS        1           193.63
            -CHECKS/DEBITS           6           233.42
            -SERVICE CHARGE                          .00
            +INTEREST PAID                           .82
            CURRENT BALANCE                      880.37

*  - - - - - - - - - - - - -INTEREST SUMMARY- - - - - - - - - - - - - - *
   INTEREST EARNED FROM  5/18/97 TO  6/18/97
   DAYS IN PERIOD                                         31
   INTEREST EARNED                                       .82
   ANNUAL PERCENTAGE YIELD EARNED                       1.01
   INTEREST PAID THIS YEAR                              8.36
   INTEREST WITHHELD THIS YEAR                           .00

*  - - - - - - - - - - - -INTEREST RATE SUMMARY- - - - - - - - - - - - -*
   DATE      RATE         DATE         RATE      DATE         RATE
   5-18      1.010

*  - - - - - - - - - - - -DAILY BALANCE SUMMARY- - - - - - - - - - - - -*
   DATE    BALANCE        DATE       BALANCE     DATE       BALANCE
   5-18     919.34        5-19       1112.97      5-21      1095.03
   5-22    1075.99        5-28       1044.02      5-29       910.55
   6-10     879.55        6-18        880.37

*  - - - -PAPER-LESS AND OTHER DESCRIPTIVE ENTRIES- - - - - - - - - - -*
   DATE      TRACER     DESCRIPTION                        AMOUNT
   5-19        16       CUSTOMER DEPOSIT                    193.63
   6-18       999       INT PMT SYS-GEN                        .82

*  - - - - - - - - - - - - -CHECKS PAID- - - - - - - - - - - - - - - - -*
   NO.    DATE       AMOUNT          NO.    DATE        AMOUNT
   759    6-10        31.00          762    5-29         38.38
   760    5-21        17.94          763    5-29         95.09
   761    5-22        19.04          764    5-28         31.97
```

FIGURE 18.9

A, Examples of bank statements. (Courtesy Sonoma Valley Bank, Sonoma, Calif.)

*PLEASE EXAMINE - IF NO ERROR IS REPORTED WITHIN 30 DAYS
STATEMENT WILL BE CONSIDERED CORRECT*

THIS FORM IS TO PROVIDE ASSISTANCE IN BALANCING YOUR CHECKING AND SAVINGS ACCOUNTS.

CHECKING

ENTER THE FINAL BALANCE SHOWN ON THE FRONT OF THIS STATEMENT $_____

AMOUNT

ADD DEPOSITS MADE TOO LATE TO APPEAR
ON THIS STATEMENT.

$ + _____

LIST THE CHECKS YOU HAVE WRITTEN, BUT HAVE NOT
RECEIVED BACK WITH THIS STATEMENT.

NUMBER	AMOUNT	NUMBER	AMOUNT	NUMBER	AMOUNT
1		9		17	
2		10		18	
3		11		19	
4		12		20	
5		13		21	
6		14		22	
7		15		23	
8		16		24	

SUBTRACT
TOTAL ▼

$ - _____

THIS AMOUNT SHOULD AGREE WITH THE FINAL BALANCE SHOWN IN YOUR CHECK-
BOOK AFTER DEDUCTING SERVICE CHARGE (IF ANY) SHOWN ON THIS STATEMENT $_____

B

SAVINGS

ENTER THE FINAL BALANCE SHOWN ON THE FRONT OF THIS STATEMENT $_____

ADD DEPOSITS MADE TOO LATE TO APPEAR ON THIS STATEMENT

AMOUNT

$ + _____

AMOUNT

SUBTRACT WITHDRAWALS NOT POSTED
ON THIS STATEMENT.

$ - _____

THIS AMOUNT SHOULD AGREE WITH THE FINAL BALANCE SHOWN IN YOUR REGISTER $_____
In case of error or questions about your statement telephone us at (707) 935-3200

Regulation E. Section 205.8(b)
IN CASE OF ERRORS OR QUESTIONS ABOUT YOUR ELECTRONIC TRANSFERS
TELEPHONE US AT (707) 935-3200
OR
WRITE US ATTENTION: OPERATIONS OFFICER, SONOMA VALLEY BANK
P.O. BOX 1228 • SONOMA, CA 95476
as soon as you can, if you think your statement or receipt is wrong or if you need more information about a
transfer on the statement or receipt. We must hear from you no later than 60 days after we sent you the FIRST
statement on which the error or problem appeared.
(1) Tell us your name and account number (if any).
(2) Describe the error or the transfer you are unsure about, and explain as clearly as you can why you
believe there is an error or why you need more information.
(3) Tell us the dollar amount of the suspected error.
We will investigate your complaint and will correct any error promptly. If we take more than 10 business days to
do this, we will recredit your account for the amount you think is in error, so that you will have use of the money
during the time it takes us to complete our investigation.
CALL COLLECT IF YOU ARE OUT OF THE TOLL-FREE AREA

Each depositor insured to $100,000

FDIC
FEDERAL DEPOSIT INSURANCE CORPORATION

FIGURE 18.9, cont'd

B, Examples of bank statements.

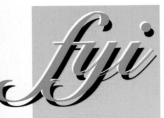

entered on the worksheet. Separately add and total the deposits not credited and the outstanding checks.

The final steps in reconciling the statement occur according to a standard procedure, which is as follows:

1. Note the ending statement balance.
2. Add the total deposits not credited.
3. Determine the subtotal of step 1 plus step 2.
4. Subtract the total checks outstanding.
5. Note the final total.

Next, identify the balance in the checkbook or on the master calendar, or with the computerized system for the last date of the month to be reconciled, subtract any service charges imposed by the bank, and adjust for any debit or credit entries made during the month. The total arrived at in step 5 should agree with the final figure arrived at in the checkbook. If they do the task is completed.

If Balances Do Not Agree

If the checkbook and bank statement balances do not agree, you must determine the source of the error. Some errors commonly are committed in reconciling bank statements; knowing what they are can help you locate the possible source of your error. First, look at the previous month's statement and crosscheck to see if all the outstanding checks noted have been listed as processed. If they have not, be sure that you have included them in the current list and total outstanding. Second, check your mathematical calculations for the outstanding checks, deposits not credited, bank statement reconciliation, and the figures carried forward on the check stubs. Third, review your figures to be sure that you have not transposed any numbers, and finally, be certain that all checks have been recorded in each check stub or in the check register. A shortcut method involves subtracting the lesser number from the greater number of the nonreconciling balances and quickly reviewing the checks, deposits, service charges, and debit and credit memos involved. However, this method will not help you locate mathematical errors or transposed numbers.

Other Banking Services

Banks supply customer services other than checking and savings accounts, including the following:

- Safe deposit boxes
- Loans
- Financial Planning
- On-line electronic banking
- Retirement funds

A medical practice may need some or all of the services available through a bank. Safe deposit boxes, available in various sizes, are used to store valuable documents such as deeds, insurance policies, and wills. An application must be submitted to the bank to obtain a box.

Once the box is acquired, the physician-owner is given a set of keys for the box and the bank retains a set for the vault slot. Both keys are needed to gain access to the box. Renters must sign a form, in the presence of a bank employee, each time they want access to the box. These measures are for the protection of the renter and the bank. You may be asked to keep a record of the contents of the box and should periodically review the list with your employer to be certain that the list is current.

The remaining bank services—loans, financial planning, on-line electronic banking, and retirement funds—are primarily the physician's responsibility. Your involvement will be minimal and may only involve retrieving tax or employee records. Any paperwork involved will be completed by the physician, the physician's accountant, and the bank.

Conclusion

Managing the banking and bookkeeping for a medical practice can affect all other aspects of the practice. Receiving and disbursing funds and maintaining records of these activities require attention to detail. Fulfilling your responsibility to these functions will put you in a position of great value.

Review QUESTIONS

1. Name the basic bank functions that you will encounter as an administrative medical assistant.

2. List and explain the 10 parts of a check.

3. List and briefly describe in your own words the six types of checks other than the basic bank check.

4. Describe four possible problems associated with checks received for accounts receivable.

5. List and describe the three most common check endorsements.

6. Complete a sample deposit slip for the following receipts:
   Cash: $14.83 ($2.83 in coins)
   Checks:

ABA Number	Amount
11-35	$ 42.00
11-1	$150.00
1-2	$ 17.80
11-35	$682.49
14-3	$ 31.27
12-1	$ 92.00

7. Describe the steps you would take on receiving a check returned from the bank marked "NSF."

8. Describe the method of preparing a voucher check for payment of a bill, including materials needed and processing of supporting documents.

9. List the five final steps in reconciling a bank statement.

SUGGESTED READINGS

American Medical Association: *The business side of medical practice,* Chicago, 1989, The Association.

Campbell T: *Principles of accounting,* San Diego, 1989, Harcourt Brace.

Fess PE: *Accounting principles,* ed 6, Cincinnati, 1989, South Western Publishing.

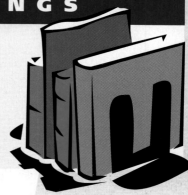

Accounting and Bookkeeping

On completion of Chapter 19 the administrative medical assistant student should be able to:

1. Define the key terms listed in this chapter.
2. Develop an effective policy for systematic bill paying.
3. Compare the three most common accounting systems used in the medical office.
4. List two bases of accounting and explain their differences.
5. List six types of accounting records.
6. Discuss the importance of a trial balance.

KEY TERMS

Account	Single financial record.
Account balance	The debit or credit balance remaining on an account.
Accounts payable	Amounts charged with suppliers or creditors that remain unpaid.
Accounts receivable	The amounts owed to the medical practice by patients and insurance carriers for services rendered.
Accrual basis accounting	Income that is recorded when earned, and expenses are recorded when incurred.
Balance sheet	A financial statement for a specific date or period that indicates the total assets, liabilities, and capital of the business.
Bookkeeping	The recording portion of the accounting process.
Cash basis accounting	Income is recorded on receipt, and expenses are recorded on payment.
Cash flow statement	A financial summary for a specific period that shows the beginning cash on hand, the income and disbursements during the same period, and the amount of cash on hand at the end of the period.
Credit balance	The amount of an overpayment on an account.
Daily journal	The ledger in which all payments and disbursements are first recorded; the general ledger or journal.
Discount	An amount a physician may designate to be forgiven on a patient's account (for example, another physician, a nurse from the hospital, or their family members; or other patients as the physician directs).
Equity	The net worth of the medical office. Equity equals the practice's total assets minus the total liabilities.

Continued

KEY TERMS

(Continued)

Invoice	A piece of paper indicating items purchased, the company from whom the items were purchased, the fee for the item(s) and tax applied, and the amount due.
Liabilities	What the medical office owes to other people.
Packing slip	The itemized list of materials or objects in the package delivered.
Payables	Amounts owed to suppliers or others.
Posting	The transferring of information from one record to another.
Receivables	The amounts owed from patients or others.
Statement	An invoice or request for payment.
Statement of income and expense	A summary of all income and expenses for a designated period.
Transaction	The occurrence of a financial event or condition that must be recorded.

*A*s in any business, financial records provide a method of monitoring the status and changes in a medical practice, and the records that are generated daily provide the foundation for all subsequent accounting records (Figure 19.1, *A* and *B*). These records involve patient relations through the billing system and provide proof of all transactions, information for financial planning, and data for tax purposes. As an administrative medical assistant you may be responsible for the basics of accounts receivable and accounts payable. You also may wish to work with the office bookkeeper or accountant to learn the skills involved in posting and balancing journals and ledgers. Depending on the size of the practice and the volume of patients, the bookkeeping record may be kept by hand or computer. Familiarize yourself with the basics of each method, and use any opportunity during your externship or career to gain experience. The additional skills will strengthen your position on the health care team.

Basic Bookkeeping Skills

The careful attention you pay to details in all aspects of your work also applies to bookkeeping functions. The time required to ensure accurate posting of entries is much less than that required to locate and correct errors. You can develop good basic bookkeeping habits by observing the following guidelines:

- Print letters and numbers correctly and legibly to decrease the possibility of errors.

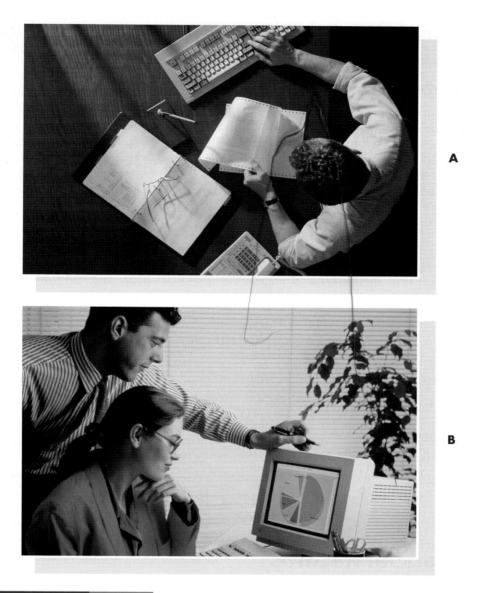

FIGURE 19.1

Financial records, kept by hand (A) or by computer (B), provide information for financial planning and data for tax purposes.

- Any entries in financial records must be made in ink, since they are permanent legal records.

- When totaling columns, you may note the amounts in pencil until they are double-checked and you are certain that they balance. Then you may superimpose the verified totals in ink.

- If errors are noted after an entry has been made, they are corrected in the same manner as a medical record; you should strike through the error with a single line, without obliterating the entry, and insert the correct information.

AT WORK TODAY

Computerized Bookkeeping

Bookkeeping is accomplished in many offices by computerized services. It saves time, especially when there are many reports to be generated. Larger offices and clinics probably invest in in-house bookkeeping software, whereas smaller offices may use the services of an outside computer service. The two basic types of outside service are (1) a "batch" service in which a courier picks up and delivers the information to and from the computer center, and (2) a telephone-linked service in which a terminal installed in your office will be connected directly with the facility so that the bookkeeping information can be entered and processed daily.

Regardless of the type of bookkeeping system used, the following rules apply:

- Fees and payments should be posted promptly.
- Checks should be endorsed with a restrictive endorsement stamp as they are received.
- Duplicate receipts should be prepared for all cash payments.
- Deposits should be prepared daily.
- All statements for accounts payable should be checked against invoices for accuracy and due date.
- All financial transactions should be conducted by check.
- A petty cash fund should be established, including a voucher system to account for expenditures.

Financial Records

Financial records provide information about the following four general areas:

- Accounts receivable
- Gross income
- Accounts payable
- Business expenses by category

Accounts receivable records contain the dollar value of services rendered daily, which are subsequently consolidated into monthly and annual totals. If the physician wishes, the data also can be developed by the type of service provided to determine the more profitable portions of the practice.

Gross income reflects the total dollars collected from practice business. The largest percentage will be from patient services, through direct payments or from accounts referred to collection agencies. Other sources of recorded business income include fees for services to professional organizations, reimbursement for expenses related to professional meetings and services, and income for complying with subpoenas and requests for medical reports.

Accounts payable details the funds expended on all goods and services necessary to maintain the practice. These business-related expenses usually are subclassified by category. Be aware of the various categories to indicate the appropriate assignment on checks when preparing them for payment. Most accounts payable can be categorized under one of the following headings:

- Automobile
- Dues and subscriptions
- Employee benefits and relations
- Insurance
- Janitorial services
- Laundry
- Licenses
- Medical-surgical supplies
- Office supplies
- Petty cash
- Professional meetings
- Public relations
- Rent
- Taxes
- Telephone

Accounting Systems

There are four types of accounting systems. They are as follows:

- Single-entry
- Double-entry
- One-write pegboard bookkeeping
- Computerized bookkeeping

Success in accounting requires a thorough understanding of the system you are using and what is to be accomplished. Accounting systems vary from the simple to the very complex. The basic principles are the same for all; only the system of recording changes.

Single-Entry

Single-entry actually is a bookkeeping function in which each dollar amount charged for services, received as income, or paid out for services is recorded in only one place in the accounting records. It is a simple, easily learned, and relatively inexpensive method of keeping records that provides the data necessary

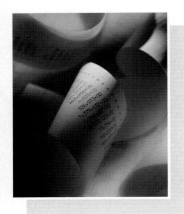

for accounting and tax purposes. It does not, however, include a built-in check system to verify all totals. It relies instead on double checks of column totals and the use of calculator tapes to check each entry by hand. The records used in a single-entry system include the following:

- General or fees journal—The log or accumulated day sheets used to enter charges for services and fees paid

- Accounts receivable journal—The total amount due or currently outstanding for all services provided to all patients. The pegboard day sheet provides a space on each sheet to record this daily, and computer systems produce the information for you automatically. Other billing systems require that you determine the totals by adding up balances due from active accounts receivable cards or statements.

- Accounts payable ledger—The checkbook is the simplest form this record can take, with the stubs and bank statements providing the necessary data. Write-it-once systems automatically produce a ledger sheet that subsequently is stored in an accounting binder, and voucher checks are recorded on a similar ledger sheet purchased for this purpose. Ancillary records in this area include payroll records and a petty cash fund.

Double-Entry

Double-entry bookkeeping systems are more sophisticated than other bookkeeping systems in that they are used by accountants to verify results and provide a built-in mechanism for the rapid identification of entry and computing errors. The fundamental principle of a double-entry system is that each entry to a debit account has a corresponding entry to a credit account and is based on the following equation:

$$\text{Assets} = \text{Liabilities} + \text{Owner's equity}$$

Any entry on the asset side must have a comparable entry in a liability account, an equity account, or in a combination of liability and equity entries equal to the asset entry. Entries from the daily journals that record services and disbursements are transferred to the appropriate accounts in the general ledger. Entries are totaled for each calendar month, and the correctness of the data is verified if the total of the debit columns equals the total of the credit columns. The next step is the transfer of monthly totals to the accounts ledger, which contains a separate page for each source of income and each category of disbursement. Verification of accuracy is again possible, because the debit and credit accounts must be equal.

One-Write Pegboard Bookkeeping

The one-write pegboard system, also known as the *write-it-once system,* generates an entry on the day sheet at the same time that a check is written. It also may include posting directly on to a ledger card for each vendor. The system includes instructions for simple checking techniques and provides balances on each day sheet to verify the totals of each column. Most mathematical or entry errors can be identified quickly. Also, this system allows control of income and receivables at a glance.

FOCUS ON THE WORKPLACE

The Superbill

When using the pegboard (write-it-once) system, the superbill can be a quick and handy tool for the front office assistant and also the patient. A "super" patient charge slip lists the examinations, procedures, and treatments a patient might receive in your medical office/clinic. They are numbered just as the receipts for the pegboard are numbered in sequence.

As a patient registers, the superbill and ledger card are layered on the day sheet (daily log). The administrative medical assistant writes the date, old balance, and patient's name on the superbill. Using the pegboard, the information automatically is transferred through all the layers using carbonized paper. The superbill then is clipped to the medical record to go into the examination room.

When the physician has completed the examination, he or she will mark the superbill to indicate the procedures, diagnosis, and any followup. The patient will take the record with the superbill to the administrative medical assistant, who will compute the charges and record them on the superbill. It then will be layered with the ledger card and day sheet to complete the day's entry. The patient will receive the superbill to be used as a receipt and for insurance purposes.

The one-write pegboard system once was one of the most popular available. This method is still used in many offices since it is easy to learn and maintain. Some physicians still prefer it for its daily access to accounts receivable information and potential control advantages. This system usually is popular in medical offices that do not have computer systems, since they eliminate the need to write the same information several times. Some offices still write their checks this way, posting them to the day sheet and later entering the information into the computer. The basic system includes the following:

- Ledger cards
- Journal page
- Checks
- Folding pegboard

You can see the advantage of having the checks preprinted; once the check is placed on the day sheet of the pegboard, you have only to write the check and the information is immediately placed on the day sheet. You need only to total the columns and confirm with the checkbook. Normally the accountant will expect that you will have balanced all day sheets before turning them over for final accounting.

Computerized Bookkeeping

Numerous computerized bookkeeping systems for accounts payable and payroll systems are available for the personal computer (PC). A practice with a PC for billing can in most cases also add an accounts payable and payroll system. The same information never has to be entered twice. You can set up a chart of accounts for the categories or the types of accounts that you pay, as well as individual vendors that you pay monthly. When you are creating checks to pay the vendors, you also are posting to the checkbook, and the information passes into the categories that you have selected. This interactive system is able to update balances instantly, reconcile your bank account in minutes, and access needed information for financial reports on whatever time frame (for example, monthly, quarterly, or yearly) that you choose as your basis. You also may use these systems with certain types of accounts receivable (for example, a payroll advance or loan to an employee). Computerized systems automatically post all of the journal entries for the accountant and provide a wide variety of reports such as profit and loss statements and balance sheets. Having a payroll module probably is one of the most time-saving portions of these programs. Working inside the payables system the payroll system calculates each employee's gross pay, plus all taxes and other deductions. It then writes the paycheck, records the transaction in the checking account, and keeps track of the tax liabilities. To do the calculations, the payroll system uses built-in tax tables, programmed by state. After you subscribe to the Tax Table Update Service, most companies will send the updates immediately when your tax rates change. Incorporating all aspects of the payroll system allows the practice to produce paychecks with accurate deductions and all tax deposits for federal Forms 940 and 941 (Figure 19.2, *A* and *B*), as well as state programs. It also creates the reports needed for the state and federal government for tax purposes, producing W-2 (Figure 19.2, *C*) and 1099 forms. In other words, this type of system can save time and effort and in general make your life much easier.

Daily Records

Whether you are using a single-entry, double-entry, pegboard, or computer system, you should balance daily. Doing so allows for fewer errors; errors that are caught earlier are easier to find than those 1 to 2 months old. If you are using a pegboard system, all columns must be totalled and proved at the end of the day. Although all bookkeeping is done in ink, it is a good idea to total in pencil and once proved, finalize in ink.

With the computer it is best if you balance with a system that forces you to correct all mistakes before finalizing the day's work. By balancing daily you will find that not only are errors easier to find but also finalizing the month and year-end totals will be easier. Daily records should include charges, payments, adjustments, and payables.

Special Account Entries

Special account entries are used in all accounting systems. They include adjustments, credit balances, refunds, nonsufficient fund (NSF) checks, and collection agency payments.

Adjustments

With today's reimbursements from the carriers, adjustments frequently are made; usually a minus adjustment is made to an account for the amount the

Form 941
(Rev. January 1997)
Department of the Treasury
Internal Revenue Service (1)

4141

Employer's Quarterly Federal Tax Return
► See separate instructions for information on completing this return.
Please type or print.

Enter state code for state in which deposits made . ► (see page 3 of instructions).

Name (as distinguished from trade name)	Date quarter ended
Trade name, if any	Employer identification number
Address (number and street)	City, state, and ZIP code

OMB No. 1545-0029

T
FF
FD
FP
I
T

If address is different from prior return, check here ►

IRS Use

1 1 1 1 1 1 1 1 1 1   2   3 3 3 3 3 3   4 4 4
5 5 5   6   7   8 8 8 8 8   9 9 9   10 10 10 10 10 10 10 10 10 10

If you do not have to file returns in the future, check here ► ☐ and enter date final wages paid ►
If you are a seasonal employer, see **Seasonal employers** on page 1 of the instructions and check here ►

1 Number of employees (except household) employed in the pay period that includes March 12th ►	**1**	
2 Total wages and tips, plus other compensation.	**2**	
3 Total income tax withheld from wages, tips, and sick pay	**3**	
4 Adjustment of withheld income tax for preceding quarters of calendar year	**4**	
5 Adjusted total of income tax withheld (line 3 as adjusted by line 4—see instructions)	**5**	
6 Taxable social security wages . . . . . **6a** $ × 12.4% (.124) =	**6b**	
Taxable social security tips . . . . . . **6c** $ × 12.4% (.124) =	**6d**	
7 Taxable Medicare wages and tips . . . **7a** $ × 2.9% (.029) =	**7b**	
8 Total social security and Medicare taxes (add lines 6b, 6d, and 7b). Check here if wages are not subject to social security and/or Medicare tax . . . . ► ☐	**8**	
9 Adjustment of social security and Medicare taxes (see instructions for required explanation) Sick Pay $ _____ ± Fractions of Cents $ _____ ± Other $ _____ =	**9**	
10 Adjusted total of social security and Medicare taxes (line 8 as adjusted by line 9—see instructions)	**10**	
11 **Total taxes** (add lines 5 and 10)	**11**	
12 Advance earned income credit (EIC) payments made to employees	**12**	
13 Net taxes (subtract line 12 from line 11). **This should equal line 17, column (d) below** (or line D of Schedule B (Form 941))	**13**	
14 Total deposits for quarter, including overpayment applied from a prior quarter	**14**	
15 **Balance due** (subtract line 14 from line 13). See instructions -	**15**	

16 **Overpayment,** if line 14 is more than line 13, enter excess here ► $ _____
and check if to be: ☐ Applied to next return   **OR**   ☐ Refunded.
- **All filers:** If line 13 is less than $500, you need not complete line 17 or Schedule B.
- **Semiweekly schedule depositors:** Complete Schedule B and check here . . . . ► ☐
- **Monthly schedule depositors:** Complete line 17, columns (a) through (d), and check here . . . . ► ☐

17	**Monthly Summary of Federal Tax Liability**		
(a) First month liability	**(b)** Second month liability	**(c)** Third month liability	**(d)** Total liability for quarter

Sign Here
Under penalties of perjury, I declare that I have examined this return, including accompanying schedules and statements, and to the best of my knowledge and belief, it is true, correct, and complete.

Signature ►   Print Your Name and Title ►   Date ►

For Paperwork Reduction Act Notice, see page 1 of separate instructions.   Cat. No. 17001Z   Form **941** (Rev. 1-97)

A

FIGURE 19.2

A, Employer's Quarterly Federal Tax Return (Form 941).

Continued

SCHEDULE B
(FORM 941)
(Rev. January 1996)
Department of the Treasury
Internal Revenue Service

5151

Employer's Record of Federal Tax Liability

▶ See Circular E for more information about employment tax returns.

▶ Attach to Form 941 or Form 941-SS.

OMB No. 1545-0029

Name as shown on Form 941 (Form 941-SS) | Employer identification number | Date quarter ended

You must complete this schedule if you are required to deposit on a semiweekly schedule, or if your tax liability on any day is $100,000 or more. Show tax liability here, not deposits. (The IRS gets deposit data from FTD coupons.)

A. Daily Tax Liability—First Month of Quarter

A Total tax liability for first month of quarter ▶ A

B. Daily Tax Liability—Second Month of Quarter

B Total tax liability for second month of quarter ▶ B

C. Daily Tax Liability—Third Month of Quarter

C Total tax liability for third month of quarter ▶ C

D Total for quarter (add lines **A, B,** and **C**). This should equal line 13 of Form 941 ▶ D

For Paperwork Reduction Act Notice, see page 2. Cat. No. 11967Q Schedule B (Form 941) (Rev. 1-96)

FIGURE 19.2, cont'd

B, Employer's Record of Federal Tax Liability, Schedule B (Form 941).

a Control number	22222	Void ☐	For Official Use Only ▶ OMB No. 1545-0008		
b Employer's identification number			**1** Wages, tips, other compensation		**2** Federal income tax withheld
c Employer's name, address, and ZIP code			**3** Social security wages		**4** Social security tax withheld
			5 Medicare wages and tips		**6** Medicare tax withheld
			7 Social security tips		**8** Allocated tips
d Employee's social security number			**9** Advance EIC payment		**10** Dependent care benefits
e Employee's name (first, middle initial, last)			**11** Nonqualified plans		**12** Benefits included in box 1
			13 See Instrs. for box 13		**14** Other
			15 Statutory employee ☐ Deceased ☐ Pension plan ☐ Legal rep. ☐ Hshld. emp. ☐ Subtotal ☐ Deferred compensation ☐		
f Employee's address and ZIP code					
16 State Employer's state I.D. No.		**17** State wages, tips, etc.	**18** State income tax	**19** Locality name	**20** Local wages, tips, etc. **21** Local income tax

Form **W-2** Wage and Tax Statement **1996**

Cat. No. 10134D

Copy A For Social Security Administration

Department of the Treasury—Internal Revenue Service

For Paperwork Reduction Act Notice, see separate instructions.

Do NOT Cut or Separate Forms on This Page

C

a Control number	22222	Void ☐	For Official Use Only ▶ OMB No. 1545-0008		
b Employer's identification number			**1** Wages, tips, other compensation		**2** Federal income tax withheld
c Employer's name, address, and ZIP code			**3** Social security wages		**4** Social security tax withheld
			5 Medicare wages and tips		**6** Medicare tax withheld
			7 Social security tips		**8** Allocated tips
d Employee's social security number			**9** Advance EIC payment		**10** Dependent care benefits
e Employee's name (first, middle initial, last)			**11** Nonqualified plans		**12** Benefits included in box 1
			13 See Instrs. for box 13		**14** Other
			15 Statutory employee ☐ Deceased ☐ Pension plan ☐ Legal rep. ☐ Hshld. emp. ☐ Subtotal ☐ Deferred compensation ☐		
f Employee's address and ZIP code					
16 State Employer's state I.D. No.		**17** State wages, tips, etc.	**18** State income tax	**19** Locality name	**20** Local wages, tips, etc. **21** Local income tax

Form **W-2** Wage and Tax Statement **1996**

Cat. No. 10134D

Copy A For Social Security Administration

Department of the Treasury—Internal Revenue Service

For Paperwork Reduction Act Notice, see separate instructions.

FIGURE 19.2, cont'd

C, Wage and Tax Statement (Form W-2).

PERSPECTIVES ON MEDICAL ASSISTING

Bookkeeping and Managed Care

Because bookkeeping is directly involved with the financial affairs of the medical office, it is vital that you understand and be aware of the differences in sources of income. A medical office's original source of income has always been whatever the patient and his or her insurance company would pay. With managed care you must be adaptable and very careful when doing accounting. Your office may have fee-for-services clients who are covered under several types of fee schedules. Your office also may be subject to capitation plans, in which a monthly fee for each patient is paid to the office. You must know which plans require copayments and what those amounts are. In addition, you must know which plans limit what they will pay. In these cases the office will need to collect any additional money owed. Some plans withhold a portion of their payments until the end of the year to encourage physicians to be thrifty. As you can see, bookkeeping can be very complicated so you may need special training in this area.

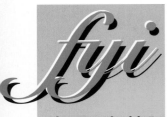

The "Receivable" Formula

When working with accounts receivable, the terms are:

1. **Credit**—A payment on an account (subtract from the account)
2. **Debit**—A charge on an account (add to the account)
3. **Adjustment**—A change added, such as a discount or write-off (entered as a credit)
4. **Balance**—The difference between the money owed and the money paid

Remember that if the balance becomes a credit balance it must be noted either by being enclosed in brackets or written in red ink.

Old balance + total charges (debits) – any payments (credits) – any adjustments = New balance

carrier (through a contract) will not pay. Adjustments also are made for professional discounts and write-offs (write-offs can either be for collection purposes or to eliminate the account). Most computer systems will have an adjustment area. However, if you are using a pegboard system, you should have an adjustment column to subtract the amount discounted or written off.

Credit Balances

Credit balances occur when the patient has paid in advance, an insurance carrier has overpaid, and sometimes an overadjustment has been made. A credit balance can be created when a patient make a partial payment and the insurance carrier pays more than expected. Thus the credit is money owed to the patient. Sometimes the patient will elect to leave the credit on account for the next service; if they do not, you must then refund the extra money.

Refunds

Refunds are made if a patient wishes to have an overpayment returned to him or her. The administrative medical assistant must then write a check for the amount owed and enter the transaction as a plus (+) adjustment. You should enter an explanation in the description area (either on the ledger card or in the computer). The balance should then be zero.

Nonsufficient Fund (NSF) Checks

Sometimes a patient gives or sends in a check without having funds sufficient to cover it; this check later is deposited to the physician's account. The bank will return the check to you marked "NSF" or "Refer to Maker." You must now perform two accounting functions:

- Deduct the amount from the checking account balance
- Add the amount back on to the patient's account balance

You may also charge the patient any fees the bank assessed for returning the check and in some states as much as three times the amount of the check.

Collection Agency Payments

When a collection agency recovers an account for the physician, the agency deducts a commission (anywhere from 30% to 50% of the amount recovered). For example, if the patient has a balance of $200 and pays it in full, the agency will send you the amount after they have deducted their commission, perhaps as high as $100. The patient currently has a balance of zero since you have written the account off for collection and it is being considered as "dead money" or noncollectible funds. To record this income you must enter a plus (+) adjustment of $200 to re-create the previous balance, subtract the $100 collection agency payment, and then make a minus (-) adjustment for the agency's fee. The balance then should again be zero.

Accounts Payable Control

A policy should be established to ensure that accounts payable are administered in an orderly and timely manner. The timetable established will depend on the size and needs of the practice. Checks can be written weekly, biweekly, semimonthly, or monthly. The schedule chosen should be followed consistently; it will allow for budgeting the funds necessary to meet the schedule. The policy also should indicate the person responsible for preparing, maintaining, and signing the checks. In some practices one signature is necessary to legally transfer funds; in others, two signatures are required for all checks or for those over a predetermined dollar amount.

You will encounter situations that require deviation from the schedule established for accounts payable or offers that make it advantageous to make an exception. Some suppliers offer a discount on their statement if the bill is paid within a certain number of days (usually 10) from the date of the statement. Others may offer a discount if payment is included when the order is placed or may require that payment be made in advance. Take advantage of the discounts offered even if it means preparing a check on a nonscheduled day. Payments required with orders also may necessitate deviation from the schedule if the order cannot be delayed.

A master calendar of recurring debts (for the pegboard system or a scheduled reminder with the computer system) will be helpful in preparing a check writing schedule and planning a budget for the practice. Certain items are predictable in that they occur monthly or periodically. These include the following:

- Rent or mortgage payments
- Janitorial services

MEDICAL ASSISTING STEP-BY-STEP

Collections

Collections are very important to the medical practice because money must come in steadily to maintain good financial health. Therefore, if a patient consistently does not pay his or her bill and does not respond to reminders or telephone calls, the office has no recourse but to turn the account over to a collection agency.

The bookkeeping procedure would be as follows:

1. The account would be written off under the adjustment column, which means it would be subtracted out of the accounts receivable balance.
2. The amount of money written off plus necessary information on the patient would be sent to the agency.
3. If the patient contacts the office and offers payment, you would refer them to the collection agency to pay.
4. Under the circumstances, if the patient calls to make an appointment, you would require cash for the visit unless the patient has been dismissed by the physician.
5. If the collection agency is successful in collecting funds from the patient, it will mail a check for the physician's share of the collection (that is, 40%, 50%, or 60% of the original amount) as agreed by contract.
6. When the check is received, add it to your adjustment column on the day sheet as a plus adjustment and then subtract the agency's fee under minus adjustment to have a zero balance.

- Telephone charges and related services
- Laundry
- Medical-surgical supplies
- Automobile payments
- Insurance policy premiums
- Taxes

By maintaining a master calendar or scheduling reminder system, you will be able to plan for the needed funds and make transfers from savings to checking if necessary.

You also will need to develop a system of storing and checking invoices and statements that are held until the scheduled payment dates. Maintaining a set of manila folders will ensure that these items are not lost or overlooked. One folder can be labeled "Invoices" and used to store the slips that arrive with supplies delivered or are left by individuals providing services for the office. Or you may choose to create a folder for each of the major suppliers for the business by placing the vendor's name on the folder. Other folders can be labeled "Statements" or labeled with specific dates if bills are to be paid on schedule, such as the fifteenth and thirtieth of each month. When a statement arrives, the appropriate invoices are retrieved and compared. The invoice numbers and the dollar amount should correspond with those listed on the statement. If there is any

AT WORK TODAY

Payroll Responsibilities

Payroll is a very important responsibility. The administrative medical assistant must ensure that wages are correct for the office and also that all records are correct and in order for the Internal Revenue Service. Because of the complex nature of payroll, some offices turn these responsibilities over to their accountant or use a service company to prepare payrolls.

Record retention is important in this process, and the following records should be kept at least 3 years (7 years for federal tax forms):

1. Employee name/Social Security number
2. Employee home address
3. Employee birth date
4. Employee sex
5. Employee occupation
6. Day and time employee work week starts
7. Employee rate of pay
8. Hours worked per day/week
9. Total weekly earnings
10. Total overtime pay
11. Total additions/deductions from pay
12. Total wages per pay period
13. Dates paid and period covered by payment

Employees must complete federal forms I-9 and W-4, which are part of the payroll record. The W-4 must be updated when the number of allowances or marital status changes.

Computer programs have become an asset in payroll because they can calculate deductions and taxes, and print necessary reports and checks. Payroll can be set up as a separate function and used only for payroll checks and local, state, and federal tax payments.

---

discrepancy, the vendor should be contacted. The statement then can be stored in the appropriate statement folder until payments are made. Invoices should be retained even after the payments are made, because they provide details of individual pricing that do not appear on statements and can be used for future comparison.

Payroll

Payroll records are considered separately because of the legal directive involved in maintaining and reporting the information. Employers are responsible for withholding income taxes from gross salaries, depositing the taxes with federal and state agencies, submitting quarterly and annual reports on taxes withheld, and providing reports needed by employees to file their annual tax reports.

When establishing a medical practice, each employer must apply for a federal and state employer's tax number that must be used on all forms and correspondence submitted to government agencies. Employees are identified, for tax purposes, by their Social Security numbers.

The first step in establishing a payroll record for each employee is the completion of a W-4 form (Figure 19.3). This form supplies the employer and the accountant with the information needed to determine the amount to withhold from the gross income of each employee. The data submitted on the employee's W-4 form are used to determine both federal and state withholding taxes. The factors that influence the amount withheld for state and federal

Form W-4 (1997)

Want More Money In Your Paycheck?
If you expect to be able to take the earned income credit for 1997 and a child lives with you, you may be able to have part of the credit added to your take-home pay. For details, get Form W-5 from your employer.

Purpose. Complete Form W-4 so that your employer can withhold the correct amount of Federal income tax from your pay. Form W-4 may be completed electronically, if your employer has an electronic system. Because your tax situation may change, you may want to refigure your withholding each year.

Exemption From Withholding. Read line 7 of the certificate below to see if you can claim exempt status. If exempt, only complete lines 1, 2, 3, 4, 7, and sign the form to validate it. No Federal income tax will be withheld from your pay. Your exemption expires February 17, 1998.

Note: You cannot claim exemption from withholding if (1) your income exceeds $650 and includes unearned income (e.g., interest and dividends) and (2) another person can claim you as a dependent on their tax return.

Basic Instructions. If you are not exempt, complete the Personal Allowances Worksheet. Additional worksheets are on page 2 so you can adjust your withholding allowances based on itemized deductions, adjustments to income, or two-earner/two-job situations. Complete all worksheets that apply to your situation. The worksheets will help you figure the number of withholding allowances you are entitled to claim. However, you may claim fewer allowances than this.

Head of Household. Generally, you may claim head of household filing status on your tax return only if you are unmarried and pay more than 50% of the costs of keeping up a home for yourself and your dependent(s) or other qualifying individuals.

Nonwage Income. If you have a large amount of nonwage income, such as interest or dividends, you should consider making

estimated tax payments using Form 1040-ES. Otherwise, you may find that you owe additional tax at the end of the year.

Two Earners/Two Jobs. If you have a working spouse or more than one job, figure the total number of allowances you are entitled to claim on all jobs using worksheets from only one W-4. This total should be divided among all jobs. Your withholding will usually be most accurate when all allowances are claimed on the W-4 filed for the highest paying job and zero allowances are claimed for the others.

Check Your Withholding. After your W-4 takes effect, use Pub. 919, Is My Withholding Correct for 1997?, to see how the dollar amount you are having withheld compares to your estimated total annual tax. Get Pub. 919 especially if you used the Two-Earner/Two-Job Worksheet and your earnings exceed $150,000 (Single) or $200,000 (Married). To order Pub. 919, call 1-800-829-3676. Check your telephone directory for the IRS assistance number for further help.

Sign This Form. Form W-4 is not considered valid unless you sign it.

A   Personal Allowances Worksheet

A   Enter "1" for **yourself** if no one else can claim you as a dependent . . . . **A** _____

B   Enter "1" if: { • You are single and have only one job; or
• You are married, have only one job, and your spouse does not work; or
• Your wages from a second job or your spouse's wages (or the total of both) are $1,000 or less. } . . **B** _____

C   Enter "1" for your **spouse.** But, you may choose to enter -0- if you are married and have either a working spouse or more than one job (this may help you avoid having too little tax withheld) . . . . **C** _____

D   Enter number of **dependents** (other than your spouse or yourself) you will claim on your tax return . . . . **D** _____

E   Enter "1" if you will file as **head of household** on your tax return (see conditions under **Head of Household** above) **E** _____

F   Enter "1" if you have at least $1,500 of **child or dependent care expenses** for which you plan to claim a credit . . **F** _____

G   Add lines A through F and enter total here. **Note:** This amount may be different from the number of exemptions you claim on your return ▶ **G** _____

For accuracy, complete all worksheets that apply. {
• If you plan to **itemize or claim adjustments to income** and want to reduce your withholding, see the Deductions and Adjustments Worksheet on page 2.
• If you are **single** and have **more than one job** and your combined earnings from all jobs exceed $32,000 OR if you are **married** and have a **working spouse or more than one job,** and the combined earnings from all jobs exceed $55,000, see the Two-Earner/Two-Job Worksheet on page 2 if you want to avoid having too little tax withheld.
• If **neither** of the above situations applies, **stop here** and enter the number from line G on line 5 of Form W-4 below. }

------------ **Cut here and give the certificate to your employer. Keep the top portion for your records.** ------------

Form **W-4**
Department of the Treasury
Internal Revenue Service

Employee's Withholding Allowance Certificate

▶ **For Privacy Act and Paperwork Reduction Act Notice, see reverse.**

OMB No. 1545-0010

1997

1 Type or print your first name and middle initial	Last name	2 Your social security number

Home address (number and street or rural route)	3 ☐ Single ☐ Married ☐ Married, but withhold at higher Single rate.
	Note: If married, but legally separated, or spouse is a nonresident alien, check the Single box.

City or town, state, and ZIP code	4 If your last name differs from that on your social security card, check here and call 1-800-772-1213 for a new card . . . . ▶ ☐

5   Total number of allowances you are claiming (from line G above or from the worksheets on page 2 if they apply)   **5** _____

6   Additional amount, if any, you want withheld from each paycheck . . . . **6** $_____

7   I claim exemption from withholding for 1997, and I certify that I meet **BOTH** of the following conditions for exemption:
   • Last year I had a right to a refund of **ALL** Federal income tax withheld because I had **NO** tax liability; **AND**
   • This year I expect a refund of **ALL** Federal income tax withheld because I expect to have **NO** tax liability.
   If you meet both conditions, enter "EXEMPT" here . . . . ▶   **7** _____

Under penalties of perjury, I certify that I am entitled to the number of withholding allowances claimed on this certificate or entitled to claim exempt status.

Employee's signature ▶ _____   Date ▶ _____ , 19____

8 Employer's name and address (Employer: Complete 8 and 10 only if sending to the IRS)	9 Office code (optional)	10 Employer identification number

Cat. No. 10220Q

FIGURE 19.3

A, Front of a federal Form W-4.

Form W-4 (1997)
Page **2**

Deductions and Adjustments Worksheet

Note: *Use this worksheet only if you plan to itemize deductions or claim adjustments to income on your 1997 tax return.*

1   Enter an estimate of your 1997 itemized deductions. These include qualifying home mortgage interest, charitable contributions, state and local taxes (but not sales taxes), medical expenses in excess of 7.5% of your income, and miscellaneous deductions. (For 1997, you may have to reduce your itemized deductions if your income is over $121,200 ($60,600 if married filing separately). Get Pub. 919 for details.)   **1** $ _____

2   Enter: { $6,900 if married filing jointly or qualifying widow(er)
 $6,050 if head of household
 $4,150 if single
 $3,450 if married filing separately   }   **2** $ _____

3   **Subtract** line 2 from line 1. If line 2 is greater than line 1, enter -0-   **3** $ _____

4   Enter an estimate of your 1997 adjustments to income. These include alimony paid and deductible IRA contributions   **4** $ _____

5   **Add** lines 3 and 4 and enter the total . . . .   **5** $ _____

6   Enter an estimate of your 1997 nonwage income (such as dividends or interest)   **6** $ _____

7   **Subtract** line 6 from line 5. Enter the result, but not less than -0- . . . .   **7** $ _____

8   **Divide** the amount on line 7 by $2,500 and enter the result here. Drop any fraction   **8**   _____

9   Enter the number from Personal Allowances Worksheet, line G, on page 1 . .   **9**   _____

10   **Add** lines 8 and 9 and enter the total here. If you plan to use the Two-Earner/Two-Job Worksheet, also enter this total on line 1 below. Otherwise, **stop here** and enter this total on Form W-4, line 5, on page 1 . .   **10**   _____

Two-Earner/Two-Job Worksheet

Note: *Use this worksheet only if the instructions for line G on page 1 direct you here.*

1   Enter the number from line G on page 1 (or from line 10 above if you used the Deductions and Adjustments Worksheet)   **1**   _____

2   Find the number in **Table 1** below that applies to the **LOWEST** paying job and enter it here . . .   **2**   _____

3   If line 1 is **GREATER THAN OR EQUAL TO** line 2, subtract line 2 from line 1. Enter the result here (if zero, enter -0-) and on Form W-4, line 5, on page 1. **DO NOT** use the rest of this worksheet .   **3**   _____

Note: *If line 1 is **LESS THAN** line 2, enter -0- on Form W-4, line 5, on page 1. Complete lines 4-9 to calculate the additional withholding amount necessary to avoid a year end tax bill.*

4   Enter the number from line 2 of this worksheet . . . . .   **4**   _____

5   Enter the number from line 1 of this worksheet . . . . .   **5**   _____

6   **Subtract** line 5 from line 4 . . . . .   **6**   _____

7   Find the amount in **Table 2** below that applies to the **HIGHEST** paying job and enter it here . . .   **7** $ _____

8   **Multiply** line 7 by line 6 and enter the result here. This is the additional annual withholding amount needed   **8** $ _____

9   Divide line 8 by the number of pay periods remaining in 1997. (For example, divide by 26 if you are paid every other week and you complete this form in December 1996.) Enter the result here and on Form W-4, line 6, page 1. This is the additional amount to be withheld from each paycheck . . . .   **9** $ _____

Table 1: Two-Earner/Two-Job Worksheet

Married Filing Jointly				All Others			
If wages from **LOWEST** paying job are—	Enter on line 2 above	If wages from **LOWEST** paying job are—	Enter on line 2 above	If wages from **LOWEST** paying job are—	Enter on line 2 above	If wages from **LOWEST** paying job are—	Enter on line 2 above
0 - $4,000	0	35,001 - 40,000	8	0 - $5,000	0	75,001 - 90,000	8
4,001 - 7,000	1	40,001 - 50,000	9	5,001 - 11,000	1	90,001 - 110,000	9
7,001 - 12,000	2	50,001 - 60,000	10	11,001 - 15,000	2	110,001 and over	10
12,001 - 17,000	3	60,001 - 70,000	11	15,001 - 20,000	3		
17,001 - 22,000	4	70,001 - 80,000	12	20,001 - 24,000	4		
22,001 - 28,000	5	80,001 - 100,000	13	24,001 - 45,000	5		
28,001 - 32,000	6	100,001 - 110,000	14	45,001 - 60,000	6		
32,001 - 35,000	7	110,001 and over	15	60,001 - 75,000	7		

Table 2: Two-Earner/Two-Job Worksheet

Married Filing Jointly		All Others	
If wages from **HIGHEST** paying job are—	Enter on line 7 above	If wages from **HIGHEST** paying job are—	Enter on line 7 above
0 - $50,000	$400	0 - $30,000	$400
50,001 - 100,000	740	30,001 - 60,000	740
100,001 - 130,000	820	60,001 - 120,000	820
130,001 - 240,000	950	120,001 - 250,000	950
240,001 and over	1,050	250,001 and over	1,050

B

FIGURE 19.3, cont'd

B, Back of a federal Form W-4.

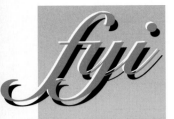

Tax Information Sources

- **State taxes/unemployment/ disability.** Telephone numbers to obtain this information vary and can be secured through your phone book or directory assistance.
- **Federal taxes/forms and payroll inquiries/instructions.** You may reach the Internal Revenue Service at 1-800-TAX-FORM. The agency's fax number is (703) 497-4150.
- **Social Security Administration (FICA).** Call your local Social Security office or dial 1-800-772-1213.

taxes are the employee's marital status, the number of allowances claimed, and the pay periods established by office policy. Employees may elect one allowance for themselves and one for each dependent. If they do not complete all appropriate information as requested, the employer will withhold taxes at the rate specified for an unmarried individual with no allowances. W-4 forms can be obtained from the Internal Revenue Service regional office on a written request. They also can be obtained from office supply stores and sometimes the local library.

Payroll accounting involves keeping a record of the gross salary, taxes withheld (including federal income tax, Social Security [FICA] tax, Medicare deduction, state income tax, and state disability insurance, if applicable), and other deductions such as insurance or retirement contributions. If the write-it-once check system is used, the task is accomplished by stating the net amount on the check and the gross amount and various amounts withheld in the appropriate columns to the right of the check. Other check-writing systems involve the transfer of data to the appropriate ledger accounts. Computerized systems detail the deductions on the lower tear-off portion of the check. Many offices prefer to maintain a separate payroll book that includes space for all necessary tax data and room to record time off for vacations, holidays, or illness. Most computerized systems can manage the same information in the database.

Be aware that many payroll services are available for a nominal fee. These services will write checks, make federal withholding deposits, produce monthly payroll records, and produce quarterly tax returns and W-2 forms. Some of these services are available to a practice with as few as two employees. These services have proved to be cost effective and reduce staff time significantly.

Payroll Taxes

Federal Income Tax

Employers are required by law to withhold and process federal taxes for each employee. The federal employer's tax guide, Circular E, is supplied to every employer with a federal identification number (EIN [employer identification number]), and includes tables for all possible combinations of variables (Figure 19.4).

FICA Tax

Several taxes, commonly known as *Social Security tax,* are covered under the Federal Insurance Contributions Act (FICA). The amount to withhold from an employee's gross income also can be determined from tables in Circular E and is calculated on a percentage of the gross salary up to an annual maximum income. FICA is different from income tax in that every dollar contributed by an employee is matched by a dollar from the employer, and the funds are used for individuals who are retired or unable to work. The Medicare contribution was once part of the FICA but has since been broken out as a separate amount to be contributed from the gross pay. Again, the information regarding the amount to deduct can be found in Circular E.

SINGLE Persons—MONTHLY Payroll Period

(For Wages Paid in 1997)

If the wages are—		And the number of withholding allowances claimed is—										
At least	But less than	0	1	2	3	4	5	6	7	8	9	10
		The amount of income tax to be withheld is—										
$2,440	$2,480	372	311	270	237	203	170	137	104	71	38	5
2,480	2,520	384	322	276	243	209	176	143	110	77	44	11
2,520	2,560	395	333	282	249	215	182	149	116	83	50	17
2,560	2,600	406	344	288	255	221	188	155	122	89	56	23
2,600	2,640	417	355	294	261	227	194	161	128	95	62	29
2,640	2,680	428	367	305	267	233	200	167	134	101	68	35
2,680	2,720	440	378	316	273	239	206	173	140	107	74	41
2,720	2,760	451	389	327	279	245	212	179	146	113	80	47
2,760	2,800	462	400	338	285	251	218	185	152	119	86	53
2,800	2,840	473	411	350	291	257	224	191	158	125	92	59
2,840	2,880	484	423	361	299	263	230	197	164	131	98	65
2,880	2,920	496	434	372	310	269	236	203	170	137	104	71
2,920	2,960	507	445	383	321	275	242	209	176	143	110	77
2,960	3,000	518	456	394	332	281	248	215	182	149	116	83
3,000	3,040	529	467	406	344	287	254	221	188	155	122	89
3,040	3,080	540	479	417	355	293	260	227	194	161	128	95
3,080	3,120	552	490	428	366	304	266	233	200	167	134	101
3,120	3,160	563	501	439	377	315	272	239	206	173	140	107
3,160	3,200	574	512	450	388	327	278	245	212	179	146	113
3,200	3,240	585	523	462	400	338	284	251	218	185	152	119
3,240	3,280	596	535	473	411	349	290	257	224	191	158	125
3,280	3,320	608	546	484	422	360	298	263	230	197	164	131
3,320	3,360	619	557	495	433	371	310	269	236	203	170	137
3,360	3,400	630	568	506	444	383	321	275	242	209	176	143
3,400	3,440	641	579	518	456	394	332	281	248	215	182	149
3,440	3,480	652	591	529	467	405	343	287	254	221	188	155
3,480	3,520	664	602	540	478	416	354	293	260	227	194	161
3,520	3,560	675	613	551	489	427	366	304	266	233	200	167
3,560	3,600	686	624	562	500	439	377	315	272	239	206	173
3,600	3,640	697	635	574	512	450	388	326	278	245	212	179
3,640	3,680	708	647	585	523	461	399	337	284	251	218	185
3,680	3,720	720	658	596	534	472	410	349	290	257	224	191
3,720	3,760	731	669	607	545	483	422	360	298	263	230	197
3,760	3,800	742	680	618	556	495	433	371	309	269	236	203
3,800	3,840	753	691	630	568	506	444	382	320	275	242	209
3,840	3,880	764	703	641	579	517	455	393	332	281	248	215
3,880	3,920	776	714	652	590	528	466	405	343	287	254	221
3,920	3,960	787	725	663	601	539	478	416	354	293	260	227
3,960	4,000	798	736	674	612	551	489	427	365	303	266	233
4,000	4,040	809	747	686	624	562	500	438	376	315	272	239
4,040	4,080	820	759	697	635	573	511	449	388	326	278	245
4,080	4,120	832	770	708	646	584	522	461	399	337	284	251
4,120	4,160	843	781	719	657	595	534	472	410	348	290	257
4,160	4,200	854	792	730	668	607	545	483	421	359	297	263
4,200	4,240	865	803	742	680	618	556	494	432	371	309	269
4,240	4,280	876	815	753	691	629	567	505	444	382	320	275
4,280	4,320	888	826	764	702	640	578	517	455	393	331	281
4,320	4,360	899	837	775	713	651	590	528	466	404	342	287
4,360	4,400	910	848	786	724	663	601	539	477	415	353	293
4,400	4,440	921	859	798	736	674	612	550	488	427	365	303
4,440	4,480	932	871	809	747	685	623	561	500	438	376	314
4,480	4,520	944	882	820	758	696	634	573	511	449	387	325
4,520	4,560	955	893	831	769	707	646	584	522	460	398	336
4,560	4,600	966	904	842	780	719	657	595	533	471	409	348
4,600	4,640	978	915	854	792	730	668	606	544	483	421	359
4,640	4,680	990	927	865	803	741	679	617	556	494	432	370
4,680	4,720	1,003	938	876	814	752	690	629	567	505	443	381
4,720	4,760	1,015	949	887	825	763	702	640	578	516	454	392
4,760	4,800	1,027	960	898	836	775	713	651	589	527	465	404
4,800	4,840	1,040	971	910	848	786	724	662	600	539	477	415
4,840	4,880	1,052	984	921	859	797	735	673	612	550	488	426
4,880	4,920	1,065	996	932	870	808	746	685	623	561	499	437
4,920	4,960	1,077	1,009	943	881	819	758	696	634	572	510	448
4,960	5,000	1,089	1,021	954	892	831	769	707	645	583	521	460
5,000	5,040	1,102	1,033	966	904	842	780	718	656	595	533	471

$5,040 and over   Use Table 4(a) for a **SINGLE person** on page 34. Also see the instructions on page 32.

Page 49

FIGURE 19.4

Page from Circular E, the federal employer's tax guide.

State Income Tax

Some states have set up a mechanism similar to that of the federal government that allows employees to withhold a portion of each paycheck for deposit on estimated annual taxes due by employees. Tables to assist employers to determine the appropriate amount are supplied by the state tax board. The only states that do not have a state employee tax are Alaska and Nevada.

State Disability Insurance

Some states have established funds to protect individuals temporarily unable to work because of illness or injury. The employee contribution is usually very limited, because the risk of needing the service is spread over many contributors.

Unemployment Insurance

Unemployment insurance is available in each state for individuals who have lost their jobs through unavoidable circumstances. The contributions and contributors to this fund vary from state to state; you will need to determine the law for your state. The possibilities include contributions only by the employer, by both employer and employee, or by employers with more than three employees. There also is federal unemployment insurance, which is a supplementary fund developed by employer contributions and intended for use after state funds have been exhausted.

Depositing Taxes Withheld

Employers are required to deposit federal taxes they withhold to a Federal Reserve Bank or authorized commercial bank on a monthly or quarterly basis. Tax deposit forms are sent annually to each registered employer and must be submitted with each deposit (the form is used to designate the quarter and type of tax, that is, income and FICA). The amount of the deposit equals the total accumulated federal income and FICA taxes withheld from employees and the matching FICA employer contribution. Deposits to the state tax board usually are done monthly or quarterly directly to the state agency and, if submitted on quarterly, are accompanied by a quarterly report that describes the required payroll information. The funds submitted include state income tax, disability insurance fees, and where applicable, unemployment insurance.

Required Reports

For tax purposes the calendar year is divided into quarters, and the mandatory quarterly reports must be submitted on or before the last day of the month that follows the end of the quarter. For example, forms for the first quarter (January, February, March) must be mailed on or before April 30. Federal and state agencies send the necessary forms during the last month of each quarter.

Annual reports involve the preparation of the W-2 forms; these are six-part forms supplied by the federal government or purchased in most office supply

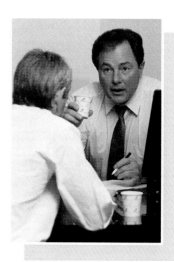

stores. Three copies of the W-2 form are given to employees. Employees need the copies to file their personal, state, and federal taxes. Another copy is given to employees to retain for their records. Employers must send one copy of the W-2 form to the federal government, one to the state, and retain one copy for office records. The federal unemployment tax is submitted with a check for the employer's contribution to the fund.

Because of their complexity, employer's personal income taxes usually are prepared by an accountant. Tax payments are made quarterly according to an estimate of the total amount due by the end of the year. The final payment for the previous year must be submitted with the annual reports by April 15 of the present year and represent any amount due over the estimated payments already made.

Computer Services

Computer services are invaluable as recordkeeping and reporting requirements become more complex. Many physician-owners and their accountants use computers. Computer services and programs are available for all accounting functions and are nearly routine today. Some of the basic advantages that computers offer are that:

- They save time
- They have built-in proofing mechanisms for the reports they produce
- They can generate all the necessary forms and reports

Some disadvantages can be cited with regard to computer services and equipment, but most of them relate to a lack of understanding of the use or potential of the system. Some basic study and research should eliminate problems related to computers, including the following:

- Fear of equipment
- Selection of inappropriate equipment and programs
- Improper use of reports

Conclusion

The management of accounting and bookkeeping systems involves a responsibility that can affect all other aspects of a medical practice. Receiving and disbursing funds and records for reporting these activities require attention to detail. The fulfillment of your responsibility to these functions will put you in a position of great value.

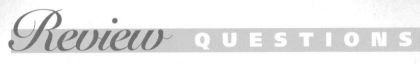

Review   QUESTIONS

1. What four general areas of information do financial records provide?

2. What is gross income?

3. List the four types of accounting systems.

4. Explain double-entry bookkeeping.

5. List types of special account entries.

6. What is the difference between a single-entry and double-entry system?

7. List and describe the basic federal and state income taxes withheld from paychecks.

8. How are taxes determined?

9. Which taxes are paid by the employer?

SUGGESTED READINGS

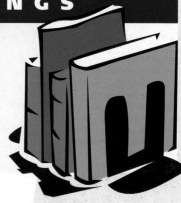

Colwell Systems: *One-write pegboard bookkeeping system,* Champaign, Ill., 1992.

Fess PE: *Accounting principles,* ed 6, Cincinnati, 1989, South Western Publishing.

Externship and Obtaining Employment

On completion of Chapter 20 the administrative medical assistant student should be able to:

1. Define key terms listed in this chapter.

2. Determine the purpose of an externship program and describe where an externship might be conducted.

3. List the three advantages of an externship program to the school.

4. State the three theoretical and two personal advantages of an externship program.

5. List the three possible personal opportunities of an externship program.

6. Define the relationship between an externship program and a course seminar.

7. Determine a method of assessing personal attributes.

8. State the primary purpose of the resume and cover letter.

9. Develop one basic and one alternative resume.

10. List the fundamental considerations in resume preparation.

11. List and describe the factors evaluated during the first-impression phase.

12. List the points evaluated in a formal application.

13. Describe the steps in preparing for an interview.

14. State the two purposes of a written follow-up to an interview.

15. List the five steps in the goal-setting process.

K E Y   T E R M S

Attitude A way of thinking or feeling; also, a body position assumed that shows the feelings or mood of an individual.

Attribute A personal trait or characteristic.

Externship A limited experience in an environment in which students can apply learned theory under supervision.

Goal The point or purpose determined to be a desirable end result.

Integrity The condition of being competent, upright, honest, and sincere.

Continued

KEY TERMS

(Continued)

Interpersonal relationship	A connection or dealings between individuals, as in business interactions.
Long-term	Far reaching or extended into the future.
Mannerism	A habitual action, gesture, or style of speech unique to or identified with an individual.
Objective	An aim or end toward which any action is directed.
Personal assessment	The act of objectively determining the value of an individual's qualities or attributes.
Perspective	The ability to view incidents in correct relation to each other; the proper relationship of things to one another.
Reference	An individual to be consulted for information regarding another person.
Resume	A synopsis or summary of an individual's education, work experience, or skills prepared as an aid in obtaining a job.
Seminar	An unstructured meeting of individuals of similar education or training to exchange ideas and theories.
Short-term	Limited, lasting for a brief period.
Theoretical	Pertaining to abstract principles; based on ideas rather than practical experience.

*A*s an administrative medical assistant you have prepared for an important position in the health care field. In this chapter the concept of an externship program and the process of obtaining a permanent position are introduced. One of the goals that you have set for yourself is to become an effective and efficient administrative medical assistant. The administrative training available through an externship program will help you attain this goal, and the guidelines presented here will help you acquire the position as an administrative medical assistant that you desire.

The Externship Experience

The externship program occurs simultaneously or soon after a theoretical foundation has been developed in the classroom. The externship program will provide you with information on and reinforcement of your skills. The externship experience also will expose you to potential employers and provide you with references for job hunting. Each subject that you have studied eventually will be put into practice.

JOB DESCRIPTION FOR RECEPTIONIST/ FRONT OFFICE ASSISTANT

Primary Responsibilities:
Primary public and staff representative of the office
Initial public contact
Public relations person

Duties:
I. Maintains Office Schedule
   A. Appointment schedule
      1. Check listing daily for proper control, that is, number new patients, consultations, necessary appointment changes, etc. Copy appointment schedule each morning for distribution to physician
      2. Note on list any reminders to obtain pertinent information
      3. Make sure that all committee meetings and other business appointments for the doctor are in the appointment schedule
II. Charts
   A. Pull charts for the next day's patients
      1. Update charts as necessary
      2. Note new information as necessary
      3. Call all patients for appointments
      4. Set up new charts with proper information
III. Greet patients on arrival to the office
      1. New patients: Obtain new patient information
      2. Established patients: Pull chart from pre-pulled file with superbill attached, place in holder, indication that patient is ready to be taken to examination room
      3. Check for any missing pertinent information, that is, MediCal card, new address, new telephone number, etc.

IV. Telephone
   A. Answer telephone first
   B. Relay messages to physician (with chart when pertaining to a specific patient)
   C. Refer drug refills to physician
   D. Make appointments by telephone
   E. Answer messages from the day before as so instructed by the physician
   F. Refer all calls regarding accounts to billing service
   G. Refer all collection calls to billing service
   H. Reschedule appointments
   I. Call missed appointments and reschedule
   J. Call and check eligibility and benefits on patients as necessary
   K. Call and make appointments for patients who need referral to a specialist, after obtaining proper authorization
V. Visitors
   A. Detail people—Refer to the physician
   B. Process servers—Refer to the physician
   C. Mail—Open daily and distribute
   D. Deliveries—Refer to back office assistant
   E. All other visitors—inform physician and leave to his or her discretion
VI. Filing
   A. Help refile charts
   B. Help file reports, letters, medical records
VII. Miscellaneous Duties
   A. Bank deposits, daily as per designation by payer
   B. Keep track of all monies—copayments, contracts, etc., on payment and adjustment sheet
VIII. Order Office Supplies

The externship program provides you with the opportunity to make a smooth transition from student to paid employee and can be viewed as a period of personal adjustment. You will be involved in new interpersonal relationships and will begin to integrate the theories and skills you have been studying. With the support of instructors who are prepared to offer guidance through the externship program, you will have the opportunity to test yourself in a receptive environment.

The externship period can be used to evaluate your skills and preferences objectively in preparation for paid employment. The opportunity to experience administrative and clinical responsibilities under "real world" conditions will allow you to develop, with your instructor's assistance, a method of evaluating

The externship experience occurs away from the self-contained environment of the classroom.

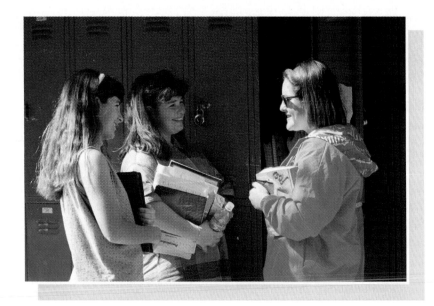

your potential. The externship period will allow you to recognize your preference, select the areas of primary interest to you, and examine the areas in which you create the most positive effect. You also will be able to determine areas in which you may need to develop further or that you may wish to study in future continuing education courses.

Many schools with programs for administrative medical assistants provide a course entitled "Externship" or "Work Experience." If the program is accredited by the American Association of Medical Assistants (AAMA), an externship is mandatory. In this course the student participates in a practical application of the theories learned in the classroom. The term *externship* is derived from the word "external," because the externship experience occurs away from the self-contained environment of the classroom (Figure 20.1). The externship experience is offered in cooperative medical offices or hospitals in the community for a predetermined period. The course may extend from several weeks to several months. It involves working in one facility or rotating to several settings 1 or 2 days each week, 3 to 8 hours each day. The externship experience is guided by an instructor, who arranges for an appropriate work setting for the student, monitors the student's adjustment and progress as an extern, and provides the student with feedback to make necessary adjustments.

Advantages to the School

Although the primary purpose of an externship program is to benefit the student, it also provides secondary benefits to the school. By working cooperatively with community facilities, the school and the medical assistant program benefit by having the use of settings and equipment not available at the school. The externship program also provides a public relations link with the community. The presence of students in community settings reminds the public that the school and the medical assistant program are available for future students and that program graduates are available for employment. In addition, the externship period gives the medical assistant program director the opportunity

PERSPECTIVES ON MEDICAL ASSISTING

What's an Externship?

An externship puts you, the student, out into the "big" world of medicine to see how you will function under "controlled" conditions. Controlled conditions mean that you will work under the supervision of a member of the medical office/clinic using skills that you have learned in the classroom. You will be evaluated on your professionalism, attitude, appearance, and job skills. In most cases the externship is a required part of the total hours of school a student must pass successfully to complete their training.

It is to your advantage to complete the externship with high marks. A successful externship can lead to a future job or recommendations for a job. It can be a rewarding learning experience and can help you decide where you would like to work, whether it is in a small office, a large office, or a clinic or hospital setting.

Just remember these bits of advice:

1. Learn to cooperate and work with the other members of the health care group.
2. Always ask for help when needed so you learn the procedures properly.
3. Be ready to assist in any task that you can. Never sit around idle or act bored.
4. Admit the errors you make and be able to accept corrections/advice from the staff.
5. Keep a positive attitude at all times; it will make a difference in your work.

to monitor community needs. This is accomplished because the externship instructors have ongoing contacts with the facilities, employers, and employees in the community. Students also will provide feedback on the observations they make in the facility at which they serve their externships. The evaluation of community needs allows the individuals responsible for the medical assistant program to make appropriate decisions when adjusting the curriculum to meet student and community needs.

Advantages to the Student

The most important concerns in an externship program are the student and the advantages to the student of working in an actual medical setting. The basic advantages of an externship program are presented here as a guide to what should be sought from the experience. Keep them in mind as you proceed through the externship process. These advantages relate both to your educational endeavors and your personal growth.

Practical Advantages

First, an externship program provides you with the opportunity to gain experience that will help you when you are ready to seek permanent employment. Second, you can begin to integrate the information learned separately in var-

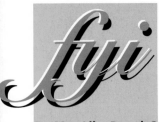

ious administrative courses by applying this information in a practical setting. Third, the real-world setting of the externship provides you with the opportunity to observe and participate in the dynamics of the various interpersonal relationships that occur in a medical facility (for example, physician-medical assistant and patient-medical assistant).

Personal Advantages

The personal advantages of the externship program include the opportunity for you to develop a base of information to help determine which type of work interests you most. You may also take advantage of this opportunity to recognize your strengths and weaknesses and develop or correct these personal characteristics as necessary.

Opportunities

When a health care facility or medical office accepts a student-extern, they are accepting an implied responsibility. This responsibility includes having staff members willing to supervise the student's activities, seeing that the student participates in a wide variety of experiences, and allowing the student to assume increasing responsibility. The willingness or the facility's health care team to work with the externship program provides the student with several opportunities. The most immediate opportunity is the chance to develop skills and test theories that were learned in the classroom in a supportive environment. This is especially important before the student ventures into a job with greater personal and medical responsibility. The supervising personnel in the health care facility will assist the student with decisions and help him or her recognize when increased responsibilities may be undertaken. The student must recognize that the office supervisor is a substitute for the school instructor and that the other personnel provide an example of teamwork in action.

A more long-term opportunity that you should keep in mind is that by working in one or more facilities during an externship, you can acquire references for future job hunting (Figure 20.2). You should approach the externship with a positive attitude and accept any guidance or responsibility offered as a learning experience. Your attitude and willingness to learn will create a positive impression of you among your externship supervisors, and this will develop potential reference sources. As your externship experience in a facility nears an end, speak frankly with your work supervisors regarding your interest in a reference. If you have established rapport with your supervisors, this will be a simple exchange that will result in a favorable reference. You may request a general reference addressed to "To Whom it May Concern" that you can take with you when you have completed your student work experience. The option is to let your supervisors know you would like to give their names as references, thereby notifying them that they may be contacted in the future by prospective employers. The first option is the most considerate choice, since your externship supervisors will need to write only one letter, which you can photocopy when references are requested. Your prospective employer can follow up with a phone call if confirmation is necessary.

A final opportunity that may develop from your externship is an offer of a permanent position at the office or facility. If the interest is mutual, your potential employer may be willing to keep the position open for you until you have

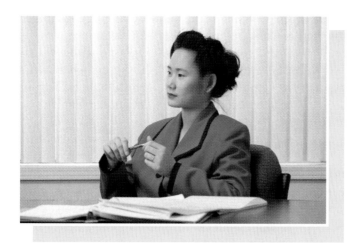

FIGURE 20.2

In addition to more training, the externship experience allows you to test your job hunting skills and provide you with references.

completed your training program, or you may be able to arrange a part-time work schedule in the interim.

Program Without an Externship

If your school does not include an externship program, you still have two options. First, you can volunteer your services in a willing medical office, hospital, or agency. Second, you can secure a part-time job in an entry-level position in a health care facility. You can use this opportunity to observe the functions of the various personnel. You also may be able to participate in activities of increasing challenge as you demonstrate your willingness and capability to assume more responsibility. A cooperative instructor in your program may be able to assist you in locating a volunteer or paid position and provide follow-up guidance when you wish to evaluate your work experience.

The Self-Supporting Student

If it is necessary for you to work during your course of study, you should be aware that your medical assistant program probably has a rule against working for pay in the same facility in which you do your externship. If there is no specific rule about this situation in your program, you should establish your own guideline. The logic behind this rule is that it is difficult to separate the paid and nonpaid (externship) times when they occur in the same setting. Isolating the externship experience allows the student, the instructor, and the externship supervisor to remain objective in evaluating the progress and development needs.

Expanding the Externship Experience

The externship process may or may not be associated with a classroom seminar. If a seminar is included, it will offer an opportunity, usually weekly, for the externship instructor and all of the students in the program to meet. The instructor provides minimal structure to the meeting and guidance or advice when necessary. The primary purpose of the seminar is to provide students with the opportunity to share experiences and observations with one another. This serves as a mechanism to reduce stress and broaden exposure, since each student is unique and is working in a different environment.

If your student work experience is not organized through your school or is not associated with a seminar, you may wish to establish an informal seminar with other students in similar situations. The result will be supportive and positive. You also may be able to enlist the help of an instructor to act as an information adviser for your group.

Whether you participate in a formal externship program organized by your school or develop one of your own, you will find externship an important and rewarding experience. What you get out of the process depends on you. Keep in mind the influence the externship experience can have on your development and future employment.

Resume Development

The resume is a common tool used in seeking employment and can be an asset to you in your job search. It should be thought of as a method of introduction, an advertisement of your skills and potential value to an employer and a facility, and a demonstration of your written communication skills. Until recently resumes tended to follow one format—the chronological resume, which is a historical account of your education and work experience, beginning with the most recent (Figure 20.3). This format may not be the most advantageous as you begin a career as an administrative medical assistant. If you are preparing for your first full-time work experience, you will only be able to record your externship in the work history section, in which employers expect to see data on paid work experience. If you are preparing for a change of career to administrative medical assisting, you will only be able to record employment information unrelated to your new career aspirations.

Alternative Resume Styles

In looking for your first position as a medical assistant, you may wish to explore some of the new, alternative-style resumes. *The Perfect Resume* by Tom Jackson is an excellent resource for learning to develop a resume that will best serve your needs. Organized in a workbook format, this reference includes step-by-step guidance in selecting and developing the resume, special notes for students and individuals reentering the job market, sample resumes of all types, and tips for handling your job search. One alternative, if you are seeking your first position, may be a skills-oriented resume (Figure 20.4).

Fundamentals

Regardless of the style of resume you choose, certain basic considerations apply to all resumes. Resumes should be clear and concise (one page maximum if at all possible), typed without error, and on a high-grade bond paper. Resumes are traditionally typed on white paper, but other soft, pleasant shades such as bone, beige, or light gray may be used. Dark or bright shades of paper should be avoided. Once you have a well-planned, well-prepared resume, you can have an

OBJECTIVE

To secure a long-term position of responsibility in a stable, progressive organization, where my skills in front office, administrative management, accounting and customer service strengths will be utilized profitably for all.

WORK HISTORY

Sept 1996-Present **TEMPORARY POSITIONS**

Nelson Human Resource Solutions: Petaluma, CA

Processed expedites in a timely manner. Sorted daily orders according to the pick locations. Picked customer orders from various locations within the warehouse, verifying the correct product number, and delivered the orders to the packing stations for final packaging. Worked at the packing stations on various days. Verified customer order was correct. Packaged orders for proper ship method according to the order form.

May 1990-Dec 1995 **OFFICE MANAGER**

Data 2000, Inc.: Cincinnati, OH

Office manager of data supplies business. Responsibilities held include invoicing and accounts receivable on Dac Easy Accounting version 4.1. Accounts payable with general ledger work. Collections on 300 plus accounts. Customer service duties ranged from answering up to six phone lines, received and placed orders, processed returns and incorrect orders. Drafted letters, created sales order, and purchase order forms, and company labels in Word Perfect version 5.1.

Nov 1986-Sep 1987 **DELIVERY & CUSTOMER SERVICE**

The New Haven Register: New Haven, Conn.

Delivered uncovered newspaper routes Saturday through Sunday. After covering routes, duties included opening the home office to answer customer service calls and delivered missed papers.

EDUCATION

Sept 1985-Jun 1988   The Hammonasset School: Madison, Conn.
General curriculum
Sept 1988-Apr 1990   The Fashion Institute of Technology: New York, N.Y.
Major: Fashion design

FIGURE 20.3

A chronological resume.

Position Desired:

Skills and Achievements:

- Multiline phones
- Basic operation of Windows95
- Excellent communication skills—both written and verbal
- Type 35 WPM
- Lotus 1-2-3
- Cash handling of large quantities
- Customer service
- Balance daily ledgers
- Data entry
- Very accurate 10-key
- Purchasing of office supplies
- Faxing documents
- Accounts receivable
- Various postage machines
- Able to establish and maintain excellent rapport with superiors and colleagues
- Independently motivated
- Excellent team player
- An enthusiastic and quick learner

WORK HISTORY:

1996-present	Transworld Systems Inc. 5880 Commerce Blvd. Rohnert Park, CA 94928
1995-1996	West America Bank 300 Rohnert Park Expressway W. Rohnert Park, CA 94928
1994-1995	Macy's 800 Santa Rosa Plaza Santa Rosa, CA 95403

EDUCATION

Present	Santa Rosa Junior College
1994	Montgomery High School
1994	Julie Nation Academy

References available upon request.

FIGURE 20.4

A skills-oriented resume.

AT WORK TODAY

The Resume

Your resume represents an important product—you!

The resume should include your current and future career goals. Education and work experience may be included, but the resume should emphasize your medical training and experience first. You may use the externship training if it was satisfactory and reflects your qualifications.

List any special honors or awards you have attained such as for perfect attendance or student of the month. You also may list any professional organizations in which you are active.

Indicate that references are available with a note on your resume that states, "References available upon request."

instructor review it for information, style, and general appearance. It is difficult to see minor flaws in a project that you have worked on so closely. To reproduce the resume, locate a copy service with a high-grade copier and have the resume copied directly onto your own paper. The copied resumes are very similar to the original, and this saves you from running off numerous copies on a laser printer (although this is a feasible option) or retyping the resume numerous times. If the resume is produced on a word processor, tell the operator to produce at least 10 copies.

The information provided in resumes today has changed from that provided in the past because of legal restrictions and the need to save space for more vital information. To avoid discrimination, the law states that you need not specify such data as age, marital status, dependents, or physical measurements (height and weight). You should not include this information on a resume. To save space you also should exclude the names and contact information of references from your resume. This information will be included on your employment application. Include those letters of reference that you have available. Preparing a resume takes time; therefore, be prepared to rewrite your resume several times to polish the finished product. It also will need to be revised over time as your experience expands and skills develop. Professional resume services are available in many cities to assist you in putting together an impressive resume.

The Cover Letter

When you send a resume to a potential employer, it must be accompanied by a cover letter. Like the resume, the cover letter should be clear and concise and attract the employer's attention. Extreme care must be taken to ensure that the potential employer's name, title, and address are accurate, with attention to spelling. Jackson's *The Perfect Resume* includes a section on cover letters, the information to include in them, and writing techniques that put you in a positive position. See Figure 20.5 for a sample cover letter.

The letter and accompanying resume will not secure you a job, but they should accomplish their primary purpose of securing the interview. Remember that the entire process of obtaining a job is salesmanship. You must convince

Date

Dear Sir/Madam:

   I was pleased to learn of your clerical position, because I am very interested in obtaining a position that will allow me to expand my skills in this field.

   With my customer service background, I feel well qualified for the position that has been described. I am accustomed to a fast-paced environment where deadlines are a priority and handling multiple jobs is normal. I would like to discuss with you how I could contribute to your organization.

   Please contact me at your earliest convenience so that I may share with you my background and enthusiasm for the job. Thank you for your time and consideration.

Sincerely,

FIGURE **20.5**

A cover letter.

prospective employers that you are exactly the individual they need. You have accomplished the first step if you are invited to interview for a position.

The Employment Search

As mentioned earlier, you are actually beginning the process of obtaining a job by beginning your current program of study. The methods used in a job search are presented in this chapter so that you may begin a personal assessment and develop the tools and skills that will assist you when you begin to look for a permanent position. As you proceed through the training period, your personal assessment will change, your skills will improve, and your tools and skills will be revised. The employment process involves two perspectives: that of the potential employee, which is presented in this chapter, and that of the employer. Both perspectives should be reviewed both as you pursue your education preparation and when you are ready to seek paid employment.

Personal Assessment

Positive attributes important for the administrative medical assistant have been presented in this textbook. You should evaluate these and other positive attributes that you identify in yourself and in other professionals during your training period. You must be honest in assessing your attributes now and in reassessing them periodically throughout the training process and your subse-

AT WORK TODAY

The Job Search

How do you find the job you want? You must put effort into the job search. First check to see if your school has job placement assistance. Be ready to send out resumes, and follow up on them. Use fax machines to put your resume at the job site quicker. Use networking. Contact friends who are working in the medical field or people you worked with during your externship. You can "direct canvas," which means to visit offices and submit your resume even though they are not advertising at the moment. You also may go to work for a "temp" service to gain more experience or contact an employment agency. Last, but not least, you can join the new world of the Internet and browse the many agencies listed there. Some maintain jobs listings; you may post your resume with others. The jobs are there, but you must be willing to work to obtain one.

quent career. Instructors and externship supervisors will be able to offer observations that can be integrated into your personal evaluation; keep in mind that these observations are intended to help you and should be accepted in the positive spirit in which they are offered.

The skills you develop in administrative and clinical areas of study also should be evaluated and periodically reassessed as you become more proficient. Accept every opportunity to practice skills in the classroom and in your externship facility. Each time you perform a skill, you improve your performance. The guidance and suggestions for improvement from instructors or externship supervisors also provide valuable feedback for improving your performance.

To assist you in establishing a format for attribute and skill analysis, you may wish to consult a reference book prepared specifically for this process. *What Color is Your Parachute?* by Richard Nelson Bolles provides an excellent collection of data on skills analysis and job-hunting techniques. It also includes an appendix that lists hundreds of resource books categorized into areas of primary concern, such as guides for college students, women, and minorities, as well as books on career planning, volunteer opportunities, and internships. Also explore bookstores in and around your school for guides to help in the evaluation process. Whatever source of assistance you choose, keep in mind that the objective evaluation of your skills and attributes is the first step in obtaining the job you want.

Sources of Employment

There are many potential sources of employment available when you are ready to enter the job market. The health care field should be viewed as a business, and the process of obtaining a job in health care requires the same approach as obtaining a job in general business. The first thing to keep in mind is that job hunting is a job and should be approached in an organized fashion using all available tools and interested individuals. You should explore all possible sources of employment. The recruiting sources that the future employer may use are listed in Table 11.2. These sources also should be reviewed and used by you. The section in Chapter 11 on recruitment and selection will alert you to what a potential employer will be evaluating when selecting an employee. Your understanding of the employer's perspective will be an asset throughout your job search. The added advantage of an externship program will round out the available sources that can be investigated for potential employment. As previously noted, your externship supervisor may be prepared to offer a permanent position after your course of study. Another opportunity that may arise during externship is that employees in your externship facility will know of possible jobs and thus be a good source of employment referral.

Interview Preparation

First Impressions

Once you have obtained an interview appointment, you should plan carefully for the interview. The first thing to remember is that your evaluation will begin the moment you arrive in the office and before you have the opportunity to speak. The factors that will be evaluated at this point include the following:

- Punctuality
- General appearance
- Dress
- Mannerisms
- Courtesy
- Attitude

Plan to arrive approximately 10 to 15 minutes before the time of your interview appointment. If you do not know the exact location of the appointment, scout it out in advance so that you are not lost and late to the appointment. By arriving early, you will have an opportunity to fill out an application (most employers wish to see your handwriting and spelling ability), compose yourself, and observe the general activity within the office or facility. You should carefully plan the time necessary to travel to the interview. However, should you encounter some unusual interference, such as automobile failure or a breakdown in the transportation system, locate a phone as soon as possible and call the interviewer's office. Briefly explain the situation, apologize for the difficulty, and request another appointment.

Your general appearance should be professional. Your hairstyle should be neat and conservative. Wear minimal jewelry, and any fragrance worn should be very subtle. If applying for a position in an allergist's office, environmental office, or holistic office, do not wear any body scents. Women should apply makeup conservatively. Men with beards or moustaches should have them carefully trimmed. Clothing should be conservative, appropriate day wear that is comfortable and well fitted. Colors should be subtle, pastels, blue, gray, or brown. Attention should be focused on the person, not on the clothing. Men should wear a suit or slacks and a complementary jacket, a dress shirt, and a tie. Men's dress shoes should be black or brown, as appropriate. Women should wear a dress or suit with a skirt. Although pantsuits may be conservative and stylish, dresses are considered to make a better initial appearance. Women's stockings should be free of flaws, and shoes should be conservative. Avoid bright colors, heels that are too high, or sandal styles. Avoid long acrylic or lacquered nails.

In preparation for the interview, you will want to evaluate yourself for the presence of distracting mannerisms. Seek the constructive criticism of observant friends or helpful instructors. Such mannerisms include excessive hand movements such as moving your hands to your face or hair, failure to make eye contact with the interviewer, frequently shifting position in the chair, chewing gum, or using redundancies of speech such as "fillers" (for example, "uhh," "you know," or "like").

Above all, be courteous and maintain a positive attitude. Your attitude is demonstrated by all of the factors that make up the potential employer's first impression of you. Your dress, general appearance, mannerisms, tone of voice, self-confidence, and courtesy demonstrate your willingness to develop a positive interpersonal relationship with the employer. Maintaining a positive attitude will require work on your part, particularly if you must participate in many interviews, before you are offered a position that you want to accept. Repeatedly answering similar questions from multiple interviewers can influence your attitude without you awareness. Being conscious of the possibility of a bored attitude or tone of voice should prevent the problem. Approach each interview as you will approach each patient in the future; each is unique and offers a special challenge. Your attitude will influence the outcome.

The Application

Filling out a preprinted application form may or may not be required at the time of the interview. It is to your advantage if you allow the time to fill out the form as completely as possible (even if you provide a resume). Smaller, private medical practices with one or two physician-employers may eliminate this step of the process. In this case your resume will serve as the application. If the potential employer has not received a resume from you before the interview, bring one with you. It will serve as a reminder of your skills and qualifications when the final selection is being made.

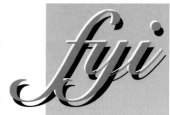

What Not to Do at the Interview!

1. Do not chew gum.
2. Try to avoid fidgeting, tugging at your clothes, stroking your face, or any other nervous gestures.
3. Do not put any belongings or your hands on the desk.
4. Do not argue, brag, or criticize.
5. Do not interrupt.
6. Do not ask too many questions.
7. Do not comment on the office furniture, artwork, and so on.

WHAT DO YOU THINK?

Jenny had completed her schooling and externship as an administrative medical assistant. She had done well in both, receiving good to excellent marks. She answered a help-wanted ad and secured an interview. This is what happened during her interview:

Jenny was 15 minutes late because she had to put gas in her car and had trouble finding a parking space. She rushed into the office and apologized for being late, then sat down, nervously chewing her gum. During the interview, she was asked to talk about herself. She spent the next 15 minutes relating the details of her life. She was nervous and out of habit kept pushing back her hair. When asked about her work experience, she explained that she had never worked in the field before and that all of her other positions had been boring, minimum-wage jobs. She thought after the interview that she had done OK.

What went wrong in this interview? Can you name the specific problems? What would you have done differently?

A

APPLICATION FOR EMPLOYMENT

PERSONAL INFORMATION: DATE:_____

NAME:_____
        LAST   FIRST   MIDDLE

PRESENT ADDRESS:_____
                    STREET   CITY   STATE   ZIP

PERMANENT ADDRESS:_____
                    STREET   CITY   STATE   ZIP

PHONE NUMBER: (_____)_____ SOC. SEC. #:_____

STATE NAME AND RELATIONSHIP OF ANY   REFERRED
RELATIVES IN OUR EMPLOY_____BY:_____

EMPLOYMENT DESIRED:

POSITION:_____

DATE YOU   SALARY
CAN START:_____ DESIRED:_____

ARE YOU
CURRENTLY EMPLOYED?_____

MAY WE CONTACT
YOUR EMPLOYER?_____

HAVE YOU EVER
APPLIED TO THIS COMPANY BEFORE?_____ WHERE?_____ WHEN?_____

EDUCATION:

SCHOOL	NAME AND LOCATION	GRADUATED		MAJOR SUBJECTS	GPA
		YES	NO		
GRAMMAR SCHOOL					
HIGH SCHOOL					
COLLEGE					
OTHER (SPECIFY)					

SUBJECTS OF SPECIAL STUDY OR RESEARCH WORK:_____

_____

SPECIAL TRAINING:_____

_____

ACTIVITIES: (CIVIC, ATHLETIC, ETC.)_____
            (EXCLUDE ORGANIZATIONS, THE NAME OR CHARACTER OF WHICH INDICATES THE RACE, CREED, SEX, MARITAL STATUS, AGE, COLOR, OR NATIONAL ORIGIN OF ITS MEMBERS.)

_____

_____

(CONTINUED ON OTHER SIDE)

LAST

FIRST

MIDDLE

FIGURE 20.6

Front (A) of an application for employment form. (Reprinted with permission from REDIFORM.)

FORMER EMPLOYERS: LIST YOUR LAST FOUR EMPLOYERS, STARTING WITH PRESENT OR MOST RECENT.

DATE MONTH AND YEAR	NAME AND ADDRESS OF EMPLOYER	SALARY	POSITION	REASON FOR LEAVING
FROM		$		
TO		PER		
FROM		$		
TO		PER		
FROM		$		
TO		PER		
FROM		$		
TO		PER		

REFERENCES: GIVE THE NAMES OF THREE PERSONS NOT RELATED TO YOU, WHOM YOU HAVE KNOWN AT LEAST ONE YEAR.

NAME	ADDRESS	BUSINESS	YEARS ACQUAINTED
1.			
2.			
3.			

IN CASE OF EMERGENCY, NOTIFY:_____
                                          NAME

ADDRESS:_____ PHONE:_____
I AUTHORIZE INVESTIGATION OF ALL STATEMENTS CONTAINED IN THIS APPLICATION. I UNDERSTAND THAT MISREPRESENTATION OR OMISSION OF FACTS CALLED FOR IS CAUSE FOR DISMISSAL. FURTHER, I UNDERSTAND AND AGREE THAT MY EMPLOYMENT IS FOR NO DEFINITE PERIOD AND MAY, REGARDLESS OF THE DATE OF PAYMENT OF MY WAGES AND SALARY, BE TERMINATED AT ANY TIME WITHOUT ANY PREVIOUS NOTICE.

SIGNED:_____DATE:_____

APPLICANT - DO NOT WRITE BELOW THIS LINE

INTERVIEWED BY:_____DATE:_____

REMARKS:_____

_____

NEATNESS:_____

ABILITY:_____

HIRED:_____DEPT:_____POSITION:_____START DATE:_____SALARY:_____

APPROVALS:

1. _____   2. _____   3. _____
        EMPLOYMENT MANAGER   EMPLOYMENT HEAD   GENERAL MANAGER

REDIFORM. 9G285
(Revised 11/90)

B

FIGURE 20.6

Back (B) of an application for employment form. (Reprinted with permission from REDIFORM.)

Application forms (Figure 20.6) are most often required in settings such as hospitals, clinics, and large group-medical practices. Be certain to answer questions briefly and clearly and in clean, neat printing. The employer will evaluate the appearance of the application as a sample of your work. Answer all appropriate questions. By law you are not required to answer questions regarding your marital status, number of dependents, religious preference, ethnic origin, and so on. You can leave these blank; no comment is necessary at this time. Even though you are not required to answer a number of questions, it is to your credit and advantage to volunteer information, particularly marital status, number of dependents, and arrangements for child care. The employer will appreciate this straightforward approach, and many times this will give you an edge over applicants who do not divulge this information. Be prepared to supply the names, addresses, and phone numbers of references at this time. You will, of course, have obtained advance permission from your reference sources and have chosen individuals who recognize your positive attributes and skills. Three references are considered the minimum. At this time you also may supply photocopies of the reference letters you may have obtained on completion of your externship.

The Interview

If you have little or no experience in seeking paid employment, anticipating an interview may be intimidating. It does not have to be! You can prepare well in advance of the actual interview. Request time in your externship seminar, or form a group of supportive friends to practice interviews. Take turns being the interviewer and the applicant; tape-record or videotape the practice, if possible. Have the interviewer and any observers report their observations. Retain the positive actions, and make any appropriate adjustments to present yourself in a better light. The tape recorder will help you objectively evaluate your speech patterns, and give you a permanent record to compare with future tapes.

Your instructor, students with interview experience, and reference books will supply you with questions that may be asked during an actual interview. Some will be very specific, such as the following:

- "What is your typing speed?"
- "What computer programs are you familiar with?"
- "What options do you have if a patient does not accept the first appointment time you offer?"
- "Which billing systems or services have you had experience with?"

Other questions may be classified as open-ended. These might include the following:

- "Tell me a little about yourself."
- "What do you consider your strengths and weaknesses?"
- "In what ways can you contribute to this practice?"
- "What are your career goals?"
- "What have you done with your life that you are proud of?"

Such open-ended questions are intended to provide the interviewer with material by which to evaluate your oral communication skills and your opinion of yourself. Both specific and open-ended questions should be answered clearly and honestly. Take time to think before answering, and answer only the specific question asked. Refrain from giving lengthy answers or volunteering information that is not requested. The interviewer may inquire about the questions you chose not to answer on the application. If you still feel that the questions are not appropriate, you should not feel pressured into answering. However, you should be careful not to reply in a hostile or defensive manner. An appropriate response might be, "I did not feel that the information was important to my professional career."

Toward the end of the interview the interviewer may ask whether you have any questions. If the opportunity to ask questions is not offered, you should request it. Asking pertinent questions demonstrates interest in the position and provides the opportunity to contribute information about yourself that did not surface in answer to the interviewer's questions. You may wish to inquire about aspects of the open position such as:

- "Do you encourage your employees to take continuing education courses?"
- "Why did the previous employee leave the position I am applying for?"
- "Do your staff members cross-train so that there is backup for each position?"

You should not begin this phase of the interview by asking about holidays, vacations, or sick leave. This would imply that your primary concern is the time you can spend being paid for time off work.

If salary has not been discussed, it should be before the interview closes. A statement in a job description or in an advertisement of "salary negotiable" is inappropriate. It should alert you to the possibility of a low salary offer. Before reporting for an interview, you should investigate the salary ranges in the area. If the potential employer states a salary that is low, politely say so, for example, "When I called several offices in the area, I did not receive information that salaries for this type of position were so low." If you are asked to state the minimum salary you accept, do not respond with a dollar amount. Instead, state that you are not interested in minimums but in a challenging career opportunity with appropriate compensation. If you know the salary ranges for the area, you may wish to name a slightly higher range. For example, if the starting salaries average $1000 to $1200 a month, you might state that you consider $1050 to $1250 an appropriate range. This way a counteroffer will still fall within the appropriate range.

As the interview is about to close you should recognize the interviewer's cue. Stand, thank the interviewer for his or her courtesy and time, and shake hands. Ask when you might hear about the final decision if the interviewer does not volunteer the information.

Interview Follow-Up

The evening of the interview you should write a brief, formal note to the interviewer thanking him or her for his or her time and courtesy. This serves two

EXAMPLE OF FOLLOW-UP LETTER

July 1, 1999

Sam D. Smith, M.D.
888 Nowhere Street, #201
Anywhere, CA 99999

Dear Dr. Smith/Name of Interviewer:

Thank you for the opportunity to interview for the Administrative Medical Assistant position today. I am truly interested in the position. It not only sounds challenging and rewarding, but will provide the opportunity for utilizing the skills I have developed through educational preparation and practical experience.

I enjoyed meeting you and your staff. There seems to be a strong sense of camaraderie between you and the staff and the patients.

Thank you for considering my application, and I look forward to hearing from you in the near future.

Sincerely,

Person's name

FIGURE 20.7

Example of a follow-up letter. (Courtesy De A. Eggers & Associates, Sonoma, Calif.)

purposes: it demonstrates your conscientiousness, and it will put your name in the interviewer's mind again (Figure 20.7).

You can usually expect to hear the outcome of the application and interview within 7 to 10 days. If the job is offered to you, take time to carefully evaluate the offer and compare the position with others that you are considering. Should you be notified that another applicant was offered the position, take the initiative to ask why in a positive manner. Make it clear that you are seeking constructive assistance for your continued job search and that you will appreciate any suggestions. Many times you will discover that the reason is that the other applicant had more experience, not that the employer had a negative impression of you. Your openness may stimulate the interviewer to become a source of leads to other positions. Do not be dismayed if the interviewer does not call. Take the initiative, call, and ask if the position has been filled. Unfortunately, many interviewers do not take the time to respond to each applicant. Consider the interviewer's point of view. In large cities a help-wanted advertisement may generate 100 applicants. The response time needed for that many people would be incredible. Call and ask. Put yourself in the forefront again.

Setting Goals

Now is also the time to set goals and objectives for your future. Some will be short-term goals, such as completing the administrative medical assistant program and passing the certifying examination, and some will be long-term goals, such as becoming an office manager within 5 years. Overall, these goals should be realistic and developed using an effective method. To set goals do the following:

- Set positive priorities and determine a goal
- Determine resources
- Develop plans and analyze barrier to goals
- Implement the plan
- Evaluate the plan periodically, adjusting and improving it when necessary

Overall, you need to develop and maintain a positive attitude toward every experience and opportunity you encounter. An optimistic approach will make you an asset in any career setting.

Conclusion

Your externship experience and preparation for a role on a health care team are, in a sense, a job in themselves. Devote careful attention to the process, and keep in mind that it is the first step to your future career. You need to develop skill in interpersonal relationships, pay serious attention to your studies in the administrative area, and identify and enhance your talents. It is in your best interest to develop a close, working relationship with your instructors. They can provide you with an objective evaluation of your development, can provide references, and are a potential source of job referrals.

Review QUESTIONS

1. Where could you work to fulfill your externship requirements?

2. How is an externship helpful to you in your theoretical courses? How is it helpful to you personally?

3. How could an externship program help you get a job?

4. List your best attributes. How will each one help you in your career?

5. What three basic considerations will you keep in mind when planning a resume?

6. Develop a basic resume based on your education and experience; develop an alternative resume.

7. Write a cover letter to a potential employer.

8. What do you expect a resume and cover letter to accomplish?

9. Prepare five questions that you would ask a potential employee if you were the interviewer?

10. Pair off with a classmate, and practice an interview as the employer. Then switch roles and repeat the interview.

11. Write an appropriate follow-up letter to a person with whom you interviewed.

SUGGESTED READINGS

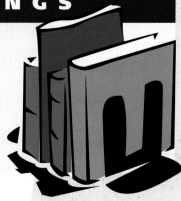

Bolles RN: *What color is your parachute?*, revised edition, Berkeley, Calif., 1991, Ten Speed Press.

Jackson T: *The perfect resume,* Garden City, N.Y., 1992, Anchor Press Doubleday.

APPENDIX A

Common Prescription Abbreviations and Symbols

Abbreviation or symbol	Meaning	Abbreviation or symbol	Meaning
a	Before	noc(t)	Night
aa	Of each	od	Daily or once a day
ac	Before meals	OD	Right eye
ad lib	As desired	oint	Ointment
amt	Amount	OS	Left eye
aq	Aqueous	OU	Both eyes
bid	Twice a day	oz	Ounce
c̄	With	℥	Ounce
cap(s)	Capsule(s)	p	After, past
cc	Cubic centimeter	per	By or with
dil	Dilute	pc	After meals
Dx or Diag	Diagnosis	po or per os	By mouth
D/C or d/c	Discontinue	prn	Whenever necessary
D/W	Dextrose in water	pt	Pint (or patient)
dr	Drain	pulv	Powder
ℨ	Dram	q	Every
ℨ	One dram	qam	Every morning
d	Day	qd	Every day
Dr	Doctor	qh	Every hour
fl or fld	Fluid	q2h or q2	Every 2 hours
gal	Gallon	q3h or q3	Every 3 hours
g or gm	Gram	qhs	Every night
gr	Grain	qid	Four times per day
gt or gtt	Drop(s)	qod	Every other day
H or hr	Hour	qs	Quantity sufficient
hs	Hour of sleep or bedtime	Rx	Take thou
IM	Intramuscular	s̄	Without
IU	International units	sc or subq or SubQ	Subcutaneous
IV	Intravenous	Sig	Directions
kg	Kilogram	sol	Solution
L	Liter	ss	One half
liq	Liquid	subling	Sublingual (under tongue)
m or min	Minimum	stat	Immediate
mgc	Microgram	tid	Three times a day
mEq	Milliequivalent	tine or tr	Tincture
mEq/L	Milliequivalents per liter	tab	tablet
mg	Milligram	tsp	teaspoon
ml	Milliliter	Tbsp	Tablespoon
mm	Millimeter	ung or ungt	Ointment
npo (NPO)	Nothing by mouth	U	units
NS	Normal saline		

525

APPENDIX B

Stratford Healthcare Management System (SHS) Software

Stratford Healthcare Management System (SHS) Software is one of the easiest and most flexible of all the medical and dental accounts-receivable software packages available. They have been Y2K ready for several years and have met all requirements of submission of electronic claims through every Medicare carrier approved by the federal government. It is almost a given that the administrative medical assistant will be working with some type of patient billing software. Developing your skills with the SHS software will assist you in learning almost any other patient billing system within a short time.

The overall software is already available through the school's system, your instructor will assign you your own account with which to work (for example, \130\206). This would work as though it is your physician's account. You will not need a separate disk; you will only need to log into your account.

Practice exercises are included in this appendix so that you may increase your knowledge and skills in assisting the practice to collect fees.

Working with the SHS

The computer system in your school may have various ways to access the SHS software. You may only have to click on an icon with the mouse, or you may need to scroll though a listing of accounts by number for each student until you locate yours (for example, Mary J. Smith [206] touch [ENTER], or you may have a prompt (C:\) at which you would enter CD\130\206 and touch [ENTER]. There are many ways to enter a program.

At the first screen in the SHS program (Figure B.1), you will touch [ENTER], which will bring up a screen asking for your password. Enter the password you created when your instructor established your account. The password will show on the screen or the instructor may simply have you type in HOME2 or DEMO2 and touch [ENTER].

Quick Start

Starting SHS

To start SHS, change to your ACCOUNTS RECEIVABLE (MAIN) DIRECTORY (Figure B.2) by typing: CD\130\200 [ENTER]
Then type BEGIN [ENTER]
The entry word may be HOME2 or DEMO2 [ENTER]

```
                         Account Number: 303546
                         Data Version: 8.2d(151)   Series 6/6
                         Date: 12/09/1998
 _\130\255-----------------------------------------------------------------

 Software                    THIS DISPLAY IS LOCKED

 -------------------------------------------------------------------------
 -----Copyright 1976-1997 All rights reserved.  A single CPU license------------
 is granted to the above user.  Any other use of this software is illegal. ------

 Stratford Healthcare Systems, Inc.    Email:mail@stratfordsoftware.com
 1346 Mitten Road                      Http://www.stratfordsoftware.com/
 Burlingame, CA 94010
 Office: (650) 692-7970
 Fax:    (650) 692-1073
 ---------------------------Physician Software----------------------------
 Please type your entry word
```

Figure B.1

```
 1.    Finished With The Patient's Receivables
 2.    Change The Report/Default Date
 3.    Patient Information (Enter,Change,Inquire)
 4.    Statement Programs
 5.    Insurance Claim Form Programs
 6.    Report Programs
 7.    Statistics and Other Information
 8.    Profile and System Management
 --\130\255----------------------------------------------------------------
    Software        ACCOUNTS RECEIVABLE (MAIN) DIRECTORY      (2) 09/02/1999
 -------------------------------------------------------------------------
 Please choose one of the above
```

Figure B.2

To Register a Patient

Select the number 3 from the ACCOUNTS RECEIVABLE (MAIN) DIRECTORY.

Type dot (period or [.])[ENTER], and the program will assign a patient account number (Figure B.3)

Assign a financial class (1=Private Pay; 2=Industrial; 3=Medicaid; 4=Medicare).

Answer the questions.

To Register an Insurance

Select the number 2 from the mini-menu at the bottom of your screen in the patient registration screen.

Select 1 to complete information for the primary insurance, and select 2 for secondary.

Select number 9 to complete the claim form questions.

To Post Transactions

Select the number 1 from the mini-menu at the bottom of your patient registration screen.

Select the transaction type (1=Charge; 2=Payment; 3=Plus Adjustment; 4=Minus Adjustment; 5=Printing Memo; 6=Non Printing Memo) (Figures B.4 to B.6) and answer the questions.

If you have loaded your fee schedule in your automatic transaction library, do not select the transaction type.

Put in your automatic transaction code now.

To Run Statements

Select number 4 from the ACCOUNTS RECEIVABLE (MAIN) DIRECTORY.

Select the type of statement you want to run.

To Run Insurance Forms

Select number 5 from the ACCOUNTS RECEIVABLE (MAIN) DIRECTORY.

Select the type of insurance form you want to run.

To Run Reports

Select number 6 from the ACCOUNTS RECEIVABLE (MAIN) DIRECTORY.

Select the type of report you want to run.

To Backup

Select number 1 from the ACCOUNTS RECEIVABLE (MAIN) DIRECTORY.

Select 1 Backup your data. If you have a Colorado jumbo tape drive, quit SHS, type CD\130\4 [ENTER].

Then type TAPSYS.

To Run Batch Processor

Select from the ACCOUNTS RECEIVABLE (MAIN) DIRECTORY.

Select 3 from the SPECIAL ITEMS directory.

To Exit Program

At the ACCOUNTS RECEIVABLE (MAIN) DIRECTORY, touch [HOME].

Other Commands

To save a window touch [CTRL+W].

To pull information previously entered touch dot (period or [.]) [ENTER].

To go from the transaction screen back to the patient information screen touch [LEFT ARROW].

Previous Balances P=Current; P1=30-59; P2=60-89; P3=90-119; P4=120-149; P5=150=179; P6=180+; M=Credit Balance.

Reorganization

Reorganization should be run at least once a week. From the ACCOUNTS RECEIVABLE (MAIN) DIRECTORY choose:

8 File and System Management; then choose:

3 Reorganize your data files (Back up your data first), then choose:

7 Complete reorganization of all files and balances

```
--\130\255----------------------------------------------------------------
    Software              PATIENT ACCOUNT INFORMATION      (2) 09/02/1999
---------------------------------------------------------------------------


You may lookup patients by name in 4 ways (Example: JOHN SMITH)

Lastname,Firstname       (Comma separator)          SMITH,JOHN
Firstname.Lastname       (dot separator)            JOHN.SMITH
Firstname Lastname       (space separator)          JOHN SMITH
First Letter of First Name+Last Name                JSMITH


                                              Enter a New Account= .

Please Enter a Social Security Number        -  -
Please Enter a Patient's Account Number or a Patient's Name
```

Figure B.3

```
Name      JOAN        SMITH              Bill To   JOAN       SMITH
Birthdate   07/17/1923 Age 75 yrs        923 COUNTRYMEADOW LANE
Social Sec# 559-22-3449 Sex F Stat D     SONOMA          CA 95476
                                   Home Ph  (707) 996-3434
CoPay     $5.00                    Work Ph
MD        CAMPBELL                 Employer
INS                                Billing  H Smts     D Stmt <None>
No 10025  VMMG                06   Main Dx  401.1
--\130\255----------------------------------------------------------------
   Software           PATIENT ACCOUNT INFORMATION      (2) 09/02/1999
-------------------------------------------------------------------------


      MEDICAL RECORDS     Notes     None
           MEDICATION     Notes     None
                VISIT     Notes     None

Date=D> <Demand Form/EDI=6>
CHOOSE <Transaction=1> <Insurance=2> <Another Patient=3> <Revision=4>
0.00
```

Figure B.4

```
Name      JOAN        SMITH              Bill To   JOAN       SMITH
Birthdate 07/17/1923 Age 75 yrs          923 COUNTRYMEADOW LANE
Social Sec# 559-55-3449  Sex F Stat D    SONOMA, CA 95476
                                   Home Ph  (707) 996-3434
CoPay     $5.00                    Work Ph
MD        CAMPBELL                 Employer
INS                                Billing  H Smts     D Stmt <None>
No 10025  VMMG                06   Main Dx 401.1
--\130\255----------------------------------------------------------------
 Srch     Dr   Date    Procedure Qty     Description   ICD-9     Amount
-------------------------------------------------------------------------
          01   08/03/99 99203     1    OFFICE/OUTPATIENT 3 401.1   120.00
          01   08/03/99               PAYMENT=THANK YOU             5.00
          01   08/24/99               VMMG PAID                    48.73-
          01   08/24/99               INSURANCE WRITE OFF          66.27-
          01   10/02/99 90724     1    INFLUENZA IMMUNIZ 3 V04.8   20.00
          01   11/12/99               VMMG PAID                     8.55-
          01   11/12/99               INSURANCE WRITE OFF          11.45-

<Chg=1> <Pmt=2> <+Adj=3> <-Adj=4> <P Memo=5> <NP Memo=6>
Please enter the Type of Transaction
0.00
```

Figure B.5

```
Name      JOAN        SMITH              Bill To   JOAN       SMITH
Birthdate 07/17/1923 Age 75 yrs          923 COUNTRYMEADOW LANE
SocSec#   559-55-3434 Sex F Stat D       SONOMA          CA 95476
                                   Home Ph  (707) 996-3434
CoPay     $5.00                    Work Ph
MD        CAMPBELL                 Employer
INS                                Billing  H Smts     D    Stmt <None>
No 10025  VMMG           06   Main Dx  401.1
--\130\255----------------------------------------------------------------
 Srch     Dr   Date    Procedure Qty     Description   ICD-9     Amount
-------------------------------------------------------------------------
          01   10/02/99 90724     1    INFLUENZA IMMUNIZ   V04.8    20.00
          01   11/12/99               VMMG PAID                     8.55-
          01   11/12/99               INSURANCE WRITE OFF          11.45-


Charge
Please enter the Rendering Provider Number
0.00
```

Figure B.6

Screens

ACCOUNTS RECEIVABLE (MAIN) DIRECTORY (see Figure B.2)

1 Finished With The Patient's Receivables
2 Change The Report/Default Date
3 Patient Information (Enter, Change, Inquire)
4 Statement Programs
5 Insurance Claim Form Programs
6 Report Programs
7 Statistics and Other Information
8 Profile and System Management
Finished With The Patient's Receivable For Now (Figure B.7)
1 Back up your data
2 Order supplies
3 Batch Processor Programs

4 Electronic Data Interchange
5 General Accounting Programs
6 Use your own Word Processing Program
7 Special Communication Program
Statement Directory (Menu choices are controlled by the user) (Figure B.8)
1 Create ALL standard 1-up Statements
2 Create ALL Open-Item Statements
3 Create ALL MEDICARE Open-Item Statements
4 Create ALL Family Account Statements
Insurance Claim Form Programs (Menu choices are controlled by the user) (Figure B.9)
1 Create ALL HCFA-1500 Private Pay
2 Create ALL HCFA-1500 Medicare
3 Create ALL 92 HCFA-1500 Private Pay
4 Create ALL 92 HCFA-1500 Industrial
5 Create ALL 92 HCFA-1500 Medicaid

```
1      Backup your data
2      Order supplies
3      Batch Processor Programs
4      Electronic Data Interchange (EDI, Electronic Claims)

6      Custom Word Processing Program
7      Custom Communication Program
8      Print/Clear the NON-EDI audits
--\130\255-----------------------------------------------------------------
 Software                        Special Items            (2)  09/02/1999
-----------------------------------------------------------------------------
 Please choose one of the above
```

Figure B.7

```
1      Create ALL Standard 1-up Statements
2      Create ALL PRIVATE PAY Open-Item Statements
3      Create ALL INDUSTRIAL Open-Item Statements
4      Create ALL MEDICARE Open-Item Statements
5      Create ALL Family Account Statements

--\130\255-----------------------------------------------------------------
 Software                     Statement Directory         (2)  09/02/1999
-----------------------------------------------------------------------------
 Print or View 2 page(s) PRIVATE PAY Open-Item Statements

 Please choose one of the above
```

Figure B.8

```
1      Create ALL Private Pay
2      Create ALL Industrial
3      Create ALL Medicaid
4      Create ALL Medicare



--\130\255-----------------------------------------------------------------
 Software                     Insurance Directory         (2)  09/02/1999
-----------------------------------------------------------------------------
 Print or View 10 page(s) Demand Private Pay

 Please choose one of the above
```

Figure B.9

6 Create ALL 92 HCFA-1500 Medicare
7 Create ALL TN/AL UB-82/92 (HCFA-1450) Dialysis Report Directory (Figure B.10)
1 Create the TRANSACTION AUDIT
2 Create a TRIAL TRANSACTION LISTING (Balance your transactions)
3 Report Gen: Collection, Recall, etc.
4 Report Generator: One at a Time
5 Reserved
6 Reserved
7 Reports: Patient: Alpha, Numeric, Aging, Service charges
8 Reports: Transaction/Production: 680/681/682/683/684/685/687/688
   Statistics Directory (Figure B.11)
1 Provider Accounts Receivable and Aging
2 Guarantor Accounts Receivable and Aging
3 Patient Accounts Receivable and Aging
4 Hardware/Software Information
5 Software/Data Entry Status, Dates, and Other Information
6 Other Information
7 Appointment Scheduling

8 Appointment Schedule Maintenance/Setup
   File and System Management Directory (Figure B.12)
1 Reinitialize the System Parameters
   Reserved
3 REORGANIZE your data files (BACKUP your data first)
4 Auto-Transactions (Enter–Change–Inquire)
5 Codes: Finical Class, Recall, Modifier, CPT, ICD, Forms, Research, User
6 Insurance Companies, Provider, Employer, Referring, UPIN, etc.
   Reserved
8 Other Special Purpose Programs
   Report Generator: One At A Time (Menu choices are controlled by the user)
1 Report Generator: 641 Label
2 Report Generator: 642 Superbill
3 Report Generator: 643 Custom
4 Report Generator: 644 Custom
5 Report Generator: 645 Custom
6 Report Generator: 646 Custom
7 Report Generator: 647 Custom
8 Report Generator: 648 Custom

```
1      Create the TRANSACTION AUDIT
2      Create a TRIAL TRANSACTION LISTING
3      Rpt Gen: Collection, Recall, etc
4      Report Generator: One at a time


Rpt Gen:  Patient   listing: code usage:    Ins Co, Employer
Reports:  Patient   : Alpha, Numeric, Aging, Codes, Service charges
Reports:  Transaction/Production:  680/681/682/683/684/685/687/688
--\130\255--------------------------------------------------------------
 Software                    Report Directory          (2) 09/02/1999
------------------------------------------------------------------------
Print or View 5 page(s) TRANSACTION AUDIT

Please choose one of the above
```

Figure B.10

```
1      Provider Accounts Receivable and Aging
2      Guarantor Accounts Receivable and Aging
3      Patient Accounts Receivable and Aging
4      Hardware/Software Information
5      Software/Data Entry Status, Dates and Other Information
6      Other Information
7      Appointment Scheduling
8      Appointment Schedule Maintenance/Setup
--\130\255--------------------------------------------------------------
 Software                    Statistics Directory      (2) 09/02/1999
------------------------------------------------------------------------
Please choose one of the above
```

Figure B.11

```
1      Reinitialize the System Parameters
2      Managed Care Programs
3      REORGANIZE your data files (BACKUP your data first)
4      Auto-Transactions (Enter-Change-Inquire)
5      Codes: Financial Class, Recall, Modifier, CPT, ICD, Forms, Research, User
6      Insurance Companies, Provider, Employer, Referring, UPIN, etc
7      EDI Related Information Programs
8      Other Special Purpose Programs (1)
--\130\255--------------------------------------------------------------
Software                  System Management Directory   (2) 09/02/1999
------------------------------------------------------------------------
Please choose one of the above
```

Figure B.12

Starting the SHS Program

At the C:\ prompt you must change directories by typing the following: CD\130\200 [ENTER]

Then type the word: BEGIN. You may type BEGIN in either upper or lower case.

You will be asked to:

Please type your entry word

Type HOME2. That will put you on entry level 2.

Enter the date and touch [ENTER]. If you touch [ENTER] without entering a date, SHS will use the computer's date. The format for the date is MMDDYYYY. You must enter two digits for the month, two digits for the day, and four digits for the year (for example, enter January 2, 2001, as 01022001).

Making a Backup

All computers must have a frequent backup. **THERE ARE NO EXCEPTIONS.** When your computer fails, and it will someday, you must have a backup or you will be forced to type all of your information again.

Daily backup

Back up your data each day you enter information (information is data).

Complete (System) backup

Do a complete system backup once a month.

From the MAIN DIRECTORY select:

1 Finished with the Patient's Receivables for Now

Remember to put in your backup medium (floppy or tape) before you give the backup command.

From the Special Item Directory select:

1 Back up your data

Moving Around in the SHS Program

You start most actions from the ACCOUNTS RECEIVABLE (MAIN) DIRECTORY, also referred to as the *main menu* or *main directory*. To get to different areas of the program you touch a number selection (1 to 8) and then touch [ENTER]. For each menu choice you make, you can be back to the previous menu by pressing [ESC]. One way to think of it is a main room with eight doors in it. If you open one of the doors and enter that room, then you touch [ESC] to leave that room. Some of the rooms also have doors in them. You can also open those doors. Some of those rooms will even have doors. The principle is the same. You make a menu choice followed by [ENTER] to open a door, or touch [ESC] to go back to the previous room. when you [ESC] back to the main room and you finish visiting, you can touch the [HOME] key to exit the main room (and thus quit the SHS program). Press the [HOME] key twice if you wish to exit faster.

In a patient account you can use the left-arrow key to go from the transaction or insurance screen back to the patient information screen.

Saving Your Work

As you enter data into the program, whether it is a new patient, an office visit, or a payment, SHS saves your data. You do not have to do a separate save command such as in word processing and other programs. For this to take place, the computer opens and closes many files on your hard disk while you enter data. Therefore it is ***absolutely critical*** that you **DO NOT** reset your computer while you are running the SHS program. This means **do not** touch [CTRL+Alt+Delete], **do not** touch the Reset button, and **do not** turn off your computer while the program is running. Doing so will damage your data files and may require you to restore from a backup!

System Defaults (Secrets)

Dot [.][ENTER]

SHS uses a dot (period or [.]) as a default. Some keyboards will have two periods, one on the number keypad and one on the typing portion of the board. When you type dot [.][ENTER] the program lets you pull in information that is already in the computer. For example, use this when you are completing the insurance screen; if the "bill to" or guarantor's name is the same as the insurer's name then type dot [.][ENTER]. The program will pull down the information. You may use dot [.][ENTER] to pull down the patient's name, address, and telephone number.

[CTRL+W] (Control Window)

If you are in the middle of entering information in a pop-up window, you have two methods of saving the information. first, you may touch [ENTER] through all the fields in the selection until you reach the last field. The contents of the widow are saved, and the window disappears. Also, you may touch [CTRL+W] to save the contents of the window without having to return through the remaining fields. For example, when you are entering the employer information, you may only want to enter the name of the employer. Instead of touch [ENTER] through these fields, you may touch [CTRL+W]. Remember that you need to hold the [CTRL] key down while you touch the letter "W". If you do not hold them down together, you will type the letter "W" instead of saving the window.

Patient Account Information—Getting Back

If you are in the Patient Transaction screen and want to go back to the Patient Account Information screen, touch [ENTER] one time. You will see a menu at bottom of the screen that states:

CHOOSE<Transaction=1><Insurance=2<Another Patient=3> <Revision=4>

Instead of making a selection, touch [LEFT ARROW]. You will be returned to Patient Account Information.

Using a Mouse

You may use a mouse with most windows. The yellow triangle on the border of the window will scroll up or down if you click on it with the mouse. Scrolling occurs in the direction in which the tip of the triangle is pointing. If you want to scroll further in the file, then you may click on the yellow diamond. By moving the diamond, you can move through a file much faster than scrolling through each line. If, for example, you move the yellow diamond to the middle of the screen, you will find yourself in the middle of the file.

To use a mouse with the SHS programs a mouse driver must be loaded. The SHS program recognizes the Windows NT mouse drive and the Windows (95) version. Make sure you are in "Microsoft Mode."

How to Make Corrections

You may make corrections by using the [BACKSPACE] or [DELETE] key. [BACKSPACE] is not the same as the [LEFT ARROW], but it can be used. [BACKSPACE] deletes from end to beginning. [LEFT ARROW] will move the cursor back or to the left. [DELETE] will delete the character that is being highlighted by the cursor. The character to the right of the cursor will then move to the left and be under the cursor.

Let's Get Started

This appendix is designed for the beginning SHS user and assumes you have little or not prior computer experience.

New users should remember five key facts. They are as follows:

1. If you learned to type a number of years ago, you were taught to use the letter "el" (l) in place of the number (1). This program distinguishes between the letter and the number; the letter "el" (l) cannot be substituted for the number (1).

2. You cannot use the letter "oh" (O) to represent the number zero (0); the program distinguishes between the letter and the number.

3. Whenever you have completed entering your answer to a question (information in a field) you must touch [RETURN] or [ENTER]. See the brackets around the word "enter" and "return"? These brackets mean that you should touch a key on your keyboard called "enter" or "return"; you are not to type in the word enter or return.

4. There are three keys on your keyboard (*Shift, Alt,* and *Ctrl*) that you will use in conjunction with other keys. For example, you may be asked to touch [CTRL+W]. For these keys, you must hold down the [CTRL] key while you touch the [W] key.

5. You should be in **Caps Lock** and **Num Lock** when using SHS. To produce a lowercase letter without removing [CAPS LOCK], just hold down the [SHIFT] key while touching the letter. If you type on the numeric keypad (usually located on the right side of your keyboard) and you do not see numbers appearing on the screen , you need to touch the [NUM LOCK] button to activate Num Lock.

Starting to Work at the Terminal

Sit in front of your display (also know as a *terminal, CRT, display,* or *VDT*). Your display and computer should always be left turned ON> Some screens darken automatically after a while (these systems have a screen saver), and others may need to have the brightness and contrast knobs turned down. First, try touch any key (it is best to use a key such as [SHIFT]). If you do not see anything on the screen, then turn both the brightness and contrast control knobs. If the terminal is not on, you will need to turn it on.

NOTE: Leaving your equipment on will cause your system to require fewer repairs. Do not worry about the computer using too much electricity. The computer and peripherals draw very little power.

Manual Notation and Other Information

A specific notation is used in this appendix to indicate what you type into each field or which keys to touch.

All the keys described in the manual, except the arrow keys, are shown in CAPITAL LETTERS and are enclosed in square brackets, for example, [ENTER]. The arrow keys are enclosed in square brackets, but the brackets will contain the words telling you which arrow key to use instead of a picture of an arrow, for example, [LEFT ARROW]. When the program asks you something, the questions will be MONOSPACED. The selection that you type or select will be in monospaced New Times Roman type and occasionally, for emphasis, **bold** type.

It is recommended that you use CAPITAL letters when you use the SHS program. If you are typing in capitals, touch the [CAPS LOCK] key. A green light will illuminate on the keyboard near the words "CAPS LOCK."

Patient Account Numbers

You may assign individual account numbers or you may let the program assign the account numbers. If you use family billing or have the same guarantor for several different patients, you can create statements by guarantor instead of by patient.

You should be at the ACCOUNTS RECEIVABLE (MAIN) DIRECTORY; if you look at the center of the screen and see the words ACCOUNTS RECEIVABLE (MAIN) DIRECTORY, then you are at the correct location. If you are not, touch [ENTER] until you arrive at this screen.

Getting to the Patient Account Information

Below are the selections in the ACCOUNTS RECEIVABLE (MAIN) DIRECTORY. Your entry word determines how many of the eight selection lines you will see. Each selection has a number in front of it. When the program asks you to "Please choose one of the above," type the number of your selection. You may select any number in the directory.

1   Finished with the Patient's Receivables
2   Change The Report/Default Date
3   Patient Information (Enter, Change, Inquire)
4   Statement Programs
5   Insurance Claim Form Programs
6   Report Programs
7   Statistics and Other Information
8   Profile and System Management

To get to the Patient Information screen from the ACCOUNTS RECEIVABLE (MAIN) DIRECTORY, select:

3   Patient Information (Enter, Change, Inquire)

Now you will see:

You may look up patients by name in 4 ways (Example; JOHN SMITH)

Lastname, Firstname   (comma separator)   SMITH, JOHN
Firstname.Lastname   (dot separator)   JOHN.SMITH
Firstname Lastname   (space separator)   JOHN SMITH
First Letter of First Name+Last Name   JSMITH
<Enter a New Account=.>
Please Enter a Social Security Number ___-__-____
Please Enter a Patient's Account Number or a Patient's Name

Entering a New Patient

To enter a new patient, you or the computer must first assign an account number to the patient. You have two choices:

- Type the account number that you want
- Let the computer assign an account number for you

If you are entering your patients from ledger cards, you should write the account number assigned by the computer or selected by you on your source document. This will help you avoid entering the same patient twice or forgetting to enter a patient.

Automatic Numbering of Patient Accounts

If you do not wish to continue your previous account numbering system or did not use patient account numbers, let the program assign the next available account number.

When the program asks you to:

You may look up patients by name in 4 ways (Example: JOHN SMITH)

Lastname, Firstname	(comma separator)	SMITH, JOHN
Firstname.Lastname	(dot separator)	JOHN.SMITH
Firstname Lastname	(space separator)	JOHN SMITH
First Letter of First Name+Last Name		JSMITH

<Enter a New Account= .>

Please Enter a Social Security Number ___-__-____

Please Enter a Patient's Account Number or a Patient's Name
_____ Touch dot [.] [ENTER]

A new sequential account number will automatically appear.

Assigning Family/Guarantor Account Numbers

If you use family account numbers instead of regular account numbers you will be able to print one statement per family.

If you have families in the practice and do not use family account numbers, then each member of the family will receive a separate statement. From a bookkeeping standpoint, it is much more accurate to have a statement created for each family member.

Family Accounts

You must assign the family account number; the program will not assign it for you. If you want the transactions of individual family members to appear on one statement, assign an account number to the family, for example, 123456. Account number 123456 would be guarantor or family number. Type your guarantor number. After you have assigned the guarantor number, fill in the rest of the account information.

Now you are ready to assign account numbers to family members. To go to another patient, when you are asked:

CHOOSE<Transaction=1><Insurance=2><Another Patient=3>
<Revision=4>

Select <Another Patient=3>

Type the number for this family member, for example, 123456, followed by a dot [.] plus up to three alpha or numeric characters for the next family member, for example, 123456.1 or 123456.AB.

When the cursor is at the first patient's name field, enter the family account number: 123456 [ENTER]. This will bring forward all information, including insurance information. All that needs to be done is to change the patient's name, birth date, Social Security number, sex, status (marital status), and if applicable, patient's relationship to insured in the insurance screen. When you reach the Enter/Revise a Guarantor section, the program will automatically pull in the name of the guarantor.

Patient Financial Class

Financial Classes

You will assign financial classes to separate patients into different groups for your management reports. You may have an unlimited number of financial classes. You may use a general category, for example, assigning the category of "Private Pay" to all patients who are not Medicare, Medicaid, or Industrial. You may want to have a separate financial class for each health maintenance organization (HMO) or preferred provider organization (PPO) if a significant number of the patients are members.

Each financial class will be aged separately on your Aged Account & Collection Report (673). If you have too many financial classes, your aged account and collection report will be divided into many small categories. You will have a difficult time getting a clear picture of your accounts receivable.

The program comes with five standard financial classes set up. If you do not remember the number of the financial class, touch [ENTER] when this field is blank and you will be presented with the "Financial classes" window. From here you can add, change, delete, or print your financial classes. A sample window follows:

Financial Classes

CODE Description
01 Private Pay
02 Industrial
03 Medicaid
04 Medicare
05 Miscellaneous

Selecting an Existing Financial Class

Use the [UP ARROW] and [DOWN ARROW] to select a financial class. When you highlight your selection, touch [ENTER].

Adding a Financial Class

To add a financial class, request the instructor to assist you with creating a new financial class. Instructions are in the SHS manual provided to the instructor.

Financial Class Code

You will be asked to:
Please enter the Financial Class Code.

Enter the next number available (or any other code you want) for your financial classes. For example, if you have four financial classes, then you may enter the number 5 as the next financial class code. The program was provided to the school with five initial financial classes.

"Private Pay" or "Miscellaneous" can include all HMOs, PPOs, and private insurance companies (for example, Aetna, Lincoln, Prudential). A private pay or miscellaneous financial classification would have a "data control code" of 1.

An "Industrial" patient would be a patient with a work-related injury. An industrial financial classification would have a data control code of 2. If you do not have industrial patients, then this financial class can be reassigned to one that is needed in your practice.

A Medicaid patient must have a data control code of 3.

A Medicare patient must have a data control code of 4. If a patient has Medicare as the primary insurance and Medicaid as the secondary insurance, you should assign Medicare as the financial class and a data control code of 4.

If you wish to separate the straight Medicare patients from the Medicare/Medicaid crossover patients, then the Medicare/Medicaid crossover patients may be placed in a different category. For example, type 04 or 04x could be labeled as Medi/Medi. Some offices accept assignment on certain procedures, but not on others. You may have two categories of Medicare patients: Medicare assigned and Medicare nonassigned. All of these Medicare financial classes must be set up with a data control code of 4.

- The data control code *must* be 1 for private pay and all other classifications that are not 2, 3, or 4
- The data control code *must* be 2 for Industrial (Workers' Compensation)
- The data control code *must* be 3 for Medicaid
- The data control code *must* be 4 for Medicare

This way the computer will know how to handle the account.

Billing Cycle

There are four choices for your billing cycle: 1=normal (a statement and insurance form may be created for the patient); 2=hold statement and insurance; 3=hold insurance; and 4=hold statement.

Patient Information (Demographics)

After you have selected the account number for the patient and the financial class, you are ready to register a patient. You will enter the patient's name, address, date of birth, Social Security number, marital status, employer, and telephone numbers. There are several optional fields such as "other information" and "main diagnosis."

Name

You will be asked:

Please enter the patient's FIRST name.

Only type the patient's first name and touch [ENTER], for example, JOHN[ENTER].

The number of available characters for the first name is 15, which means that you can type beyond what appears to be the end of the field.

These questions will follow:

Please Enter the Patient's MIDDLE initial. Type the middle initial and [ENTER], for example, A [ENTER].

DO NOT put a period after the middle initial because there is only one space available for the initial. If you put in a period, you will see a period for the middle initial.

If the patient lacks a middle initial, touch [ENTER] to bypass the question.

Type the last name followed by [ENTER], for example, SMITH [ENTER]. The field for the last name has 25 characters.

Birth Date

Please enter the Patient's BIRTH DATE. Type the birth date of the patient using the format MMDDYYYY (MM=month, DD=day, YYYY=year), for example, 01011963, which signifies January 1, 1963. You are required to use the full year, that is 1891, 1963 or 2001. The program will automatically calculate the patient's age. DO NOT insert slashes or dashes when you type the birth date.

Social Security Number

Please enter the Patient's SOCIAL SECURITY NUMBER. **Do not** insert dashes or spaces; the program will do this.

Sex

Please enter the Patient's SEX (M or F). You may enter "M" for male and "F" for female, or the number "1" for male and the number "2" for female.

BOX B-1

Priscilla says: "I am confused. What is the difference between data control codes and financial classifications and financial classes? Did you dream this up just so you could make a very simple program seem more complicated? Why do I have to learn this stuff?"

SHS Answer: The computer knows what the "data control code" means and will use it to decide how to do the billing. You do not need to do or know anything about data control codes, really. SHS just put this discussion here for those customers who want to customize the program and have a more detailed production breakdown at the end of the month. Most customers do not wish to add or change the system.

Marital Status

When the program asks you to "Please enter the Patient's Marital Status" you will see a small pop-up window:

Marital
1 Single
2 Married
3 Widowed
4 Divorced
5 Unknown

You may choose a number from 1 to 5 or you may scroll with the arrow key and touch [ENTER] for the highlighted selection.

Other Information Lines

Four optional lines are available to use as you need them for more information about the patient. It is important that you use them consistently since information entered on each line can be used in special reports. For example, line 1 can be used to remind you of the amount of the copayment due from the patient. The first information line would show: COPAY $10

The second information line could show:
REF BY DR. A. SCHULTZ
The third information line might show:
ALLERGIC TO PENICILLIN

Guarantor

The guarantor is the person who is responsible for the bill. Even if you are only billing the insurance company, you would still fill in the patient's name. If the billing or guarantor's name is the same as the patient's name, touch dot [.][ENTER] and the patient's name will be copied into the slots labeled as "First Name," "Middle," "Last Name". If the guarantor is a different person from the patient type the name.

Type the street address. You enter it just as you would like it to appear on the statement or insurance form. When you reach the line that asks for "CityStZip," you may enter only the Zip code of the city in the slot that is labeled "city." The computer will pull in the name of the city, state, and Zip code for you from the Zip code index. If there is more than one city for that Zip code, a listing window will pop up showing the city, state, Zip code. Touch [ENTER] if the highlighted city is the one you wish to use.

If you do not know the Zip code of the city and would like to see the Zip codes available for that city, type a dot [.] before the name of the city. A pop-up widow will appear with all the Zip codes for that particular city. You must select the correct Zip code; the computer can only give you the selections.

NOTE: When you are entering an industrial account; the programs will ask you for the insurance company's name and address instead of the guarantor's name and address.

Telephone Numbers

Two lines are available for telephone numbers. When you enter the patient's home telephone number and work number, you do not need to put in the area code. The program has Zip code index that cross-references area codes. The only time you need to enter the area code is if it is different or has changed from the default code.

NOTE: Do not insert dashes, parentheses, or spaces in the telephone numbers; the program will fill these in for you.

Employer

Enter the name of the employer.

Address 1

Enter the address of the employer. You have two lines to use for the street address. One line could be used for an attention line.

Address 2

This is the second address line, which may or may not be used.

City State Zip

The Zip code lookup is active in this line. If, instead of entering the city, you enter its Zip code, the computer will pull in the city, name and state.

Telephone

Enter the telephone number of the employer.

Other

This is a data field. You can enter an extension or a telephone number.

ID Number

The Employer ID Code is the federal tax number or Social Security number of the employee. Enter the Social Security number of the employee. You may enter dashes or punctuation; this field is a free text.

Contact

You may enter the name of a contact person and if you have enough room, you may wish to include his or her telephone extension.

Comment

You may put whatever information you wish in this section.

Changing the Employer Information

Touch [C] (**do not** touch [ENTER] to change the highlighted employer). The "Enter/Revise an Employer" window will appear. You may use your arrow keys to make your changes.

Billing Cycle

This section will automatically be filled in for you because when you set up financial class you specified the billing cycle. When you select <Revision=4> you will see the summary window:

Billing Control
Billing Cycle
1 Normal

2 H Smts&Ins
3 H Ins
4 H Smts

"Normal" means that you want a statement and insurance form created if they are appropriate for that patient. "H Smts&Ins" means Hold Statements and Insurance forms. H Ins means "Hold Insurance forms" (will not automatically print the form) even if you have entered insurance information. "H Smts" means "Hold Statements."

Dunning

Y=OK to have dunning messages (default)
NM=No dunning messages on statements

Open Item Posting

Y=Open item posting is required for this patient
N=DO NOT set up budget billing for this patient (default)

Main Diagnosis Codes

This field is optional; it is not used for billing insurance. You would use this if you see the same patient repeatedly with the same diagnosis. This can save you time later when you are posting your transactions (charges).

You may enter up to four separate ICD-9 codes in this section. You make look up the diagnosis either by code of by name.

If you do not wish to complete this section, skip it by touching [ENTER]

Entering Diagnosis Codes by Number

All the current ICD-9 codes from the Government printing Office have been loaded in an index. When the Diagnosis Code window pops up, you can look up the ICD-9 code by number or by name. For example, if you type number 410 the index will pull in the description "Acute Myocardial Infarct".

Entering Diagnosis Codes by Description

If you do not know the ICD-9 number, you can type up to 26 letters of the description of the disease and a pop-up window will show you the nearest match. You must use the same description as in the ICD-9 code book. Using the [UP ARROW] or [DOWN ARROW] you may scroll through the list. If you wish to scroll faster, you can use the [PAGE UP] and [PAGE DOWN] keys. Once you have found the disease that you want, touch [ENTER] and your selection will be entered.

Statement

There is an item named "stmt <None>"; when you enter a new patient this section will have the word <None> because you have not yet created a statement for this patient. When you create a statement, the computer will fill in the date that the statement was created. The date in this section will always be the last statement date.

Industrial Account Information

Entering the patient information for an industrial account is the same as entering information for a private patient. The guarantor window is used for the company or corporate name and address.

Three additional fields must be filled in for an industrial account. After entering or bypassing the main diagnosis field a "Workers' compensation" window appears:

Workers' Compensation
Date of Injury
Claim Number
Attention

To enter the date of the initial injury, use the "MMDDYYYY" format.

Next enter the claim number for the case. **Remember** the dot [.] If the claim number contains the patient's Social Security number you can enter the dot [.] where the number would go. The last field in the window is for entering the name of the claim adjuster or your contact person at the insurance company.

Revision or Making Corrections

We have now completed the PATIENT ACCOUNT INFORMATION screen. If you wish to correct any errors, select <Revision=4> and each of the fields will have a number next to it. Choose the number of the field that you wish to change.

Backing Up to the Previous Question

If you wish to make a correction before you have answered the last question (Main Dx), you may back up one step by touching [ESC]. It is very easy to correct your errors or to make changes in the information entered.

You may also use your arrow keys to move backward and forward. This is a great correction tool to use when entering information.

Note Windows

The instructor will determine whether the student will use the Note Windows. Should the instructor choose to utilize this portion of the program he or she will draw the information from the SHS Master Manual.

Copying Patient Information

Once you have entered the information for one patient, you may copy the information to another patient's account.

First you must select your new account number in the usual way, either dot [.] [ENTER] if you wish to let the computer pick the number (this reduces the number of duplicate accounts), or you may type a number.

Enter the patient's financial class. To copy information from another account, instead of entering the patient's first name in the name field, you enter the account number of the patient whom you want to copy. For example, you have set up a patient account 100 and you want to copy the information from patient 100 to 101. When the program asks you to:

Please enter the patient's FIRST NAME

You would enter the number 100. The program will now copy the information from account number 101.

Patient Lookup

Now that the patient has been entered you may look up the patient by name, by account number, or by Social Security number.

Alphabetical

When you see this screen:

You may look up patients by name in four ways (example, JOHN SMITH)

Lastname, Firstname	(comma separator)	SMITH,JOHN
Firstname.Lastname	(dot separator)	JOHN.SMITH
Firstname Lastname	(space separator)	JOHN SMITH
First Letter of First Name+Last Name		JSMITH

<Enter a New Account=>

Please Enter a Social Security number ___-__-____

Please enter a patient's Account Number or a Patient's Name

_____

If you enter a comma in the entry field:

1. The program will assume that the letters to the left of the comma are all or part of the patient's last name.
2. The program will assume that the letters to the right of the comma are all or part of the patient's first name.

The search is on the last name so if the program finds more than one match, then you will see a window sorted by last name and then first name.

If you enter a dot [.] in the middle of some letters (not at the beginning of the field):

1. The program will assume that the letters to the left of the dot are the patient's first name.
2. The program will assume that the letters to the right of the dot are all or part of the patient's last name.

This search is on the first name so if the program finds more than one match, you will see a window sorted by the first name and then the last name. This lookup is most useful in finding patients for whom you do not know the spelling of the last name and for those with two first names, such as the name JIN SOON KIM. By putting the [.] after the JIM SOON, you are telling the computer that KIM is the last name rather than SOON KIM.

If you enter a space in the middle of some letters (not at the beginning of the field):

1. If you enter more than one space, the program will only see the last (right-most) space.
2. The program will assume that the letters to the left of the space are the patient's last name.

This search is on the first name, so if the program finds more than one match, you will see a window sorted by the first name and then the last name. This lookup is most useful in finding patients for whom you do not know the spelling of the last name and for those with two first names, such as the name JIN SOON KIM. The right-most space after the JIN SOON tells the program that KIM is the last name rather than SOON KIM.

You may enter from 1 to 41 characters of a patient's name, and the computer will display patient accounts that match your entry. You may scroll through them until you find the account you want.

The computer will ignore apostrophes and spaces when trying to find a match. For example, it will find O'Brien if you type either of the following:

OBRIEN

O'BRIEN

The computer will not distinguish between upper and lower case. For example, it will find de la TORRE if you enter "dela", "DELA", "deLA", and so on.

If you enter only one character, the computer will assume that it represents the first letter of the last name.

If you enter more than one character, the computer will assume that the first letter of your entry represents the first letter of the first name; and all additional letters of your entry represent the last name.

If you do not know the first name of the patient and you want to make a selection based on just the last name, enter a space followed by the first letter of the last name followed by a comma and then touch [RETURN]. For example, if you enter _GRAY, the computer will display information for the following accounts:

GRAY, BARRY

GRAY, NANCY

GRAYSON, FRED

GRAYVILLE, GINA

Social Security Number

If you wish to look up a patient by Social Security number, touch the [UP ARROW]

Now you will see:

You may look up patients by name in 4 ways (example, JOHN SMITH)

Lastname, Firstname	(comma separator)	SMITH,JOHN
Firstname.Lastname	(dot separator)	JOHN.SMITH
Firstname Lastname	(space separator)	JOHN SMITH
First Letter of First Name+Last Name		JSMITH

<Enter a New Account= .>

Please Enter a Social Security Number ___-__-____

Please Enter a Patient's Account Number or a Patient's Name

_____

and you will be placed at the question that asks

Please Enter a Social Security Number ___-__-____

Enter the patient's Social Security Number.

Account Number

If you know the patient's account number you may enter it in the space for an account number.

Guarantor Account Status

You are able to look at the account balance for a particular guarantor. You will be able to see the account numbers, names, and the individual balances for each patient. To see this information on your screen select:

7 Statistics and Other Information
   from the ACCOUNTS RECEIVABLE (MAIN) DIRECTORY
   Then select:
2 Guarantor Accounts Receivable and Aging
   Then the program will ask you to:

Please enter the guarantor's account number

When you enter the account number, you will see the aging.

Insurance Company Registration

There are two parts to registering insurance. The first part involves entering the basic insurance information. The second part involves completing the claim questions. This section will teach you how to enter the basic insurance company information for your patients.

SHS can complete six general insurance forms: the new HCFA-1500, the old HCFA-1500, the 40-1C and 15-1C (Medicaid), PM-160 (CHDP), and US-82/92.

Registering insurance company information will be a relaxing experience with SHS. The school receives updates to keep the insurance programs current.

Getting to the Insurance Screen

To get to the insurance screen (Figure B.13) from the ACCOUNTS RECEIVABLE (MAIN) DIRECTORY select:

3   Patient Information (Enter, Change, Inquire)

There are three ways to display a patient's information. You may enter (1) the patient's account number, (2) the first initial of the patient's first name and up to eight letters of the last name, or (3) the patient's Social Security number. If you look up the patient by name, the program takes you to the alphabetical lookup screen. The name you entered will be highlighted. If the highlighted name is correct, touch [ENTER]. You are now in "Patient Account Information."

From the Patient Account Information Screen

From the Patient Account Information screen, select:
<Insurance=2>

Now you are in the insurance information menu. Initially there are three choices: (1) empty slot for primary insurance, if any, and (2 and 3) insurance claim questions. Some health care specialties will have an additional selection for filling out information required to bill electronically (for example, ambulance and durable medical equipment [DME]). The program will ask you to "Choose One". In selection 1 (primary insurance), answer the questions about the patient/subscriber's name and address; whether the doctor accepts assignment; the

identification number of the patient, the group number, and so on. If there is a secondary insurance, you would then go to selection 2. You can have up to eight separate insurance companies per patient. The program has eight slots reserved for basic insurance company information. If you choose:

9   Insurance Claim Questions

you will see a pop-up window with the "Form Information" menu.

Entering Insurance Company Information

Select:
1   Empty Slot for Primary Insurance, if Any
The heading in the middle of the screen will be
Insurance Information

The questions that the program asks you on the insurance registration screen are based on the financial class you selected when you entered the patient.

NOTE: You can only enter this information once. It is not necessary to re-enter the information each time you wish to produce insurance forms for the patient.

You will see the following pop-up window:

Insurance Information
Lookup code
Name
Address1
Address2
CityStZip
Telephone   Other
Payer ID
ClmOffcID
MediGapID
Contact
Comment
InsCoName
Insurance Company Name

Type the name of the insurance company (for example, CIGNA). If this is a Medicare patient, the word MEDICARE (capital letters) will be entered automatically when you touch [ENTER]. The name

```
Name      JOAN        SMITH        Bill To   JOAN           SMITH
Birthdate 07/17/1923                923 COUNTRYMEADOW LANE
Soc Sec#  559-55-3434               SONOMA,          CA 95476
                     Home Ph  (707) 996-3434
CoPay     $5.00      Work Ph
MD        CAMPBELL   Employer
INS                  Billing   H Smts        D    Stmt <None>
No 10025  VMMG       06  Main Dx 401.1
--\130\255-------------------------------------------------------------
Software                  INSURANCE INFORMATION        (2) 09/02/1999
----------------------------------------------------------------------
Name      VMMG SECURE HORIZONS       Relation  Self
          PO BOX 1486                PtSigInf  Release information
          SONOMA         CA 95476    PtSigPay  Pay Provider
Pays%     0.0                        AccAsign  Assign is accepted
Name      JOAN        SMITH          Subsc ID  3833809-01 NSS
          923 COUNTRYMEADOW LANE     SubscGrp  SH
          SONOMA         CA 95476    FormType  511
          7079963434   07/17/1923 F
Address   923 COUNTRYMEADOW LANE     Date Ins Reg:  08/06/1998
          SONOMA         CA 95476    Last Print:    10/27/99

<Date=D> <Demand Form/EDI=6>
CHOOSE <Transaction=1> <Insurance=2> <Another Patient=3> <Revision=4>
```

Figure B.13

and address of the insurance company must be located in the insurance index to be pulled into the name field. The insurance index is a listing of some insurance companies and addresses provided to you as part of your SHS program. SHS will compare the insurance company name you enter against the insurance index. If there is an exact match, the address will automatically be entered. If there is more than one match or no name that matches, a window will pop up with the closest match highlighted. Select the one you want using your arrow keys and by touching [ENTER].

Insurance listing

Code	Insurance Company Name	Address	City/State
AARP	AARP GRP HEALTH CLAIMS	PO BOX 1011	MONTGOMERY, AL
ATHP	AETNA HEALTH PLAN	PO BOX 2404	FRESNO, CA
AET	AETNA LIFE & CASUALTY		
ATHECA	AETNA LIFE AND LCAM W102	151 FARMINGTON	HARTFORD, CT
ATAP	AETNA LIFE INS CO	3541 WINCHESTER	ALLENTOWN, PA
ATLICV	AETNA LIFE INS CO	PO BOX 91555	ARLINGTON, VA
ATLICS	AETNA LIFE INS CO	PO BOX 810	SEATTLE, WA

Press [A] to add an Insurance Co.
Press [C] to change the highlighted Insurance Co.
Press [D] to delete the highlighted Insurance Co.
Press [P] to print list.

If you are in the insurance listing window and you wish to move across the screen to look at the information, you may either use your right and left arrow keys or use the [TAB] key to move the cursor to the right across the screen one field at a time. To move to the left with the [TAB] key, hold down the [SHIFT] key and simultaneously touch [TAB].

NOTE: If your computer is equipped with a mouse, you may expand the insurance company window to fill the entire screen. Using the mouse, move your cursor to the three small yellow lines (if you have a color monitor) in the upper right-hand corner of the window. Click one time and the window will expand. To shrink the window put the cursor over the three lines again and click. To close the window click on the upper left box or touch [ESC].

Adding an Insurance Company

If you look at the bottom of the insurance company window, you will notice a small menu. If your insurance company is not on the index and you wish to include it, touch [A] to add an insurance company. Do not touch [ENTER] after you have touched [A]. Another window will pop up and it will be labeled "Enter/Revise an Insurance."
Enter/Revise an Insurance
Enter the Lookup Code   AETNA
Name
Address1
Address2
CityStZip
Telephone   Other
Payer   ID
ClmOffcID
MediGapID
Contact
Comment
    The first question that you will be asked is to enter the lookup code. You may enter an abbreviation of the insurance company name or you

may enter a number or combination of alphabetical or numeric characters. Once you have assigned a code to the insurance company, you may retrieve the company by name or by code. It is not necessary to memorize the code. The computer will pull in the name you originally typed into the insurance company name field. At this time you can accept the name by touching [ENTER] or modify it by typing additional characters or letters.

Several other fields are available in this window. You are not required to fill out each field; just enter the information that you consider to be important. Next, you should enter the street address or post office box of the insurance company. Note that four lines are available in which to enter the address for the insurance company. If you enter the Zip code in the spot where the computer asked you to enter the city, the computer will pull in the city, state, and Zip code. The next three fields are used for electronic data interchange (EDI). Refer to that section of the manual for more information. You may type in the name of the contact person at the insurance company. The comment line is free text.

NOTE: If you do wish to complete all the insurance window information at this time, touch [CTRL+W]. The program will save the window without your having to touch [ENTER] in the remaining fields.

If you want to back out of the insurance window, you may select [ESC] and you will be backed out one step at a time. The [UP ARROW] and [DOWN ARROW] keys will move you back and forth through the fields. You may add, change, delete an insurance company or print a list of insurance companies.

Changing Insurance Company Information

You can touch [C] to change the highlighted insurance. A window named "Revision of an Existing Insurance" will appear.

Deleting Insurance Company Information

You can touch [D] to delete the highlighted insurance. The "Delete an Existing Insurance" window will appear. The program will ask you: Are you sure you want to delete this insurance Y or N?

Printing Insurance Company Information

Touch [P] to create a list of insurance companies. You will see a pop-up window labeled "Sort". You may sort by code or by name. To print or view your insurance company listing, go back to the ACCOUNTS RECEIVABLE (MAIN) DIRECTORY and select:
8 File and System Management
Then select:
6 Insurance Companies, Provider, Employer, Referring, UPIN, etc.
Then select:
9 Print or view 11 page(s) INSURANCE COMPANY LISTING
    You will have the choice to print or view the insurance company listing.
    NOTE: If you do not wish to complete the insurance information at this time, you can [ESC] and back out of the window with the insurance listing. There are additional markings on the screen that look like small diamonds, small triangles, and dashes. These markings are for individuals using a mouse. Using the mouse, move your cursor to the three yellow bars in the upper right-hand corner of

your screen. Click one time and the window will expand to fill the entire screen. If you click again the window will contract. You may put your cursor on the scroll bars (the small triangles) if you wish to scroll up or down.

Subscriber Information

When you reach the "Subscriber" name field, you will see the following pop-up window:
Subscriber Information
First Name
Address 1
CityStZip
Telephone
Birth Date
Sex
Employer
   NOTE: If the subscriber information is the same as guarantor information, dot [.][ENTER] will bring it down.

Patient Address
Please enter patient address.
Please enter patient city.
Please enter patient state.
Please enter patient Zip code.
   NOTE: If patient information is the same as guarantor information, dot [.][ENTER] will bring it down.

Relation
Relation to subscriber
You will be asked to:
Please enter the patient's relationship to insured (1/2/3/4).
A window will appear. Fill in the correct option by using your arrow keys or selecting the number:
1   Self
2   Spouse
3   Child
4   Other
5   Leave this box blank
For example: 2   Spouse

PtSigInf
Patient signature information
The program will ask you to:
Please enter if signature to release information is on file.
The three selections for Information Release are:
Information Release
1   Release information
2   DO NOT release information
3   Leave this box blank
   You must chose 1, 2, or 3 or use your arrow keys and touch [ENTER] at the highlighted selection.

PtSigPay
Patient Signature Payment To Provider
The program will ask you to:
Please enter if signature to pay provider is on file.
You will see a pop-up window with the following selections:
Payment to Provider
1   Pay Provider
2   DO NOT pay Provider
3   Leave this box blank

You must chose 1, 2, or 3 or use your arrow keys and touch [ENTER] at the highlighted selection that you want.

AccAsgin
Accept Assignment
The program will ask you to:
Please enter if provider accepts assignment.
The selections for completing the accept-assignment box are:
Accept Assignment
1   Assign is accepted
2   Assign NOT accepted
3   Assign accepted ONLY on lab
4   Leave this box blank

Subsc ID
Subscriber ID Number
Type the subscriber's identification number unless it is the same as the Social Security number. to pull down the Social Security number, you may touch dot [.][ENTER].
For example:
247402840
If the subscriber's ID number is the Social Security number followed by a letter(s) or number(s), enter a dot [.] plus the letter(s) or number(s). For example,
.A   [ENTER]
and you will get
247402840A
for the subscriber ID number.
   If you ask the program to pull down the Social Security number, the computer will take out the dashes between the numbers when it enters the numbers on the insurance information screen. If you type the subscriber ID number and type the number with the dashes, your insurance form will print the number with dashes. The program removes the dashes when you submit the claim electronically.

SubscGrp
subscriber's Group No. (Or Group Name)
Type the group number or location (for example, A070-01).

Form Type
If you touch [ENTER], the computer will select the correct form type only for primary insurance. Additional insurance's will require you to enter the form type if you want the computer to create a form.
   The available form types are:

Code	Description
511	Private Pay
512	Industrial
513	Medicaid
514	Medicare
515-9	User definable: HCFA-1500, UB92, or ADA
522	Doctor's First Report (California)
551	PM 1605/90 CHDP Form
561	Private Pay
562	Industrial
563	Medicaid
564	Medicare
565-9	User definable: HCFA-1500, UB92, or ADA

Other less common forms are available.

Date Ins Reg
Date Insurance Registered
The program will automatically fill in the date you entered the insurance information.

Last Printing of Insurance

When you create your insurance forms, the program will fill in the last date that you created an insurance form for a particular insurance company.

NOTE: SHS assigns a three-digit number for private insurance, HMO/PPO (511, 561), industrial insurance (512, 562), Medicaid (513, 563), and Medicare (514, 564).

DO NOT FORGET TO ANSWER INSURANCE CLAIM FORM QUESTIONS NO. 9 (covered in another section of this appendix).

Industrial Insurance Information

Most of the information is the same as that just given. The exceptions and additions are provided below:

Subscriber Information: When you reach the subscriber name field you will see the following pop-up window:

Subscriber Information

Employer

Address1

CityStZip

Telephone

NOTE: If employer information is entered into the patient account information and in the employer file index, dot [.][ENTER] will bring in the information.

Medicaid Insurance Information

InsCoName

Insurance Company Name

When you choose 1 to add the primary insurance, the name "Medicaid" will be pulled in by the computer if you set up the patient as a Medicaid financial class.

Use this section to enter basic insurance information for Medicaid and CHDP patients.

Insurance Information

Lookup code MCAL

Name	MEDICAI
Address1	
Address2	
CityStZip	
Telephone	Other
Payer ID	MEDI
ClmOffcID	
MediGapID	
Contact	
Comment	

PtAddress

Patient Address

Touch dot [.][ENTER], and the computer will pull down the address information from the "bill to" section.

PtIDNo

Patient ID Number

Please enter the patient's identification number.

You may enter the number with or without the dashes. The program will remove the dashes if the number is going to be sent to Medicaid by EDI.

Form Type

The program will fill in the correct form type. The program number will be 513 or the default you have set up. Just press [ENTER] when you reach this field.

NOTE: If the Medicaid form is a cross-over, (for example, Medicare/Medicaid) the program will not put in a form type. The program will create one form with all the information for Medicare only.

Date Ins Reg

Date Insurance Registered

The program will automatically fill in the date you registered the insurance information.

Last Print

The program will automatically fill in the last date that you created your forms for this patient.

DO NOT FORGET TO ANSWER INSURANCE CLAIM FORM QUESTIONS SELECTION NO. 9.

Medicare Insurance Information

InsCoName

Insurance Company Name

When you choose 1 to enter the primary insurance, the name "Medicare" will be pulled in by the computer if you set up the patient as a Medicare financial class.

Below are some additions/changes/deletions from the private pay insurance screen.

No subscriber information

No relation question

No group number

CrossOver

The program will ask:

Please enter Y/N if this insurance is a "Crossover."

"Crossover" in this question refers to the patient's second insurance being Medicaid or other insurance that you want Medicare to send ("crossover") the charge and payment information. Enter [1] or [Y] if it is a crossover or [2] or [N] if it is not.

CHDP Form PM-160

You complete the basic insurance information for CHDP just as you complete the information for the Medicaid form. There is a separate set of claim questions for this form. Set up the patient as a Medicaid financial class. When you reach the question for form type, enter 551. Then PM160 5/90 CHDP form is form type 551 in SHS.

Deleting An Insurance Company

To delete an insurance company from within a patient's account, go to the insurance information screen. Select the number of the insurance company that you wish to delete. Then select:

<REVISION=4>

In the field labeled insurance company name 01, type the word DELETE. If there are any letters remaining on this insurance name line, you must use the delete key to erase them before touching [ENTER]. This does not delete the insurance from the lookup file.

Creating Insurance Forms

Insurance forms may be created from three locations: the insurance menu (selected off the ACCOUNTS RECEIVABLE (MAIN) DIRECTORY), from the patient screen, and from the batch processor. Insurance forms call all be created at the same time (cycle billing) or they may be demanded (created one at a time).

Insurance Directory

From the ACCOUNTS RECEIVABLE (MAIN) DIRECTORY, select:
5   Insurance Claim Form Programs

You will see a display similar to the one below. The selections that you see on your insurance directory will depend on where you are located. Your insurance directory might not look like the sample following.

1   Create all HCFA=1500 Private Pay
2   Create ALL HCFA=1500 Medicare
3   Create ALL 92 HCFA=1500 Private Pay
4   Create ALL 92 HCFA=1500 Industrial
5   Create ALL 92 HCFA=1500 Medicaid
6   Create ALL 92 HCFA=1500 Medicare
7   Create ALL Tn/Al UV-82/92 (HCFA=1450) Facility (Dialysis)

At the bottom of the screen the program will ask you to "Please choose one of the above." From the Insurance Directory select the number of the insurance program that you wish to run. The program will look at the status codes and find all the transaction lines preceded by a lowercase letter I. The program will create an insurance form for each patient who has transaction lines with the lowercase I. When the program has created the form it will change the lowercase I to an uppercase I. See the Transaction Entry section of this appendix for more information regarding these status codes.

The creation of the form and the printing are separate operations. In other words, you may create a form and print it later.

Printing Insurance Forms

Once you have created the form, under the wording "Insurance Directory" you will see the word "print" preceded by a number, for example:
9   PRINT 1 page HCFA=1500 Medicare
To print this form you would select
9
The following pop-up window will appear:
Print or view Selection
1   PRINT this file: M6R504.LST
2   VIEW the field on the screen
If you just want to look at this file choose
2   VIEW the file on the screen
A window will pop up and show the top half of the form. Below this window, it will tell you the name of the file and to [ESC] to stop viewing it.
After you [ESC] you will be asked if you want the file erased, answer Y/N.
If you want to print the file you would choose:
1   Print this file

Several print windows will appear; just answer the appropriate questions. The first window will ask:
Is the correct paper loaded?
Did you check the alignment?
Is the printer ready to print?
Please enter: <Y=YES> <N=NO>
If you answer YES, the next window will ask:
Do you want to print a test form?
Please enter: <Y=YES> <N=NO>
If you answer NO, then you will be asked:
Do you want to print all forms now?
Please enter: <Y=YES> <N=NO>
If you answer YES, then you will be asked:
How many copies do you want to print?
Enter the number of copies that you want to print. The number 1 is the default number of copies.

Demanding Insurance Forms

Once you have printed a charge on an insurance form, the charge will not be picked up automatically again. If you want to print it on a form again, for any reason, you must DEMAND a new form. For example, if a patient called you and told you that the insurance company never received the insurance form, then you could print another one for the same period as the lost form. You must be in the patient's account to demand an insurance form.
Select the appropriate patient's account. Select:
<Demand Forms=6>
Then select:
2   Demand Insurance

You will see a pop-up window named "Insurance Selection." Use your arrow keys to select the insurance company, if there is more than one insurance company registered. Touch [ENTER] for the computer to read your selection.

Date Range for Demand Forms

You will be asked to choose the BEGINNING and ENDING DATES. Enter one of the following:
- To create an insurance form with ALL DETAIL that is available in the computer for that account, touch [ENTER] when the program asks you for both the BEGINNING and ENDING DATES. The program will ask:
  Are you satisfied with these dates Y/N?
- To create an insurance form for one day's activity only, enter the SAME DATE, using the format MMDDYYYY, for both the BEGINNING and ENDING DATES.
- To create an insurance form for a specific period, when the program asks you for the BEGINNING DATE, enter the date for the oldest transaction that you want. When the program asks you for the ENDING DATE, enter the date of the most recent transaction.

The computer will then itemize all transactions within those dates.
For example:
BEGINNING DATE 040499
ENDING DATE 043099

Printing Demand Forms

The computer will ask if you would like to print the demand forms now. If you type YES, the computer will print all demanded forms of the same form type you are demanding (such as all 511 forms). If you answer NO to this question at this place in the program, you must go to the Insurance Directory to print the forms. Follow the same directions as the previous printing section (see Printing Insurance Forms).

Insurance Program Operation Detail

The computer will produce an insurance form for each insurance that you have registered for a patient.

Charges will automatically print on an insurance form once. The transaction line status code will show a capital letter "I" when a charge has appeared on an insurance form.

You **must** spell MEDICARE correctly when registering your insurance, or the insurance program will not pick up that insurance for EDI!

Normally, only charges will appear on the insurance form. If you want a Printing Memo Line to print on an insurance form, you have two choices. First, you can revise that memo and answer YES to "Print on Insurance Claims & EDI (Y or N)." Your second choice is to build an auto-transaction, perhaps named INSMEMO, designate it as a printing memo, answer "Y" to "Print on Insurance," and leave the description blank.

Insurance Claim Questions

This section will teach you how to complete your insurance claim questions. Several different screens of claim form questions are covered in this section: HCFA-1500, HCFA-1450 (UB-82/92) and the PM-160, and Doctor's First Report. Note that some reference will be made to the 15.40-IC forms since this program still supports them. These forms are obsolete and will probably not be mentioned in future manuals.

Claim Form Questions

To get to the claims form question menu from the patient account information screen or transaction entry screen, select:

    <Insurance>

Then select:

9   Insurance Claim Questions

A pop-up window will appear with the following selection:

1   HCFA=1500
2   15/40-IC (being eliminated)
3   HCFA 1450 (UB-82/92)
4   Doctor's First Report
5   PM=160

This is where you answer the questions about hospitalization, authorization numbers, facility name and number, referring provider name and number, and so on. There are claim form questions for different types of insurance forms:

- The HCFA-1500 (the universal form used for private insurance, HMOs, PPOs, and Medicare)
- The UB-82/92 (the form used by facilities, dialysis units, and some surgical centers)
- The PM-160 (used for CHDP)

If you register insurance information and you choose a normal or HSmt (hold statement) billing, the program will automatically produce a standard insurance form with the patient charge. It is important that you register an insurance when you have the registration information available. If you do not put in insurance information, you will not get an insurance form.

NOTE: If you do not want an insurance form for a patient, do not entry any insurance information. If you want to enter the insurance information but do not want a form, enter the insurance information and select H Ins (hold insurance) for the billing cycle. You may also leave the form type blank.

If a patient is billing his or her insurance by a charge slip or superbill, DO NOT register their insurance. (you may want to record the information by noting it on the other information lines).

HCFA-1500 Claim Form Questions

Select:
1   HCFA 1500

from the Form Information window. You will see a screen like the one below. It is unlikely that you would answer more then just a few questions. The numbers after the abbreviated words are the revision numbers. If, for example, you want to enter the information about the outside lab, select the number 17.

HCFA=1500 Claim information

Program 01	ChmpusSp11	Outs Lab17	DtTtDFr24
EmpStat 02	BrhOfsrv12	Lab Chg 18	DtTt1DTo 25
EmpInCvr03	EmergChk13	Dtof Ill19	DtPt1DFr26
EmployR04	EPSDT 14	DtofCns120	DtPt1Dto27
AccidOth05	Fam Plan15	DtSmI1Fr21	DtHospFr28
AccidAuto06	PrAuthNo16	DtSmI1To22	DtHospTo29
AA Place07			
RefPers08		Ref Id#	Box 10d30
Facility09		Fac Id#	Box 11d31
Lab Name10			

Please enter the number to revise.

Depending on the requirements of the specific insurance carrier, these claim questions are available for you to complete:

Program 01

Applicable program block to check (top of form)

    Type of Program
1=Medicare
2=Medicaid
3=CHAMPUS
4=CHAMPVA
5=Group Health Plan
6=FECA Blk Lung
7=Other
8=Leave Blank

EmpStat 02

Employment Status

Please Enter Patient's Employment Status

    Patient Status
1=Employed
2=Full time student
3=Part time student
4=Leave blank

EmplnCvr 03

Employer Insurance Coverage

Please enter (Y/N) Insured is covered by employer health plan

EmployR 04

Employment Related

Please enter (Y/N) was this related to employment?

AccidOth 05

Accident Other

Please enter (Y/N) was this related to an accident other than auto?

AA Place 07

Accident Place

Please enter Auto Accident: PLACE (State)

Ref Pers 08

Referring Person

Please enter the referring person lookup code

    Referrer Information

Lookup Code

Name

Address1

Address2

CityStZip

Office Phone   Emerg

State License Number

Tax ID/SSN Number   EIN

Medicaid Number

Medicare (PIN)

Medicare (UPIN)

Blue Shield Number

Title   Specialty Code

When you select this field, a window named "Referrer Information" will appear and ask you to enter the referring person. If you have already entered the information, the program will fill in the blanks for you. If it is the name of a new referrer, another window will pop up and ask for the lookup code. You must enter a number or code. The program will ask you to fill out the address, city, state, and Zip code. If you just put I the Zip code, the program will pull in the city, state, and Zip code automatically. The ID number should be filled in if you have it available. After you have completed the information, touch [ENTER] and the program will pull the information into your HCFA-1500 Claim Information Screen

Entering a New Referrer Name

If the name of the referrer matches a name already in the referrer name index, then the computer will pull in the information. If there is no match, you will get a Referrer listing window. Touch [A] (DO NOT) touch [ENTER] to add a referrer.

A window will pop up that says:

Enter/Revise a referrer

You will be asked to enter the lookup code. Complete the address, city, state, Zip code (remember that you may use the Zip code window), telephone and ID number, contact, and comment fields.

NOTE: When entering referring doctor information, make sure the referring doctor's UPIN number is entered in the field Medicare (UPIN) and *not* in the State License Number field or your claims may be rejected. UPINs are in the format A00000.

Next, you will get another blank pop-up window so that you can complete the referrer information for another referrer at this time if you wish. If you only want to enter the information for one referrer,

then touch [ESC] and you will be put back in the referrer listing. Select [ENTER] and the referrer name and referrer ID will be pulled in from the information entered on the window.

NOTE: If you do not know the Zip code of the city, you may put a dot [.] before the name: for example, entering .New York tells the computer that you do not know the Zip code of the city but would like to see the available selections. If for some reason you want to type the city and state without a Zip code, or you wish to override the index, then you would type the information field by field.

NOTE: Touch [CTRL+W] if you do not want to complete all the information asked for in the window. [CTRL+W] saved the information you entered.

Changing Referrer Information

Touch [C] (DO NOT) touch [ENTER] to change the highlighted referrer. Use your arrow keys to reach the field that you wish to change.

Deleting a Referrer Name

Touch [D] [ENTER] to delete the highlighted referrer.

You will be asked:

Are you sure your want to delete this referrer Y or N.

You may not delete a referrer name if it is in use by a patient.

Creating the List of Referrers

Touch [P] to create the list Do not touch [ENTER].

Facility 09

Facility Information

Please enter the facility lookup code

    Facility Information

Lookup Code

Name

Address1

Address2

CityStZip

Telephone   Other

ID Number

Contact

Comment

Entering a New Facility Name

If the name of the facility matches a name already in the facility name index, then the computer will pull in the information. If there is no match, you will get a facility listing window. Touch [A] (DO NOT touch [ENTER]) to add a facility. A window will pop up that states, "Enter/Revise a Facility".

You will be asked to enter the lookup code. Complete the address, city, state, Zip code (remember that you may use the Zip code window), telephone and ID number, contact, and comment fields. Then you will get another blank pop-up window so that you may complete the facility information for another facility at this time if you want. If you only want to enter the information on one facility, then touch [ESC] and you will be put back in the Facility Listing. Touch [ENTER] and the facility name and facility ID number will be pulled in from the information entered on the window.

NOTE: If you do not know the Zip code of the city, you may put a dot [.] before the name; for example, .New York tells the computer that you do not know the Zip code of the city but would like to see the available selections. If for some reason you want to type the city and state without a Zip code, or you wish to override the index, then you would type the information field by field.

NOTE: Touch [CTRL+W] if you do not want to complete all of the information asked for in the window. [CTRL+W] saves the information you entered.

Changing Facility Information

Touch [C] (DO NOT touch [ENTER]) to change the highlighted facility. Use your arrow keys to reach the fields that you wish to change.

Deleting a Facility Name

Touch [D] [ENTER] to delete the highlighted facility. You will be asked:
Are you sure you want to delete this facility Y or N?
You may not delete a facility name if it is in use by a patient.

Creating the List of Facilities

Touch [P] to create the list. Do not touch [ENTER].
Lab Name 10
Laboratory Information
The following pop-up window will appear:
    Laboratory Information
Lookup Code
Name
Address1
Address2
CityStZip
Telephone   Other
ID Number
Contact
Comment

Entering a New Laboratory Name

If the name of the laboratory matches a name already in the laboratory name index, then the computer will pull in the information. If there is no match, you will get a laboratory listing window. Touch [A] (DO NOT touch [ENTER]) to add a laboratory. A window will pop up that states, "Enter/Revise a laboratory".

You will be asked to enter the lookup code. Complete the address, city, state, Zip code (remember that you may use the Zip code window), telephone and ID number, contact, and comment fields. Then you will get another blank pop-up window so that you may complete the laboratory information for another laboratory at this time if you want. If you only want to enter the information on one laboratory, then press[ESC] and you will be put back in the laboratory listing. Touch [ENTER] and the laboratory name and laboratory ID will be pulled in from the information entered on the window.

NOTE: If you do not know the Zip code of the city, you may put a dot [.] before the name; for example, .New York tells the computer that you do not know the Zip code of the city but would like to see the available selections. If for some reason you want to type the city

and state without the Zip code, or you wish to override the index then you would type the information field by field.

NOTE: Touch [CTRL+W] if you do not want to complete all of the information asked for in the window. [CTRL+W] saves the information you have entered.

Changing Laboratory Information

Touch [C] (DO NOT touch [ENTER]) to change the highlighted laboratory. Use your arrow keys to reach the fields that you wish to change.

Deleting a Laboratory Name

Touch [C] (DO NOT touch [ENTER]) to delete the highlighted laboratory. You will be asked:
    Are you sure you want to delete this laboratory Y or N?
    You may not delete a laboratory name if it is in use by a patient.

Creating the List of Laboratories

Touch [P] to create the list. Do not press [ENTER].
ChampusSp 11
Champus Sponsor
Please enter the Champus Sponsor Status:
1=Active; 2=Retired; 3=Deceased
BrhOfSrv 12
Branch of Service
Please enter the branch of service.
EmergChk 13
Emergency Check
Please enter (Y/N) Check if emergency?
EPSDT 14
Please enter (Y/N) Is this related to EPSDT?
Fam Plan 15
Family Planning
Please enter (Y/N) Is this related to family planning?
PrAuthNo 16
Preauthorization Number
Please enter the preauthorization number.
Outs Lab 17
Outside Laboratory
Outside Lab
1   Yes, work was performed outside office
2   No, work was NOT performed outside office
3   No purchased tests
4   Leave blank
Lab Chng 18
Laboratory Charge
Please enter the amount the outside lab charged the provider.
Dt of Ill 19
Date of illness (beginning date)
Please enter the date the illness began.
DtofCnsl 20
Date of First Consultation
Please enter the date of first consultation.
DtSmllFr 21
Date Similar Illness (beginning date)
Please enter the date the similar symptoms began.
DtSmllTo 22
Date Similar Illness, End

Please enter the date the similar symptoms ended.

DtRetWk 23

Date Return to Work

Please enter the date the patient may return to work.

DtTtlDFr 24

Date Total Disability, Begin

Please enter the date the total disability began.

DtTtlDTo 25

Date Total Disability, End

Please enter the date the total disability ended.

DtPtlFr 26

Date Partial Disability, Begin

Please enter the date the partial disability began.

DtPtlDTo 27

Date Partial Disability, End

Please enter the date the partial disability ended.

DtHospFr 28

Date Hospitalization, Begin

Please enter the date the hospitalization began.

DtHospTo 29

Date Hospitalization, End

Please enter the date the hospitalization ended.

Box 10d 30

Please enter data reserved for local use (not Medicare special requirements). If you answer with a dot [.] then you will bring up a menu of possible choices required by Medicare of you may enter what you want to print in box 10d.

Box 10d

1=MSP (4,7,11)

2=2MSP (4,7,11,At)

3=MG (9,9a-9d)

4=MSP/MG (4,7,11,At)/(9,9a-9d)

5=2MSP/MG (4,7,11,At)/(9,9a-9d)

6=MSP/MG/SP (4,7,11,At)/(9,9a-9d)

7=SP (9,9a-9d)

8=MSP/SP (4,7,11,At)/(9,9a-9d)

9=MG/SP (9,9a-9d)/(At)

A=MCD (9,9a,9b)

B=MSP/MCD (9,9a,9b)

C=MG/MCD (9,9a-9d)/(11,11a)

D=MSP/MG/MCD (4,7,11 add:At)/(9,9a-9d)/(At)

Leave Box 10d Blank (HCFA 12/90 form)

Box 11d 31

1 Yes, there is another plan

2 No, there is not another plan

3 leave blank

4 Another Plan

5 Use computer's defaults

If this question is not answered, it will automatically be answered "N" for private insurance claims and left blank for Medicare (as per special bulletin dated summer of 1992). If Medicare changes these requirements, the programs will reflect the changes as necessary on the regular or supplementary updates that are available.

Automatic Transaction Library

In this section you will learn how to enter charges, payments, adjustments, and memo lines into your automatic transaction library. You will also learn how to load your fee schedule(s) into your automatic transaction library. The automatic transaction library lets you eliminate all of your repetitive typing.

The section Transactions will teach you how to enter transactions in the transaction screen of your program. We shall briefly cover material in this section related to the transaction screen.

Building Your Automatic Transaction Library

If your office uses the same transactions repeatedly, these may be loaded in your automatic transaction library. You may access the library from the patient transaction screen or from the SYSTEM MANAGEMENT DIRECTORY.

To pull in an automatic transaction, just enter the code (alpha or numeric) that you have selected for this transaction. Your automatic transaction code may be the same as your procedure code. For example, if you want to select the charge for an office visit, you could enter 99212 as the automatic transaction code. The code 99212 will select the same procedure code with the description, place of service, and your fee. The automatic transaction code must have at least two digits if you want to use a number. If you use letters, you may have one or more letters.

You also may have the same auto-transaction code listed several times with different fee for each one specifying the financial class for the auto-transaction code. To access the automatic transaction library, select a code that is not in the library. The Auto-Transaction Library window will pop up. At the bottom of the window will be the following selections:

Touch [A] to add an auto-transaction

Touch [P] to print list

Touch [C] to change the highlighted auto-transaction

If you select [A] or [C], you will see the following pop-up window:

Enter/Revise Auto-Transactions

Enter Auto-Trx Code

Type of Transaction

Use for Financial Class

Print on Insurance

Research Code

Provider Code

Procedure Code

Modifier

Quantity

Description

Place of Service

Type of Service

Diagnosis Code

Amount

You may use your up and down arrow keys to move through the field if you are changing an automatic transaction. If you do not want to complete all the information in the window, touch [CTRL+W].

If you touch [P] to print the list you will see the following pop-up window:

Sort

1 Sort by code

2 Sort by description

Setting Up Auto-Transactions

Using Multiple Fees for the Same Procedure

If the financial class field is blank, the default will be ALL financial classes. For example:
You want the same price for all Medicare patients but different from private pay.

1 Make an auto-transaction with 04 for the financial class.
04 will work for 04, 04X, 04T, 04XT, etc.
04X will not work for 04 but will work for 04X and 04XT.

2. After all the transactions are set up for specific financial classes, set up a default auto-transaction with a blank financial class for the all the rest.

Chaining Auto-Transactions

A chained auto-transaction automatically calls one or more auto-transactions.

Why use it?

If you always enter four transactions together, this will allow you to link them so you enter the first and the other three are automatic. You are allowed a maximum of 10 transactions, including the main transaction.

1. If you use provider numbers, all lines will default to the first transaction.
2. The date will default to the first transaction.
3. If the first transaction is a charge, all linked transactions will default to the diagnosis codes in the first transaction unless you enter specific diagnosis codes in the linked automatic transactions.

How do you make it work?

1. Put the number 1 (remember, "1" means YES) in the master table Cm_chain.
2. The auto-transaction window will then ask you for the next transaction lookup code. For example:
first code: 80059 hepatitis panel
second code: 82520 assay blood bilirubin
third code: 84455 assay transaminase (SGOT) and so on
Now when you enter 80059 as an auto-transaction code, all three auto-transactions will appear in order.

Special Uses for Chained Auto-Transactions

Auto-transactions may be used for many special situations. For example, the California Medicaid program has unique procedure codes that you must use instead of the standard CPT-4 code. To avoid needing to have the user learn these unique codes, set up two auto-transactions with the standard CPT-4 s the lookup code. Have the first auto-transaction limited to the Medical financial class with the unique procedure code in the auto-transaction setup. Have the second auto-transaction setup with the standard CPT-4 code. This way, when you enter the CPT-r code while working in a Medicaid patient account, you will get the standard CPT-4 code.

Transactions

In this section you will learn how to enter charges, payments, adjustments, and memo lines. You also will learn how to load your fee schedule(s) into your automatic transaction library to eliminate repetitive typing. After you have entered your transactions, you may create your statements and insurance forms.

The computer will expect you to keep a total on each type of transaction that you enter. The computer will want to compare YOUR totals with its totals for EACH type of transaction (charges, payments, plus adjustments and minus adjustments). The section on How to Balance Your Transactions will teach you how to check your entries for the day.

Methods of Posting

Transactions may be posted using two methods: "balance forward" and "open-item." You select the method you want to use when you set up your financial classes.

Balance Forward Posting

"Balance forward" is the method in which you post your payments and adjustments against the patient's account balance. Using balance forward, the oldest unpaid charges are paid first; however, you will not know which line items have been paid; you will only know the patient's account balance. When the patient's account balance is zero, you will know that all the line items have been paid.

Open-Item Posting

If you wish to apply payments and adjustments to specific line items, you will want to post "open-item." You set up open-item posting when you set up the financial class. You can have open-item posting for one financial class and balance forward posting for another. When you set up your financial classes you will be asked:
Force Open-Item Posting
You will answer [Y] for yes.
When you are setting up your financial classes, you will see a pop-up window that has the following selections:
    Enter/Revise Financial Classes
Please enter the Financial Class code
Description
Billing Cycle
Allow Dunning
Force OpnItemPost   Yes
Budget billing
Aging Period—days
Ins Form Default
Data Control Code

When you are in the transaction screen (after you have entered a charge), you will see another field located after the description of the procedure. In this field there will be a number (in yellow if you have a color screen) That represents the balance for each line item. When you enter a payment or adjustment against a line item, the open item balance will reflect your entry. Your payments or adjustments will appear under the charge line item, regardless of the date of the payment or adjustment. When you look at the screen you will see the related items sorted together. The charges are listed chronologically with the related payments or adjustments appearing immediately under the charge before you see the next charge. As always in the SHS programs, you will see up to the last 10 transaction line items on the screen when you choose to see the transactions one line at a time using your arrow keys or a page of 10 transactions at a time using the [PAGE-UP] or [PAGE-DOWN] keys.

Methods of Entering Transactions

There are two methods for entering transactions. If you have set up auto-transactions you may simply enter the auto-transaction code in place of the normal choices for transactions and your auto-transaction will be entered in to the transaction file. You will be prompted to enter the date of transaction plus any information that you left blank when you created the auto-transaction. If any other auto-transactions are chained to the first auto-transaction, then the also will be entered with the same date and provider number (if any).

You also can manually enter your transactions. Simply choose one of the menu items (1 for a charge, 2 for a payment, 3 for a minus adjustment, 4 for a plus adjustment, 5 for a printing memo, or 6 for a nonprinting memo). The computer will prompt you for all the needed transaction information.

Charges, How to Enter

Srch (Research Field)

Research Code

The research code is not used for most types of health care billing (exception: UB82/92 form). This field usually is used for reporting purposes in which the procedure code, diagnosis code, and other required fields do not allow the user to obtain the desired information. For example, you are an orthopedic surgeon and you want to know how many hip replacements you perform on left legs. You could code the left and right legs with this field. You could also use this field in minus adjustment transactions for tracking certain types of write-offs. You must activate the research code listing in the Main Variable Control if you want to be able to enter this information If you have activated the field, the program will stop on this selection to let you fill in the research number. If the field is not activated, the program will skip this selection.

If you enter a research number that has already been defined, the program will accept it and move to the next field. If you enter a new number, a small window will pop up that will have the heading research code listing description. The cursor will highlight one research code. If this is the code that you want, then press [ENTER] and that choice will be selected. At the bottom of the window are three selections. Touch [A] to add a research code. Touch [C] to change the highlighted research code. Touch [D] to delete the highlighted research code. Touch [P] to create a listing of your codes suitable for printing.

You must enter a number for the research code. You cannot enter a alphabetical characters. We refer to this as *numeric*.

The program has a field named RESEARCH information (Srch). Facilities (for example, dialysis units) enter their revenue codes in this field. Medical practices use this field to create reports. The user defines the research code. You may use any number from 1 to 999. For example, you may identify all patients who have had an injection by the procedure code. You may use the research code to give you a report that can show you which patients had a specific injection. You may assign a different code to each kind of injection.

You can get a special report that includes all the information that you entered with all RESEARCH codes, or with a specific RESEARCH CODE.

You can include the SRCH information when first entering a transaction line or you can later REVISE the line to include a research code.

Activating the Research Code Field

To activate the research code field, go to the ACCOUNTS RECEIV-
ABLE (MAIN) DIRECTORY; select:
8 Profile and System Management
Then select:
1 Reinitialize the System Parameters
Then select:
2 Set the Main Control Variables

You will see a pop-up window named "System Variable Listing." Using the [DOWN ARROW], move to the field Cm_rsentry and put the number 1 next to that field. Touch [CTRL+W] to save your changes. To go back to the ACCOUNTS RECEIVABLE (MAIN) DI-RECTORY, touch [ESC] until you reach it. This will allow research codes for all transactions. If you only want research codes for charges, put a number 1 in cm-rschg, NOT in cm-rsentry.

Dr

Provider Number Listing

Your must activate the provider name listing (listed as "Cm-pventry") in the main control variables if you want to be able to enter this information. When you reach this field, you will see a pop-up window with the heading "Provider Name." The choices at the bottom of the window are the same as the procedure code listing window. Touch [A] to add a provider. Touch [C] to change the highlighted provider. Touch [D] to delete the highlighted provider. Touch [P] to print the list. Provider 00 is the corporation or group name or solo practitioner. You will be able to choose to set provider 00 as an individual or group practice.

If you select [A] to add or [C] to change the highlighted provider you will see the following window:

Enter/Revise a Provider

Enter the Lookup Code
Name
Address1
Address2
CityStZip
Office Phone   Emerg
State license   Number
Tax ID/SSN Number
Medicaid Number
Medicare (PIN) Number
Blue Shield Number
Title   Specialty Code

If you are entering a new provider, put in the requested information. If you are changing the provider information, use your up and down arrow keys to reach the field(s) you wish to change.

You may have up to 9999 providers in each accounts receivable.

Activating the Provider Field

To activate the provider field, go to the ACCOUNTS RECEIVABLE (MAIN) DIRECTORY and select:
8 Profile and System Management
Then select:
1 Reinitialize the System Parameters
Then select:
2 Set the Main Control Variables

You will see a pop-up window named "System Variable Listing."

Using the [DOWN ARROW] move to the field Cm_pventry, put the number 1 next to that field. If you only want a provider number on charges, enter "1" next to cm_pvchg and NOT next to cm_pventry. Touch [CTRL+W] to save your changes. To go back information to the ACCOUNTS RECEIVABLE (MAIN) DIRECTORY, touch [ESC] until you reach it.

Date of Service

Then you will be asked:
Please enter the date of service.

You may automatically pull in the system date by touching dot [.][ENTER] or you may pull down the date in the transaction above by touching [ENTER]. As always you have the option to type the date (using the format MMDDYY). DO NOT use dashes or slashes when you type the date.

Procedure Code

You will be asked to enter the procedure code. If you do not know the correct code, type the description of the procedure and a window will pop up to help you.

Procedure Code Window

When you reach the procedure field, you may enter the procedure number (CPT-4 code or HCPCS code). If the number you enter is invalid or does not match a number in the index, a window will pop up and the cursor will highlight the nearest match. If you do not know the procedure code number for the procedure you want, you may type the description of the procedure. If you know a portion of the number of the procedure, you may type as much of the number as you know. After you type the number you will see a pop-up window. The cursor will be located on the description you typed in if it finds a match. If the program cannot find that description, the cursor will be on the nearest match. If the cursor is on the code you want, touch [ENTER] to choose that one.

At the bottom of the procedure code listing window you have several choices. Touch [A] to add a procedure code. Touch [C] to change the highlighted procedure code. Touch [D] to delete the highlighted procedure code.

NOTE: Using the letter "U" for "unspecified" in place of a procedure code will allow you to skip passed that field.

Quantity

If you touch [ENTER] when you reach this field, the quantity will be zero. When you use the automatic transaction library you may have a completed transaction line with the unit value ($) and zero quantity entered. When you are in the transaction screen, the program will stop on the quantity field. When you enter a quantity the program will automatically multiply that quantity times the unit value you entered. Remember to enter the value for one unit in your automatic transactions if you want to use this feature.

Description

The description and procedure code are linked. When you pull the procedure code you will also pull the description. You may change the description if you wish.

Place of Service

You will be asked:
Please Enter the Place of Service
Use the original AMA codes
    Place of Service

1	Inpatient Hospital	
2	Outpatient Hospital	
3	Office	
4	Patient Home	
5	Day Care Facility/Psych Facility	
6	Psychiatric Residential Treatment Center	
7	Nursing Home/Nursing Facility	
8	Skilled Nursing	
A	Independent Laboratory	
B	Ambulatory Surgery Center	
C	Residential Treatment Center/Substance Abuse	
D	Specialized Treatment Center/Intermediate Care	
E	Comprehensive Outpatient Rehab Facility	
F	Independent Kidney Disease Treatment Center	
G	Emergency Room (Hospital)	
H	Birthing Center	
I	Military Treatment Center	
J	Custodial Care Facility	
K	Hospice	
L	Ambulance (Air or Water)	
M	Inpatient Psychiatric Facility	
N	Community Mental Health Center	
O	Other (use the letter O, not zero)	
P	HMSA, Inpatient Hospital	*use 1 with modifier*
Q	HMSA, Outpatient Hospital	*use 2 with modifier*
R	HMSA, Office	*use 3 with modifier*
S	HMSA, Patient's Home	*use 4 with modifier*
T	HMSA, Nursing Home	*use 7 with modifier*
U	HMSA, Skilled Nursing Facility	*use 8 with modifier*
V	HMSA, Other	*use letter O*
W	HMSA, Ambulatory Surgical Center	*use letter B*
X	Comprehensive Inpatient Rehab Facility	
Y	State or Local Public Health Clinic	
Z	Rural Health Clinic	

The computer will convert this code to the required code when it prints the form. You do not have to learn the nonstandard codes for the place of service. If you are using your automatic transactions, you may put in the place of service. The program usually will default to the correct place of service.

Diagnosis Code

You will be asked:
Please Enter the Diagnosis Code.

You may enter the ICD-9 code. If the code you enter matches a code in the ICD-9 index, that code and the description will be pulled into the field. If you do not know the ICD-9 number you may enter up to a 16-letter description of the diagnosis. A window will pop up with the diagnosis code and description highlighted. If there are multiple matches, then the nearest match will be highlighted.

NOTE: Using the letter "U" for "unspecified" in place of a diagnosis will allow you to skip passed that field.

Transaction Amount

Enter the amount of the charge. The program assumes that you are entering whole-dollar amounts unless you put in a decimal. If you want to enter $10.00 you enter "10" without the dollar sign, the decimal point, or the two zeroes. If you want to enter $10.50 you enter 10.50 or 10.5.

Charges, Correcting Mistakes

If you have just passed the field that you want to correct you may use the [LEFT ARROW] or {ESC} keys to move back one field at a time. If you have completed the entire line you must make changes by choosing:

<Revision=4>

When you answer the last question that the program asks while you are entering a new transaction, the program automatically saves that transaction permanently. It then asks you if you want to enter another transaction for this patient. If you have no more transactions to enter for this patient, touch [ENTER]. If you note an error, select:

<Revision=4>

and choose the number of the line containing the error. Then select the number of the field that you wish to change.

Payments, How to Enter

Select <Transaction=1> if you are not in the transaction screen.

Select <Pmt=2> if you want to enter the payment field by field.

Enter the automatic transaction instead of selecting <Pmt=2> if you want to use a payment from your automatic transaction library.

Srch (Research Field)

Research Code

If you have activated the research code for payments, the program will stop at this field.

If not the program will skip this field.

Dr

Provider Number

If you have activated the provider number, the program will stop at this field. If not, the program will skip this field.

Description

Put in the description of the payment, for example "Medicare payment".

Bank Number/Other

You will be asked:

Please enter the bank number or <Cash=1><M/Ch=2><Visa=3> <Other=4>

The bank number refers to the ABA number, and you must enter the dash between the two sets of numbers. To speed up your data entry, use a dot [.] instead of dash in you ABA number. The program will change the period into a dash.

Amount

Enter the amount of the payment. The program assumes that you are entering whole-dollar amounts unless you put in a decimal. If you want to enter $10.00 you would enter 10 without the dollar sign, the

decimal point, or the two zeroes. If you want to enter $10.50 you would enter 10.50 or 10.5.

Plus Adjustments, How to Enter

From the transaction screen, enter <+Adj=3>

You will be asked Is this a REFUND (Y or N). The default is NO. If the adjustment is not a refund, touch [ENTER].

Srch

Research Code

If you have activated the research code for plus adjustments, the program will stop at this field. If not, the program will skip this field.

Dr

Provider Number

If you have activated the provider number, the program will stop at this field. If not, the program will skip this field.

Description

Put in the description of the plus adjustment (for example, Refund).

Amount

Enter the amount of the plus adjustment. The program assumes that you are entering in whole dollar amounts unless you put in a decimal. If you want to enter $10.00 you would enter 10 without the dollar sign, the decimal point, or the two zeroes. If you want to enter $10.50 you would enter 10.50 or 10.5.

Minus Adjustments (Write-Off), How to Enter

From the transaction screen, enter:

<-Adj=4>

Srch

Research Code

If you have activated the research code for minus adjustments the program will stop at this field. If not, the program will skip this field.

Dr

Provider Number

If you have activated the provider number, the program will stop at this field. If not, the program will skip this field.

Amount

Enter the amount of the minus adjustment. The program assumes that you are entering whole-dollar amounts unless you put in a decimal. If you want to enter $10.00 you would enter 10 without the dollar sign, the decimal place or the two zeros. If you wanted to enter $10.50 you would enter 10.50 or 10.5.

Printing Memo Lines, How to Enter

A Print Memo is a message that will appear on your video display screen very much like a charge or payment and will be printed on your statements and reports. The option exists to print the message on your insurance forms. For example, you may use a Print Memo as a reminder to the patient in collections work.

From the transaction mini-menu select:

<P Memo=5>

Srch

Research Code

If you have activated the research code for print-memo line, the program will stop at this field. If not, the program will skip this field.

Dr

Provider Number or Code

If you have activated the provider number, the program will stop at this field. If not, the program will skip this field.

Description

Put in the description of the printing memo line.

Non-Print Memo, How to Enter

A Non-Print Memo is a message that will appear on your video display screen, but it will not be printed on your statements or on your insurance forms. It will appear on your reports.

You may use a Non-Print Memo as your reminder (one that you would not want the patient to see). For example, you might want a non-print memo that shows when you contacted a patient about payment on an overdue account. You may use your non-print memos to note when you sent an account to collection or when you made a claims inquiry.

From the transaction mini-menu select <NPMemo=6>

Srch

Research Code

If you have activated the research code for non-print-memo, the program will stop at this field. If not, the program will skip this field.

Dr

Provider Number

If you have activated the provider number, the program will stop at this field. If not, the program will skip this field.

Description

Put in the description of the non-print memo line.

Printing Transactions and Memo Lines

When you revise a charge, adjustment, or memo line you will have several options. You will be able to delete the transaction (this can only be done before you audit). You can make the charge, adjustment, or memo line change from printing to non-printing. You can choose to have a memo line print on a statement and on an insurance form.

Whenever you enter a printing memo line, the default selection is for the line to print on the statement. If you want the memo line to print on the insurance form:

Select <Revision=4> and select the line you want to revise.

A window named Status/Control will pop up and ask you:

Do you want to make this line non-printing?

Do you want to DELETE this transaction YES/NO?

Do you want this transaction to Print on Statements?

Print on Insurance Claims & EDI (Y or N)

Transaction Scrolling Controls

You can see 10 transaction lines at a time on your screen. When there are additional lines on an account, you will need to use your arrow keys. When you see the mini-menu:

Choose <Transaction=1><Insurance=2><Another Patient=3> <Revision=4>

Use the [UP ARROW] to scroll backward and the [DOWN ARROW] to scroll forward. The [LEFT ARROW] takes you back to the patient information screen and the [RIGHT ARROW] takes you back to the ACCOUNTS RECEIVABLE (MAIN) DIRECTORY.

Transaction Status Codes

Each transaction line will have a set of STATUS CODES on the far left side of the transaction line. The program used letter codes to show you which forms (statements, insurance forms, reports, and so on) have printed each transaction. If the code is a lowercase letter, you have not created the form. If the code is an uppercase letter, you did create the form or report.

You will learn how to do the "magic trick" of changing small letters to big letters as you learn more about auditing and printing of reports. We call it "changing the little I to a big I."

The code definitions are as follows:

A or a = Audit or reconciliation of transactions

S or s = Statements

I or i = Insurance forms

C or c = Refund check

\ = Designates nonprinting

- = Payment or write off

n = No insurance registered

Balancing Your Transactions

The computer keeps track of each transaction that you enter and it expects YOU to keep track of each transaction, too! The computer will want to know the total amount of charges, payments, plus adjustments and minus adjustments. When you reconcile with the computer daily, it is easy to keep your books balanced. This is also an excellent way to detect errors in posting and data entry.

Creating a Day Sheet

The purpose of balancing your transactions is to create a day sheet (batch audit). Let's see how you work with the computer to complete the required audit of your books.

When you enter a transaction for a patient, you begin to turn on the BRIGHT LIGHTS. The bright lights show on each directory to signal you that you have unfinished business or transactions that MUST be audited.

When you look at the ACCOUNTS RECEIVABLE (MAIN) DIRECTORY, you see that

6   Report Programs

now appears in BRIGHT LIGHTS. This is the computer's way of reminding you that you have entered transactions that you have not audited. Let's find out how to audit your transactions, and turn down the BRIGHT LIGHTS. When you check the dollar amounts you posted against the computer's totals, you are auditing your accounts.

From the ACCOUNTS RECEIVABLE (MAIN) DIRECTORY select:

6   Report Programs

Your ACCOUNTS RECEIVABLE (MAIN) DIRECTORY will look like the following if your "entry level" is 3 or lower:

1   Finished with the Patient's Receivables

2   Change the Report/Default Date

3   Patient Information (Enter, Change, Inquire)

4   Statement Programs

5   Insurance Claim Form Programs

6   Report Programs

7   Statistics and Other Information

8   Profile and System Management

NOTE: A highlighted sentence indicating the number of unbalanced transactions should appear in the lower part of the screen.

Balancing Your Entries

From the REPORT DIRECTORY select:

2   Create a TRIAL TRANSACTION LISTING

A line at the bottom of the screen will tell you the number of unbalanced transactions.

The computer will ask you:

Please Enter the Amount of Charges

At the top of the screen you will see:

Transaction Count

Charge Count

Payment Count

+Adjustment Count

−Adjustment Count

Print Memo Count

Non-Print Memo Count

Type the total amount that you have entered for each transaction type and touch [ENTER].

If you have not kept track of the amounts you entered for charges, payment, and adjustments, you will have no way to verify that your data entry was accurate. You will have to accept the numbers entered into the computer. You will eventually find any errors that you made during data entry. You will be required to post adjustments to them. If you wish to accept the numbers entered into the computer as accurate, you will need to do the balance procedure. Just touch [ENTER] when it asks you for the amount of each type of transaction. The computer will beep at you for each item that is not zero. You must write down the totals given by the computer, then run through the balancing procedure again and this time enter the correct numbers. The best method for balancing is still to keep track of all data entry so that you can have an accurate day sheet.

Viewing Your Unbalanced Transactions

If the amount that you type does not agree with the computer's total, the program will let you try another time. If on the second try you still do not agree with the program's total, the program will display your entry, its total, and the difference between the two totals. You have the option to view your transactions off the screen, if you answer YES to the question:

Would you like to view your transactions?

If you want to view your transactions, a window will pop up showing you the unbalanced transactions. Use your arrow keys to move up and down through the listing and then touch [ENTER].

Creating a Trial Transaction Listing

The program will ask:

Would you like to have a trial transaction listing created for you?

If you answer yes, one will be created.

To print it, select the number in front of the trial transaction listing.

A trial transaction listing is an edit sheet that gives you a printout of the transactions you entered. Creating a trial transaction listing is not the same as balancing. You still must balance. You will notice that:

2   Create a TRIAL TRANSACTION LISTING (Balance your transactions) is still highlighted.

Until this selection is not longer highlighted you have not balanced.

Balanced Entries, Next Step

If your charge amount agrees with the computer charge amount, enter the amount for the payments, plus adjustments, minus adjustments. If all the amounts agree, the program will create a transaction/deposit slip audit for you. When you print this out you will have your day sheet.

The program will ask, Would you like to audit these transactions now?

NOTE: If you want to create a "TRANSACTION AND DEPOSIT SLIP AUDIT" you must successfully balance your data entry totals against the computer's totals.

Printing the Transaction and Deposit Slip Audit

To print the TRANSACTION AND DEPOSIT SLIP AUDIT (601), you must be working at Entry Level 3 or lower. To print:

Select:

9   Print or View 1 page(s) Transaction Audit

A pop-up window will appear:

Print or View Selection

1   PRINT this field: (M6R601.LST) or (M6R602.LST)

2   View the file on screen

Then you will be asked:

Is the correct paper loaded?

Did you check the alignment?

Is the printer ready to print?

Please enter: <Y=YES><N=NO>

Then you will be asked:

Do you want to print these forms now?

Please enter: <Y=YES><N=NO>

You will be asked:

How many copies do you want to print?

Follow the directions on the screen, and the 601 Report will be printed.

Deposit Slip

Each practice has the option of setting up deposit slips to be created automatically after each Transaction and Deposit Slip Audit (601).

This deposit slip will be a condensation of all payments that you included in the preceding audit.

1. Cash payments will be itemized and sub-totaled separately from checks/money orders/travelers checks.
2. Your total deposit will consist of the sum of your cash and checks/money orders/travelers checks.
3. Credit card payments will broken out from your deposit separately since most banks require the credit card payments to be deposited separately.
4. Your total payments will equal the sum of your cash/checks deposit and your credit card deposit.

NOTE: We suggest you post and audit large Medicare or Medicaid checks in a separate batch from your regular deposit. Your total check will be itemized on your deposit slip as SEPARATE payments from EACH PATIENT.

Statements

In this section you will learn how to create and print statements. Only the patients that you have designated will receive statements. You have several statement types available with options for printing each type. You may create a balance forward statement, an open item statement, and a family account statement. You may select the patient financial classes that you want to receive a statement.

Statement Directory

From the ACCOUNTS RECEIVABLE (MAIN) DIRECTORY choose:

4   Statement Programs

You will see a menu similar to the following:

1   Create ALL Standard 1-up Statements
2   Create ALL Private Pay Open-Item Statements
3   Create ALL Industrial Standard Statements
4   Create ALL MEDICARE Open-Item Statements
5   Create ALL Family Account Statements

You set up the frequency between your statements (also called *billing cycle*) on your System Variable Listing. For example, if you set this variable to 30 days between statement, a patient will receive a statement at intervals no less than 30 days no matter how often you run your statements. The program puts in the date it created the last statement to a patient in the Patient Account Information Screen.

You may override the 30-day waiting period for the next statement by creating a demand statement.

You also have control over how far back statements are itemized. If you run open-item statements, all "open" charges are shown on the statement. If you run "Standard 1-up" statements, charges are only itemized for a period defined in the system variable cm-tritmsm. This variable is set to 30 days "from the factory," but you may change it to any number you wish (including 999,999) "Thirty" means the last 30 days of activity will be itemized on the statement. Any balance prior to 30 days will be listed as "Previous Balance."

NOTE: You must always create statements in the following order: Open-item statements first, then standard 1-up, and then family account statements. If you run the family statements first it will create a family statement for all patients and you will not be able to create open items or 1-ups.

Changing the Statement Frequency

From the ACCOUNTS RECEIVABLE (MAIN) DIRECTORY select:

8   Profile and System Management

From the SYSTEM MANAGEMENT DIRECTORY select:

1   Reinitialize the System Parameters

Then select:

2   Set the Main Control Variables

A warning will appear:

THIS IS YOUR ONLY WARNING!
That you MUST NOT change
any of these variable unless
you are sure you know what
you are doing. SHS may not be able
to help you recover EVEN WITH A BACKUP

At the bottom of the screen you will see:

Are you sure you want to change this master control file?

If you answer YES the following screen will appear:

Control Variables

1   Entry Variables Listing

2   Program Labels Listing
3   Form Control Variable Listing
4   Internal Numbering Variable Listing
5   All Variables

Choose:

3   Form Control Variable Listing

Use the [DOWN ARROW] to reach Cm_mintmsm, which stands for "minimum days between statements." Type the number of days you want between your statements. Type your new number over the old number.

Standard 1-Up Statements

The standard 1-up statement is a balance-forward statement. The statement will itemize the transactions one time. On the next statement you will see a previous balance for the older charges and itemization for the transactions that are appearing on the statement for the first time.

You may set the length of time you want to see itemization.

Once you have created the statements you will see:

9   Print or View 1 page(s) Demand 1-up Statements

To print or view the statements, select the number 9. You will see a pop-up window like the following:

Print or View Selection

1   PRINT this file: (M6D401.LST)
2   VIEW the file on screen

Enter 1 or 2 or use your arrow keys to make your selection. If you view the file, use your arrow keys to scroll through the file if it is larger than your screen. When you have finished viewing the file, touch [ESC] to exit from the file.

If you chose to print, the following pop-up window will appear:

Is the correct paper loaded?
Did you check the alignment?
Is the printer ready to print?
Please enter: <Y=YES> <N=NO>

If you chose [Y] for Yes the program will ask you:

Do you want to print a test form?
Please enter: <Y=YES><N=NO>

If you answer [N] for NO it will ask you:

Do you want to print these forms now? Please enter: <Y=YES> <N=NO>

If you print the file you will see a print menu. In this menu you can choose the number of copies that you want to print.

Private Pay Open-Item Statements

When you create open-item statements you will see each line item that does not have a zero balance. Each line item listed will tell how much is still owed for that service. To be able to create open-item statements, you must post your transactions "open item."

NOTE: You may post your transactions open item and produce a balance-forward statement, but you cannot post balance forward and then get an open-item statement. To get a balance-forward statement on an open-item patient, you must demand it from inside the patient's account or use the "doopenitm=yes" variable in the statement control file.

Select:

2   Create ALL Private Pay Open-Item Statements

Once the statements are created you will see a highlighted selection on the menu. When you look at the selection, you will be able to tell how many statements you created. You may either view or print the statements. To print or view the statements select:

9 Print or View Page(s) Standard 1-up Statements

When you make this selection you will see a pop-up window:

Print or View Selection

1 PRINT this file: (M6R401.LST)

2 VIEW the file on the screen

Enter 1 or 2 or use the [DOWN ARROW] and [UP ARROW] to make your selection. if you view the file, touch [ESC] to stop viewing. If you choose to delete, the data file is still marked and these statements will be destroyed. You will be asked:

Do you want me to delete (erase) this file for you? (Y or N)

You do not have to print your statements at this time. You may create them and print them later. You will see:

4 Statement programs

highlighted on your ACCOUNTS RECEIVABLE (MAIN) DIREC-TORY, just to remind you that you have statements that you have not printed. This selection will remain highlighted until you print statements.

Industrial Open-Item Statements

If you select:

3 Create ALL INDUSTRIAL Standard Statements

the statements will be processed for industrial patient accounts only.

Medicare Open-Item Statements

To add the Medicare Open-Item Statement to the Statement Directory, select:

8 Profile and System Management

Then select:

5 Codes: Financial Class, Recall, Modifier, CPT, ICD, Forms, Research, User

Then select:

6 Form Type Setup: Statement, Insurance, Report, EDI, Other

Then select:

1 Statement Form Setup

The Form Code Listing window will pop up.

Select "A" to add form code 434.

When you enter code 434, you will see a window that looks like the following:

Enter/Revise Forms

Form Code	434
Description	Medicare Open-Item
Maximum Entry Level	5
Ask Patient Number	P
Ask Beginning Date	B
Ask Ending Date	E

If you touch [ENTER] at the end of the screen, another Enter/Revise Forms screen will appear so you can enter more. Touch [ESC] or [ENTER] if you would like to return to the Form Code Listing Screen.

The difference between regular Open-Item Statements and Medicare Open-Item Statements is that on the Medicare Open-Item Statement only the items that have had charges posted against them will show up on the statement. This feature is optional and can be controlled through the main control variables.

Create All Family Account Statements

A family account statement, also called a *guarantor statement,* is one in which "bill to" (the person paying the bill) is not necessarily the patient. The "bill to" could be a parent, in the event the patient is a child. All the transactions for the patients assigned to a guarantor will be printed on one statement addressed to the guarantor. For example, in a pediatric practice, you might want the parent to get one bill with all the transactions for all of the children.

NOTE: Even if a guarantor is paying the bill, each patient still has a separate account in order to bill insurance.

You may have a situation in which you are billing an institution (for example, a hospital or nursing home) for patients whom you have seen. The statement would be address to the hospital or nursing home, and each patient would be listed on the bill.

To get this type of statement you must enter the guarantor in the "Bill to" field.

To run this program select:

5 Create All Family Account Statements from the Statement Directory. Once you have created the statements you may view or print them.

Reprinting Statements

What if you make a mistake and print the statements on the wrong form? What if the printer jams and ruins your forms? You can reprint the statements without having to re-create them. The statement field has a file name. To reprint the statements you would exit from the SHS program and go to the:

C:\130\200 (prompt) and type:

COPY M6R401.LPT1 (this would resend the latest 401 statements to the printer to reprint)

You can substitute the three-digit number part of the file name for any other form type, such as 431, and substitute LPT2 if you wish to send to another printer.

Insurance Creating and Printing

In the Insurance section you entered the basic insurance information and completed the insurance claim questions. In this section you will learn how to create and print your insurance forms.

Creating Insurance Forms

From the ACCOUNTS RECEIVABLE (MAIN) DIRECTORY select:

5 Insurance Claim Form Programs

You will see the Insurance directory, which may look like this:

1 Create ALL HCFA-1500 Private Pay

2 Create ALL HCFA-1500 Medicare

3 Create ALL 92 HCFA-1500 Private Pay

4 Create ALL 92 HCFA-1500 Industrial

5 Create ALL 92 HCFA-1500 Medicaid

6 Create ALL 92 HCFA-1500 Medicare

7 Create ALL Tn/Al UB-82/92 (HCFA-1450) Facilities (Dialysis)

At the bottom of the screen the program will ask you:

Please choose one of the above.

Select the form that you want to create.

Once the form is created you will see a listing of the forms that are ready to be printed. For example, if you select

1   Create ALL HCFA-1500 Private Pay

You will see:

9   Print or View 97 page(s) HCFA-1500 Private Pay

Each form created will have a number in front of is so you will be able to tell how many forms have been created.

When you select the number of the form you want to view or print, you will see a small pop-up window. Use the up and down arrow keys to choose whether you want to view or pint it.

Print or View Selection

1   PRINT this file: (M6R501.LST)
2   VIEW the file on the screen

To decide which transactions to put on an insurance form the program will look at the transaction status codes and find all the transaction lines preceded by a lowercase letter "I". The program will create an insurance form for each patient who has transaction line(s) with the lowercase "I". When the program has created the form it will change the lowercase "I" to an upper case "I".

The creation of the form and the printing are separate operations. In other words, you may create a form and print it later.

Printing Insurance Forms

Once you have created the form you will see:

9   PRINT 1 page(s) HCFA-1500 Private Pay

To print this form you would select:

9

Several windows will appear with questions. The first window looks like this:

Print or View Selection

1   PRINT this file: (M6R501.LST)
2   VIEW the file on the screen

Touch [ENTER] if you want to print.

Is the correct paper loaded?

Did you check the alignment?

Is the printer ready to print?

Please enter: <Y=YES> <N=NO>

The next window will ask:

Do you want to print a test form?

Please enter: <Y=YES><N=NO>Y

If you answer NO then you will be asked:

Do you want to print all forms now?

Please enter: <Y-YES> <N=NO> Y

Touch [ENTER] if you want to print.

How many copies do you want to print? 1

Enter the number of copies that you want to print. The number 1 is the default number of copies.

Demanding Insurance Forms

From Patient Account

Once you have printed a charge on an insurance form, the charge will not be picked up automatically again. If you want to print it on a form again, for any reason, you must DEMAND a new form. For example, if a patient called you and told you that the insurance company never received the insurance form, then you could print another one for the same period as the lost form. You must be in the patient's account to demand an insurance form.

Select the appropriate patient's account. Select:

<Create Demand Form=6>

Select:

<Insurance=2>

You will see a pop-up window named "Insurance Selection." Use your arrow keys to select the insurance company if more than one insurance company is registered.

Date Range for Demand Forms

You will be asked to choose the BEGINNING and ENDING DATES. Enter one of the following:

1. To create an insurance form with ALL DETAIL that is available in the computer for the account, touch [ENTER] when the program asks you for both the BEGINNING and ENDING DATES.
2. To create an insurance form for one day's activity only, when the SAME DATE, using the format MMDDYYYY, for both the BEGINNING and ENDING DATES.

The computer will then print all charges within those dates.

Beginning=oldest date

Ending=recent date

For example:

BEGINNING DATE 04011999—old

ENDING DATE 04301999—recent

Printing Demand Forms

To print demand forms you have some options. After demanding the form, your program will ask if you would like to "print the demand forms now?" If you answer YES it will print all the forms you have demanded and not printed. If you answer NO you can demand more forms or print the forms from the Insurance Directory.

Insurance Program

The computer will produce an insurance form for each insurance that you have registered for a patient.

Charges will automatically print on an insurance form once. The transaction line status code will show when a charge has appeared on an insurance.

You MUST spell MEDICARE correctly when registering your insurance, or the EDI program will not pick up that insurance as a Medicare!

Normally, only charges will appear on the insurance form. If you want a Printing Memo Line to print on an insurance form, you must set the status for that transaction.

Electronic Data Interchange (Electronic Claims Submission)

This mini-manual will not address actual submission of electronic claims (Figure B.14), since the school does not have access for this type of submission. This information is available in the master manual that your instructor maintains.

Business Financial Reports

You can create many standard reports with the SHS program. You should keep the two reports that constitute your audit trail, the Day Sheet (Transaction and Deposit Slip or 601) and the End of Month Report (Periodic Transaction Listing or 680). The end of month report is the report that your accountant will want to review.

Report Directory

To reach the Report Directory select:
6 Report Programs from the ACCOUNTS RECEIVABLE (MAIN)" DIRECTORY
The Report Directory will look like this:
1 Create the TRANSACTION AUDIT
2 Create TRAIL TRANSACTION LISTING
3 Rpt Gen: Collection, Recall and so on
7 Reports: Patient: Alpha, Numeric, Aging, Codes, Service Charges
8 Reports: Transaction/Production: 680/681/682/683/684/685/687/688

There are two types of reports: standard and custom. To run a standard report, pick the report you want to run from the directory. If you need more information than you would get on a standard report, you can set up custom report.

Day Sheet (601)

In the SHS system this report is named the "Transaction and Deposit Slip Audit." When you balance and audit your transactions, you will automatically create this report. To create the day sheet select:

6 Report Program from the ACCOUNTS RECEIVABLE (MAIN) DIRECTORY
Then select:
2 Create a TRIAL TRANSACTION LISTING from the Reports Directory

Day Sheet

- Lists all transactions posted since last day sheet
- Creates a deposit slip
- Breaks out payments by type: cash, check, credit card
- Shows beginning and ending accounts receivable
- Total charges, adjustments, and payments
- Can be compared with appointment schedule to make sure all patient visits have been entered into computer
- Makes dollar amounts posted permanent to protect practice from embezzlement

Deposit Slip

The program will create a deposit slip on the right-hand side of the day sheet. You have the option of getting an additional deposit slip on a separate page that prints after the day sheet. You may attach the additional deposit slip to your bank deposit. To activate the additional deposit slip, you must set up a deposit template file by the name of DPSLIP.DAT in your account.

Aged Account and Collection Report by Financial Class (673)

To create the aged account and collection report, select:
6 Report Programs from the ACCOUNTS RECEIVABLE (MAIN) DIRECTORY
Then select:
7 Reports: Patient: Alpha, Numeric, Aging, Codes, Service Charges
Then choose:
3 Create an AGED PATIENT LISTING by Financial Class
The name of the file is M6R673.LST
- Keeps track of past due accounts
- Easily identifies slow-paying patients

```
Name      JOAN        SMITH       Bill To   JOAN         SMITH
Birthdate 07/17/1923 Age 75 yrs   923 COUNTRYMEADOW LANE
SocSec#   559-55-3434 Sex F Stat D SONOMA           CA 95476
                      Home Ph     (707) 996-3434
CoPay     $5.00       Work Ph
MD        CAMPBELL    Employer
INS                   Billing     H Smts        D Stmt <None>
No 10025  VMMG        06  Main Dx  401.1
--\130\255-----------------------------------------------------------------
Software                  DEMAND FORM/EDI CREATION     (2)  09/02/1999
-------------------------------------------------------------------------
Form Selection
Demand Statement
Demand Insurance
Select Insurance
Eligibility EDI
Select Report
Label
Superbill

0.00
```

Figure B.14

- Tracks Medicare, Medicaid past due accounts
- Tracks HMO, PPO past due accounts

By getting a financial class aging instead of an alphabetical aging, you will be able to easily identify the patients who owe the most money for the longest period. Once you have identified the problem accounts, you will be certain that your collection person targets those accounts first.

This is also an excellent way to track PPOs and HMOs.

Alphabetical Aged Patient Listing (674)

This report has the same information as the AGED PATIENT LISTING by financial class except that the program sorts the patients alphabetically.

From the ACCOUNTS RECEIVABLE (MAIN) DIRECTORY
    select:
6   Report Programs
From the Report Directory select:
7   Reports: Patient: Alpha, Numeric, Aging, Codes, Service Charges
Then Choose:
4   Create an ALPHABETICAL AGED PATIENT LISTING
The name of the file is M6R674.LST

- Keeps track of past due accounts
- Clearly shows date of last payment
- Gives patient's telephone number
- Gives aging of your total accounts receivable

Aging by Insurance (675)

This report has the same information as the AGED PATIENT LISTING by financial class except that the program sorts the patients by insurance company.

From the ACCOUNTS RECEIVABLE (MAIN) DIRECTORY
    select:
6   Report Programs
From the Report Directory select:
7   Reports: Patient: Alpha, Numeric, Aging, Codes, Service Charges
Then choose:
3   Create an AGED PATIENT LISTING by Insurance Company
The name of the file is M6R675.LST

- Keeps track of past due accounts
- Clearly shows date of last payment
- Gives patient's telephone number
- Gives aging of your total accounts receivable

Listing by Transaction Codes (677)

This is a standard report that search for information requested by the user.
From the ACCOUNTS RECEIVABLE MAIN DIRECTORY select:
4   Report Programs
From the Report Directory select:
7   Reports: Patient: Alpha, Numeric, Aging, Codes, Service Charges
Then choose:
7   Create a Patient Listing Using ICD, CPT-4, Research Codes, Providers Dates
The name of the file is M6R677.LST.

Questions for a Transaction Code Report

Beginning Date	01011999	
Ending Date	01111999	
	First	Last

Research Code
Provider Code
Procedure Code
Diagnosis Code

This report can be run from the batch processor. The program will remember the code values that you used last and run the report that way. You will be asked for the beginning and ending dates at the time you set up the report to process.

End of Month Report (680)

The name of the file is M6R680.LST.

- Monthly audit of accounts receivable
- Calculates figures for accountant quickly

This report is the second report in your audit trail. The first report is the day sheet. With the day sheet and the end of month report you should be able to reconstruct your entire accounts receivable. It is important that you keep these reports. This report cannot be re-created, when you run the report the transactions are flagged and will only appear on the report one time. You may run this report from the Report Director or from the batch processor.

This report provides a printed copy of the month's financial activity. It will be listed in alphabetical order by patient. The following information is included on this report:

Patient Account Number
Patient Name
Guarantor Name
Billing Address
Primary Phone Number
Account Balance
Financial Class
Previous Balance
Date of Last Statement (Produced)
Date of Last Insurance (Form Produced)
Aging (*=30 days, **=60 days, *** =90 days)
Provider Number
Date of Service
Research Code (if any)
Procedure Code
Transaction Description
Bank Number (Payments)
Diagnosis Code (Changes)
Amount (Charges, Payments, Adjustments)

Comprehensive Transaction Listing (683)

This report lists all transactions by patient that have been entered into the computer. It is formatted identically to the 680 report. This report can be very large and take a very long time to print. At the ACCOUNTS RECEIVABLE (MAIN) DIRECTORY select:
6   Reports Programs
Then select:
8   Reports: Transaction/Productions:
    680/681/682/683/685/687/688

Next select:
4   Create a COMPREHENSIVE TRANSACTION LISTING

Production Report (By Provider) (685)

When you run your end of month report you will automatically get a provider production report. You may also run this as a stand-alone report. It provides the following information:

- Totals for charges, payments, adjustments per provider
- Tracks cash flow
- Tracks payment history of insurance carriers
- Sorts by financial class

At the Accounts Receivable directory select:
6   Reports Programs
Then select:
8   Reports: Transaction/Production:
    680/681/682/683/684/685/687/688
Next select:
6   Create a PRODUCTION REPORT (by Provider) 685
When prompted, supply the beginning and ending date of the report.

Note the section that discusses the batch audit (601). You may get a production report by provider with each batch audit. This batch audit production report has similar information to this provider production (685) report.

Production Report (By CPT) (687)

When you run your end of month report you will automatically get a procedure production report. You may also run this as a stand-alone report. It provides the following information:

- Totals occurrences, billed amount, and percent of all charges for each procedure
- Gives above totals for each provider and percent of all providers
- Lists totals for all providers
- Sorted by financial class

At the ACCOUNTS RECEIVABLE (MAIN) DIRECTORY select:
6   Reports Programs
Then select:
8   Reports: Transaction/Production:
    680/681/682/683/684/685/687/688
Next select:
7   Create a PRODUCTION REPORT (by CPT) 687
Supply the beginning and ending date when prompted.

Alphabetical Patient Listing (671)

You may run an alphabetical patient listing at any time. It provides the following information:

- The stars tell you whose accounts are past due
- Identify patients on "hold statement"
- See which patients are set to be recalled for future visits and reason for visit
- Find out the next sequential account number

To run this report, at the ACCOUNTS RECEIVABLE (MAIN) DIRECTORY select:
6   Reports Programs
Then select:
1   Create an ALPHABETICAL PATIENT LISTING

The Alphabetical Patient Listing is a quick reference to the status of your patient's accounts. This report can provide a valuable link between the billing office and those who deal with the patients at the front desk.

You may run this report from the batch processor by selecting:
1   Finished with the Patient's Receivables for Now
from the ACCOUNTS RECEIVABLE (MAIN) DIRECTORY.
Then select:
3   Batch Processor Programs
Next choose:
1   Set Up the Batch Processor (choose programs to run)
Then enter the program to run, in this case type "671".

Patient Listing by Diagnosis, Procedure, (And Other) Codes

You may wish to get a list of all patients in your practice who have a certain diagnosis code.

- Tracks patients with a certain diagnosis code
- Selects a diagnosis code range that you want to track.

To run this report select:
6   Report Programs
from the ACCOUNTS RECEIVABLE (MAIN) DIRECTORY
Then select:
7   Reports: Patient: Alpha, Numeric, Aging, Codes, Service Charges
Next select:
5   Create a listing using ICD, CPT-4, research codes, providers, dates
You will be asked to:
Please enter the beginning date: MMDDYYYY
When you are asked:
Are you satisfied with these dates Y/N
answer YES
The following screen appears:

Beginning date	01/25/98
Ending Date	01/30/98
Research Code	
Provider Code	
Procedure Code	
Diagnosis Code	

This screen will let you enter a range of research codes, provider codes, procedure codes, and diagnosis codes. The first field is the lowest (minimum/first) occurrence and the second is the highest (maximum/last) occurrence possible in the range. If you want a report for a single code, then enter that code as both the minimum and the maximum.

Recalls

Recalls are used for several reasons. One reason is to remind patients that is time for to make a follow-up appointment. In the case of a serious diagnosis, the doctor may have a legal obligation to see that his or her patient is getting continuing care. Documented recalls can help to meet this responsibility. Recalls also are used to generate income. A yearly reminder of a history and physical or gynecological exam mailed to every appropriate patient will certainly generate many more appointments than just leaving it to the patient to remember to call on his or her own.

The recall program is very flexible. You can have as many types of recalls as you wish. You might keep it simple and use only one recall that asks the patient to call for an appointment. You might use the recall program to produce superbills, collection letter, and return-visit notices.

Self Mailers

SHS sells a multipart self mailer that is half page in length. The mailer separates, supplying you with a sealed notice that is ready to mail to your patient, as well as a copy to keep for your records. Contact SHS if you would like a sample of this form.

Definitions

Recalls as used in SHS refer to the letters or other forms created by the recall program.

"Recall Code" is the alpha-numeric code used within SHS to refer to a particular template. For instance, Recall Code "HP" could refer to a reminder mailed to a patient to call for a physical examination.

"Recall Date" is the date you wish SHS to create a letter/form for a particular patient. Every recall code "TWO" requires two file names: "M6RTWO.DAT" and M6STWO.DAT".

Files used in this section refer to the files that contain the information/template used by SHS in creating the recall forms. These files must contain the recall code in their names. Recall code "TWO" requires two files names: "M6RTWO.DAT" and "M6STWO.DAT".

Request Codes are encase in brackets that tell SHS to go to each patient account to pull in certain information. An example is [*13*], which tells SHS to pull the patient's account number into the recall.

Recall Files

For reach recall code you need two files. How you name the files is critical. The names contain within them the first five characters of the individual recall code. This is best described by showing you some example codes and their corresponding file names. For instance, if you use recall code "HP," the corresponding files are: M6RHP.DAT and M6SHP.DAT.

More examples are as follows:

Recall code	File name	
APPT	M6RAPPT.DAT	M6SAPPT.DAT
1	M6R1.DAT	M6S1.DAT
10	M6R10.DAT	M6S10.DAT
6MONTH	M6R6MONT.Dat	M6S6MONT.DAT

The following will not work because the first five characters of each recall code are not unique:

Recall code	File names	
LETTER1	M6RLETTE.DAT	M6SLETTE.DAT
LETTER2	M6RLETTE.DAT	M6SLETTE.DAT

For your files, the M6R . . . DAT files is the header file. If you are using the SHS recall forms, this file should be an empty file because there is no header. All that is needed is for the file to exist. If you are using the recall program to create a recall report, you may want to include a header to appear at the top of the first page. Using a text editor such as DOS EDIT you can create any header you wish. Never use tabs when creating your text file.

The M6S . . . DAT file is the body of the recall and must be the same length as the requested letter/document. This field contains your entire recall message and any request codes for information that you want pulled in from the patient database in the format [*01*]. If you have multiple recall reasons, then all the M6S*.DAT files must be the same length. If you use the standard SHS snap-apart recall forms, you must be aware that they are *exactly* 33 lines long. If you use DOS EDIT or another text editor that shows line and character position, you want to set up your file so that:

- the doctor's address starts at line 5, character 15
- the body of the message starts at line 11, character11 and runs through to line 25, character 80

The patient's address starts at line 27, character 11. If you use the recall for creating reports instead of recall forms, you are not really limited to the spacing. Just remember that the neater you create the report, the easier it will be to read and interpret. A standard piece of $8^1/_2 \times 11$ paper is 66 lines in length and approximately 80 usable characters wide if you use a standard dot matrix printer. If you use a laser printer the measurements may be different depending on the font, proportional spacing and so on. You cannot use a laser printer with a snap-apart form. This type of form requires an "impact" printer. A laser printer does not "hit" the paper; it "coats" the paper like a copy machine so the image is only on the top copy.

In the \130\1 subdirectory is a sample file named RECALL.TEM that can be copied from \130\1 into your data account to use as a starting template. The command to copy this file into your account is: COPY\130\1RECALL.TEM\130\200\M6SHP.DAT

Print the sample file and study how it is set up.

The next step is to use your favorite text editor to make appropriate changes. Request codes can be used to pull in specific information on each patient. For instance, [*25*] will cause the patient's account balance to print. This would be useful in a collection letter. The RECALL.TEM file uses the following request codes:

[*10*]
[*11*]
[*12*]

to pull in the guarantor name, street, address, and city-state-Zip code, respectively. You can find a complete list of request codes at the end of the CUSTOM REPORT section.

Once you have edited your recall, save the file as a DOS text or an ASCII file. Be sure to test your recalls before using them for a complete run.

Building Your Recall Codes

To build your recall codes you must first get to the RECALL CODE LISTING directory.

From the ACCOUNTS RECEIVABLE (MAIN) DIRECTORY choose one of the following:

8 Profile and System Management

Then choose:

5 Codes: Financial Class, Recall, Modifier, CPT, ICD, Forms, Research, User

Then select:

2 Patient Recall Setup

This will bring you to the RECALL CODE LISTING where you can add, change, print, and delete recall codes.

Remember that the recall code must match its corresponding template file names.

Assigning a Recall Code to a Patient

The first step to assigning a recall code is to enter the patient you wish to recall.

Once you are in the patient's account and at the "Patient Account Information" screen, choose:

<Revision=4>

Choose the highlighted "09" and a window will appear that will allow you to enter up to four recall dates and codes. You may enter the date in the usual manner, or you may let the computer calculate the date. To let the computer assign the recall date, type a dot [.] and the number of months. For example, a recall date 6 months in the future could be entered as .6, or a 12-month recall could be entered as .12. You may also enter **"m"** with the number of months: **m9** to calculate a date 9 months in the future. You may also enter **"d"** with the number of days: **d45** to calculate a date 45 days in the future. You may also enter **"y"** with the number of years: **y3** to calculate a date 3 years in the future. The month and year calculations will give a date that is the same day of the week as the date you have chosen at the main directory.

Generating Your Recalls

Recalls are created by choosing in order from the ACCOUNTS RECEIVABLE (MAIN) DIRECTORY:

6   Report Programs

Then select:

3   Rpt Gen: Collection, Recall, and so on

Then choose:

5   Report Generator: 635 (recalls)

If the patient has a recall date that is equal to or less than 30 days from the "system" date, the program will create the appropriate recall for that patient. As with all reports, the recall program can be run by the batch processor, just request report number 635.

Appointment Scheduling

In this section you will learn how to set up the appointment scheduler and how to make appointments. Once you have entered your appointments you may print out your appointment schedule. You may sort the appointments by date, provider, or by patient.

Activating the Appointment Schedule Module

If you select a patient and you see:

<Appointment=A>

at the bottom of your screen, your appointment scheduling module is activated.

If you do not see:

<Appointment=A>

at the bottom of your screen, you must activate the scheduler.

To activate your scheduler select:

8   Profile and System Management

from the ACCOUNTS RECEIVABLE (MAIN) DIRECTORY.

Then select:

1   Reinitialize the System Parameters

from the SYSTEM MANAGEMENT DIRECTORY. Then select:

2   Set the Main Control Variable

You will see a warning:

THIS IS YOUR ONLY WARNING!
That you MUST NOT change
any of these variables
unless you are sure you
know what you are doing.
SHS may not be able to help
You recover EVEN WITH A BACKUP

The bottom of the screen will state:

Are you sure you want to change this master control file?

If you type YES then this pop-up window will appear:

Control Variables

1   Entry Variables Listing
2   Program Labels Listing
3   Form Control Variable Listing
4   Internal Numbering Variable Listing
5   All Variables

Choose:

1   Entry Variables Listing

Type the number 1 next to the CM_appt variable. To exit, touch [CTRL+W]. You may touch [RETURN] until you reach the ACCOUNTS RECEIVABLE (MAIN) DIRECTORY.

Setting Up the Calendar

Before you can start making appointments, you must set up your appointment calendar. To reach the calendar, start at the ACCOUNTS RECEIVABLE (MAIN) DIRECTORY.

Select:

7   Statistics and Other Information

From the STATISTICS DIRECTORY select:

8   Appointment Schedule Maintenance/Setup

A window labeled "Appointment Schedule Maintenance" will pop up.

Appointment Schedule Maintenance

Appointment Calendar Begin Date   01081999
Enter the Appointment Calendar End Date   12312001

Enter the starting date for your appointment book; then enter the appointment calendar end date. Your appointment scheduler is ready to use. If you touch [ENTER] the program will select today as the beginning date. If you touch [ENTER] the program will select a date, 1 year away, as the ending date.

Checking Available Appointment Times

With the SHS appointment scheduler, you may book multiple appointments at the same time. To check to see which times are available, select:

7   Statistics and Other Information

from the ACCOUNTS RECEIVABLE (MAIN) DIRECTORY.

From the STATISTICS DIRECTORY select:

7   Appointment Scheduling

You will see a large pop-up window named "Appointment Listing." You may scroll through that window with your up and down arrow keys to see which time slots are available. Touch [A] to add an appointment. Touch [C] to change the highlighted appointment. Touch [D] to delete the highlighted appointment. Touch [P] to print schedule.

Making an Appointment

You may go to a patient account to make the appointment. If you have activated your appointment scheduler, you will see a selection:

<Appointment=A>

at the bottom of your patient account information screen.

Select A to make your appointment. You will see a pop-up window named Appoint Add/Revise.

You will then be asked to fill in the following information:

Appointment Date

Appointment Time

Provider Number

Appointment Length

Enter Appointment Notes Y/N

Enter through the screen to make another appointment or touch [CTRL+2] to get back to the Appointment Listing Screen

If you have only one provider activated in your program, you will not be required to enter a provider number.

Printing the Appointment Schedule

After you have made the appointment, you can print the appointment schedule. The selections at the bottom of the Appointment Listing are:

- Press [A] to add an appointment
- Press [C] to change the highlighted appointment
- Press [D] to delete the highlighted appointment
- Press [P] to print schedule

When you press [P] you will see a pop-up window named "Print Appointment Schedule". You will then be asked to fill in the following information:

Enter the Beginning Date

Enter the Ending Date

Enter the Provider Number

Enter the Sorting Order

You will see a small pop-up window like this:

   Print Sorting

Date

Provider

Patient

   Move the cursor using the arrow keys to highlight the sorting sequence that you want. The program will create your appointment schedule.

Changing an Appointment

When you are in the patient's account looking at the Appointment Listing, press [C] to change the highlighted appointment. You will see the following window with the appointment information you previously entered:

   Appointment Revise

Appointment Date   01/09/1999

Enter the Appointment Time   10:00

Enter the Provider Number   01

Enter the Appointment Length   15

   Use your arrow keys to make your change. Touch [CTRL+W] to save the window, or touch [ENTER] until you pass each field in the window. If you select a patient by mistake and decide that you do not want to make any changes, touch [ESC] to get back to the appointment listing.

Deleting an Appointment

You may display the appointment listing window by selecting:

<Appointment=A>

Select [D] to delete the highlighted appointment.

The "Delete and Existing Appointment" pop-up window will appear.

   Make sure this is the appointment you want to delete.

The program will ask you:

Are you sure you want to delete this Appointment Y or No?

APPENDIX C

AAMA Role Delineation Chart

ADMINISTRATIVE

Administrative Procedures

- Perform basic clerical functions
  Whole book
- Schedule, coordinate, and monitor appointment
  Chapter 7
- Schedule inpatient/outpatient admissions and procedures
  Chapter 7
- Understand and apply third-party guidelines
  Chapter 16
- Obtain reimbursement through accurate claims submission
  Chapter 16
- Monitor third-party reimbursement
  Chapters 14, 15, 16
- Perform medical transcription
  Chapter 9
- Understand and adhere to managed care policies and procedures
  Chapter 15
- Negotiate managed care contracts (advanced)
  Chapter 15

Practice Finances

- Perform procedural and diagnostic coding
  Chapters 13, 14
- Apply bookkeeping principles
  Chapters 16, 19, 20
- Document and maintain accounting and banking records
  Chapters 19, 20
- Manage accounts receivable
  Chapters 16, 17, 19
- Manage accounts payable
  Chapter 20
- Process payroll
  Chapter 20
- Develop and maintain fee schedules (advanced)
  Chapter 16
- Manage renewals of business and professional insurance policies (advanced)
  Chapter 14
- Manage personnel benefits and maintain records (advanced)
  Chapters 11, 19

GENERAL (TRANSDISCIPLINARY)

Professionalism

- Project a professional manner and image
  Chapters 4, 11
- Adhere to ethical principles
  Chapter 3
- Demonstrate initiative and responsibility
  Chapters 1, 5
- Work as a team member
  Chapters 1, 5, 11
- Manage time effectively
  Chapters 1, 5
- Prioritize and perform multiple tasks
  Chapter 20
- Adapt to change
  Chapter 1
- Promote the CMA credential
  Chapters 1, 2, 3
- Enhance skills through continuing education
  Chapters 1, 11

Communication Skills

- Treat all patients with compassion and empathy
  Chapters 3, 5, 6
- Recognize and respect cultural diversity
  Chapter 5
- Adapt communications to individual's ability to understand
  Chapters 5, 6
- Use professional telephone technique
  Chapter 6
- Use effective and correct verbal and written communication
  Chapter 5
- Recognize and respond to verbal and nonverbal communications
  Chapters 5, 6
- Use medical terminology appropriately
  Chapters 5, 12
- Receive, organize, prioritize, and transmit information
  Chapters 5, 6, 7
- Serve as liaison
  Chapters 5, 6, 7
- Promote the practice through positive public relations
  Chapters 5, 6

Legal Concepts

- Maintain confidentiality
  Chapters 2, 3, 4, 9
- Practice within the scope of education, training, and personal capabilities
  Chapters 1, 2, 3
- Prepare and maintain medical records
  Chapters 2, 4, 9
- Document accurately
  Chapter 9
- Use appropriate guidelines when releasing information
  Chapters 4, 9
- Follow employer's established policies dealing with the health care contract
  Chapters 14, 15, 16
- Follow federal, state, and local legal guidelines
  Chapters 12, 14
- Maintain awareness of federal and state health care legislation and regulations
  Chapter 14
- Maintain and dispose of regulated substances in compliance with government guidelines
  Chapters 11, 12
- Comply with established risk management and safety procedures
  Chapters 11, 12
- Recognize professional credentialing criteria
  Chapters 2, 3
- Participate in the development and maintenance of personnel, policy, and procedure manuals
  Chapter 11

GENERAL (TRANSDISCIPLINARY)

Instruction

- Instruct individuals according to their needs
  Chapter 7
- Explain office policies and procedures
  Chapter 5
- Teach methods of health promotion and disease prevention (advanced)
- Locate community resources and disseminate information
  Chapter 5
  - *Orient and train personnel (advanced)*
  - *Conduct continuing education activities (advanced)*

Operational Functions

- Maintain supply inventory
  Chapters 11, 12
- Evaluate and recommend equipment and supplies
  Chapter 11
- Apply computer techniques to support office operations
  Chapters 17, 18
  - *Supervise personnel*
    Chapter 11
  - *Interview and recommend job applicants*
    Chapter 11
  - *Negotiate leases and prices for equipment and supply contacts*
    Chapter 11

Adapted from the 1998 American Association of Medical Assistants (AAMA) Medical Assistant Role Delineation Chart.

Index